The Role of Anesthesiology in Global Health

Ram Roth • Elizabeth A.M. Frost
Clifford Gevirtz
Editors

Carrie L.H. Atcheson
Associate Editor

The Role of Anesthesiology in Global Health

A Comprehensive Guide

Springer

Editors
Ram Roth
Department of Anesthesiology
Icahn School of Medicine at Mount Sinai
New York, NY, USA

Elizabeth A.M. Frost
Department of Anesthesiology
Icahn School of Medicine at Mount Sinai
New York, NY, USA

Clifford Gevirtz
Department of Anesthesiology
LSU Health Sciences Center
New Orleans, LA, USA

Associate Editor
Carrie L.H. Atcheson
Oregon Anesthesiology Group
Department of Anesthesiology
Adventist Medical Center
Portland, OR, USA

ISBN 978-3-319-09422-9 ISBN 978-3-319-09423-6 (eBook)
DOI 10.1007/978-3-319-09423-6
Springer Cham Heidelberg New York Dordrecht London

Library of Congress Control Number: 2014956567

Printed on acid-free paper

Springer is part of Springer Science+Business Media (www.springer.com)

To Aren, who encouraged me to go on my first surgical mission many years ago and inspires me every day. Only two of many reasons that I love you.

R.R.

To my many friends and colleagues around the world who continue to amaze and humble me by how much they achieve, often with much less than I have.

E.A.M.F.

To my beloved wife, Alison, and my sons, Theo and Graham, who are a constant source of inspiration; to Elizabeth Frost, a teacher, colleague, and friend who has always given me brilliant perspective and wisdom; and to my patients who teach me every day, meliora.

C.G.

To my husband, Eric, whose love of the written word and commitment to service make him my constant companion and inspiration.

C.L.H.A.

Foreword

Ram Roth and his coeditors have created a unique book. Anesthesiology is focussed on the relief of acute and chronic pain and the preservation and enhancement of life in all aspects of medical care. Despite this, many people, both medical and lay, would not realize this wide spectrum of care and would consider those who practice in our specialty as physicians who merely remain in the operating theatre. Medical knowledge has developed in different civilizations at different times. While many currently affluent societies were rigidly blaming illnesses on personal sin and treating with complex herbal mixtures and prayer, other currently less affluent areas had sophisticated therapeutics and surgery based on sound physiological knowledge.

This persistent inequality in access to medical care has changed from country to country as civilizations come and go, but in today's world, appalling inequality still exists. If the mortality purely from anesthesia in, say, London is around 1:200,000, that in parts of West Africa right now is 1:150. This is not acceptable and has to be changed.

Humanity has always had individuals who want to make a difference. Initially, these might have been medical missionaries who combined teachings about their faith with simple improvements in healthcare. Soon this was associated with travelling surgeons and nurses; with the advent of modern anesthesia, this, too, would be added into the travelling mix. In the early days, this provision of pain relief would be part of the surgical remit, but as anesthesia developed and became specialized, slowly, anesthetists started to travel and teach.

Early medical missions went to areas and built hospitals, taught locally, and stayed for the rest of their lives. Often, however, their deaths resulted in a loss of service and a return to "the old ways." As time passed, all countries started medical schools and local doctors emerged, but anesthesiology has always been regarded by many as a "low-quality" speciality. This is now changing, but not fast enough.

Nowadays, there is a very confusing picture of humanitarian aid throughout the less affluent world. Some NGOs have found it difficult to demonstrate that donated funds reach those most in need. Many "aid workers" go into an area and do tremendous surgical or medical interventions but then depart without any thought of leaving a legacy beyond those individual lives they have changed. There is almost a sense of medical tourism for some, with the collecting of photographs of terrible pathology and beautiful landscapes for what almost seems like the "entertainment" of people back home.

It is now obvious what needs to be done to improve essential surgical and anesthesia care around the world. Governments can see what could be done and they need to allocate appropriate resources to make this happen. Those who travel to teach need to "teach the teachers" and leave a legacy on which further developments can be built. At this time, the WHO realizes that death from infectious diseases is falling, while death from essential surgery and anesthesia is rising. They, too, will seek to influence governments. The WFSA will seek to assist them in this work.

This book describes many sound ways forward. It is a great start, but the finish will come when inequality in care is abolished.

David J. Wilkinson, L.R.C.P., M.R.C.S., M.B., B.S.
World Federation of Societies
of Anaesthesiologists (WFSA)
London, UK May 2014

Preface

No man is an island entire of itself … any man's death diminishes me, because I am involved in mankind.

John Donne, *Devotions upon Emergent Occasions,* 1624.

Anesthesiologists provide acute and critical medical care to patients as well as the necessary infrastructure to enable surgeons to implement dramatic, life-changing interventions around the world. In and around any operating room anesthesiologists are the professionals who provide preoperative evaluation, consult with the surgical team, and create a plan tailored to each individual patient—including airway management, intraoperative life support, pain control, and postoperative management. It is in this capacity as perioperative physicians that anesthesiologists improve the safety and efficacy of surgical interventions for underserved patients in low- and middle-income countries.

When we first embarked on this project to identify the role of anesthesiology in global health, we knew that many organizations around the world were already involved in medical missions. We came to this task with different perspectives, from resident to senior practitioner, and diverse experiences, gained over the years from travels, consultations, and basic care in many countries. We suspected that anesthetic care providers would identify common areas of concern and similar difficulties. What we have learned from writing this book is so much more. Through reports from so many mission providers, we learned that many of the problems are the same … lack of basic supplies, education, infrastructure, and communication. A need to understand that more can indeed be done with less is a recurring theme. The difficulties have all been identified succinctly and on many occasions, but no common solutions have been determined. Moreover, in diverse corners of the world anesthesiologists have developed programs that they individually believe to be unique but in fact are mirrored to a greater or lesser extent by other practitioners. Thus, the need for a collaborative effort and true development of a global health strategy is underscored. Can this be done by one entity such as a government or medical school or international organization? Probably not! Rather, as some of our authors present, representatives and leaders from among the ranks of health care professionals should put aside different agendas to develop a workable health program that is truly global. The resources are there: organizing and harnessing those resources is the next step in the process. If readers find that there is duplication in some chapters, they are correct. We have deliberately left it that way to underscore the need for closer alliances and communication. It is our hope that with this text we might, in some small way, help jump-start the process of globalization in anesthetic services.

We are fortunate that we have been able to incorporate the experiences of many professionals from around the world in this text; we are grateful to them for sharing so much of their time, experience, and efforts. Our thanks go also to the staff at Springer, especially Jeff Taub and Shelley Reinhardt, for their continuing assistance.

New York, NY, USA Ram Roth
New York, NY, USA Elizabeth A.M. Frost
New York, NY, USA Clifford Gevirtz
Portland, OR, USA Carrie L.H. Atcheson

Acknowledgment

We would like to thank Ms. Shelley Reinhardt and Ms. Joanna Perey from Springer Science+Business Media, LLC for their support and help in bringing this project to fruition.

Ram, Elizabeth, Cliff, and Carrie

Contents

Contributors

Helen Akinc, M.B.A NavyBrat LLC, Winston-Salem, NC, USA

Natasha Anushri Anandaraja, M.B.Ch.B., M.P.H. Arnhold Global Health Institute, Mount Sinai Medical Center, New York, NY, USA

Departments of Preventive Medicine & Medical Education, Icahn School of Medicine at Mount Sinai, New York, NY, USA

Alberto E. Ardon, M.D., M.P.H. Department of Anesthesiology, University of Florida, Jacksonville, FL, USA

Carrie L.H. Atcheson, M.D., M.P.H. Oregon Anesthesiology Group, Department of Anesthesiology, Adventist Medical Center, Portland, OR, USA

Anis Baraka, M.D., F.R.C.A. (Hon.) Department of Anesthesiology, American University of Beirut Medical Center, Beirut, Lebanon

Curtis L. Baysinger, M.D. Department of Anesthesiology, Vanderbilt University School of Medicine, Nashville, TN, USA

John Benjamin, M.D. Department of Anesthesia, Walter Reed National Military Medical Center, Bethesda, MD, USA

Steven Dale Boggs, M.D., M.B.A The James J Peters VA Medical Center, Bronx, NY, USA

The Icahn School of Medicine at Mount Sinai, Manhattan, NY, USA

Debbie Chandler, M.D. Department of Anesthesiology, LSU School of Medicine Shreveport, Shreveport, LA, USA

Nicholas W. Chee, M.P.H. Hospital for Joint Diseases, NYU Langone Medical Center, New York, NY, USA

Kathryn Chu, M.D., M.P.H. Eerste River Hospital, Eerste River, South Africa

Jason Cone, B.A. MSF-USA, New York, NY, USA

Lena E. Dohlman, M.D., M.P.H. Department of Anesthesia, Critical Care, and Pain Management, CHA/MGH, Boston, MA, USA

Marcel E. Durieux, M.D., Ph.D. Department of Anesthesiology, University of Virginia, Charlottesville, VA, USA

Ebby Elahi, M.D. The Icahn School of Medicine at Mount Sinai, New York, NY, USA

Angela Enright, O.C., M.B., F.R.C.P.C. Department of Anesthesia, University of British Columbia, Royal Jubilee Hospital, Victoria, BC, Canada

Charles James Fox, M.D. Department of Anesthesiology, LSU School of Medicine Shreveport, Shreveport, LA, USA

Jeffrey S. Freed, M.D., M.P.H., F.A.C.S. Department of Surgery, Icahn School of Medicine at Mount Sinai, New York, NY, USA

Elizabeth A.M. Frost, M.B., Ch.B. DRCOG Department of Anesthesiology, Icahn School of Medicine at Mount Sinai, New York, NY, USA

Dorothy Gaal, M.D. Department of Anesthesiology, Yale University School of Medicine, New Haven, CT, USA

Ronald B. George, M.D., F.R.C.P.C. Department of Women's & Obstetric Anesthesia, IWK Health Centre, Halifax, NS, Canada

Erin Gertz, M.D. Global Women's Health Division, Department of Obstetrics, Gynecology and Reproductive Sciences, Icahn School of Medicine at Mount Sinai, New York, NY, USA

Clifford Gevirtz, M.D., M.P.H. LSU Health Sciences Center, New Orleans, LA, USA

Somnia, Inc., New Rochelle, NY, USA

Gabriel M. Gurman, M.D. Professor Emeritus, Anesthesiology and Critical Care, Ben Gurion University of the Negev, Beer Sheva, Israel

Natalie F. Holt, M.D. Yale School of Medicine, 333 Cedar Street, TMP 3, P.O. Box 208051, New Haven, CT, USA

Grace Hsu, M.D. Department of Anesthesiology and Critical Care Medicine, The Children's Hospital of Philadelphia, Philadelphia, PA, USA

Monique James, M.D., M.P.H. Icahn School of Medicine at Mount Sinai, Mount Sinai Hospital, New York, NY, USA

Laurent Jouffroy, M.D. French Society of Anesthesia and Intensive Care, Anesthesiology and Critical Care, Ambulatory Surgery Unit, Clinique du Diaconat, Strasbourg, France

Patricia Kahn, Ph.D. MSF-USA, New York, NY, USA

Alan David Kaye, M.D., Ph.D. Department of Anesthesiology, LSU School of Medicine, New Orleans, LA, USA

Yenabi Keflemariam, M.D. Department of Anesthesiology, LSU School of Medicine Shreveport, Shreveport, LA, USA

Philip J. Landrigan, M.D., M.Sc., F.A.A.P. Department of Preventive Medicine, Icahn School of Medicine at Mount Sinai, New York, NY, USA

V. Lekprasert, M.D., M.S. Department of Anesthesiology, Ramathibodi Hospital, Mahidol University, Bangkok, Thailand

Kate M. Liberman, M.D. Department Anesthesiology, Perioperative and Pain Medicine, Brigham and Women's Hospital, Boston, MA, USA

K.A. Kelly McQueen, M.D., M.P.H. Department of Anesthesiology, Vanderbilt University Medical Center, Nashville, TN, USA

Ofer Merin, M.D., M.H.A. Shaare Zedek Medical Center, Jerusalem, Israel

Miodrag Milenovic, M.D. Department of Anesthesiology and Intensive Care Medicine, Clinical Center of Serbia, Belgrade, Serbia

Medge Owen, M.D. Wake Forest University, Winston-Salem, NC, USA

Kybele, Inc., Winston-Salem, NC, USA

Somsri Pauswasdi, M.D. Department of Anesthesiology, Ramathibodi Hospital, Mahidol University, Bangkok, Thailand

Maria Eugenia Interiano Portillo, M.D. Hospital Leonardo Martinez Valenzuela, San Pedro Sula, Honduras

Peter M.J. Rosseel, M.D. Department of Cardiothoracic Anesthesia and Intensive Care, Amphia Hospital, Breda, The Netherlands

Ram Roth, M.D. Icahn School of Medicine at Mount Sinai, New York, NY, USA

John Rotruck, M.D. Department of Anesthesia, Walter Reed National Military Medical Center, Bethesda, MD, USA

Jodi Sherman, M.D. Department of Anesthesiology, Yale School of Medicine, New Haven, CT, USA

B.M. Shrestha, M.B.B.S., D.A., F.R.C.A.T. Department of Anaesthesia and Intensive Care, Kathmandu Medical College Teaching Hospital, Sinamangal, Kathmandu, Nepal

Lester Silver, M.D., M.S. Division of Plastic and Reconstructive Surgery, Icahn School of Medicine at Mount Sinai, New York, NY, USA

Peter J. Taub, M.D., F.A.C.S., F.A.A.P. Division of Plastic and Reconstructive Surgery, Icahn School of Medicine at Mount Sinai, New York, NY, USA

Carrie Teicher, M.D., M.P.H. Epicentre, Paris, France

Miguel Trelles, M.D., M.P.H., Ph.D. MSF-Belgium, Brussels, Belgium

Fiona Turpie, M.D., F.R.C.P.C., D.T.M.H. Department of Anesthesiology, Pain Management, and Perioperative Medicine, Dalhousie University, Halifax, NS, Canada

Theogene Twagirumugabe, M.D. National University of Rwanda, Rwanda, Africa

Ivan Velickovic, M.D. Department of Anesthesiology, State University of New York Downstate Medical Center, University Hospital of Brooklyn, Brooklyn, NY, USA

Julia L. Weinkauf, M.D. Department of Anesthesiology, University of Virginia, Charlottesville, VA, USA

Part I

Evolution and Development of Missions

1 Medical Missions: A Short History from There to Here

Elizabeth A.M. Frost

> Gross ignorance, superstition and fanaticism, caste, social habits and national prejudices are barriers which the mere missionary finds difficult to overcome and which may compel him to remain for years in isolation and shunned, if not despised and thus the opportunity of doing good for which he yearns is utterly denied him, whilst, to the missionary physician, the hovel and the palace are alike opened to his approach, suspicions are allayed, prejudice is disarmed, caste distinction for the time at least is over come: even the harem where the brother may not intrude is not too sacred for the "infidel." John Lowe 1903.

Thus was the difference between the missionary and the medical missionary defined.

But the words for healing and salvation are closely linked. Healing, and hence health, denote a state of well-being and salvation indicates deliverance from suffering. The word "salve" means to soothe like a curative ointment and a means to achieve a better existence. Thus it is hardly surprising that these two concepts have been linked to religious organizations for centuries—a healing of the body and mind with deliverance to a higher power. The main codification of Jewish law, the Shulchan Arukh, compiled in the sixteenth century, states that the Torah gives the physician permission to heal, adding that this is a religious precept, included in the category of saving life (Yoreh Deah, no. 336). Many well-known Rabbis of the Talmudic period were also physicians. As late as the Middle Ages it was still common for the positions of physician and Rabbi to be held by the same person. Talmudic scholars, including translators, could use the practice of medicine to earn a living. Indeed it is thanks to Jewish physicians that many Arab and Greek medical treatises were translated into Latin and Hebrew and vice versa [1].

First mentioned by Isaiah, the coming of a Messiah who would bring physical and spiritual healing was heralded by the prophet who wrote "the spirit of the Lord God is upon me because the Lord has anointed me to preach good tidings to the needy. He has sent me to bind up the brokenhearted, to proclaim freedom to the captives by opening of the prison to them that are bound… to comfort all who mourn… to bestow on them beauty for ashes, the oil of gladness instead of mourning and a garment of praise for the spirit of despair" [2]. Some 600 years later during a sermon in a synagogue in Nazareth, a prophet named Jesus Christ read the same passage aloud to the congregation and confirmed that it was his mission [3].

This close association between medical missions and religious teaching from earliest times is clear. While the intention may well have been to bring relief to suffering peoples, the relationship often resulted in zealous crusading and evangelical spreading of Christian beliefs, practices often regarded with grave suspicion by the people of "invaded" countries.

E.A.M. Frost, M.B.,Ch.B. DRCOG (✉)
Department of Anesthesiology, Icahn School of Medicine at Mount Sinai, New York, NY, USA
e-mail: elzfrost@aol.com

R. Roth et al. (eds.), *The Role of Anesthesiology in Global Health: A Comprehensive Guide*,
DOI 10.1007/978-3-319-09423-6_1, © Springer International Publishing Switzerland 2015

Earliest Missions

Again in the Bible, Luke recorded; "Now when the sun was setting, all they that had sick with divers diseases brought them unto him: and he laid his hands on every one of them and healed them" [4]. Maimonides, (Fig. 1.1) (1135–1204) the great Spanish (Cordoban) philosopher, Rabbi and physician spent most of his life in Egypt where he carried out a very busy clinical practice in Cairo, disapproved of charms and incantations and spoke against believing things which were not objectively attested. At variance with earlier traditions that healing was a religious obligation and thus should be done free, he earned his living from the practice of medicine among Jews and Gentiles [5]. He also strenuously attacked the growing commercialism of Rabbinic learning and the increasing numbers of "quacks" who used superstition and magic arts on a gullible population. His teachings were further advanced by the fifteenth century Jewish philosopher, Isaac Arama, who preached that man must not rely on Providence alone or on miracles when it comes to healing and sickness [6].

During the Middle Ages, Catholicism became dominant in the religious world. Much of the responsibility of the care of the sick fell to monastic orders. Unlike in the Jewish tradition, monks, while learned, were not usually physicians and had not studied anatomy or completed an apprenticeship with a medical teacher. In addition, the Roman Catholic Church declared that the shedding of blood was incompatible with holding holy office (the *Ecclesia Abhoret a Sanguine* edict of 1163). Henceforth, monks, the educated class, were prohibited from performing surgery. But up to that point, following in the Greco-Roman tradition and the teachings of the Talmud, many operations such as wound care, lithotomy, amputations, reduction of dislocations, and even Cesarean sections had been carried out in monasteries. The barbers who had shaved the monks' heads and who had often assisted the monks took over the practice of surgery often with disastrous results [7]. Monks were left to rely on herbal and other ancient methods of care. For example, leprosy was endemic in medieval Europe. While avoidance of contact with the sick and their isolation had been advocated both in the Bible and by Jewish law, in 1313, Philip the Fair of France ordered that all lepers should be burned [8]. Fortunately, before this edict could be fully executed, some 17,000 monasteries of Saint Lazarus (a brother of Martha and Mary who is said to have been raised from the dead by Christ, Fig. 1.2) were set aside for these victims who were then cared for, mostly in complete solitude by monks, who were themselves lepers. These facilities were known as lazarettos and numbered over 19,000 in Europe alone. By the end of the sixteenth century, the pestilence had died out in that part of the world and lazarettos were abolished by Louis XIV in 1656, the proceeds from their sale used to build hospitals [8].

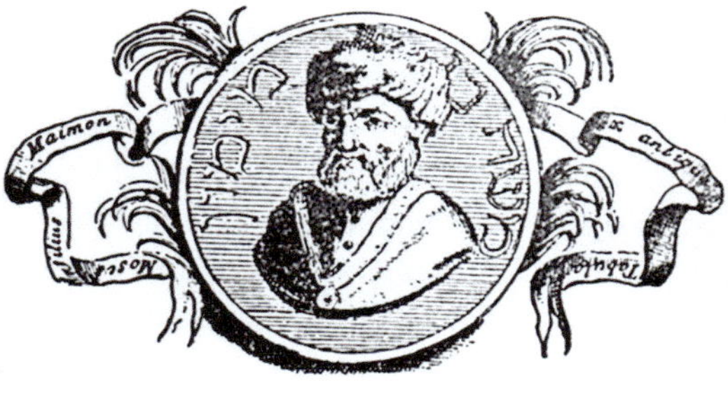

Fig. 1.1 Maimonides eighteenth-century portrait of Maimonides, from the *Thesaurus antiquitatum sacrarum* by Blaisio Ugolino (Wikipedia accessed March 11th 2014)

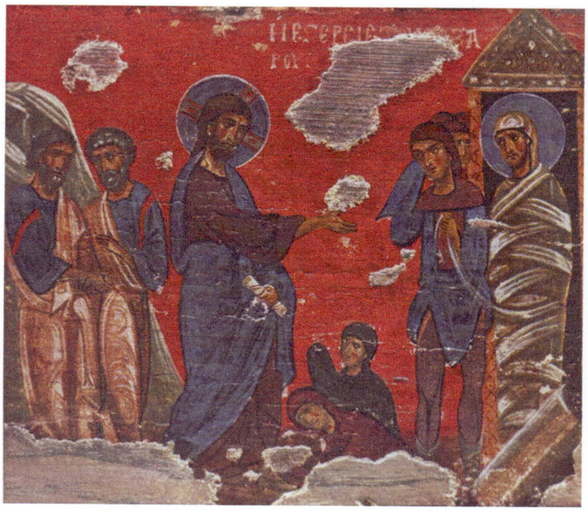

Fig. 1.2 Christ Raising of Lazarus, Athens, twelfth to thirteenth Century (From Wikipedia accessed March 11th 2014)

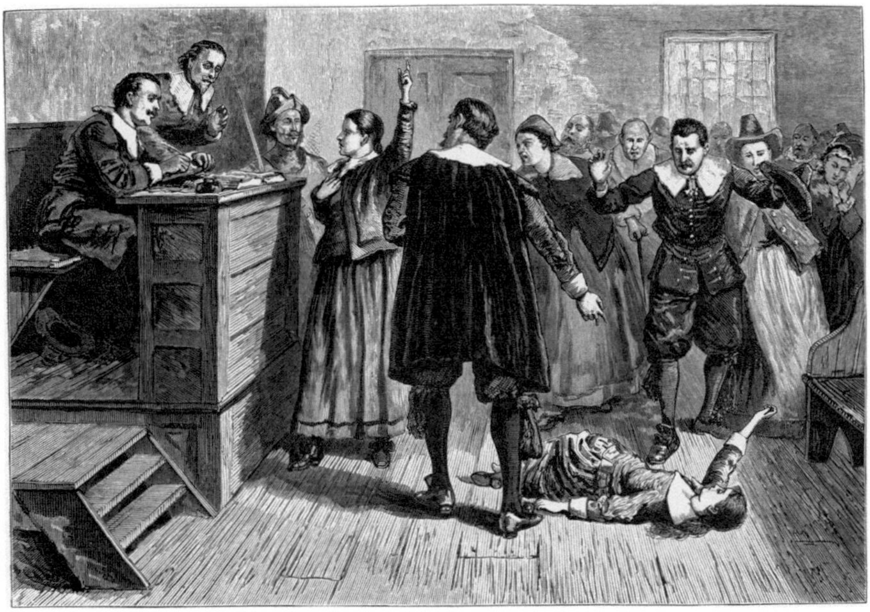

Fig. 1.3 The Salem witch trials were a series of hearings and prosecutions of people accused of witchcraft in colonial Massachusetts between February 1692 and May 1693. These trials resulted in 20 people being executed, most of them women. The central figure in this 1876 illustration of the courtroom is usually identified as Mary Walcott (from Wikipedia accessed March 11th 2014)

Several other diseases were assigned to saints and adopted by specific monastic orders. The order of St. Anthony was founded in the eleventh century to take care of sufferers of acute ergot poisoning which was named St. Anthony's fire [9]. Midwives had also used controlled amounts of ergot to induce abortions for centuries. St. Anthony's fire was later determined to be due to tainted rye and the convulsions associated with consumption of the bread have been claimed to be the accusations of bewitchment that spurred the Salem witch trials between 1692 and 1693 (Fig. 1.3). There was said to be an abundance of rye in the region [10, 11]. The association of a saint to a disease was often determined by the manner in which the saint died. St. Appolonia had her teeth and jaw shattered and it was to her that one prayed for relief of toothache. St. Vitus' dance (Sydenham chorea) was named after the patron saint of dance. St. Agattin who suffered a double mastectomy was the patron saint of nursing women and St. Valentine oversaw the care of epileptics. For cure of these and many other disorders, pilgrimages to the designated monasteries where they where cared for by monks who where proclaimed to have special knowledge of the respective disorders.

Eighteenth to Late Nineteenth Centuries

In its earliest stages, the missionary movement from the West mainly centered on enlightened views of healing and incorporated them into theology and practice. In essence, Western medicine was brought to a world beyond the west, often for the first time and became established as the main source of health care for the region. Common remedies and purges might be dispensed, programs for community hygiene commenced, anesthesia introduced, planning for medical facilities started, and research established into finding the cause for diseases. But while medical knowledge and new means of treatment were advanced, people on missions found out that they were exposed to and often in conflict with other concepts of the causes of illnesses. Radically different modes of treatment and contrary understanding of what constitutes human wellness were difficult notions to embrace. In addition, the economics of missions changed. Ethical and theological issues arose as to how or if treatment should be paid. Medical missions changed many assumptions as to how hospitals should function and what role women should play.

Although monasteries were declining as a center for healing, major achievements were made by many medical missionaries dispatched and funded often by religious organizations or governments in the United Kingdom and other parts of Europe. Perhaps one of the first physicians sent from a Protestant Church and sponsored by Germany and Denmark was Dr. Kaspar Gottleib Schlegemilch in 1790. Sadly he died of dysentery in India only a month after his arrival and thus was able to achieve little [12]. He was followed by other Dutch and German doctors who did not stay long or also died of tropical diseases [12]. But many more physicians and other healthcare providers travelled to distant lands, some with little medical training. Missions usually lasted for years, the health of the provider often the determining factor. During this time, clinics and facilities were established and supply lines set up. Only within the past few decades have missions been arranged for days or weeks to areas where infrastructures already exist.

The need for medical training was slowly becoming realized, but not all missionaries were so enlightened. The Rev Halvor Ronning, his wife, Hannah, and sister Thea went to China from the United States (Later they became Canadian citizens) in 1891 to found a Lutheran mission in the interior of China in the city of Fancheng in Hubei Province. Once there they established a school and had great success extending medical care to the indigent, including abandoned female newborns and breaking the boundaries of outmoded traditions by offering "modern" education to young men and especially to women. Hannah would not permit girls with bound and broken feet into the school which went on to become the largest establishment in the area. Although they had no medical training they quickly learned from the two doctors (who also had no more than 2 years instruction) and some nurses who joined them at the mission site how to dispense medicines, apply dressings, and instill eye drops among other simple procedures (Audrey Ronning Topping, personal communication).

Rev John Lowe the secretary of the Edinburgh Medical Missionary Society in the nineteenth century wrote a handbook on the place and power of medical missions, first published around 1903. Therein he set out some of the requirements for a successful mission. First of all, the missionary's professional education should be thorough and comprehensive. He emphasized the need for surgical training, pointing out that "natives almost everywhere have a kind of intuitive knowledge of the medicinal virtue of indigenous plants and although they are as a rule, utterly ignorant of the diseases they presume to treat, yet much confidence is placed in the native doctors and their nostrums, and, somehow they do at times appear to effect wonderful cures; but they can do nothing whatever in surgery, even in the simplest cases" [13]. Rev Lowe eschewed any private practice as a means to improve the circumstances of medical men, nor should they be paid more than ordinary missionaries, ideas that were generally not well received. Fluency with the native language was a prerequisite and having overcome that obstacle, the medical missionary should open a dispensary in as central a locality as possible, "associating himself with an earnest, intelligent, judicious native evangelist." Patients could then be followed up in their homes by the associate. Lowe goes on to say; "Two or three intelligent native Christian youths should as soon as possible be selected and trained as assistants. They will soon be able to dispense medicines, serve as dressers and do all the drudgery of dispensary work and thus much of the medical missionary's time will be set free for more important duties." A hospital, on a small scale, perhaps for 2–3 patients only was to be opened as soon as possible.

Later on Lowe remarks on the practices of women "doctors" of the Madi or Moru tribe of Central Africa. These women treated all cases except wounds, accidents, and snake bites (left to male doctors). Management was the same for most diseases: a double magic wand about a foot long, one part filled with small stones and the other empty was waved and rattled over the affected part accompanied with incantations. The lady "doctor" then placed her hand into the empty tube and extracted the disease [14]. Several other spells were also commonly used and predictions made as to whether the patient should live or be killed. Séances often terminated in convulsions for the healer who upon recovery collected her fee, usually of a small domestic animal.

It is not difficult to see that many areas of the world would welcome practitioners with some better grounding in medical matters and improved chances of success. A few of the early medical missionaries and the work they accomplished are mentioned:

John Thomas

In 1793, Dr. John Thomas who had already been in Calcutta was in England seeking funds for a return mission to India. He met William Carey, known as the "father of modern missions." Carey was one of the founders of the Baptist Missionary Society and as a missionary in the Danish colony, Serampore, India, he translated the Bible into Bengali, Sanskrit, and numerous other languages and dialects. The two travelled to India together where they established the first Protestant mission [15].

John Scudder

Dr. John Scudder, the first American medical missionary, went to Ceylon in 1819 and later travelled to India. Apart from providing medical care, he established schools and a college. He had seven sons, many of them also physicians who served as medical missionaries. His granddaughter, Dr. Ida Sophia Scudder, became a third-generation American medical missionary in India of the Reformed Church in America [16] (Fig. 1.4). She dedicated her life to the plight of Indian women and the fight against bubonic plague, cholera, and leprosy. In 1918, she started one of Asia's foremost teaching hospitals, the Christian Medical College and Hospital, Vellore, India.

Peter Parker

In 1834, The American Board of Commissioners for Foreign Missions sponsored Dr. Peter Parker to travel to China in 1834 where he had the distinction of being the first full-time Protestant medical missionary [17] (Fig. 1.5). Trained as a surgeon at Yale Medical School and ordained as a Presbyterian minister also at Yale, he performed many of the first surgical procedures in China. In 1835, he opened the Ophthalmic Hospital in Canton, which later became the Guangzhou Boji Hospital (the Canton Hospital). Although Parker

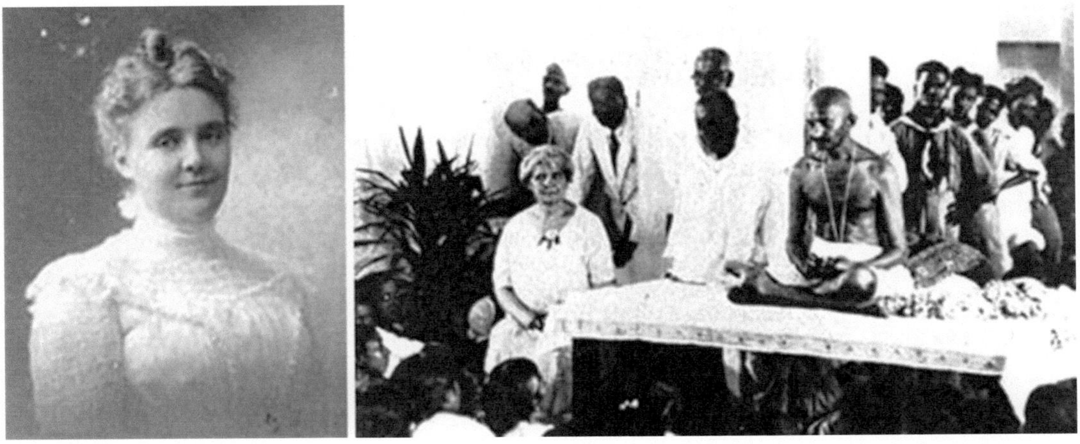

Fig. 1.4 Ida S. Scudder as a young Woman (accessed from Wikipedia March 12th 2014) and later with Mahatma Gandhi

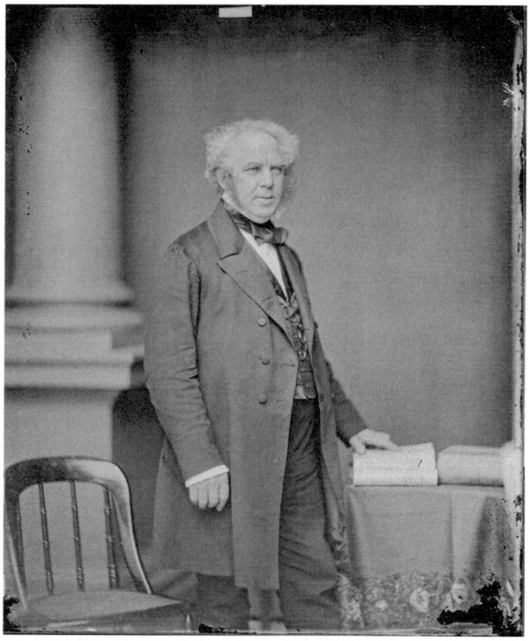

Fig. 1.5 Dr. Peter Parker, photograph by Mathew Brady (this is a file from the Wikimedia Commons. Accessed March 12, 2014)

specialized in diseases of the eye, including cataracts, and also resected tumors it soon became apparent that many other maladies required care. Over 2,000 patients were admitted the first year. Parker also introduced Western anesthesia in the form of sulfuric ether and instructed Chinese students before the establishment of medical schools. Later, Parker served as the main interpreter and negotiator of the Treaty of Wanghia with the Qing Empire. In 1845 he became a secretary and interpreter to the new embassy from the United States, while still keeping the hospital in operation. It was said that Parker "opened China to the gospel at the point of a lancet."

Asahel Grant

The first American missionary to Persia and Turkey was Dr. Asahel Grant [18]. Born in Marshall, New York in 1807, he seemed to be destined to be a farmer, before slicing his foot with an axe. After a stint teaching in a country school, he studied medicine with Dr. Seth Hastings in Clinton, New York. His further medical training included auditing a chemistry class at Hamilton College and a few medical lectures in Pittsfield, Massachusetts. He did not receive a formal college degree. Despite the establishment of several medical schools by the early nineteenth century, most "doctors" assumed the title after apprenticeship to local physicians and may never have attended any medical lectures. In Utica Dr. Grant became involved with the Presbyterian Church and also set up practice as a general practitioner. In 1835, at the age of 27, and sponsored by the American Board of Commissioners for Foreign Missions he sailed with his wife, age 20 and also a missionary, to the Middle East. Within days of arrival he became ill with cholera, a disease from which he never fully recovered. Nevertheless, both he and his wife were able to build up a stellar reputation for the quality of medical care they provided and for the many schools they opened and supervised. Sadly his wife and twin children died of malaria within 5 years. He continued his work, both in providing medical care and in his many attempts to convert the Nestorians (Assyrians), a fierce isolated people who lived in the mountains of Hakkari across the border in Ottoman Kurdistan. He died of malaria and cholera in 1844 at the age of 37. His success as a physician not only saved his life on several occasions (he travelled with a lancet and bled himself frequently, treatment believed to be beneficial at that time), but opened the way for missionary successors.

Paul Brand

Only towards the end of the nineteenth century did some Protestant denominations start to provide some basic medical training for missionaries before they left their native countries. Not infrequently, these people were the only "doctors" available in the areas to which they were assigned. Dr. Paul Brand's parents were missionaries in India and with little training and very limited supplies, for many years they were the only source of care for many remote villages. Brand, himself, was born in India in 1908 where he sustained frequent bouts of dysentery and malaria [19]. Back in the United Kingdom, he received 12 months of

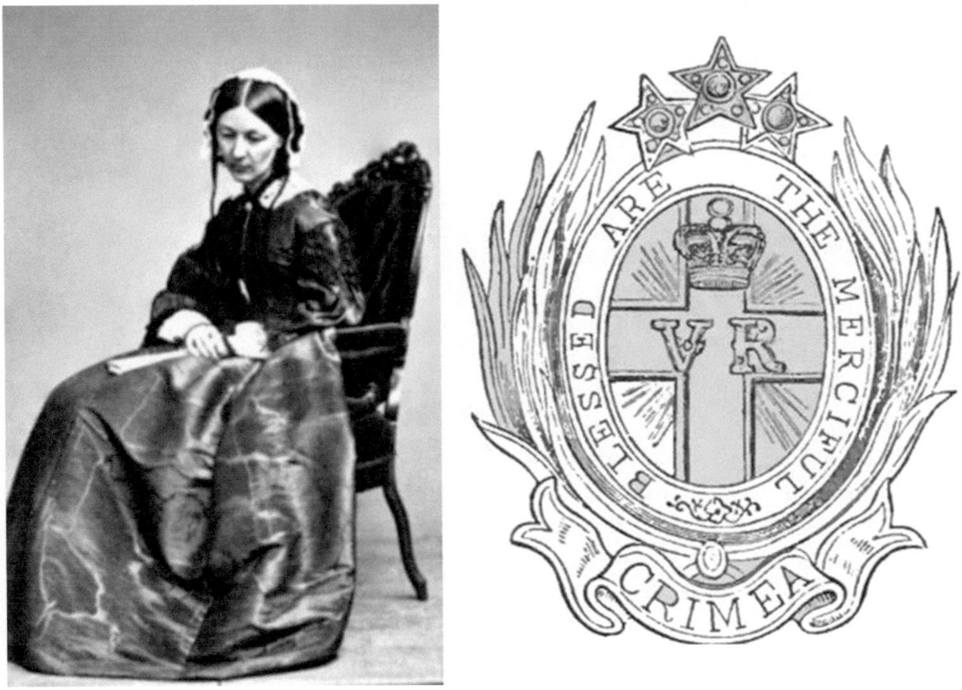

Fig. 1.6 Florence Nightingale and the medal she received from Queen Victoria (from Wikipedia; accessed March 13th 2014)

medical training and then returned to India as a builder. During the second World War, he studied medicine at the University College Hospital in London and as a surgeon, went back to India where he pioneered reconstructive work in leprosy, especially tendon transplants.

Nurses and Medical Missions

Undoubtedly the best known nurse in medical missions is Florence Nightingale (Fig. 1.6). Born to a very wealthy family in Florence, Italy in 1820, she resisted her family's efforts to require her to conform to their gentrified ways. Rather she persisted in her desire to study nursing. A celebrated social reformer and statistician, and the founder of modern nursing, she came to prominence when she was sent to serve as a nurse during the Crimean War [20]. With 38 volunteer nurses that she had trained and 15 nuns she went to Scutari, a large and densely populated district and municipality in Turkey, where the death rate from cholera, typhoid, and typhus was ten times that of battle wounds. Enlisting the help of the British Government she was able to reverse these statistics and, on her return to England, set standards for hospital management and nursing care, emphasizing the use of pie charts as a visual means to understand data [21]. She established the Nightingale Training School for nurses at St. Thomas' Hospital in 1860.

Apart from or as an extension of her ideas of social reform, Nightingale was as early promoter of medical tourism. During 1856, she sent several letters back to her family and friends in the United Kingdom describing spas in the Ottoman Empire. She had interviewed and overseen the care of several patients in these facilities and was impressed with the excellent health conditions, physical plants, general well-being, and dietary care. She noted especially that the treatment was much less expensive than in Switzerland where rich families tended to send their members, often for the care of tuberculosis. She opened the Nightingale Training School at St. Thomas

Hospital on 9 July 1860. A few years later, she mentored Linda Richards, who was to be recognized as "America's first trained nurse," and enabled her to return to the United States with adequate training and knowledge to establish her own, high-quality nursing schools. Linda Richards went on to become a great nursing pioneer not only in the United States but also in Japan.

Several other nurses have also contributed in major fashion to medical missions. Elizabeth Bernard, who had been trained as a nurse and served in the US army from 1918 to 1920, went to China in 1933 to care for the sick and orphans. She stayed there in Hong Kong until her death in 1972 [12]. Alvin and Georgia Hobby had been missionaries in Northern Rhodesia. They returned to the United States in 1962 and after finishing nursing training, returned to Zambia where they stayed for almost 40 years and established a clinic at the Namwianga Christian School, which remains in operation [22].

Kate Marsden also a nurse was a British missionary, explorer, and writer. Born in London in 1859, her interests in nursing developed early (she was a nurse by age 16). She first went to Bulgaria with others to nurse Russian soldiers wounded in Russia's war with Turkey in 1877. There she met two lepers and became convinced that it should be her mission to study this disease and care for its victims [23]. But restrained by family ties she first went to New Zealand to nurse her consumptive sister until the latter died. She then became Lady Superintendent at Wellington Hospital, an institution primarily for the Maoris where she claimed to have treated lepers although it was not a disease indigenous to those people. Before she returned to England she established the first New Zealand branch of the St. Johns Ambulance Brigade.

She continued to work as a nurse but finally left England to treat leprosy. After obtaining the support of Queen Victoria and Princess Alexandra, she went to Russia hoping to obtain funding from the Russian Royal family. On the way she met an English doctor in Constantinople who told her of the curative properties for leprosy of an herb found in Siberia. Now with support also of Empress Maria Fedorovna, she travelled from Moscow to Siberia to find this magical cure. Her journey took her some 11,000 miles (17,000 km) across Russia, by train, sledge, on horseback, and by boat (Fig. 1.7). As she recorded in her memoirs, "Riding through Siberia": [24].

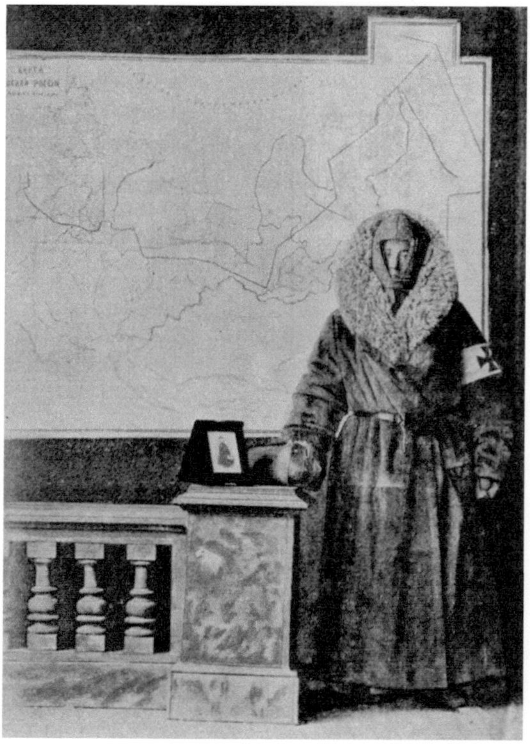

Fig. 1.7 Kate Marsden showing the clothing she wore with a map of her journey (Wikipedia: 3/13/14)

> During the summer the mosquitoes are frightful, both in the night and in the day; and when you arrive at a yourta [yurt], which serves as a post-station, the dirt and vermin and smell are simply disgusting; bugs, lice, fleas, etc., cover the walls, as well as the benches on which you have to sleep. Even on the ground you will find them, and, as soon as a stranger comes in, it seems as if the insects make a combined assault on him in large battalions; and, of course, sleep is a thing never dreamed of. After a few days the body swells from their bites into a form that can neither be imagined nor described. They attack your eyes and your face, so that you would hardly be recognised by your dearest friend. Really, I think the sufferings of this journey have added 20 years to my age. But I would willingly do it ten times over to aid my poor lepers who are placed in the depths of' these unknown forests. You are always running the risk

> of being attacked by bears here, so that we always kept our revolvers ready at our side or under our heads; and two Yakuts as sentinels, with large fires at each end of the little encampment, we were obliged to travel in the night, because our horses had no rest in the day time from the terrible horse-flies that were quite dangerous there. They instantly attacked the wretched beasts, so that it was an awful sight to see our horses with the blood running down their sides, many of them becoming so exhausted that they were not able to carry our luggage.

Along the way she was noted for helping prisoners, especially women. At Yakutsk she obtained the herb that she believed might be the cure. Although the herb did not bring the success she had hoped for, she continued to work amongst the lepers in Siberia where she created a leper treatment center.

Yet another example of nursing involvement in missions was the enormous efforts of Mrs. Francis Piggott who proposed the Colonial Nursing Association in 1895 to supply the colonies and dominions of the United Kingdom with trained nurses. Between 1896 and 1966 when the Association was terminated over 8,400 women supported the health of white colonists abroad. The mission was to use personal and public hygiene mainly to create physical and cultural boundaries around white patients and thus put colonists apart from the colonial setting [25].

Albert Schweitzer

Physician, philosopher, organist, missionary, and theologian, Albert Schweitzer (Fig. 1.8) was born in the province of Alsace-Lorraine, at that time part of the German Empire [26]. He received the 1952 Nobel Peace Prize for his philosophy of "Reverence for Life," and is probably most famous for founding and sustaining the Albert Schweitzer Hospital in Lambaréné, now in Gabon, west central Africa (then French Equatorial Africa) [27]. At age 30, he embarked on a 3 year course towards the degree of a Doctorate in Medicine, a subject in which he had little knowledge. He planned to spread the Gospel by healing, rather than preaching. In June 1912 he married Helene Bresslau.

As a gifted musician he was able to raise sufficient funds to equip a small hospital and with his wife and infant son he travelled to Lambaréné, in Gabon in the spring of 1913. During the rest of that year, he and his wife treated more than 2,000 patients for diseases such as yaws, malaria, sleeping sickness, tumors, and hernias. They also dealt with fetishism and cannibalism among the Mbahouin. Their first hospital was a shed, built as a chicken hut. By the autumn of 1913, they relocated to a corrugated iron structure with two rooms (examination room and an operating room). They also built a dispensary and an area for sterilizing equipment as well as a dormitory and waiting room, constructed like native huts out of unhewn logs.

Schweitzer's wife, Helene, (Fig. 1.9) had studied history, art, philosophy, nursing, and theology. She acted as an anesthetist for her husband's surgeries although it is unclear if she had any training in the specialty, probably using open drop ether [28]. She was an avid skier but had broken her back in a skiing accident. Later she developed tuberculosis but despite her physical disabilities she continued to work with Schweitzer for many years. She returned to New York in 1937 to raise money and tell the United States about their work with the hospital. Back in Lambaréné, by 1940, she spent WWII at the hospital, before leaving Africa in 1946. She returned only once in 1956 before her death in 1957 [26].

Later, accusations were made in Europe of unsanitary conditions at the hospital. On the day of Schweitzer's death, an African contended: "How do they (Europeans) know? They have never come here to see us. The grand Doctor, he came here and stayed for most of his life and gave us all he had to give, and that was a great deal" [26].

After Schweitzer died in 1965 at the age of 90, administration of the hospital was handed over to his daughter, Mrs. Rhena Eckert. The hospital is now supported by the Albert Schweitzer Fellowship, which was founded during 1940 in the United States [29]. It remains the primary source of health care for a large

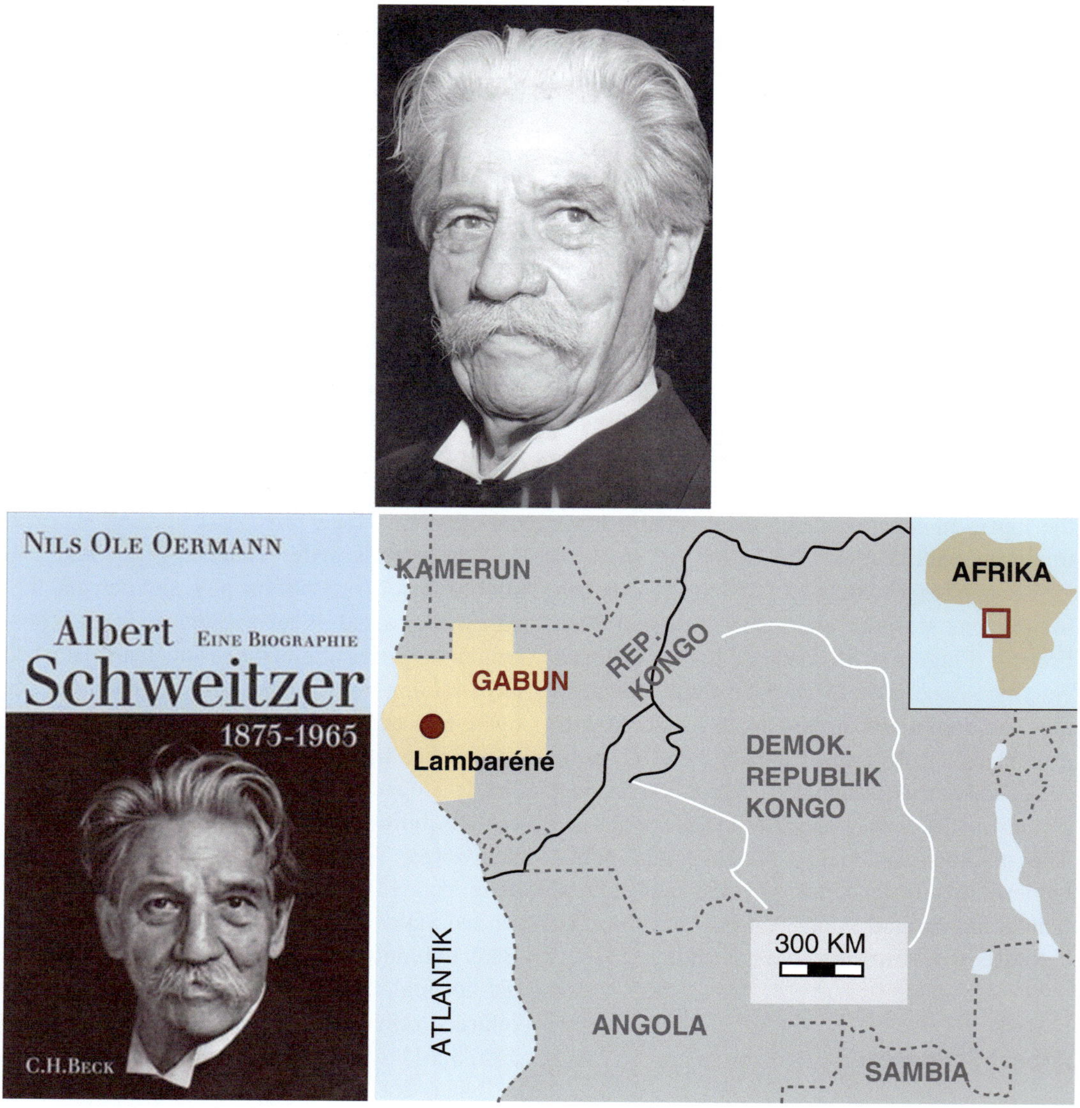

Fig. 1.8 Albert Schweitzer (accessed from Wikipedia; 3/13/14). (**a**) Dr. Albert Schweitzer and a map of Gabon, indicating his clinic

surrounding region. Over 35,000 outpatient visits and more than 6,000 hospitalizations occur annually. Two surgeons and their teams carry out some 2,200 operations every year. There are 160 members on staff. The current facility includes two operating rooms, a dental clinic, and inpatient wards for pediatric, adult medicine, surgical, and obstetrical patients. The National Institute of Health has recognized the hospital's research laboratory as a leading facility engaged in studies of malaria, HIV/AIDS, and tuberculosis and children with severe malaria at the Schweitzer Hospital have the lowest mortality rates in Africa.

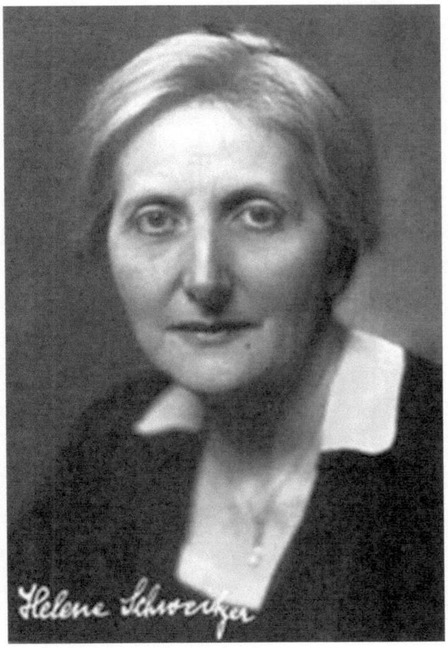

Fig. 1.9 Mrs. Helene Schweitzer Breslau

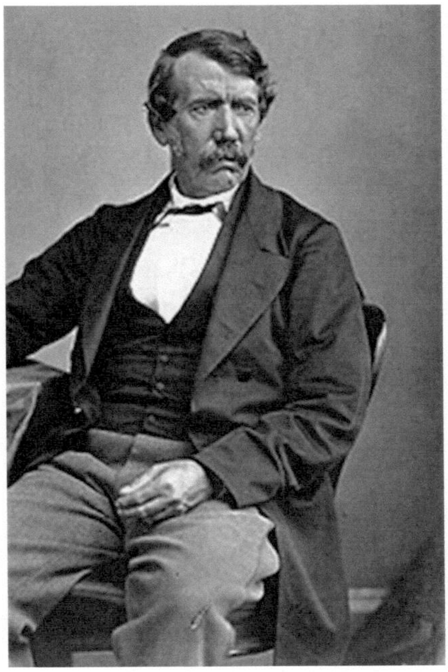

Fig. 1.10 Dr. David Livingstone (accessed Wikipedia 3/13/14)

David Livingstone

Born in a single-end (a one room flat), in Blantyre near Glasgow in 1813 David Livingston(e) (his family name had no "e" but after his medical certificate was issued with the letter, he used it thereafter) became one of the greatest of the Victorian pioneers and medical missionaries (Figs. 1.10 and 1.11) [30]. Employed as a piecer (a person who joins the ends of broken threads) at the local mill by the age of 10, his further schooling was during the 2 h that followed after his 12 ½ day shift, 6 days a week. On Sundays, he was required to attend church in nearby Hamilton. At one of these services, his father found a pamphlet written by Karl Friedrich August Gützlaff. Gützlaff, was a German missionary to the Far East, and one of the first Protestant missionaries in Bangkok (1828), China, and Korea (1832) [31]. What impressed the young Livingstone, now 20 years old, was a new idea presented by Gutlaff that missionaries should be trained as physicians. For the next 2 years Livingstone studied medicine at the Anderson's College in Glasgow and later continued his medical studies in London. He wanted to go to China but the opium wars prevented that journey. He applied to the London Missionary Society (LMS), at that time the major

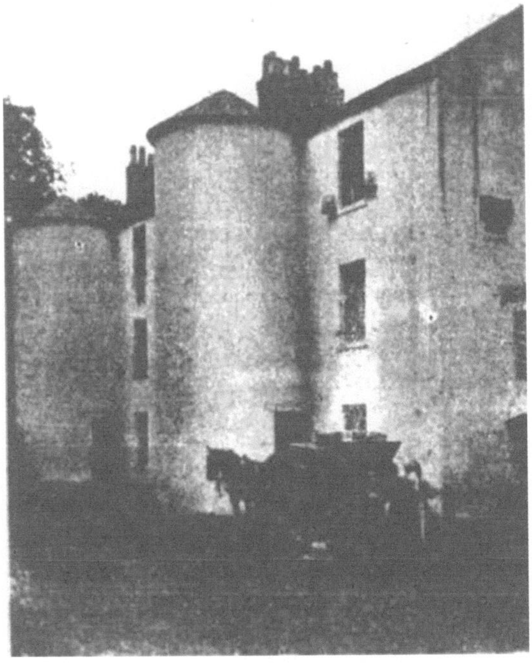

Fig. 1.11 Dr. Livingstone's birthplace in Blantyre, Scotland

mission society in the United Kingdom for an appointment. The LMS was, also, the only society open to him as the other Anglican, Baptist, and Methodist societies were clearly denominationally defined [30]. The LMS, founded in 1795, was rooted in the tradition of Evangelicalism, believing that denomination was secondary for converted Christians [32–34]. It continues today as the Council for World Missions.

In London, Livingstone met Dr. Robert Moffat, who was in England to create interest in his South African mission. Livingstone learned of "a vast plain to the north where he had sometimes seen, in the morning sun, the smoke of a 1,000 villages, where no missionary had ever been." He decided that Africa was his destiny. On December 8, 1840, he sailed for that mainly unknown continent, going out by way of Brazil and the Cape of Good Hope, learning on the way how to use the quadrant for navigation and take nautical observations, useful skills for his later journeys [29].

As an explorer he obsessed with discovering the sources of the River Nile a goal that he never reached. Nevertheless, his travels covered one-third of the continent, from the Cape to near the Equator, and from the Atlantic to the Indian Ocean. On November 15th 1855, he was probably the first European to reach the falls on the Zambezi River, known by the Africans as "the smoke that thunders" or Mosi-oa-Tunya and which he named the Victoria Falls, in honor of the Queen. During his explorations he drew the attention of the world to the horrors of the African slave traffic showing that the African was "wronged" rather than depraved, and slavery must be outlawed. He saw a cure for injustice in Christianity and commerce and inspired enterprises such as the African Lakes Company. After him came European settlements and the colonial rush to Africa with many of the tensions that followed.

Recognizing the constant threat of tropical diseases, especially trypanosomiasis and malaria and the need to provide an array of medical care, Livingstone maintained a kind of mail order education, arranging for papers, books, and lectures on advances in medicine to be sent to him at frequent intervals. A long list of books he ordered from John Snow of Paternoster Row in 1853 indicates his continuing intellectual interests. He also learned to use chloroform, quinine, and even arsenic in small doses [30].

Before Livingstone, Africa's interior was almost entirely unknown to the outside world. Vague notions prevailed about its geography, fauna, flora, and human life. Livingstone dispelled much of this ignorance and opened up Africa's interior to further exploration. No one made as many geographical discoveries in Africa as Livingstone, and his numerous scientific observations were quickly recognized [35].

He received many honors including the Gold Medal of the Royal Geographical Society of which he became a fellow. The London Missionary Society honored him; he was received by Queen Victoria; and the universities of Glasgow and Oxford conferred upon him honorary doctorates [34]. In November 1857 his first book, "Missionary Travels and Researches in South Africa," including a sketch of 16 years residence in the interior of Africa, was published by John Murray, Albemarle Street, London [36].

Twentieth Century

With the advent of the twentieth century it was clear that good medical care and especially anesthetic management was far from universally available. The Unitarian Service Committee (USC) Medical Missions was established in 1940 as a standing committee of the American Unitarian association, a nonsectarian voluntary agency with a mission to promote human welfare and justice [37]. Between 1945 and 1956 teams were organized to teach the latest developments to many countries around the world. Distinguished anesthesiologists were sent to 13 different countries including Drs. Beecher, Cullen, Dillon, Dripps, Kohn, Krayer, Morris, Robbins, Rovenstein, Saklad, Straus, Visscher, Volpitto, Wassermann, and White [38]. In 1950, medical missions to Tokyo and Osaka-Kyoto helped establish the new specialty of anesthesiology in Japan.

The origins of anesthesia in Japan can be traced back to 1804 when Sieshu Hanaoka gave anesthesia [39]. Also, in 1860, the Tokugawa Shogunate dispatched a group of Japanese, headed by Masaoki Niimi, the ambassador to Washington to ratify a treaty of commerce and amity. After the ratification, the group visited Baltimore and Philadelphia to see other institutions. Three Japanese medical doctors observed a lithotomy operation by Dr. Samuel Gross at the Jefferson Medical College and ether administration by Dr. William Morton, who had demonstrated his anesthetic technique in Boston on October 16th 1846 [40]. Neither of these opportunities appear to have benefitted or furthered the specialty of anesthesia in Japan. Such modern advances did not take hold until two programs from the USC were initiated in the 1950s, both supported by the US government [37].

At the end of World War II there was no organized anesthesiology service in Japan until the University of Tokyo founded an independent department of anesthesia in 1952. Before that, anesthesia was given by junior surgeons and there was not one physician trained in anesthesiology in all of Japan. There was little or no anesthetic equipment and less than 10 % of cases were done with general anesthesia. Death from local anesthetic toxicity was not uncommon. Libraries were bare because regulations prohibited Japanese currency as a medium for foreign exchange limiting subscriptions to foreign medical journals.

The first mission to Tokyo comprised physicians from several specialties with Dr. Meyer Saklad from Rhode Island representing anesthesiology. He presented many lectures and joint sessions with his colleagues. The mission then journeyed to Osaka and Kyoto and repeated the educational endeavors and also arranged for the donation of desperately needed books. A second mission was organized in 1951. This time Dr. Volpitto from the Medical College of Georgia spearheaded the anesthesia section. Four teams visited 12 medical schools, giving lectures, round table, and panel discussions and clinical demonstrations. A third mission, this one initiated by Japanese physicians, was again invited from the USC. Presentations now related mainly to research projects.

The effects of these three missions have been to enable an orderly transition to an American style medical system, especially in anesthesiology and to shape the specialty in Japan. Many Japanese have travelled to the United States and returned to their country where they have become leaders in their departments. From 2002 to 2007 Japanese anesthesiologists presented over 300 papers at the annual meetings of the American Society of Anesthesiologists.

Founded by a Buddhist nun, Dharma Master Cheng Yen in 1966, the Tzu Chi is a global service network of over 5,500 licensed doctors and nurses who serve as volunteers [41]. Based on the concept of "educating the rich to help the poor; inspiring the poor to realize their riches," the foundation's mission has expanded from its beginnings in the remote area of Hualien in Taiwan to all 5 continents with chapters and offices in 47 countries that provide aid to 70 countries and over one million people. Starting with charity, and quickly understanding that charity provide at best a temporary solution to a problem while sickness leads to poverty, the organization extended to medical care, including surgery, education, and the building of schools and humanistic culture. The Tzu Chi Medical Association with the vision of "Curing Sickness, Healing People, Healing Hearts" was later expanded to "Tzu Chi International Medical Association" or TIMA. Rather than a religion, Buddhism seeks to instill a way of life, marking its goals aside from many of the earlier missionary works. Some of the most important efforts have been realized during disasters when members of the Tzu Chi Disaster Relief committee travel to the stricken areas to treat the sick and wounded and provide support to devastated relatives (recently to the relatives of Malaysia Fl 370, lost March 8th 2014).

A Reverse Mission

Lady Mary Wortley Montagu, born in England in 1689, was an English aristocrat and writer (Fig. 1.12) [42]. Early in 1716, her husband, Edward Wortley Montagu, was appointed

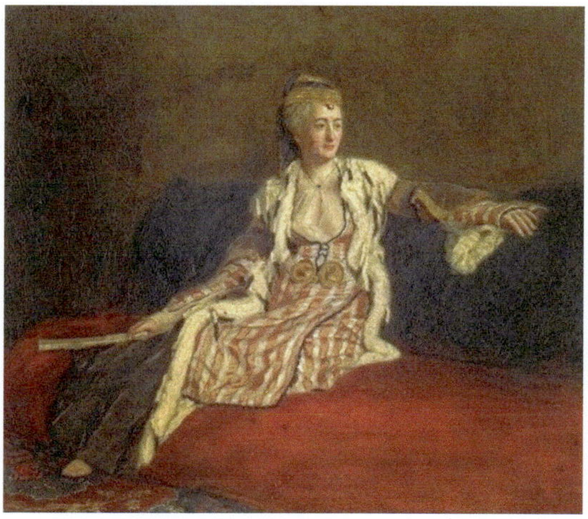

Fig. 1.12 Lady Mary Wortley Montague (from Wikipedia; 3/13/14)

Ambassador at Istanbul. Over some inadvertently circulated satirical remarks concerning members of the Royal family, Lady Mary was disgraced at court and thus accompanied her husband to Turkey. He was recalled in 1717, but they remained in Istanbul until 1718. During her stay in that city, she became acquainted with many of the customs of the local women, specifically their practice of inoculation against smallpox—variolation (from varus, Latin for pimple)—which she termed engrafting, and she wrote home about it [3]. She herself had suffered from smallpox and her brother had died of the disease. Variolation involved live smallpox virus in liquid form taken from a blister in a mild case [44]. She had her son inoculated while in Turkey. When she returned to London, she promoted the procedure, but encountered resistance from the medical establishment, because it was an "Oriental" process. A smallpox epidemic struck England in 1721 and Lady Mary also had her daughter inoculated. She then persuaded a Royal to authorize the process on seven condemned prisoners (in exchange for their lives) as well as six orphans. They all lived.

But in another household, six servants became ill with smallpox after a child was inoculated. Clergymen then announced that trying to prevent the illness was against God's will. Indeed inoculation carried about a 3 % risk of dying while contracting the disease had a 20–40 % mortality rate. But inoculation gained acceptance and in 1754, 8 years before her death, Lady Mary was recognized for bringing the practice to Britain [43].

Concluding Statement

Medical missions have spanned many centuries and changed dramatically in scope and practice. From bands of evangelists who travelled for years to establish churches and hospitals, often with no medical training, few supplies, and little support it is now common practice for highly trained specialists to mount well financed and organized enterprises for a few days or weeks with excellent support mechanisms and the aim to introduce and teach new methods of care needed and applicable to the country thus allowing local healthcare teams to become self-sufficient.

References

1. Collins K. Go and learn. Aberdeen: Aberdeen University Press; 1988. p. 3–4. ISBN 0 08 036408-X.
2. The Holy Bible. King James Version Isaiah. 61:1–3.
3. Ibid. Luke. 4: 14–30.
4. Ibid. Luke 4: 40.
5. Baron AW. A Social and Religious History of the Jews, vol. 8. New York, NY: Columbia University Press; 1958. p. 233–4. ISBN ISBN-10: 0231088450 ISBN-13: 978-0231088459.
6. Jakobovits I. Jewish medical ethics. New York, NY: Bloch Publishing Co; 1975. p. 4. ISBN ISBN-10: 0819700975; ISBN-13: 978-0819700971j.
7. Silen W, Frost EAM. Surgery before and after the discovery of anesthesia. In: Eger EI, Saidman LJ, Westhorpe RN, editors. The wondrous story of anesthesia. New York, NY: Springer; 2014. p. 167–8. ISBN 978-1-461-8440-7.
8. Haggard HW. Devils, drugs and Doctors. New York, NY: Blue Ribbon; 1929. p. 194–5.
9. Ibid. p. 216–7.
10. Caporael LR. Ergotism: the satan loose in Salem. Science. 1976;192(4234):21. doi:10.1126/science.769159. Bibcode: 1976 Sci…192…21C. PMID 769159.
11. Matossian M. Ergot and the Salem witchcraft affair. Am Sci. 1982;70(4):355. Bibcode: 1982 Am Sci.. 70.. 355M. PMID 6756230.
12. Boyd HG. A brief history of medical missions gospel advocate. 1990;132(12):14–5.

13. Lowe J. Medical missions their place and power. 5th ed. Oliphant Anderson and Ferrier: Edinburgh; 1903. p. 41–50.
14. IBID. p. 165–8.
15. Dodd EM. The gift of the healer. New York, NY: Friendship; 1964. p. 14.
16. Wilson DC. *The story of Dr. Ida Scudder of Vellore*. New York, NY: McGraw-Hill; 1959. p. 18. ASIN: B002AT0OT6.
17. Gulick EV. Peter Parker and the opening of China. Cambridge: Harvard University Press, Harvard Studies in American-East Asian Relations; 1973. p. 3. ISBN 0-674-66326-8.
18. Taylor G. Fever and thirst. An American doctor amid the tribes of Kurdistan, 1835–1844. Chicago: Academy Chicago Publishers; 2005. p. 1–13. ISBN 978-0-89733-572-0.
19. Anderson GH. Biography of Paul Wilson brand. Cambridge: Wm B Eerdmans Pub Grand Rapids and Cambridge; 1999. p. 86. ISBN 978-0-8028-4680-8.
20. Gill CJ, Gill GC, Gill GC. Nightingale in scutari: her legacy reexamined. Clin Infect Dis. 2005; 40(12):1799–805. doi:10.1086/430380. ISSN 1058-4838. PMID 15909269.
21. Nightingale F. Preface. In: Nightingale F, editor. Notes on nursing: What it is and what it is not. Glasgow & London: Blackie & Son Ltd.; 1974. First published 1859. ISBN 0-216-89974-5.
22. Eichman P (2014) Medical missions among the churches of Christ. History of medical missions Chapter 2. 2nd ed. 2002. P. 3–6. http://bible.ovu.edu/missions/medical/medbook2.htm. Accessed 5 Mar 2014.
23. Bessonov Y (2014) An outstanding journey of a British nurse to the Yakut Lepers in Siberia. J Nurs. http://rnjournal.com/journal-of-nursing/an-outstanding-journey-of-a-british-nurse-to-the-yakut-lepers-in-siberia. Accessed 5 Mar 2014.
24. Mission of Mercy, Long Riders Guild. http://www.thelongridersguild.com/marsden.htm. Accessed 5 Mar 2014.
25. Howell J, Rafferty AM, Wall R, et al. Nursing in the tropics: nurses as agents of imperial hygiene. J Public Health (Oxf). 2013;35(2):338–41. doi:10.1093/pubmed/fdt016.
26. Cousins N. Albert Schweitzer's mission. New York, NY: Norton; 1985. p. 11–4. 68–70, 302. ISBN 0-393-02238-2.
27. Nobel Peace Prize 1952 Award Ceremony Speech. The Nobel Peace Prize 1952. Albert Schweitzer. Nobelprize.org (1953-12-10). Retrieved on 6 Mar 2014.
28. http://www.findagrave.com/cgi-bin/fg.cgi?page=gr&GRid=34278577. Accessed 6 Mar 2014.
29. http://en.wikipedia.org/wiki/Albert_Schweitzer_Hospital. Accessed 6 Mar 2014.
30. Ross A. David Livingstone: mission and empire. London: Hambledon; 2001. p. 2–26. ISBN 1 85285 285 2.
31. Lutz JG. Opening China: Karl F.A. Gützlaff and Sino-Western relations, 1827–1852. Grand Rapids, MI: William B. Eerdmans Pub. Co.; 2008. ISBN 080283180X.
32. Wadsworth KW. Yorkshire United Independent College: two hundred years of training for Christian ministry by the congregational churches of Yorkshire. London: Independent; 1954.
33. Parker I. Dissenting academies in England: their rise and progress, and their place among the educational systems of the country. Cambridge: Cambridge University Press; 1914. p. 140. ISBN 978-0-521-74864-3.
34. Lovett R. The history of the London Missionary Society, 1795–1895. London: Henry Frowde; 1899.
35. Swinton WE. Physicians as explorers. David Livingstone: 30 years of service in darkest Africa. CMA J. 1977;117:1435–40.
36. Ross A. David Livingstone: mission and empire. London: Hambledon; 2001. p. 118. ISBN 1 85285 285 2.
37. Ikeda S. The Unitarian service committee medical mission. Anesthesiology. 2007;106(1):178–85. PMID:17197860.
38. Ikeda S. American anesthesiologists' contribution to post world war ll global anesthesiology. J Clin Anesthesia. 2011;23(3):244–52. doi:10.1016/j.jclinane.2010.08.013. PII: S0952-8180(11)00118-8.
39. Ikeda S. American contributions to Japanese anesthesiology-a historical view. Masui. 2013;62(6):761–9. PPMID: 23815010.
40. Matsuki A. New study on the history of anesthesiology-three Japanese doctors who observed William TG Morton's ether anesthesia at the Gross Clinic in 1860. Masui. 2005;54(2):202–8. PMID 15747522.
41. http://www.tzuchimedicalfoundation.org/index.php?option=com_content&view=article&id=14&Itemid=96.
42. Grundy I. Lady Mary Wortley Montague. Oxford: Oxford UP; 1999. p. 103.
43. Lady Mary Wortley Montagu (1689–1762): Smallpox Vaccination in Turkey Lady Mary Wortley Montagu, Letters of the Right Honourable Lady Mary Wortley Montague: Written During her Travels in Europe, Asia and Africa…, vol. 1 (Aix: Anthony Henricy, 1796), p. 167–69; letter 36, to Mrs. S. C. from Adrianople, n.d. Modern History Sourcebook: Fordham University.
44. Case CL, Chung KT. Montagu and Jenner: the campaign against smallpox. SIM News. 1997;47(2): 58–60.

Further Reading

Cousins N. Albert Schweitzer healing and peace. New York, NY: Norton; 1985. ISBN 0-393-02238-2.

La Berge AF. Mission and method the early 19th century public health movement. Cambride: Cambridge University Press; 1992.

Ross A. David Livingstone: mission and empire. London: Hambledon; 2001. ISBN 85285 285 2.

Topping AR. china mission a personal history form the last imperial dynasty to the people's republic. Baton Rouge: Louisiana State University Press; 2014.

Taylor G. Fever and thirst an American doctor among the tribes of Kurdistan 1835–44. Chicago: Academy Chicago Publisher; 2005.

Lowe J. Medical missions: their place and power (1903). 5th ed. Ithaca: Cornell University Library; 1903. Digital Collection from Oliphant, Anderson and Ferrier, Edinburgh and London.

2 The Evolution of Surgical Humanitarian Missions

Ofer Merin

Abbreviations

FMTs Foreign medical teams
NGOs Nongovernmental organizations

Introduction

International aid agencies have traditionally focused on infectious diseases in resource-limited settings. Global health initiatives, however, are now increasingly addressing surgical conditions as well. A growing awareness of the heavy burden of surgically treatable diseases and conditions has led to extensive involvement of both public and public resources in surgical international humanitarian missions, which perform and teach surgery in order to improve healthcare worldwide [1, 2]. These services can be in the form of a preplanned mission to an underserved region, or an acute response in the aftermath of a major disaster or humanitarian crisis. The latter is provided by medical and surgical units, collectively referred to as "foreign medical teams" (FMTs). A "global burden of surgical disease working group" was established in 2008, and it arrived at a strategy consensus of how to measure the burden of surgical conditions and the unmet needs for surgical care [3].

Every year thousands of physicians and nurses travel to developing countries, with stays ranging from days to years. The increased ease of world travel and transport and the heightened interest in international matters have led to greater numbers of healthcare providers involved in these humanitarian efforts. Humanitarian assistance can be in the form of a single individual, a group, part of a nongovernmental organization (NGO), a government agency, or under the auspices of a United Nations (UN) Organization, such as the World Health Organization (WHO).

This chapter will briefly describe the history of surgical missions, update the current situation and identify the main global players, and then focus on the main challenges and dilemmas faced by these missions. The benefits will be balanced against any potential harm resulting from their deployment. Some of those challenges will be described in greater detail than others. Just as little guidance exists on how to measure the benefits of outreach trips, even less is known about what harm they might cause or how to deal with that harm. This chapter will conclude with a vision for the future.

History

Before World War II (WWII), two institutions dominated international health development: The Pasteur Institutions (functioning mainly in

O. Merin, M.D., M.H.A. (✉)
Shaare Zedek Medical Center,
P.O. Box 3235, Jerusalem 9103102, Israel
e-mail: merin@szmc.org.il

R. Roth et al. (eds.), *The Role of Anesthesiology in Global Health: A Comprehensive Guide*,
DOI 10.1007/978-3-319-09423-6_2, © Springer International Publishing Switzerland 2015

the Far and Middle East and Africa) and the Rockefeller Institute (functioning mainly throughout Latin America). Their efforts were largely directed to the control or eradication of major infectious scourges, such as malaria, typhoid, plague, and other tropical and sanitation-based public health problems. Basch characterized international health after WWII as having evolved through four distinct stages [4]:

1. 1945–1950: Period of general international stability with intergovernmental cooperation for reconstruction.
2. 1950–1970: Development of various UN agencies largely around a medical model focused on eradication of diseases.
3. 1970–1980: UN agencies' development of a series of "agendas," such as primary health care, community empowerment, and women's issues.
4. 1980–1990: The World Bank, the International Monetary Fund (IMF), and various NGOs focusing more on underlying health and societal system-level issues as obstacles to optimum health.

The publication of the Global Burden of Disease Report in 1996 [5] has increased the awareness of the impact of chronic diseases and injuries on the overall health burden, leading to recognition by international development agencies that more attention must be directed toward them. Remarkably little attention was drawn to surgical missions throughout this entire period.

The Present

Global health policy in the developing world traditionally emphasized primary prevention and categorical vertical programs aimed at communicable disease, maternal health, perinatal and child health, and nutritional deficiencies. Such categorical health initiatives have achieved considerable success in developing countries [6]. They emphasize healthcare delivery at the primary care level, and provide preventative measures, health promotion activities, and essential primary care services. Their premise is that "an ounce of prevention is worth a pound of cure." It makes sense to focus on communicable and infectious diseases, since about 25 % of deaths in developing countries are secondary to those diseases compared to only 3–4 % in developed countries. It became evident over the last decade, however, that global epidemiologic and demographic shifts have been changing the burden of disease in all societies. Developing countries are now facing a dramatic increase in noncommunicable diseases, including injuries and chronic illnesses [7]. This change is gradually producing a parallel shift in the focus of healthcare provision in terms of individual patients vs. cohorts/populations. Today, surgeons and anesthesiologists are becoming involved in humanitarian efforts to a much greater extent than ever before.

Although there is an increasing awareness of the importance of unmet needs for surgical care worldwide, it is still estimated that up to one-half of the world's population lacks access to basic surgical needs [8]. The burden of surgical care is potentially enormous. It was estimated that 2–3 billion people (approximately one-third to one-half of the world's population) have no access to basic surgical care [9, 10]. Despite this clear imbalance around the world, surgery is still "the neglected stepchild of global health" as noted by Farmer and Kim [11]. There are probably many reasons for this, one of which is that international health was dominated for decades by those concerned with communicable diseases, from smallpox to AIDS. Another reason is that surgery is much more complex and more expensive to deliver than vaccinations [11].

The international projects that aimed to fill the gaps in surgical needs may be classified into three types: clinical, relief projects, and developmental projects.

Clinical: These are preplanned delegations that deal mainly with chronic conditions and diseases, often targeted to a specific disease. Humanitarian missions to underserved areas throughout the world aim to relieve specific surgical conditions. Examples include plastic surgical procedures [12, 13], pediatric cardiology surgery [13, 14], ophthalmology (mainly cataract surgery) [15, 16], pediatric neurosurgery [17], and combined specialties, such as otorhinolaryngologists and plastic surgeons who repair facial deformities [18], among others.

Relief: These include surgical teams that respond to needs that result from natural disasters or wars (see Chap. 11). They are "acute" missions, organized within a short time frame, and frequently deal with many uncertainties. Their aim is to alleviate a time-limited crisis. These include foreign medical teams (FMTs) that respond in the aftermath of sudden impact disasters, either to substitute or complement the local medical system. They have three distinct purposes [19]:

1. Early emergency care. This period lasts up to 48 h following the onset of an event.
2. Follow-up care for trauma cases, emergencies, and routine health care (from day 3 to day 15). During this phase, the local health services are progressively overwhelmed by the need for secondary or maintenance care for the trauma victims. The primary roles of the FMTs are to temporary fill the gaps in emergency medical assistance resulting either from a large number of casualties or the inability of the local health services to respond to the usual emergencies.
3. Act as a temporary facility to substitute for damaged local facilities during the rehabilitation phase until a permanent solution (reconstructive phase) is available. This phase usually starts from the second month and can last up to several years.

Developmental: These are organized for a long-term framework and their aim is to create or augment local capacity to address the burden of surgical disorders. There is an increasing understanding that short-term medical missions cannot substitute for a continuing investment in the local health infrastructure and staff training that will allow low- and middle-class countries to develop their own long-term surgical capacity [20]. Training programs, when carefully considered and implemented, can be mutually beneficial and provide a sustainable and lasting solution to the unmet health needs of the developing world. The outcome of such a training program should be reasonably self-sufficient local surgeons who are able to cope with most of the surgical problems in district hospitals in the developing world.

Major Players in Humanitarian Assistance

The total number of humanitarian aid workers around the world was 210,800, as calculated in 2008 by the Active Learning Network for Accountability and Performance in Humanitarian Actions (ALNAP), a network of agencies working in the humanitarian system [21]. The last decade has witnessed increasing involvement in the provision of humanitarian aid: it is estimated that the humanitarian fieldworker population has been increasing by approximately 6 % per year [21]. Those workers include medical students, residents, senior and retired surgeons who were involved in short-term missions and physicians/nurses who devoted longer periods (months/years) in order to treat the needy and train local health providers.

The involvement of medical students in this system has been increasing. For example, 22 % of US medical students had completed an international educational experience in 2004 [22], and 47 % of accredited MD-granting medical schools had established initiatives, centers, institutions, or offices of global health by 2008 [23]. All of the plastic surgery residents who participated in such missions reported that this experience had an important impact upon their life and career [13]. Two-thirds of responders to an American College of Surgeons (ACS) survey asked to be placed on a mailing list of surgeons interested in volunteerism [24]. Similar responses were received to a questionnaire of the American Association of Thoracic Surgeons [25].

The major participants in humanitarian assistance typically fit into one of the five following categories [26]:

1. United Nations (UN) organizations and other international organizations. Included are the UN High Commissioner for Refugees (UNHCR), the WHO, and the International Committee of the Red Cross (ICRC).

These organizations typically provide the oversight, coordination, and funding for NGOs and program implementers.

2. Governmental organizations. Various industrialized countries maintain funding agencies dedicated to relief and development. Examples include the US agency for International Development and the relief and disaster branch, the United Kingdom's Department for International Development, The European Commission Humanitarian Aid Office, the Canadian, Danish, and Australian Agencies for International Development, and many more. These governmental agencies set priorities for funding and provide financial support for implementing partners through grants and contracts.
3. NGOs and private voluntary organizations. The World Bank defines NGOs as being private, independent organizations that initiate activities to relieve suffering, promote the interests of the poor, provide basic social services, and/or undertake community development [27]. These organizations are the primary implementers of relief assistance. Today, there are over 40,000 actively engaged NGOs [28]. They can be large or small, local or international, religious or secular, and have a wide range of expertise. In some countries, like Haiti, NGOs account for over 70 % of the total healthcare delivery. The need for external governments not to be seen as directly intervening in another sovereign territory is one cause for the NGO's expansion. Government-funded NGOs generally work from a position of neutrality and impartiality and are therefore regarded as being free of political influence. Their ability to gain easier cross-border access and attract less attention and scrutiny than governmental agencies has motivated major funding from governmental donors and spurred their global growth. This increased funding has promoted the growth of some well-known established international agencies, such as the Medecins Sans Frontiers (MSF: Doctors without Borders). The MSF received the 1999 Nobel Peace Prize in recognition of its members' continuing efforts to provide medical care in acute crises, as well as raising international awareness of potential humanitarian disasters. Other large organizations include the International Rescue Committee, CARE International, Catholic Relief Services, and World Vision.
4. Private industry, consulting firms, and academic organizations. There has been a significant growth in the participation of for-profit organizations and consulting firms in humanitarian aid and post-disaster reconstruction. Similarly, greater numbers of academicians in the various fields of medicine, public health, human rights, epidemiology, and social services have been providing assistance. Universities, such as Johns Hopkins, Harvard, Tufts, Columbia, and others, have academic programs in various aspects of humanitarian aid. The American College of Surgeons (ACS) has also become involved in volunteer activities by establishing the volunteer initiative, Operation Giving Back (OGB) [29].
5. The military. Various military branches are involved in important humanitarian aid in the form of security, communications, and logistic operations, as well as the provision of medical assistance, food, shelter, and public health around the globe. The Office for the Communication of Humanitarian Affairs developed a set of guidelines for the use of military assets in non-conflict relief operations known as the "Oslo guidelines" [30].

Challenges

A foreign team is parachuting into a foreign environment. Medical care in underserved and under-resourced areas is provided in a difficult environment for a foreign medical team. Primary care is often not available in many of these areas, and therefore many medical conditions are underdiagnosed and undertreated. Surgeons on overseas missions will wrestle with challenges that are a far cry from their usual clinical practice, sometimes to the point of appearing surreal.

Surgeons on humanitarian missions are inarguably engaged in a noble cause, but good intentions alone cannot ensure success. The principle of non-malfeasance, often defined as the obligation to "do no harm," must be rigidly upheld under all conditions. Many medical initiatives automatically focus on what and how to provide appropriate medical/surgical care. Equally imperative, however, is what *not* to offer. One has to be aware of the risk in conducting a mission that provides temporary, short-term solutions but fails to take in the entire picture.

It is impossible to establish clear-cut guidelines before embarking upon humanitarian missions in foreign countries, but it is important to take appropriate precautions when planning and executing such missions. The line between an exemplary voluntary humanitarian effort of altruistic health providers that has an important positive impact and a mission criticized and labeled as "neocolonialism," "surgical safari," "medical tourism," and "short-term overseas work in poor countries by clinical people from rich countries" [31] is sometimes not clear enough. Not infrequently, and despite the best of intentions, mistakes are made in attempts to help others. Groups must be aware of and avoid, as much as possible, "the seven sins of humanitarian medicine" [32] and the potential pitfalls [33, 34].

The following *Ten Commandments* are proposed to describe some of the unique challenges in planning and executing surgical humanitarian missions. They are based on accounts in the literature as well as on personal insights after responding to disaster areas around the globe:

1. *Careful selection of cases and of the most appropriate anesthesia.* One important surgical challenge in these short-term missions is to perform the right procedure. It is a common temptation to perform complex surgery when indicated. However, once the short-term mission leaves, the local physicians will have to deal with any complications from surgeries which they themselves cannot perform, or do not have the knowledge or expertise to properly treat. It is sometimes better to do a simpler procedure within the abilities of a given local system. Better to leave with hope than with desperation. When choosing the proper procedure the best interest of the patient, the hospital, and the local physicians should clearly prevail. According to Welling et al., "One good rule is to offer the types of procedures that are minimally invasive, relieve immediate discomfort, and require little follow-up care, especially for missions that are short term" [32]. Complications may be inevitable, but when they affect an impoverished patient in a developing country who was treated by a volunteer physician, the situation can be politically as well as emotionally charged [35].

   Choosing the most appropriate anesthetic technique is another challenge. It should be tailored to the kind of care, monitoring, and skills that will be available postoperatively. It is sometimes better to choose a different approach from what one might usually employ (our preference is to use regional/local anesthesia, instead of general anesthesia, if at all possible).
2. *Follow-up.* Short-term missions provide clinical/surgical care for patients who may never be seen again by the foreign team. Continuum of care which is a basic and essential part of surgical treatment is lacking. The local community sometimes criticizes this failure to provide follow-up care. One example was the accusation of Operation Smile volunteers by local surgeons of "dumping" their complications once their mission was over. The organization refuted this charge [35], but one should bear in mind that this can be a sensitive issue. When it is not possible to provide long-term follow-up care, it is recommended that chronic care medications and elective surgery be avoided.
3. *Cultural competence.* This item refers to the ability of healthcare providers to deliver effective services to racially, ethnically, and culturally diverse patient populations. A culturally competent physician is aware of different cultural beliefs or concepts of illness and health and has the skills to explore how and whether these beliefs are relevant to a specific individual [36]. There are several models available that emphasize the important concepts of cross-cultural communication

process. One such example is the RESPECT model, developed by the Boston University Residency Training Program in Internal Medicine, Diversity Curriculum Taskforce [37]. The RESPECT model stands for: Respect, Explanatory model, Sociocultural context, Power, Empathy, Concerns and fears, Therapeutic alliance/trust. Personnel involved in such work should understand and respect the local culture and be aware of the local customs. How we dress, how we act, what we drink, and other behaviors will define us to our hosts. Miscommunication and misunderstanding may lead to potential harm. Therefore, one should establish an effective method of communication and become familiar with cultural norms before departure. Awareness of a given culture's beliefs and practices is important because it fosters an environment of trust and mutual respect, which may translate to better compliance and greater effectiveness of medical treatment [38].

4. *Informed consent.* The principle of informed consent is aimed at the legality of health assistance and reflects the concept of autonomy and of decisional auto-determination of the patient. Operating even in a disaster scenario does not allow another individual to decide for a conscious and coherent patient. The same rules apply as they do within the United States. The World Medical Association (WMA) 1994 statement on medical ethics in the event of disasters states there may not be enough time for informed consent to be a realistic possibility in a disaster response situation [39]. This may also apply when responding to disasters in one's own country, but we believe that a different approach should be taken when one arrives to a foreign country as a relief delegation. Our team, which has vast experience in response to natural disasters, is very strict about this issue. We never operate or perform an invasive procedure on a patient without his/her consent (or consent of a surrogate) after a clear explanation by a local interpreter. It should be borne in mind that cultural and religious differences may exist, and that relief workers are at risk of delivering culturally inappropriate services.
5. *Cooperation with local authorities.* Foreign healthcare teams are supposed to support and reinforce the national health system, not replace it. Every attempt should be made to collaborate with the local system. By ignoring local healthcare providers, many volunteer programs undermine the local infrastructure, create new barriers to care, and cause harm. Local practitioners who must earn a living in the community cannot compete with volunteers who donate their services. While assisting the Philippine people after the 2013 typhoon, it was the decision of our group to integrate our team with the local hospital, creating one coordinated facility [40]. Collaboration with local surgeons is especially critical in surgical missions since the latter need to provide follow-up care and treat complications after the guest surgeons' departure.
6. *Triage and ethical dilemmas.* Mass casualty triage needs to be implemented when available resources are insufficient to meet the needs of all patients in a disaster situation. The basic principle is to do the maximum good for the most casualties with the least amount of resources. Disasters require physicians to shift to "utilitarian-based ethics" in which medical decisions are based on available resources, much in the way that a triage system prioritizes victims who are predicted to have the best chance of survival [32]. The WMA statement on medical ethics in disasters recognizes these unique situations and noted "The physician must act according to the needs of patients and the resources available. He/she should attempt to set an order of priorities for treatment that will save the greatest number of lives and restrict morbidity to a minimum" [39]. Such situations will inevitably lead to serious ethical dilemmas. Efforts will be needed in order to achieve a balance between individual and collective rights. There is generally a conflict between autonomy of the individual and the desire to

protect and promote public health. This "dual loyalty" also exists in many disaster situations. It is necessary to develop a system that identifies patients by their medical/surgical needs and the likelihood of benefit, especially in the context of disaster response, but also during short-term initiatives. Because of the complexity of triage in such conditions, the basic concept underlying the process should be decided before departure. In addition, the process must be fair, transparent, and meet the principles of distributive justice [41]. Triage can conflict with human rights legislation, and even with humanitarian laws, but "accountability for reasonableness" can temper the disagreements on the setting of priorities. Triage in a disaster setting, however, requires a basic change in thinking. Of necessity, this adjustment includes dealing with ethical dilemmas for which there is little preparation [42, 43]. Among the many proposed approaches to triage, perhaps the most common is the utilitarian notion of doing the most good for the most people. Our personal recommendation after dealing with ethical and triage issues while responding to the Haiti earthquake is that it is imperative to establish and strictly follow clear-cut guidelines [44].

The ethical "code of conduct" of the International Red Cross (ICRC)/Red Crescent seeks to outline the principles of conduct of foreign teams responding to a disaster [45]. The main ethical principles in the provision of health services during an event and during the early response phase of disasters pertain to non-malfeasance, beneficence, justice, and the respect of autonomy.

7. *Licensure, credentialing, and malpractice issues*. Unlike country/state licensure and hospital accreditation which is standardized, there is no comparable international system, and this is an area that causes much concern for surgeons. These issues cannot be dealt with before departure to disaster areas. Recent discussions have highlighted the difficulties and concerns with using untrained volunteers to deliver care in international settings. International humanitarian volunteers have different levels of knowledge, medical education, and levels of competence. Medical personnel in resource-poor locations are subject to the same ethical principles of their own countries. Licensure is important since it may serve as restraint against unethical conduct [46]. Although medical negligence lawsuits are not currently a significant problem for humanitarian medical/surgical groups [47], many of them are becoming more concerned that such lawsuits may soon have an impact upon their missions [48].
8. *Mutual expectations*. A key to success is to promise less than what can be delivered, and to deliver more than what was promised. Accordingly, humanitarian aid providers should avoid creating false or unreasonable expectations on the part of the recipients.
9. *Standard of care*. Volunteers should not provide medical services beyond their level of expertise. Personnel must be aware of the pitfalls in practicing beyond their abilities. Alarmingly, medical students and residents often view medical missions to developing countries as opportunities to gain unrestrained exposure to techniques and procedures they are not qualified to perform in their home countries [49]. One has to find the right balance in this twofold goal: allow residents an opportunity to both learn and serve. Visiting physicians sometimes feel compelled to treat patients outside their specialty, simply because no specialist is available, even though lowering the standard of care for patients in developing communities is unprofessional, unsafe, unethical, and oftentimes illegal [50]. Healthcare providers working in humanitarian missions should be able to recognize their limitations and act accordingly. Humanitarian missions can have an important role in modern surgical training, but they should never turn into a self-serving opportunity for the visitor at the expense of the recipient nation which could feel that it is being treated as an experimental guinea pig.
10. *Know and understand what is unique to the operating zone*. Diseases can be encountered

with unfamiliar presentations and with unexpected patient profiles. All of these factors should have direct implication on clinical decision-making. Members operating in remote areas should be familiar with endemic local pathology. We encountered patients in Haiti, and later on in the Philippines, who presented with abdominal pain which we initially considered as being caused by an acute abdomen (with which we were familiar), but which turned out to be typhoid fever (which we had never seen before). In resource-poor countries, one may encounter higher rates of malnutrition and underweight in children, and of low plasma protein concentration and anemia in adults. Thus, patients treated by members of a surgical mission may be more prone to wound infection, wound dehiscence, and other related complications, factors that have to be taken into account when offering surgical care.

The Future

More and more individuals and teams are involved in surgical humanitarian aid with understandably varied levels of quality. Questions concerning the competence of some of the deployed medical teams have recently been raised. These findings have promoted the international community to call for "greater accountability, stringent performance oversight, reporting, and better coordination" [51]. In the coming years, we will be seeing a trend toward better and closer control in some of the following areas:

1. Classification and accreditation of FMTs. The foreign medical teams working under the auspices of the global health cluster and the WHO recently (2013) commissioned a document entitled: "Classification and minimum standards for foreign medical teams in sudden onset disasters" [52]. It introduces a simple classification, minimum standards, and a registration form for FMTs that arrive to provide surgical and trauma care in the aftermath of a sudden disaster. These guidelines can also serve as tools to improve the coordination between foreign medical teams, and be the reference to registration on arrival. According to this document, the foreign medical teams are expected to declare to which of three distinct categories they belong according to their capacity and capabilities. Once an FMT declares its capability to offer a specific type of care and any additional services, it is expected to comply with the technical standards related to those services. The next step will be registration of that FMT [53]. This concept of an international registration process could be a first step toward future accreditation of FMTs.
2. Operational guidelines. The WHO/Pan-American Health Organization (PAHO) published essential guidelines for the FMTs as follows [19]:
   - Be fully operational within 3–5 days.
   - Be self-sufficient with minimal need for support from the local communities.
   - Have basic knowledge of the health situation and language and respect for the culture.
   - Include health professionals in selected specialties.
   - Ensure capacity for sustainability, including appropriate technology costs.

   Of the 44 FMTs responding within the first month after the Haiti earthquake, only 11 adhered to essential deployment requirements and none followed all the requirements of WHO/PAHO [54]. Volunteer efforts need to be preplanned in order to respond within an adequate time frame. Individuals interested in taking part should belong to a designated team ready to be deployed. One example is the Disaster Medical Assistance Teams (DMATs), which are groups of medical personnel set up to respond to disasters or unusual events. Composed of about 35 individuals or more, they are rapid responders and provide primary care or augment local staff [55].
3. Sustainability. Suchdev et al. [33] suggested a model for sustainable short-term international medical trips. They identified seven areas of focus: developing a clear mission, collaborating with the local community, educating travelers and the local community, making the commitment to serve the needs of the local

community, engaging in teamwork, having sustained capacity building, and developing a system for periodic evaluation. The benefits of these medical initiatives should extend beyond the presence of foreign medical assistance. Sub-specialized surgical care may be best addressed with visiting teams, but a much more preferred expanded model of sustainable delivery of surgical care, which emphasizes empowerment of local healthcare practitioners through education, equipment support, and quality benchmarks, has been described [56].

4. Accountability. There is no single official definition of accountability in the humanitarian context. Accountability per se is defined as having three components: transparency, responsiveness, and compliance [19]. Accountability is mainly at the organization level, but there is also a component of individual accountability. We should expect that missions would use evidence-based medicine as the benchmark, although it is difficult to come up with a single set of outcome measures and levels that fits all the different environments in which these missions operate. Working with its partners, disaster survivors, and others, Humanitarian Accountability Partnership International (HAP International) produced the HAP 2007 Standard in Humanitarian Accountability and Quality Management. This certification scheme aims to provide assurance that certified agencies manage the quality of their humanitarian actions in accordance with the HAP standard [57].
5. Data collection. Humanitarian missions deliver health care in especially difficult environments where patients may be more prone to complications. This makes the evaluation of these different programs of utmost importance. Only a few groups have collected data, and even fewer have evaluated those data or statistics [58]. Our group has developed a specially tailored information technology solution which is implemented in the field hospital we deploy in disasters [59]. This solution includes a hospital administration system as well as a complete electronic medical record and a lightweight picture archiving and communication system (PACS). Patient transfers within the hospital are noted, and an online command dashboard screen is generated. Patient care is delivered by means of an electronic medical record. Digital radiographs are acquired and transmitted to stations throughout the hospital. The system helps to introduce order into an otherwise chaotic situation and enables adequate utilization of scarce medical resources by continually gathering information, analyzing it, and presenting it to the decision-making command level. The establishment of electronic medical records promotes facilitated continuity of care. Based on our experience, we encourage disaster response teams and agencies to consider the use of information technology as part of their contingency plans.

A 2011 Davos global health risk forum conference reviewed emergency surgical findings to date and called for improved data collection [60]. There is a consensus of a strong need to establish an international standardized reporting format. A proposed standard data collection form for sudden onset humanitarian crisis and natural disasters was suggested [61]. Multiple FMTs were mobilized following the recent large-scale disasters specifically, the 2010 Haiti earthquake. Thousands of surgical procedures were performed to alleviate pain, save lives, and allow rehabilitation and recovery. Many of these FMTs provided high-quality care, but they lacked basic medical record-keeping. In the absence of systematic information management and data collection, it is unlikely that the true impact, both positive and negative, of FMTs in a crisis setting will ever be known. It is disappointing to note that the massive medical response, presumably at immense cost, is inadequately documented. Without basic outcome data, there can be neither accountability nor a report of lessons learned.

Some groups recently began to collect and report outcome measures. In 2005, Operation Smile International (OSI) implemented an electronic medical record system that helps monitor a number of critical indices that are essential for quality assurance reviews of surgical missions. In one retrospective analysis of more than 8,000 cases (mostly cleft palate procedures in children), the complication rates were similar to those reported in the United States and United Kingdom [62]. This finding is in accordance with other reports. In an analysis of data from three otology surgical missions conducted in Paraguay and Honduras from 2003 to 2006, the authors concluded that the results fall within those expected in developed nations [63]. The information in these reports are testimony to the importance of precise record-keeping and self-monitoring which would be invaluable to the efforts of organizing and regulating surgical humanitarian aid the world over.

Concluding Remarks

Humanitarian aid is a young science. The medical/surgical care provided in disasters or remote areas is unique and different than that of routine practice in the industrialized countries. Adaptability to the different scenarios is essential. As more and more medical personnel become involved, we may see these missions turning into a separate medical specialty. Toward that end, Farmer et al. [64] described a novel concept of creating a global health equity residency at Harvard's Brigham and Women's Hospital. Those of us involved in surgical humanitarian aid are acutely aware of the shortcomings of current practices and are actively striving to overcome them. We are optimistic that the next decade will witness major improvements in all of the areas that were described in this report, in full recognition of our responsibilities to provide care for the victims of global disasters that we are powerless to prevent.

References

1. Global Burden of Surgical Disease Working Group. Need and impact of surgical services in low-resource countries unaccounted for. Available at: http://www.globalhealthdelivery.org/blog/2008/05/global-burden-of-surgical-disease-working-group-need-and-impact-of-surgical-services-in-low-resource-countries-unaccounted-for/.
2. Ozgediz D, Jamison D, Cherian M, McQueen K. The burden of surgical conditions and access to surgical care in low- and middle-income countries. Bull World Health Organ. 2008;86:646–7.
3. Bickler S, Ozgediz D, Gosselin R, Weiser T, Spiegel D, Hsia R, et al. Key concepts for estimating the burden of surgical conditions and the unmet need for surgical care. World J Surg. 2010;34:374–80.
4. Basch PF. Textbook of international health. 2nd ed. New York, NY: Oxford; 1999.
5. Murray CJ, Lopez AD. The global burden of disease: a comprehensive assessment of mortality and disability from diseases, injuries and risk factors in 1990 and projected to 2020, Global burden of disease and injury series, vol. I. Cambridge, MA: Harvard School of Public Health; 1996.
6. Lee JW. Global health improvement and WHO: shaping the future. Lancet. 2003;362:2083–8.
7. Smith J, Haile-Mariam T. Priorities in global emergency medicine development. Emerg Med Clin North Am. 2005;23:11–29.
8. Gosselin RA, Gyamfi YA, Contini S. Challenges of meeting surgical needs in the developing world. World J Surg. 2011;35:258–61.
9. Taira BR, Kelly McQueen KA, Burkle Jr FM. Burden of surgical disease: does the literature reflect the scope of the international crisis? World J Surg. 2009;33:893–8.
10. Contini S. Surgery in developing countries: why and how to meet surgical needs worldwide. Acta Biomed. 2007;78:4–5.
11. Farmer PE, Kim JY. Surgery and global health: a view from beyond the OR. World J Surg. 2008;32:533–6.
12. Bermudez LE. Operation smile: plastic surgery with few resources. Lancet. 2000;356:S45.
13. Campbell A, Sherman R, Magee WP. The role of humanitarian missions in modern surgical training. Plast Reconstr Surg. 2010;126:295–302.
14. Kalangos A. "Hearts for all": a humanitarian association for the promotion of cardiology and cardiac surgery in developing countries. Ann Thorac Surg. 2002;73:341–2.
15. Johns AW. The role of international non-governmental organizations in dealing with cataract blindness in developing countries. Doc Ophthalmol. 1992;81:345–8.
16. Klauss V, Schaller UC. International initiatives for the prevention of blindness. Ophthalmologe. 2007;104:855–9.
17. Mainthia R, Tye GW, Shapiro J, Doppenberg EM, Ward JD. A model for neurosurgical humanitarian aid based on 12 years of medical trips to South and Central America. J Neurosurg Pediatr. 2009;4:4–9.
18. Abenavoli FM. Operation smile humanitarian missions. Plast Reconstr Surg. 2005;115:356–7.
19. WHO-PAHO guidelines for the use of foreign field hospitals in the aftermath of sudden-impact disasters.

http://www.who.int/hac/techguidance/pht/FieldHospitalsFolleto.pdf.
20. Bae JY, Groen RS, Kushner AL. Surgery as a public health intervention: common misconceptions versus the truth. Bull World Health Organ. 2011;89:394.
21. Harvey P, Stoddard A, Harmer A, Taylor G. State of the humanitarian system report. ALNAP. 2010, downloaded from the ALNAP website www.alnap.org.
22. Drain PK, Primack A, Hunt DD, Fawzi WW, Holmes KK, Gardner P. Global health in medical education: a call for more training and opportunities. Acad Med. 2007;82:226–30.
23. Crump JA, Sugarman J. Ethical considerations for short-term experiences by trainees in global health. JAMA. 2008;300:1456–8.
24. Thompson MJ, Huntington MK, Hunt DD, Pinsky LE, Brodie JJ. Educational effects of international health electives on U.S. and Canadian medical students and residents: a literature review. Acad Med. 2003;78:342–7.
25. Godkin M, Savageau J. The effect of medical students' international experiences on attitudes toward serving underserved multicultural populations. Fam Med. 2003;35:273–8.
26. VanRooyen M, Venugopal R, Greenough PG. International humanitarian assistance: where do emergency physicians belong? Emerg Med Clin North Am. 2005;23:115–31.
27. Non-governmental organizations: research guide. http://docs.lib.duke.edu/igo/guides/ngo/.
28. http://www.ngo.in/.
29. http://www.operationgivingback.facs.org/.
30. Guidelines on the use of foreign military and civil defence assets in disaster relief: "Oslo Guidelines" Updated November 2006. Available at http://www.ifrc.org/docs/idrl/I634EN.pdf.
31. Bezruchka S. Medical tourism as medical harm to the third world: why? for whom? Wilderness Environ Med. 2000;11:77–8.
32. Welling DR, Ryan JM, Burris DG, Rich NM. Seven sins of humanitarian medicine. World J Surg. 2010;34:466–70.
33. Suchdev P, Ahrens K, Click E, Macklin L, Evangelista D, Graham E. A model for sustainable short-term international medical trips. Ambul Pediatr. 2007; 7:317–20.
34. The importance of avoiding pitfalls in global health & development, in http://www.uniteforsight.org/pitfalls-in-development/.
35. Wolfberg AJ. Volunteering overseas: lessons from surgical brigades. N Engl J Med. 2006;354:443–5.
36. Sarfaty S, Arnold LK. Preparing for international medical service. Emerg Med Clin North Am. 2005;23: 149–75.
37. Mostow C, Crosson J, Gordon S, Chapman S, Gonzalez P, Hardt E, et al. Treating and precepting with RESPECT: a relational model addressing race, ethnicity, and culture in medical training. J Gen Intern Med. 2010; 25 Suppl 2:S146-54. Erratum in. J Gen Intern Med. 2010;25:1257.
38. Nguyen GC, LaVeist TA, Harris ML, Datta LW, Bayless TM, Brant SR. Patient trust-in-physician and race are predictors of adherence to medical management in inflammatory bowel disease. Inflamm Bowel Dis. 2009;15:1233–9.
39. World Medical Association statement on medical ethics in the event of disasters. Adopted by the 46th WMA General Assembly Stockholm, Sweden, September 1994 and revised by the WMA General Assembly, Pilanesberg, South Africa, October 2006. Available at: http://www.wma.net/en/30publications/10policies/d7/index.html.
40. Merin O, Kreiss Y, Lin G, Pras E, Dagan D. Collaboration in response to disaster: Typhoon Yolanda and an integrative model. N Engl J Med. 2014;370:1183–4.
41. O'Laughlin DT, Hick JL. Ethical issues in resource triage. Respir Care. 2008;53:190–7.
42. Society of Critical Care Medicine Ethics Committee. Consensus statement on the triage of critically ill patients. JAMA. 1994;271:1200–3.
43. Pesik N, Keim ME, Iserson KV. Terrorism and the ethics of emergency medical care medical care. Ann Emerg Med. 2001;37:642–6.
44. Merin O, Ash N, Levy G, Schwaber MJ, Kreiss Y. The Israeli field hospital in Haiti: ethical dilemmas in early disaster response. N Engl J Med. 2010;362:e38.
45. Code of Conduct for the International Red Cross and Red Crescent Movement and Non-Governmental Organizations (NGOs) in Disaster Relief. http://www.icrc.org/eng/resources/documents/publication/p1067.htm.
46. Jesus JE. Ethical challenges and considerations of short-term international medical initiatives: an excursion to Ghana as a case study. Ann Emerg Med. 2010;55:17–22.
47. Uejima T. Medical missions and medical malpractice: the current state of medical malpractice overseas. ASA Newsletter. 2011;75:22–4.
48. Lund DW. Medical liability in the developing world. In: http://www.aaos.org/news/aaosnow/oct08/managing8.asp.
49. Shah S, Wu T. The medical student global health experience: professionalism and ethical implications. J Med Ethics. 2008;34:375–8.
50. Banatvala N, Doyal L. Knowing when to say "no" on the student elective. Students going on electives abroad need clinical guidelines. BMJ. 1998;316:1404–5.
51. Registration and coordination of Foreign Medical Teams responding to sudden onset disasters. Foreign Medical Team Working Group. http://www.who.int/hac/global_health_cluster/fmt_way_forward_5may13.pdf.
52. Classification and minimum standards for foreign medical teams in sudden onset disasters. http://www.who.int/hac/global_health_cluster/fmt_guidelines_september2013.pdf.
53. Redmond AD, O'Dempsey TJ, Taithe B. Disasters and a register for foreign medical teams. Lancet. 2011;377:1054–5.

54. Gerdin M, Wladis A, von Schreeb J. Foreign field hospitals after the 2010 Haiti earthquake: how good were we? Emerg Med J. 2013;30:e8.
55. Marmot M. Inequalities in health. N Engl J Med. 2001;345:134–6.
56. Tollefson TT, Larrabee Jr WF. Global surgical initiatives to reduce the surgical burden of disease. JAMA. 2012;307:667–8.
57. http://www.hapinternational.org.
58. Baiden F, Hodgson A, Binka FN. Demographic surveillance sites and emerging challenges in international health. Bull World Health Organ. 2006;84: 163.
59. Levy G, Blumberg N, Kreiss Y, Ash N, Merin O. Application of information technology within a field hospital deployment following the January 2010 Haiti earthquake disaster. J Am Med Inform Assoc. 2010;17:626–30.
60. Emergency Surgery Workshop Davos 2011 emergency surgery during disaster relief activities surgery under critical environmental conditions. http://www.grforum.org/de/risk-academy/former-workshops-courses/emergency-surgery-workshop-davos-2011/.
61. Burkle Jr FM, Nickerson JW, von Schreeb J, Redmond AD, McQueen KA, Norton I, et al. Emergency surgery data and documentation reporting forms for sudden-onset humanitarian crises, natural disasters and the existing burden of surgical disease. Prehosp Disaster Med. 2012;27:577–82.
62. McQueen KA, Magee W, Crabtree T, Romano C, Burkle Jr FM. Application of outcome measures in international humanitarian aid: comparing indices through retrospective analysis of corrective surgical care cases. Prehosp Disaster Med. 2009;24:39–46.
63. Horlbeck D, Boston M, Balough B, Sierra B, Saenz G, Heinichen J, et al. Humanitarian otologic missions: long-term surgical results. Otolaryngol Head Neck Surg. 2009;140:559–65.
64. Farmer PE, Furin JJ, Katz JT. Global health equity. Lancet. 2004;363:1832.

The Global Burden of Surgical Need

3

K.A. Kelly McQueen

Abbreviations

BoSD	Burden of surgical disease
GBD	Global burden of disease
LMIC	Low- and middle-income countries
NCD	Noncommunicable disease
DALY	Disability adjusted life years
POMR	Perioperative mortality rate

Defining Surgical Need

The global health community defines *need* based on measureable population outcomes, primarily disability and premature death. The *burden* of disease, or the contribution of a disease, group of diseases, or conditions to the overall disability and premature death in a population, is a complex estimation reported in Disability Adjusted Life Years (DALYs). One DALY is equal to 1 year of healthy life lost due to death or disability from a disease process. The global burden of disease (GBD) is a dynamic estimate of global health and is influenced by acute and chronic disease patterns as well as by the interventions that impact or avert disease burden. These interventions include vaccines, medicines, and surgery [1]. (Figures 3.1 and 3.2)

Surgical disease is specifically defined for the purposes of communicating with the global health community, and the burden of surgical disease is described as the disability and premature death that is prevented or potentially averted by surgical intervention [2]. Similarly surgical interventions, or operations, are identified and the provision of anesthesia is included as necessary for a majority of operations. The inclusion of safe anesthesia as a necessary element for meeting surgical need is essential [3].

Early estimates of the burden of surgical disease (BoSD) suggested that 11 % of the overall GBD could be prevented or averted by surgical intervention [4]. In the years since this pivotal chapter by Debas et al., the epidemiologic shift in GBD from communicable disease to noncommunicable disease (NCDs) has been recognized [5] and this has led to new estimates that surgical intervention and safe anesthesia comprise up to 38 % of GBD [6]. The BoSD is equal to the total surgical need in a community, including the *met need* (i.e., that proportion of surgically treatable conditions that are seen and treated), the *unmet need* (i.e., that proportion of surgically treatable conditions that remain unseen and untreated), and the *unmeetable need* (i.e., that proportion of potentially surgically treatable conditions that are so severe that death and/or disability could not be averted even with adequate access to quality surgical care) [7].

K.A.K. McQueen, M.D., M.P.H. (✉)
Department of Anesthesiology, Vanderbilt Institute for Global Health, Vanderbilt University Medical Center, 1301 Medical Center Drive, #4648 TVC, Nashville, TN 37232, USA
e-mail: kelly.mcqueen@vanderbilt.edu

R. Roth et al. (eds.), *The Role of Anesthesiology in Global Health: A Comprehensive Guide*, DOI 10.1007/978-3-319-09423-6_3, © Springer International Publishing Switzerland 2015

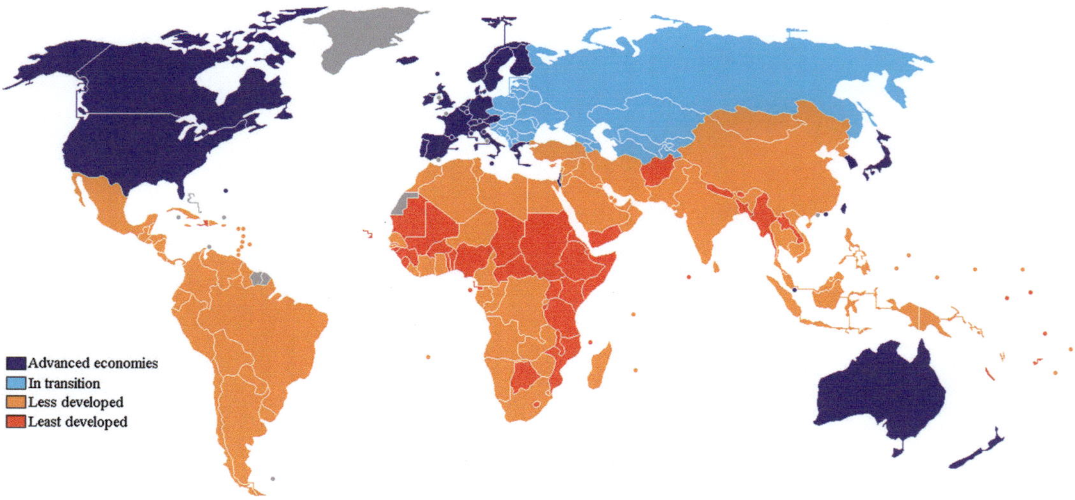

Fig. 3.1 Country Development based on World Bank GDP Status. Countries with less economic development (Less in *orange* and Least in *dark orange*). Developed Countries are also those with the greatest unmet surgical needs: Greatest need in *dark orange* ≫ High need in *orange*

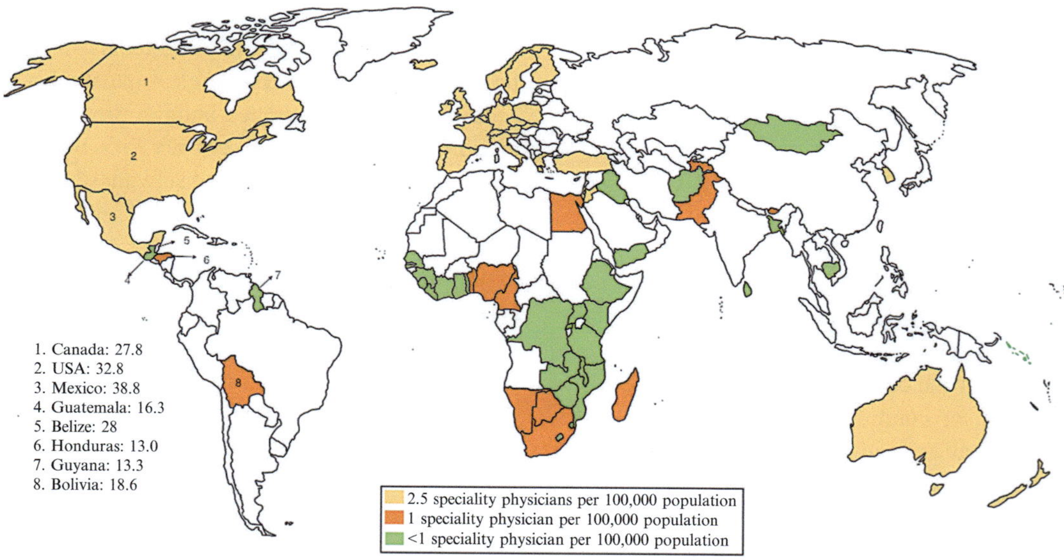

Fig. 3.2 Countries surveyed by infrastructure surveys [41] by physicians per 100,000 [38] and cesarean section rates

Global unmet surgical need is large and growing, with a majority of the need existing in the poorest countries with the fewest healthcare resources for surgery and anesthesia. In 2010 it was estimated that two billion people worldwide had no access to emergency or essential surgery [8], with the greatest burden and fewest resources in Africa [9].

The Elements of Unmet Surgical Need

Surgical intervention and safe anesthesia for noncommunicable diseases (NCDs) including cardiovascular disease and trauma are grossly underserved in LMICs. Importantly, surgical and anesthesia capacity are similarly underserved for obstetric emergencies in LMICs [10]. Unmet surgical need will only be addressed when surgical and anesthesia capacity are increased in tandem, and when appropriate technology, education and training, and access to equipment, essential medicines, and blood products are uniform [11]. Perioperative outcomes are dependent upon timely surgical intervention and safe anesthesiology. Currently, successful surgical outcomes are critically limited by absent or unsafe anesthesia practices in the countries in greatest need [12]. In the following section, each of these related areas of unmet surgical need is explored in more detail.

Table 3.1 Anesthesia-related and perioperative mortality in high-income countries (HICs)

	Prior to 1970	Since 1990
Anesthesia-related mortality per million population	357	34
Perioperative mortality per million population	10,600	1,170

Perioperative Mortality in HICs has improved dramatically over the past 40 years, demonstrating that with adequate professional training, appropriately directed healthcare resources, and application of evidence-based interventions, undergoing anesthesia can be very safe

Adapted from Bainbridge D, Martin J, Arango M, Cheng D, Evidence-based Peri-operative Clinical Outcomes Research Group. Perioperative and anaesthetic-related mortality in developed and developing countries: a systematic review and meta-analysis. Lancet 2012;380:1075–81

Safe Anesthesia Care

The global anesthesia crisis [13] limits access to emergency and essential surgical intervention, and contributes to poor patient outcomes. The survey data among practitioners in LMICs shows that a lack of education, limited training, and dwindling interest in the specialty have contributed to a lack of or absence of trained anesthesia providers [13]. Unpredictable access to essential medications and limited safety equipment has resulted in unsafe conditions for the provision of anesthesia and surgical intervention [13].

The contribution of anesthesia to unmet surgical need is difficult to quantify and measure [3]. Evidence from developed countries confirms that acceptable surgical outcomes—including mortality rates—depend on safe anesthesia practice, and safe anesthesia practice can only occur when trained anesthesia providers, safety equipment, essential medicines for anesthesia, and systems for pain control and resuscitation are available [14]. With this in mind, surgical burden, inclusive of both met and unmet surgical need, is predicated on lack of anesthesia care. In LMICs the scarcity of anesthesia resources may limit the provision of surgical intervention, but unfortunately, more often the intervention proceeds without appropriate anesthesia care. The resulting high anesthesia-related mortality rates are doubly tragic in the context of patient suffering [15–18]. Therefore, in order to impact the BoSD, a healthcare system must build capacity in all areas: physical infrastructure, surgeons, anesthesiologists, nurses, and technicians.

Anesthesia in resource-rich countries is very safe [14, 19]. Adequate numbers of physicians, supervision of nonphysician personnel, the continuous use of required safety monitoring, as well as an ample supply of medications, equipment, and blood products contribute to the safety and successful outcomes in developed countries. Outcomes related to anesthesia and surgery have steadily improved in these countries since the 1970s (Table 3.1).

Too little is known about anesthesia resources and practices in LMICs but the mortality rates reported in a few countries tell the shocking truth [15–18, 20]. Deaths attributable to anesthesia in most LMICs result from limited training and education, including continuing education, as well as limited or absent resources, especially safety monitoring. Published reports reveal mortality attributed to anesthesia as high as 1 in 133 anesthetics [15], with other reports of avoidable anesthesia-related death rates as high as 1 in 144 [16] and 1 in 504 anesthetics [17]. Of even greater concern is that many of the preventable anesthesia deaths occurred in otherwise young, healthy patients, many of whom were women undergoing cesarean delivery [20].

Essential Medicines

The WHO Model List of Essential Medicines [21] guides procurement of medications for governments internationally and includes a wide variety of pharmaceuticals for treatment or therapeutic uses—including anesthesia and pain management. The first Model List of Essential Medications was published in 1977, and since 2007, the list has been updated every two years. The anesthetic and analgesic medications from the 18th edition released in 2013 are listed in Table 3.2. The WHO's process of selection utilizes a relatively small number of experts and who meet over a short period of time; in 2011, 20 experts met for 5 working days. Their goals are to "satisfy the health care needs of the majority of the population" while ensuring cost-effectiveness and promoting quality [22]. The list lacks many medications routinely used in HIC, many of the medicines not included are hotly debated annually, and the medicines within each category are included because they fulfill a specific function, are least expensive, or most consistently available.

Consistent with many guidelines provided by the WHO, country-level adherence to the essential medicine guidelines is influenced by resources as well as weighted prioritization within the health-care system and Ministry of Health. Despite this planning and strategizing, in many LMICs the availability of medicines is inconsistent, especially in the first referral hospitals in LMICs. For example, oxygen, considered requisite to safe anesthesia, was only added to the WHO Essential Medicine list in 2013, and is available consistently in only 45.2 % of district hospitals and is unavailable in 35.0 % of these primary referral hospitals [23]. In addition, rescue medicines for hypotension and dysrhythmias are not consistently available. Finally, the paucity of narcotic pain medicines for treating acute and chronic pain in many of the poorest countries is of great concern. Regulatory issues, misinformation, and too few heath care practitioners providing access to these important medications contribute to this disparity[1] [24].

Table 3.2 The World Health Organization's list of essential medicines for anesthesia and pain management

Medication class	Specific medication listed
Inhaled gas	Oxygen, halothane, isoflurane, nitrous oxide
Muscle relaxant	Suxamethonium, atracurium
Sedative/hypnotic	Ketamine, propofol or thiopental, midazolam, diazepam
Narcotic	Morphine, codeine
Local anesthetic	Lidocaine, bupivacaine
Anti-inflammatory	Ibuprofen Paracetamol
Antiemetic	Ondansetron
Chronic pain relief	Amitriptyline
Reversal agent	Neostigmine Naloxone
Rescue medicines	Epinephrine, atropine, ephedrine

The anesthetic and analgesic medications included in the 2013 WHO Model List of Essential Medicines were selected for their unique pharmacologic contribution to balanced and safe anesthesia, cost-effectiveness, and wide availability. Interestingly oxygen was included for the first time in 2011

Adapted from WHO Model List of Essential Medicines 2013. www.who.int/topics/essential_medicines/en

Blood Banking and Blood Products

The ability to cross-match and transfuse blood to patients with symptomatic anemia or hemorrhage was a great medical advance that has positively impacted surgical and anesthetic outcomes globally over the past 40 years [25]. The ability to collect, match, and test blood for infectious disease is considered a prerequisite for surgical, obstetric, and trauma programs [26] but even as surgical care advances in LMICs, solutions for the provision of a safe and predictable blood supply are not obvious. The limitations of blood banking in LMICs primarily relate to basic issues of electricity and refrigeration, as well as the unavailability of pathology services [27]. Inexpensive and rapid blood typing and infectious disease screening are available [28], but the widespread use of this technology is often underutilized due to the greater issues of predictable, constant electricity necessary for refrigeration. Uninterrupted electricity is only available in 59 % of primary referral hospitals in Africa and

[1] See the chapter entitled "The Global Burden of Acute and Chronic Pain" in this text for a more in-depth discussion of this topic.

Asia [23]. Utilizing "walking" or "living" blood banking—the practice of either formally or informally tracking blood types among community members with organized collection of whole blood and transfusion on demand—remains a viable practice in low-resource settings [26, 29]. However, even this practical solution is limited by the spread of misinformation, especially within the countries ravaged by the HIV pandemic, about the relationship of the donating and receiving blood products [30, 31].

Table 3.3 Anesthesiology workforce

Country	Number of anesthesiologists	Population (in millions)
Afghanistan	9	32
Bhutan	8	0.7
Rwanda	0	8
Uganda	13	27
United Kingdom	12,000	64

The number of trained physician anesthesiologists in five countries representing the extremes of the disparity in anesthesiology workforce for 2001–2010. (Adapted from ref. 40)

Surgical Capacity

The challenges of developing sufficient surgical capacity—the personnel, infrastructure, and systems—to meet surgical need in LMICs are many. Most advanced medical care including surgical procedures, diagnostic testing, and specialty care is centralized in LMICs [9]. At the first referral hospital where many patients in LMICs access health care there is limited infrastructure and few human resources. These primary care hospitals, often referred to as "district hospitals," indicate regional hospitals, but transportation is limited, and even regional hospitals in the poorest countries have limited capacity to provide emergency and essential surgery [10, 11].

In the past decade many reports from LMICs have documented the extent of limited infrastructure, lack of anesthesia and surgical providers, and unpredictable availability of essential medications, monitors, and safety equipment; studies have also documented how these conditions impact access to surgery and anesthesia creating the unmet need for surgical intervention for a spectrum of disease [32–36].

The surgical and anesthesiology workforce is one area of well-documented disparity. It is estimated that a ratio of 7 surgeons per 100,000 people is needed to meet the surgical needs of a population. In the United States, there are 5.8 surgeons per 100,000 population (with more in urban and less in rural areas), but in many LMICs there is less than one surgeon per 100,000 people [37, 38]. The anesthesiology workforce is even more disparate (see Table 3.3) [39].

Many of the emergency and essential surgical interventions that address unmet surgical need in LMICs are cost-effective [40–43] as is the provision of safe anesthesia [44–47]. Ample documentation in the literature, as cited above, has brought attention to the issue, but such emphasis has not yet led to improved access or patient safety.

Surgical Outcomes

Too little is known about the longitudinal patient outcomes of surgical and anesthesia interventions in LMICs or about outcomes related to the absence of emergency surgery or late access to surgery. Improving data collection and reporting is a critical component of addressing surgical need.

An absence of surgical and anesthesia outcome data limits the investment of resources into surgical infrastructure and safe anesthesia in LMICs. Little is known about the incidence of mortality directly attributed to lack of surgical access especially in LMICs where death certificates are often not issued and most patients die at home where data collection is sparse [48]. In a majority of operating theaters in LMICs the only documentation of a serious operative complication or death is the paper logbook of the operating theater [49]. Little outside of the logbook is known about the perioperative mortality rate (POMR) of the hospital, region, or country. Follow-up of patients after surgery is limited to the time they are hospitalized, and once discharged to home few patients are followed [50].

Additional information about surgical and anesthesia outcomes would provide information about patient safety in LMICs and may also allow benchmarking from a baseline quality indicator such as the POMR if routinely collected and reported [49]. The POMR is nonspecific, and similar to the Maternal Mortality Rate (MMR) is easy to collect and the trend over time allows for analysis of interventions and system changes. If the POMR is stratified for ASA status, age, and gender the rate will become increasing valuable [50]. Measuring a baseline and following mortality rates even while access to surgery and safe anesthesia is limited is important. Tracking a health indicator such as POMR brings awareness to the issue of unmet surgical need and anesthesia safety, and allows the impact of interventions to be prospectively evaluated.

Meeting Surgical Need in LMICs

Progressing from the description of the BoSD and unmet surgical needs in LMICs to the implementation of appropriate surgical services is the next step in the continuum of responding to the projections of the 2010 GBD [5], and planning for the Post-2015 Development Goals [29, 30]. The Millennium Development Goals, which emphasized MMR, HIV, and other pressing health concerns of 2000, significantly impacted and improved the related health indicators due to the increased attention and funding received secondary to the UN focus on ten goals. The success of improving access to surgical intervention in LMICs will only be realized when investments are made for the totality of surgical care—from early diagnosis through treatment and from infrastructure to patient safety and outcome monitoring [49, 51].

Emergency surgery is embraced as a necessary component of a healthcare system, and, yet many LMICs lack the ability to provide emergency surgery including cesarean sections and trauma surgery outside of the largest regional hospitals [5]. The World Health Organization recommends cesarean delivery rates to be 5–10 % of the live birth rates, which corresponds to adequate access to operative deliveries for indications such as obstructed labor and eclampsia; in many low-income countries the rates are less than 5 %, and even 1 % [52]. This low rate corresponds with high maternal mortality rates, and likely also corresponds with the inability to provide emergency surgery in general. Interventions could focus on only one service line, such as obstetric surgery. Building infrastructure for one group of surgical services will increase the overall ability to provide surgical intervention and anesthesia due to the overlap in equipment, medicines, and personnel.

Table 3.4 Cost-effective emergency and essential surgical interventions recommended for all LMICs

	Emergency and essential surgery at first referral hospitals
Emergency	Cesarean Section/D&C
	Appendectomy/Ex Lap
	Anesthesia/Emergency Airway
	ORIF/I&D
Essential	Hernia
	Cataract
	Cleft Lip/Club Foot

Essential or elective surgery is underserved as well in LMICs. The growing evidence for the cost-effectiveness of essential surgery encourages global health and national governments to increase infrastructure and therefore access to basic essential surgery, including surgery for hernia, congenital malformations, cancer, and cataracts [53]. Debates regarding the inclusion of surgical interventions on the "essential list" have been ongoing for more than a decade; however inclusion of these effective and appropriate operations is inclusive to the basic right to health [54]. The prioritization of surgical interventions has been considered for LMICs based on cost-effectiveness, prevalence, burden, and the success of the intervention (see Table 3.4) [14, 55]. The initial ability to provide safe surgery and anesthesia for any basic operation is likely to increase access to an increasing number of surgical services over time (see Table 3.5) [5, 56].

Increasing access to safe anesthesia and surgical intervention in any hospital, country, or region must begin by engaging, working with,

Table 3.5 Disability and death potentially averted with surgical interventions and safe anesthesia

Surgical disease type	Potentially averted with intervention (28 % of GBD) (%)
Trauma	38
Malignancy	19
Congenital anomalies	9
Pregnancy and perinatal	10
Cataracts	5

During the course of many surgical diseases, there is an opportunity for surgical intervention that would result in an increase in DALYs for the population. Listed are those surgical diseases for which improved surgical capacity would result in averted disease burden and improved quality of life

Adapted from Surgical Intervention Impact on Global Burden of Disease (GBD). Murray CJ. The Global Burden of Disease Study. Lancet 2012;380:2053–260

and building upon the existing structure of surgical care. Trained anesthesia providers are the rate-limiting step for access to surgery, and are also a contributor to poor outcomes, including death [16–18]. LMICs with small numbers of local physician anesthesiologists will benefit from functional groups of technicians providing anesthesia. Improving the ability of technicians to provide safe anesthesia while simultaneously increasing the delivery of anesthesia through nurse and physician providers is practical and beneficial to the population. Physician leadership for training, education, certification, and oversight cannot be discounted, but in LMICs the practicalities of meeting surgical needs will require a diverse workforce including nurses and technicians [57, 58].

Conclusions

Surgical disease significantly contributes to premature disability and death. Low- and middle-income countries suffer with the largest BoSD and are dramatically underserved with respect to diagnostic services, surgical intervention, and safe anesthesia. Documentation of the cost-effectiveness of emergency and essential surgery and safe anesthesia is in place, and awareness of these unmet needs is growing. Hope is on the horizon for the effective treatment of the growing burden of surgical disease in LMICs.

References

1. Murray CJ, Lopez AD. Global mortality, disability and the contribution of risk factors: global burden of disease study. Lancet. 1997;349:1436–42.
2. Bickler S, Ozdegiz D, Gosselin R, et al. Key concepts for estimating burden of surgical conditions and unmet need for surgical care. World J Surg. 2010; 34(3):374–80.
3. McQueen KA. Anesthesia and the global burden of surgical disease. Int Anesthesiol Clin. 2010;48(2): 91–107. PMID: 20386230.
4. Debas HT, Gosselin R, McCord C, Thind A. Surgery. In: Disease Control Priorities in Developing Countries, vol. 1. 2nd ed. New York, NY: Oxford University Press; 2006. p. 245–60.
5. Murray CJ. The global burden of disease study. Lancet. 2012;380:2053–260.
6. Debas H, Mock C, Kruk M. "Essential Surgery" Disease control priorities in developing countries, 3rd ed. Advance online publication: http://www.dcp-3.org/chapter/essentialsurgery. Accessed 14 May 2014.
7. Ozdegiz D, Hsia R, Weiser T, et al. Population metric for surgery: effective coverage of surgical services in low-income and middle-income countries. World J Surg. 2009;33(1):1–5.
8. Funk L, Weiser T, Berry W, et al. Global operating theater distribution and pulse oximetry supply: an estimation from reported data. Lancet. 2010;376(9746): 1055–61.
9. Ozdegiz D, Jamison D, Cherian M, McQueen K. The burden of surgical conditions and access to surgical care in low and middle income countries. Bull World Health Org. 2008;86(8):646–7.
10. Hogan M, Foreman K, Naghavi M, et al. Maternal mortality for 181 countries, 1980–2008: a systematic analysis of progress toward millennium development goal 5. Lancet. 2010;375(9726):1609–23.
11. Lebrun DG, Chackungal S, Chao TE, Knowlton LM, Linden AF, Notrica MR, Solis CV, McQueen KA. Prioritizing essential surgery and safe anesthesia for the post-2015 development agenda: operative capacities of 78 district hospitals in 7 low- and middle-income countries. Surgery. 2014;155(3): 365–73.
12. Notrica MR, Evans FM, Knowlton LM, Kelly McQueen KA. Rwandan surgical and anesthesia infrastructure: a survey of district hospitals. World J Surg. 2011;35:1770–80.
13. Dubowitz G, Detlefs S, McQueen K. Global anesthesia workforce crisis: a preliminary survey revealing shortages contributing to undesirable outcomes and unsafe practices. World J Surg. 2010;34(3):438–44.

14. Bainbridge D, Martin J, Arango M, Cheng D. Evidence-based peri-operative clinical outcomes research G. Perioperative and anaesthetic-related mortality in developed and developing countries: a systematic review and meta-analysis. Lancet. 2012; 380:1075–81.
15. Walker IA, Wilson IH. Anaesthesia in developing countries: a risk for patients. Lancet. 2008;371:968–9.
16. Hodges SC, Mijumbi C, Okello M, et al. Anaesthesia services in developing countries: defining the problems. Anaesthesia. 2007;62:4–11.
17. Ouro-Bang NA, Maman AF, Tomta K, Ahouangbevi S, Chobli M. Deaths associated with anaesthesia in Togo, West Africa. Trop Doc. 2005;35:220–2.
18. Hansen D, Gausi SC, Merikebu M. Anaesthesia in Malawi: complications and deaths. Trop Doc. 2000; 30:146–9.
19. Buck N, Devlin HB, Lunn JN. The report of a confidential enquiry into perioperative deaths. London: Nuffield Provincial Hospitals Trust and the King's Fund Publishing House; 1987.
20. Enohumah K, Imarenglaye C. Factors associated with anesthesia-related maternal mortality in a tertiary hospital in Nigeria. Acta Anaesthesiol Scand. 2006;50:206–10.
21. World Health Organization. Model essential medicines. Available at www.who.int/topics_essential-medicines/en. Accessed 10 May 2014.
22. Manikandan S, Gitanjali B. National list of essential medicines of India: the way forward. J Postgrad Med. 2012;4(4):199–200.
23. McCunn M, Vo D, Cherian MN. Anesthesia capacity in 22 low and middle income countries. J Anesth Clin Res. 2012;3(4):207. doi:10.4172/2155-6148.1000207.
24. Jackson TP, Stable V, McQueen K. The global burden of chronic pain. ASA Newslett. 2014;78(6):24–7.
25. Farmer PE, Kim J. Surgery and global health: a view from beyond the OR. World J Surg. 2008;32:533–6.
26. Hrezo RJ, Clark J. The walking blood bank: an alternative blood supply in military mass casualties. Disaster Manag Response. 2003;1(1):19–22.
27. Lee HH, Allain JP. Improving blood safety in resource poor settings. Vox Sang. 2004;87:176–9.
28. Marwaha N. Whole blood and component use in resource poor settings. Biologicals. 2010;38(1): 68–71. doi:10.1016/j.biologicals.2009.10.020.
29. Kushner A, Cherian M, Noel L, et al. Addressing the millennium development goals from a surgical perspective: essential surgery and anesthesia in 8 low- and middle-income countries. Arch Surg. 2010;145(2):154–9.
30. Gosselin R, Gyamfi Y, Contini S. Challenges of meeting surgical needs in the developing world. World J Surg. 2011;35:258–61.
31. Doorley S, Doohan N, Kodali S, McQueen K. Social determinants of the impact of surgery on health. Trop Med Surg. 2013;1:113.
32. Lebrun DG, Saavedra-Pozo I, Agreda-Flores F, Burdic ML, Notrica MR, McQueen KA. Surgical and anesthesia capacity in Bolivian public hospitals: results from a national hospital survey. World J Surg. 2012;36(11):2559–66. PMID: 22864566.
33. Lebrun DG, Dhar D, Sarkar MI, Imran TM, Kazi SN, McQueen KA. Measuring global surgical disparities: a survey of surgical and anesthesia infrastructure in Bangladesh. World J Surg. 2013;37(1):24–31. PMID: 23052803.
34. Knowlton LM, Chackungal S, Dahn B, Lebrun D, Nickerson J, McQueen K. Liberian surgical and anesthesia infrastructure: a survey of county hospitals. World J Surg. 2013;37(4):721–9.
35. Solis C, León P, Sanchez N, Burdic M, Johnson L, Warren H, Iddriss A, McQueen K. Nicaraguan surgical and anesthesia infrastructure: survey of ministry of health hospitals. World J Surg. 2013;37(9): 2109–21.
36. Thind A, Mock C, Gosselin RA, McQueen K. Surgical epidemiology: a call for action. Bull World Health Org. 2012;90(3):239–40.
37. Hoyler M, Finlayson SR, McClain CD, Meara JG, Hagander L. Shortage of doctors, shortage of data: a review of the global surgery, obstetrics, and anesthesia literature. World J Surg. 2014;38(2):269–80.
38. Lynge DC, Larson EH, Thompson MJ, Rosenblatt RA, Hart LG. A longitudinal analysis of the general surgery workforce in the United States, 1981–2005. Arch Surg. 2008;143(4):345–50.
39. Cherian M, Choo S, Wilson I, Noel L, Sheikh M, Dayrit M, Groth S. Building and retaining the neglected anaesthesia health workforce: is it crucial for health systems strengthening through primary health care? Bull World Health Org. 2010;88: 637–9.
40. Corlew DS. Estimation of the impact of surgical disease through economic modeling of cleft lip and palate care. World J Surg. 2010;43(3):391–6.
41. Shillcutt SD, Clarke MG, Kingsnorth AN. Cost-effectiveness of groin hernia surgery in the Western Region of Ghana. Arch Surg. 2010;145:954–61.
42. Shillcutt SD, Sanders DL, Teresa Butron-Vila M, Kingsnorth AN. Cost-effectiveness of inguinal hernia surgery in northwestern Ecuador. World J Surg. 2013;37:32–41.
43. Malalasekera AP, Ariyaratne MH, Fernando R, Perera D, Deen KI. Cost accounting in a surgical unit in a teaching hospital: a pilot study. Ceylon Med J. 2003; 48:71–4.
44. McKenzie AG. A plea for "low flow" anaesthesia in Zimbabwe. Cent Afr J Med. 1993;39:175–6.
45. Chi X, Chen Y, Liao M, Cao F, Tian Y, Wang X. Comparative cost analysis of three different anesthesia methods in gynecological laparoscopic surgery. Front Med. 2012;6:311–6.
46. Vaz FA, Abreu RA, Soarez PC, Speranzini MB, Fernandes LC, Matos D. Cost-effectiveness analysis on spinal anesthesia versus local anesthesia plus sedation for loop colostomy closure. Arq Gastroenterol. 2010;47:159–64.

47. Paletta Guedes RA, Paletta Guedes VM, Chaoubah A, Montesi Pereira F, Montesi Pereira P, Pereira Da Silva AC. Topical versus peribulbar anesthesia in non-penetrating deep sclerectomy. A cost-effectiveness analysis. J Fr Ophtalmol. 2011;34:629–33.
48. Mathers CD, Fat DM, Idoue MF, et al. Counting the dead and what they died from: an assessment of the global status of cause of death data. Bull World Health Organ. 2005;83:171–7.
49. McQueen K. Global surgery: measuring the impact. World J Surg. 2013;37:2505–6. doi:10.1007/s00268-013-2198-4.
50. Watters DA, Hollands MJ, Gruen RL, Moate K, Perndt H, McDougall RJ, Morriss WW, Tangi V, Casey KM, McQueen KM. Perioperative Mortality Rate (POMR): a global indicator of access to safe surgery and anaesthesia. World J Surg. 2014. Published ahead of print. doi: 10.1007/s00268-014-2638-4.
51. Lipnick M, Mijumbi C, Dubowitz G, et al. Surgery and anesthesia capacity-building in resource-poor settings: description of an ongoing academic partnership in Uganda. World J Surg. 2013;37:488–97.
52. World Health Organization. WHO statistical information system [Internet]. 2010. Available from: http://www.who.int/whosis/en/index.html. Accessed 22 Mar 2014.
53. DCP3. Disease control priorities, 3rd ed. http://www.dcp-3.org/volume/9/essential-surgery. Accessed 19 May 2014.
54. McQueen K, Ozdegiz D, Riveillo R, et al. Essential surgery: integral to the right to health. Health Hum Rights. 2010;12(1):137–52.
55. Mock C, Cherian M, Juliard C, et al. Developing global priorities in addressing surgical conditions-furthering the link between surgery and public health. World J Surg. 2010;34:381–5.
56. Weiser TG, Regenbogen SE, Thompson KD, et al. An estimation of the global volume of surgery: a modeling strategy based on available data. Lancet. 2008; 372(9633):139–44.
57. Chu K, Rosseel P, Gielis P, Ford N. Surgical task shifting in sub-Sahara Africa. PLoS Med. 2009; 6(5):e1000078.
58. Ozgediz D, Kiljambu S, Galukande M, et al. Africa's neglected surgical workforce crisis. Lancet. 2008;371(9613):627–8. doi:10.1016/S0140-6736(08)60279-2.

4 Anesthesia Disparities Between High-Income Countries and Low- and Middle-Income Countries: Providers, Training, Equipment, and Techniques

Steven Dale Boggs and Nicholas W. Chee

> A person is a person because he recognizes others as persons.
>
> Desmond Tutu, 7 September 1986.

The stark inequities in economic benefits that are spread among the members of the world's community highlight how the place of one's birth in large part determines one's fate. To address this imbalance, the Millennium Summit of the United Nations in 2000 [1] set out three broad categories for improving the welfare of the world's peoples: human capital, infrastructure, and human rights (social, economic, and political) with the intent of increasing living standards. More specifically, eight Millennium Development Goals were established:

1. To eradicate extreme poverty and hunger.
2. To achieve universal primary education.
3. To promote gender equality and empowering women.
4. To reduce child mortality rates.
5. To improve maternal health.
6. To combat HIV/AIDS, malaria, and other diseases.
7. To ensure environmental sustainability.
8. To develop a global partnership for development.

These eight factors are inextricably linked, with at least three of these goals specifically dealing with health care. More specifically, Thomas LaVeist of the Bloomberg School of Public health [2] has identified six key factors that cause healthcare disparities: socioeconomic conditions, social and physical environments, access to quality care, cultural competency, health literacy, and empowered healthcare consumers. These factors are inextricably linked. To provide excellent healthcare, each factor must be optimized.

As is seen in the USA at present, funding alone is not sufficient for the delivery of efficient and high-quality healthcare. However, in low- and middle-income countries (LMIC), the problems are both lack of funding and also knowing where to start to address the multitude of medical problems. This chapter will outline several issues that impede the provision of surgical and anesthetic care in LMICs. Included is a discussion of the global disparities in access to surgical and anesthetic care, the differential risk of anesthesia in high-income countries (HIC) and LMICs, the distribution of anesthesia providers worldwide, and how certain anesthetic techniques and methods have been adapted for situations with limited access to providers and adequate infrastructure.

S.D. Boggs, M.D., M.B.A. (✉)
The James J Peters VA Medical Center, Bronx, NY, USA

The Icahn School of Medicine at Mount Sinai, Manhattan, NY, USA
e-mail: steven.boggs@va.gov

N.W. Chee, M.P.H.
Hospital for Joint Diseases, NYU Langone Medical Center, New York, NY, USA

R. Roth et al. (eds.), *The Role of Anesthesiology in Global Health: A Comprehensive Guide*, DOI 10.1007/978-3-319-09423-6_4, © Springer International Publishing Switzerland 2015

Essential Surgical and Anesthesia Services

In its most recent report [3], the UN Millennium Development Goals Report (2013), striking successes have been noted. The proportion of people living in extreme poverty has been halved at the global level. Over two billion people gained access to improved sources of drinking water despite significant population growth. Remarkable gains have also been made in the fight against smallpox, malaria, and tuberculosis. The hunger reduction target is within reach and the proportion of undernourished people in developing regions decreased from 23.2 % in 1990–1992 to 14.9 % in 2010–2012. New HIV infections are declining. From 1990 to 2011, 1.9 billion people gained access to a latrine; globally the maternal mortality ratio declined by 47 % over the last two decades, from 400 maternal deaths per 100,000 live births to 210 between 1990 and 2010; and worldwide the mortality rate for children under five dropped by 41 %—from 87 deaths per 1,000 live births in 1990 to 51 in 2011.

While these successes are admirable, they also underscore the problem of global inequitable access to safe surgery and anesthesia. Historically, world health has focused on the treatment and prevention of communicable disease. Surgery and anesthesia have been viewed in the past as high technology solutions that do not yield sufficient return on investment and therefore as being interventions that would be addressed when primary care systems were in place. Yet, data from the World Health Organization (WHO) now suggest that by the year 2026 the global burden of disease from malaria, tuberculosis, and HIV will be eclipsed by surgical disease [4].

There is a need to prioritize surgical care globally, especially in LMICs. Six years ago, Paul Farmer, a physician well known for his historic focus on bringing general medical care to and combating HIV in disadvantaged communities, observed that surgery is the neglected stepchild of global health [5]. Surgical disease is among the top 15 causes of disability, and inadequate surgical conditions account for up to 15 % of total disability adjusted life years (DALYs) lost worldwide (see Appendix). Urbanization and industrialization have seen an increase in the number and severity of traffic accidents, in part because road quality has not improved at a commensurate rate. By 2030, road traffic accidents are expected to be the seventh leading cause of mortality and the fourth cause of DALYs in Low-Income Countries. The most severely affected age group are those between 5 and 14 years and those in the age range between 5 and 59 account for almost 75 % of those killed—that is, a population in the most productive years. Injuries in general kill more than five million people globally and account for one out of every ten deaths [6].

The WHO began to examine global disparities in the delivery of surgical and anesthetic care by hosting the first WHO Global Initiative for Emergency and Essential Surgical Care (GIEESC) Biennial Meeting in 2005 Geneva, Switzerland [7]. Subsequently, there have been four more of these conferences, the most recent in October 2013. The GIEESC meetings have focused on six areas (below), which in many ways reflect the problems Médecins Sans Frontières have been addressing for years [8] (Table 4.1).

These definitions do require some care, however. Certain conditions that should be classified as surgical—for example long bone traction—may not be so classified because no anesthetic or operating suite is involved. Conversely, other conditions that do not require a surgical incision but are also on the spectrum of surgical care—fluid resuscitation and emergency airway management—may also be misclassified [9].

While surgery does require significant input in terms of skilled labor (e.g., surgeons, anesthetists, and nurses) and is technologically intensive (surgical and anesthetic equipment, dedicated operating room space), the presented evidence suggests that the return in quality life years for selected patients can exceed the expenditure. For example, emergency obstetric care at a rural hospital in Bangladesh was calculated to be US$10.93 per DALY averted [10–12].

Table 4.1 Medical and surgical issues facing LMICs

Group	Injuries	Infectious disease	Cancer	Pregnancy-related complications	Disasters and emergencies	Congenital disease
WHO GIEESS [7]	Optimal management starts at first-referral facility EESC works to strengthen essential surgical care	High-HIV transmission risk in Africa EESC works to improve safety of clinical procedures	EESS works for early detection	1/3 of all pregnancy-related complications can be treated with surgery	Timely access reduces death rate and disability EESC works with partners to provide guidance for disaster preparedness and response	50 % of congenital abnormalities can be treated with surgery EESC promotes cost-effective and disability-preventative measures
Médecins Sans Frontières [8]		Chagas Cholera Leishmaniasis Malaria Measles Meningitis Tuberculosis Trypanosomiasis		Women's health Obstetric fistulae	Natural disasters Armed conflicts	
Debas (author) four Sig. types of surgery [91]	Provision of competent care to injury victims Reduce preventable deaths Decrease personal dysfunction Decrease burden on families	HIV		Handling of obstetric complications: – Obstruction of labor – Hemorrhage		Elective care of simple surgical conditions: – Hernia – Clubfoot – Cataract – Hydrocele – Otitis media
WHO data [92–94]	5,000,000 deaths per year due to injuries 1,200,000 deaths per year due to road accidents 50,000,000 injured due to road accidents			287,000 deaths per year due to pregnancy-related complications 800 deaths per day 2,000,000 obstetric fistulae per year		100,000 children born annually with club feet

No exact counterpart the classification system that Debas uses for categorizing surgical management of abdominal and extra-abdominal emergent and life-threatening conditions

Disparity in Access to Surgical Care

Before analyzing discrepancies in surgical care between HIC and LMICs, the framework utilized to make these comparisons must be understood. The WHO classifies member countries depending on both Gross National Income and Region, based on World Bank criteria [13].

WHO Member States are grouped into six regions (2012) including the African Region, the Region of the Americas, the Eastern Mediterranean Region, the European Region, the South-East Asia Region, and the Western Pacific Region. WHO Member States are grouped into four gross annual income groups (GNI) per capita (low, lower middle, upper middle, and high) based on the World Bank list of economies for the year 2011 (released July 2012) (Table 4.2).

In the USA, annual per capita healthcare spending (2011) is on the order of $8,608 [14, 15]. Of this, roughly US$4,400 is spent by the government. At the other extreme Eritrea, Ethiopia, Central African Republic, Madagascar, the Democratic Republic of the Congo and Niger all spend less than $20 USD per capita annually on health care (Table 4.3), which is extremely low, even when calculated in terms of purchasing power parity (PPP).

Data from the World Bank [16]. PPP is used in international comparisons based on currencies to estimate what market basket of goods a currency could purchase. They are used in economics to eliminate distortions that can occur when comparisons are made on the basis of market exchange rates.

Table 4.2 World Bank categories of countries by income group

Gross income groups	Criteria (per capita)
Low income (LI)	Less than $1,035
Lower middle income (LMI)	$1,036–$4,085
Upper middle income (MI)	$4,086–$12, 615
High income (HI)	Greater than $12,616

Table 4.3 Purchasing power parity, total healthcare expenditure, and healthcare expenditure as a percentage of GDP, 2012 data (World Bank)

Rank	Country	Region	$PPP	THE	% GDP
3	Qatar	[a]	80,470	1,707	1.9
8	Singapore	[a]	60,110	2,787	4.6
	USA	[a]	52,610	8,608	17.9
140	Mongolia	East Asia and Pacific	5,020	251	5.3
168	Nigeria	Sub-Saharan African	2,450	139	5.3
170	Yemen, Republic	Middle East and N. African	2,310	152	5.5
186	Zambia	Sub-Saharan African	1,590	99	6.1
187	Afghanistan	South Asia	1,560	50	9.6
187	Tanzania	Sub-Saharan African	1,560	107	7.3
191	Nepal	South Asia	1,470	68	5.4
194	Rwanda	Sub-Saharan African	1,320	135	10.8
196	Haiti	Latin American and Caribbean	1,220	94	7.9
199	Uganda	Sub-Saharan African	1,120	128	9.5
200	Ethiopia	Sub-Saharan African	1,110	52	4.7
207	Togo	Sub-Saharan African	900	80	8.0
208	Niger	Sub-Saharan African	760	39	5.3
209	Malawi	Sub-Saharan African	730	77	8.4
210	Liberia	Sub-Saharan African	580	112	19.5
211	Burundi	Sub-Saharan African	550	52	8.7
211	Eritrea	Sub-Saharan African	550	17	2.6
213	Congo, D.R.	Sub-Saharan African	390	32	8.5

[a]Not classified by region—data not available + nurses and midwives

Table 4.4 Physicians, nurses, and hospitals beds

Rank	Country	Region	Physicians per 1,000	Nurses[+] per 1,000	Hospital beds per 1,000
3	Qatar	[a]	2.80	7	1.2
8	Singapore	[a]	1.90	6	2.7
13	USA	[a]	2.40	10	3.0
140	Mongolia	East Asia and Pacific	2.80	4	6.8
168	Nigeria	Sub-Saharan African	0.40	2	–
170	Yemen, Republic	Middle East and N. African	0.20	1	0.7
186	Zambia	Sub-Saharan African	0.10	1	2.0
187	Afghanistan	South Asia	0.20	0	0.4
187	Tanzania	Sub-Saharan African	0.00	0	0.7
191	Nepal	South Asia	–	–	5.0
194	Rwanda	Sub-Saharan African	0.10	1	1.6
196	Haiti	Latin American and Caribbean	–	–	1.3
199	Uganda	Sub-Saharan African	0.10	1	0.5
200	Ethiopia	Sub-Saharan African	0.00	0	0.4
207	Togo	Sub-Saharan African	0.10	0	0.7
208	Niger	Sub-Saharan African	0.00	0	–
209	Malawi	Sub-Saharan African	0.00	0	1.3
210	Liberia	Sub-Saharan African	0.00	0	10.8
211	Burundi	Sub-Saharan African	–	–	1.9
211	Eritrea	Sub-Saharan African	–	–	0.7
213	Congo, D.R.	Sub-Saharan African	–	–	0.8

[a]Not classified by region—data not available + nurses and midwives

As the above tables show, there are dramatic funding disparities from country to country. However, even if funding were to be increased in sub-Saharan Africa—the most concentrated, impoverished region—there would be major issues of healthcare delivery because there is no established infrastructure coupled with a large deficit of healthcare providers here and in other LMICs. In Table 4.4, we also see the significant variation in the distribution of physicians, nurses, and available hospital beds when countries are ranked by PPP. Regional variation again is striking, with sub-Saharan Africa having the greatest shortages in all categories.

As seen in Table 4.4, LMICs have fewer physicians, nurses and midwives, and hospital beds per capita compared to more affluent countries. Exacerbating this discrepancy however is the fact that compared to population growth rates, most-sub-Saharan African nations have an actual negative annual growth rate in the number of physicians produced [17]. Because of the hardships of practice in these locations, better reimbursement for competing professions (engineering) and the employment opportunities in countries which spend more money per capita on healthcare, many individuals in LMICs either choose alternative professions or if they do enter medicine, they are induced to migrate elsewhere for better wages and living conditions.

A study of healthcare workers in Ghana revealed a marked preference for migration to ODEC countries [95]. For healthcare workers, this was of particular concern because their training is generally publically funded. One model found that for the United Kingdom, the country had a net overall gain by the importing of foreign physicians, the exact opposite was seen in the exporting country. Although only 1.91 % of the total population migrated, this was reflective of 8.07 % of the total expenditure on education of the current population.

Access to surgery, operating suites, and trained anesthesia personnel is even more starkly imbalanced between HI countries and those of sub-Saharan and other LI countries. Weiser et al. [18]

found that the global volume of major surgery was between 187 and 281 million cases, which is equivalent to one operation for every 25 people living in 2004. These researchers further found that countries spending less than USD $100 (2004) per person only had 295 major surgeries per 100,000 people. In contrast, countries spending more than USD $1,000 (2004) per person had surgical incidences of 11,110 per 100,000 people.

Weiser et al. also showed that MI and HI countries accounted for 30.2 % of the world's population but received 73.6 % of the surgical operations, whereas poor expenditure countries (less than or equal to USD $100 per person) accounted for 34.8 % of the global population and received only 3.5 % of all surgical procedures. This striking difference is not primarily due to nonessential surgical care. For example, in the USA in 2010 there were 51.4 million procedures performed on inpatients. Some of these procedures were endoscopies and cardiac catheterizations, but for the most part the procedures are those typically associated as "surgical" [19]. The number of aesthetic surgical procedures performed in the USA in 2012 was 289,000 [20]. Consequently, it can be seen that even with cosmetic and other procedures, the bulk of surgical interventions in the USA and other HI countries is not solely the result of nonessential intervention. Rather, what these data emphasize is that the extremely low volume of surgery performed in LMICs underscores a lack of access to surgical services in these locations. With this large, unaddressed surgical disease burden worldwide, measurement of surgical outcomes and public health evaluations in surgical disease are warranted.

In HI countries, mortality from anesthesia was found to be on the order of 6.4 deaths per 10,000 anesthetics by Beecher and Todd in 1954. By 1980, the mortality rate from anesthesia had decreased to 2 deaths per 10,000 anesthetics and current data indicates that anesthetic mortality is on the order of 1 death per 100,000–200,000 [21]. Major morbidity occurs in 3–16 % of cases. In contrast, in developing countries, the death rate remains 5–10 %, which is 500–1,000 deaths per 10,000 administered anesthetics [22] (Table 4.5). These data suggest that while affluent portions of the world have benefited from advances in anesthesia over the past six decades, with risk from dying from anesthesia being on the order of 1:200,000 anesthetics, LMICs have not seen any improvement. Anesthetic-related mortality in these environments is worse than experienced in the developed world since the inauguration of the age of anesthesia in the nineteenth century [23].

Table 4.5 Current comparative mortality rates in the UK and selected LMICs

Study	Mortality rate	Reference(s)
UK confidential enquiry for perioperative death	1:185,000	[26, 86]
University teaching Hospital, Zambia	1:1,925	[87]
Central Hospital, Malawi	1:504	[88]
District Hospital, Zimbabwe	1:482	[9]
Teaching Hospital, Nigeria	1:387	[89]
Teaching Hospital, Togo	1:133	[90]

Differences in frequency of surgical procedures could perhaps be explained by availability of surgical resources. Funk et al. [24] noted that there are more than 14 operating theaters per 100,000 people in high-income countries and 1–25 per 100,000 in middle to low-income countries. Moreover, almost 20 % of operating rooms worldwide were not equipped with pulse oximeters and this was not the case in high-income countries. Pulse oximeters are not the only equipment-related resources missing in LMICs. As seen below, simple things such as functional operating table are frequently not available. And, basic infrastructure requirement—such as electricity and water—cannot be guaranteed (Table 4.6).

Workforce

Differences in the availability of human resources are also striking. In the USA (2011), there were approximately 35,000 anesthesiologists, an equal number of certified registered nurse anesthetists (CRNA), and 1,300 anesthesia assistants (AA) actively practicing in the USA [25]. This yielded a trained anesthesia provider for every 4,295 individuals in the USA. In the UK, the ratio is on the order of 1 anesthetist for every 5,333 persons (2007) [26].

Table 4.6 Unavailability of requirements for administration of anesthesia

% Unavailable	*Anesthesia specific*
74	Pulse Oximeter
59	No spinal solutions available at all times
23	Tilting operating room table
22	Oxygen source
21	Appropriately sized endotracheal tubes
	Facility Specific
80	Electricity not always available
44	Running water not always available
30	Fluids not always available

In contrast to high-income countries, in a 2006 study in Uganda [27], questionnaires were distributed to attendees at a national anesthesia refresher course sponsored by the Ugandan Society of Anaesthesia, the Association of Anaesthetists of Great Britain and Ireland (AAGBI), and the World Federation of Societies of Anesthesiologists (WFSA). Of the 91 attendees, only one was a physician anesthetist in the group (all called anesthetists in this study). The vast majority of providers had attended a course in the administration of anesthesia of 1–2 years duration. Fewer than half had their own textbooks of anesthesia. In the UK, for 60 million people, there are roughly 12,000 anesthetists while in Uganda with a population of 27 million, there are 13 medical anesthesiologists and 330 nonphysician anesthesia providers. These figures are also seen in Afghanistan, with nine physician anesthetists for a population of 32 million and Bhutan with eight for a population of 700,000 [28].

In this study, only 23 % of the Ugandan anesthesia providers had the minimum requirements in their facilities for the safe administration of general anesthesia, only 13 % of anesthetists were able to provide safe anesthesia to children, and only 6 % of anesthetists in this study could provide safe anesthesia for a C-section with either a general or spinal anesthetic.

Dubowitz et al. provides some explanation of a relationship between economic rank and anesthesia availability [94]. Using a descriptive questionnaire mailed to the LMICs from the WHO, ministries of health, the following significant findings emerged:

1. Most LMICs surveyed had ratios of 1 or less physician or nonphysician anesthesia provider per 100,000 populations.
2. Inadequate nursing and surgical staff and limited hospital beds are also critical issues.
3. These discrepancies translate into low average life expectancy, high infant mortality, and high under-five mortality rates.
4. Again, as noted above, anesthesia-related mortality is extremely high.

Lack of funds and training are not the only problems, however. Even if appropriate funding were available, other problems for the provision of healthcare services–especially anesthesia service–remain. There is poor infrastructure, inadequate equipment or equipment that is frequently in disrepair, long and harsh working conditions, bureaucratic roadblocks [29] and lack of professional recognition. There are also incentives for trained personnel to migrate to urban settings or transnationally [30].

Within LMICs, most surgical and anesthesia providers cluster in urban environments, especially treating patients with the financial resources to pay for care [31]. For example, if one looks at the statistics for the entire country of Haiti before the 2010 earthquake, low-end estimates of maternal mortality are 523 per 100,000 live births. Community-based surveys have placed this number for the country as a whole at 1,400 per 100,000 live births [32]. This is in stark contrast to the much lower C-section rates and maternal mortality rates seen in Haitian cities, which approach those seen in the US. The maternal mortality ratio in other LMIC countries is 240 per 100,000 births versus 16 per 100,000 in HI countries with large disparities within countries, between people with high and low income, and between people living in rural and urban areas [33].

Delivery of Anesthesia Care

In general, three types of clinical personnel administer anesthesia globally: anesthesiologists, anesthesia assistants, and nurse anesthetists or surgical nurses. Anesthesiologists are medical professionals who have received medical degrees and appropriate training. Anesthesia assistants are trained professionals that specifically assist anesthesiologists. Nurse anesthetists are nurses who receive specialized training related to anesthesia, which may include drug administration. In certain countries, surgical nurses are trained to administer and/or monitor anesthesia. Thus, the specialty of nurse anesthetist does not exist. Each country has various restrictions that govern the practice of each type of clinical personnel.

The level of training of personnel allocated to administering anesthesia seems to be directly related to a country's total expenditures on healthcare. On one hand, nations, like the USA and the UK, that spend considerably more on healthcare tend to rely on anesthesiologists to administer anesthesia-related care. On the other hand, nations, like Rwanda and those in Sub-Saharan Africa, which spend less on healthcare, tend to rely on nurse anesthetists, surgical nurses, and/or less-trained clinical personnel.

Comparatively, in 2011, approximately 35,000 anesthesiologists practice in the USA; while Rwanda in the same year had a total of nine physicians who practice anesthesia [34]. Similarly, when the survey was conducted in 2007, researchers found that a total of 121 anesthesiologists served the French-speaking part of Sub-Saharan Africa compared to 665 nurse anesthetists and midwives. Researchers also found that in this region more than 80 % of anesthesia was provided by nurse anesthetists or midwives. In the UK, there are approximately 12,000 physician anesthetists for 64 million people [26]. In contrast, Uganda has 330 non-physician anesthetists to help fill needs for anesthesiology, a number that still remains insufficient [27].

In the African region, the supply of physician is estimated at 2.5 per 10 000 population and in the Southeast Asia region, it is 5.5 per 10,000 population. These figures are much lower compared to those in the Americas where there are 20.4 physicians per 10,000 population [35].

In Mongolia [36], roughly half of the population lives in rural areas, difficult to access. In these regions, availability of surgical or anesthetic care is limited. While Mongolia's absolute supply of physicians (2.8 per 1,000) appears adequate, their distribution is homogenous. In Ulaanbaatar there are 17.3 physicians per 1,000, while in rural areas the ratio is much lower. No primary level hospitals had a full-time surgeon or anesthesiologist. In primary facilities, 23 % had anesthesia administered by non-physician providers and 11 % had anesthesia administered by general physicians administering anesthesia. There were no anesthesiologists reported in the 44 sites sampled in the study.

Lack of trained personnel to administer anesthesia seems not to be explained by a lack of demand for surgeries. In surveyed hospitals in Rwanda, over 45,000 surgical cases occur each year [34]. However, this lack of trained personnel is not restricted to LMICs. A RAND study examining data from 2007 showed shortages of both anesthesiologists and nurse anesthetists in the USA [38]. In most simulations, researchers projected that it is likely there will be a shortage of anesthesiologists and a surplus of nurse anesthetists by 2020. Like in the USA, Europe has been experiencing shortages of anesthesiologists, which has induced demand for nurse anesthetists [38].

In terms of care delivery, a number of different kinds of models can be found internationally. Popularly in the USA, a "team" approach is used, where an anesthesiologist supervises nurse anesthetists and/or anesthesia assistants; and they collaboratively implement an anesthesia care plan. Switzerland also uses a collaborative approach given its lengthy historical use of nurse-administered anesthesia [38]. This is not to say, however, that nurses and physicians do not have conflicting views in these countries. For instance, anesthesiologists and nurse anesthetists in the USA continue to debate scope of practice [39]. In other countries, like the UK and Germany, where nurse anesthesia is a relatively new discipline, anesthesia care remains more restricted to anesthesiologists [40]. In contrast, primarily due to lack of supply of anesthesiologists, many LMICs have used nurses and midwives to administer anesthesia-related care as stated previously.

Current Training for Healthcare Professionals in Anesthesia

Both how anesthesia care is delivered and how human resources are available when comparing high-income countries to LMICs centers on how

Table 4.7 Educational training of physicians and nurses for careers in anesthesia

Country	Anesthesiologist education characteristics	Nurse anesthetist education characteristics
United States [39, 41, 42]	• Undergraduate college degree • Four years of medical school (3–4 years) • Four years of residency program • Pass Medical Licensing Exam • Most pass the American Board of Anesthesiology Exam	• Bachelor of Nursing or equivalent degree (3–4 years) • One year in acute care setting • Pass Nursing Licensing Exam • Two to three years of anesthesia graduate program • Pass national certification exam
United Kingdom [43, 44]	• Five to six years undergraduate medical training • Two years foundational training in hospitals • Seven to eight year anesthesia training program • Optional additional training in anesthesia	• Complete foundational nursing education courses • Secure employment as a nurse in a UK Hospital • Become a Band five nurse • Complete 6–12 month university education courses in anesthesia
France [45, 46]	• Two years undergraduate studies and pass exam at end of first year • Four years of master's program study including clinical training and passing several exams • Three to five years of residency training for specialty and thesis defense	• Three years of nursing education • Two years of practical experience • Two years of nurse anesthesia program (clinical practice and coursework)
Australia [45, 47, 48]	• Five to six years undergraduate degree or four years graduate degree • Two years internship • Five years anesthesia training	• Bachelor of Nursing • One year postgraduate study in anesthesia

medical and nurse professionals are trained and educated. In high-income countries, like the USA and the UK, educational standards for anesthesiologists and nurse anesthetists are fairly established. Standards for both professions are determined by a combination of government entities and professional societies. Table 4.7 summarizes educational characteristics for both professions for the USA, the UK, France, and Australia.

From these countries, one can see significant similarities when comparing physician education requirements. Students across these countries need approximately 11–15 years to complete physician education, are subjected to rigorous examinations, and must complete practical training.

While these countries all require some kind of postgraduate study, significant variation exists in education for nurse anesthetists. France and the USA seem to have the lengthiest requirements: 7 years, which is substantially shorter than anesthesiologist education durations. In contrast, the UK has historically trained nurses through hiring students at a hospital. Practical training and education led by clinical staff at the hospital then commences. Global agencies, such as the International Federation of Nurse Anesthetists, attempt to reduce these inconsistencies and promote educational standards for nurse anesthesia [46].

LMICs, however, face the summation of many different problems including fragmentation in medical and nursing education. For instance, Bird and Newton summarize the problems facing increasing the anesthesia workforce in Africa [49]:

> The lack of adequate numbers of training programs; the insufficient numbers of graduates of medical schools in LICs [Low Income Countries] who choose anesthesia; the shortage of proper training materials, including anesthesia books and training modalities; the lack of academic educational partnerships between resource-rich and resource poor countries; the lack of adequate basic medical infrastructure that would promote an anesthesia educational center; and the lack of alternative anesthesia care provider training models would each individually, but certainly collectively, contribute to the overall lack of anesthesia care necessary for the millions of patients in LICs.

Moreover, Greysen et al. report that research available on how specialists are trained compared to generalists in Sub-Saharan Africa is fragmented, which in turn creates difficulties for making improvements to the physician and healthcare workforce [50].

Advancing Training in Anesthesia in LMICs

A number of efforts on the international stage have been implemented to help LMICs train more anesthesiologists and nurse anesthetists. For example, the WHO and World Bank actively works with LMICs to reform national health policy involving medical and nursing education, such as efforts in Myanmar [51] and Nepal [52].

Other global agencies, such as the World Federation of Medical Education (WFME), have also attempted to create some standardization in medical education internationally [53]. For instance, the WFME has created medical education standards as well as guidelines for creating medical education accreditation bodies. As an example for adoption, the European Society of Anesthesiology offers the European Diploma in Anesthesia and Intensive Care, which is an examination to qualify as a specialist anesthesiologist [54]. Passing this exam grants European-educated anesthesiologists more freedom to practice throughout Europe. Accreditation procedures for medical and nursing schools along with standardization of education requirements could bolster the quality of overall education provided in many LMICs. As of 2011, only 7 of 35 African countries with medical schools have accreditation procedures [54].

The WHO has compiled a "Guide to Infrastructure and Supplies at Various Levels of Healthcare Facilities—Emergency and Essential Surgical Care (EESC)" for anesthesia which discusses the anesthetic requirements for Level 1 (Small Hospitals), Level 2 District (Provincial Hospitals), and Level 3 (Referral Hospitals). This document gives recommendations for procedures to be undertaken in each type of facility, the training of the personnel staffing these facilities, medications to be utilized, and specific anesthetic equipment and disposable equipment [55].

For the administration of anesthesia, WHO recommends paramedical staff without formal anesthesia training at Level I facilities, one or two trained anesthetists in Level 2 facilities, and clinical officers and specialists in anesthesia for Level 3 facilities. These recommendations seem to be consistent with past programs in LMICs.

For example, one of the common tactics implemented to help reduce anesthesia-related complications and deaths is to provide training to nurses and other non-physician personnel at hospitals. Médecins Sans Frontières has trained nurse anesthetists for over 10 years in Haiti [56]. In this program, in the 10-year period from 1998 to 2008, 24 students completed the program, 19 continued to work as anesthetists at the time of publication (2010) and 5 emigrated. When these anesthetists administered emergency care following Haiti's disastrous hurricane, the mortality rate was 0.3 % in 330 cases (one death). Additionally, significant amounts of their cases involved administering anesthesia independent of physician assistance.

Other tactics involved the training of physicians. In Nepal, in 1985 a 1-year diploma in anesthesia (DA) training program for physicians was created by the ministry of health (MOH) with the support of the Canadian Anesthesiologists' Society International Fund [57]. Forty-three (43) individuals graduated this course. Subsequently, in 1996, a 3-year anesthesia residency program was established. Following the establishment of the residency program, the ministry of health discontinued the recognition of the DA program. Nineteen (19) of those graduates worked for the MOH at the time of publication (2006), 11 are in private hospitals and 13 have left Nepal. However, in the period of time when the program was functioning, anesthesiologist (DA) were available at the ten hospitals outside the Kathmandu valley.

A similar situation existed in Rwanda. In 1996, an anesthesia-training program was initiated at the Kigali Health Institute for high school graduates who had studied health-related topics. If admitted, these individuals had a 3-year training program in anesthesia. From 1996 to publication (2007) there were 96 graduates of this program. In 2003, though, the National University of

Rwanda collaborated with the Canadian Anesthesiologists' Society and the American Society of Anesthesiologists Overseas Teaching Program to develop their own residency program. Tactically, however, some errors were made. Residents had to complete all of their training in country. This was not popular. In addition, trying to develop de novo an academic culture was not easy. As in all LMICs, availability of equipment and support was, and remains challenging.

Unsurprisingly, many individuals, groups, and practitioners in HICs recognize the urgency of this situation. For decades, groups such as ReSurge (formerly Interplast), Operation Smile, ORBIS, Health Volunteers Overseas, and countless others have been working in LMICs to provide otherwise unavailable surgical treatment and necessary education and training for local clinical staff. The US Department of State and the American Medical Association's International Health Database can provide a registry of health-oriented volunteer organizations [58].

In spite of these successes in directly educating clinical staff in LMICs, there have been some observations that detract from programs' sustainable progress. For example, there has been growing concern about the costs versus benefits of medical volunteerism [59]. Maki et al. evaluated 543 medical mission trips that conducted 6,000 annual short-term programs [95]. The average expenditure was $50,000 per mission, giving a minimal estimate of $250 million per year for just those programs. Significantly, there was a lack of standardization to evaluate patient safety, quality control, and mission impact, so determining optimal performance was impossible. These authors developed a tool to evaluate short-term surgical (and medical) mission on six criteria: Cost, Efficiency, Impact, Preparedness, Education, and Sustainability.

Moreover, further evidence from sub-Saharan Africa questions current models of health volunteerism. Laleman et al. [60] reviewed the comments of in-country experts (medical officers from sub-Saharan African countries). They had more negative than positive views of International Health Volunteers (IHV). The cost per expatriate volunteer was calculated to be US$36,000–US$50,000 annually. This study found that there were not more than 5,000 full-time equivalent IHV working in the region in 2005, of which not more than 1,500 of these were physicians (complicating this study). The surveyed country experts did state that IHVs were defendable as a temporary measure. Similar concerns were voiced by Acherman as it related to the training of healthcare workers for HICs in LMIC locations [96].

Another problem is the issue of medical migration, or physicians who train in a country and relocate to another country [49]. The negative effects of medical migration are particularly severe for LMICs. In fact, one in eight physicians trained in Sub-Saharan Africa is lost to medical migration [63]. Also, physician emigration is attributed to 6 of 47 Sub-Saharan African countries that lose over 60 % of their physician workforce [62, 63].

Several criticisms highlight important areas for future surgical and anesthesia training programs to consider in reducing the surgical burden of disease in LMICs:

- Education and training of the local workforce is imperative if any long-lasting change is to occur.
- Local authorities and other significant parties must feel that they are part of a lasting relationship.
- Metrics must be utilized to assess impact, outcomes, and cost-benefit.
- Volunteer staff should have an understanding of the community's culture.
- Trained workforce are given incentives to stay in aided communities.

Along these lines, the Bloomberg School of Public Health has developed an ethics curriculum for short-term global health trainees [64]. As observed with the WHO checklist, standardization promulgates norms for medical and surgical care worldwide, in this case including such issues as appropriate informed consent, ensuring sustainability, and not exceeding the provider's level of training.

Groups, such as CapaCare (Capacity Building and Training of Medical Staff), furnish examples of what can be accomplished in rural areas. With annual surgical production in the government

(1,700 cases) and an unknown number in the private/military and nongovernmental organization (NGO) sector in 2008, CapaCare committed itself as an organization to train 30 non-physician or young physicians to handle the most common life-threatening obstetrical and surgical emergencies in Sierra Leone. Volunteer surgeons, nurses, and anesthesiologists do two (2) to six (6) week rotations, giving both didactic and practical training. The WHO Integrated Management for Emergency Essential Surgical Care program is an essential component of the training. Collaboration with other NGO facilities is encouraged. Furthermore, CapaCare has a timeline to evaluate costs in 2014 and quality in 2015. This program includes all essential elements of a sustainable program that will be cost-effective.

Innovations in Anesthetic Techniques

In addition to improving training and access to anesthesia providers and availability of anesthetic equipment, anesthetic techniques must be adapted to particular situations in LMICs. Ideally, patients in these locations will ultimately be afforded the same anesthetic choices that patients in HICs receive. However, that is to ignore the current situation. Surgeons and those who have administered anesthesia in LMICs historically have relied quite heavily on both local anesthesia and sedation for pain relief. Vo et al. [28] found that regional anesthesia was offered by 56 % of facilities surveyed, spinal anesthesia was offered by 65.5 %, ketamine by 71.5 %, and general inhalational anesthesia was offered by 58.5 %.

The concept of pain—both chronic and also acute surgical—has significant cultural overtones and suffers from social constructs. In an editorial entitled, "Pain Management in Low and Middle Income Countries—Just Put Up With It?," Goucke and Morris [65] note that nociception from the periphery to the brain is the same in all humans, irrespective of where they live. There are innumerable benefits that accrue with treatment of surgical and chronic pain, including early mobilization, ability to self-care, and quicker hospital discharge. It could be argued that these factors are even more important in LMICs. It can appear that people in LMIC accept pain as an unavoidable part of life [64]. Patients often appear stoic and medical and nursing staffs may either not have treatments to offer or may believe that pain is a part of the natural history of the disease.

Tobias et al. [67] pointed out that premedication is frequently not administered, either intentionally not given or forgotten. However, particularly in difficult cultural situations, premedication may be highly desirable.

Local anesthesia, while not always the ideal technique, may be the only option in certain circumstances until anesthesia providers become more readily available. In extreme situations, even a C-section can be performed under local anesthesia [68]. Hemorrhoidectomies [69] and urethrotomies [70] have also been performed successfully under local anesthesia, perhaps as much a testament to the surgical skill of the providers as to the fortitude of the patients.

Ketamine [71] has been an invaluable agent in LMICs. It offers multiple routes of administration (intravenous, intramuscular, oral, rectal, subcutaneous, epidural, and transnasal routes) and its ability to function as a preoperative sedative, intraoperative anesthetic, and a postoperative analgesic is unique. Moreover, it preserves cardiorespiratory function, a critical asset in regions without reliable infrastructure for cardiopulmonary resuscitation.

Spinal anesthesia is not used as frequently as it could be, primarily due to limitations in availability of medications and equipment, especially spinal needles [36]. In addition, heretofore, training in regional has not been emphasized.

Improvements in Basic Infrastructure and Equipment

The provision of safe surgery and anesthesia in LMICs is limited by the fact that a significant proportion of operating suites do not have reliable sources of fresh water, electricity, or technicians to maintain equipment. Most modern surgical equipment assumes the existence of such infrastructure to run operating rooms. However, advances to overcome gaps in LMICs' infrastructures are being made.

Electricity and Water

In the instance of electricity, there are a number of innovations that use alternative energy. One such example is We Care Solar's [72] "solar suitcase" which provides reliable DC electricity for any kind of environment where access to power is critical but unavailable. It is self-contained and comes with everything needed to provide instantaneous power right out of the box. Current pricing is $1,495 and for $1,595, a fetal Doppler is included.

Other innovations include devices that use little electrical energy. For instance, students at the University of Utah [73] have also developed a surgical light that uses LED lights, a simple metal frame, and a battery backup. At present, this device can produce 70 % of the light recommended by international standards for illumination in operating suites and the inventors believe that 100 % of recommended levels is achievable. Another example is the solar-powered autoclave. Resources dedicated to sterilization of surgical equipment are often scarce or in repair in LMICs. Solar-powered autoclaves, which can be cost-effective, can help fill this need until a more developed and reliable electrical infrastructure is created.

In the case of water, sometimes distilled or deionized forms must be available. In small quantities, specialized water is not an obstacle. However, continuous sources are not typically available. The lack of water [74] is often associated with a lack of public infrastructure such as good roads, because in many cases, all water to remote locations is distributed via household service, vehicle, truck, or bottled water. In addition, to demonstrate how relatively inexpensive water can be provided for a hospital, a Canadian-Forces led project to build three water tanks was completed at HEAL Africa's tertiary hospital in Goma, DRC [75] in August 2010. The tanks ensure the hospital has a reliable source of clean water for drinking, sanitation, and surgical procedures. The total budget for the project was $61,266. Before the project, the hospital was buying at least three truckloads of water per week at $90 per truckload. Since the implementation, no disruptions in healthcare delivery because of lack of water have occurred.

Oxygen

The hospital choice between relying on tank oxygen or oxygen concentrators is also illustrative of how dependent decisions are upon external factors such as road quality. To deliver oxygen to a patient from an oxygen cylinder, the hospital must have a vehicle to get the cylinder, fuel for the vehicle, roads that can support the vehicle, a factory (reasonably close by) that produces the oxygen to fill the cylinder, and, of course, the money to acquire the tanked source. Largely because of a lack of public infrastructure, as much as 75 % of the developing world has no oxygen supply, relying on oxygen concentrators.

However, in all resource-poor countries, interruption of supply occurs. In a WHO analysis [76], it was suggested that if power is reliable, oxygen concentrators are preferable while if the power supply cannot be made reliable and if road transport is reliable, tank supplies are advantageous.

Medical Equipment

The WHO has estimated that 50–80 % of medical equipment in LMICs is out of service [77] while another study suggests that the figure is closer to 40 % [97]. In comparison in HICs less than 1 % of medical equipment is out of service [78]. In a comprehensive document, the Tropical Health and Education Trust (THET) [79] reviews the complex decisions associated with the donation of medical equipment to LMICs.

- Deciding whether to donate.
- Planning the donation.
- Supplying the equipment.
- Verifying the equipment's quality and safety.
- Storing packing and shipping.

- Receiving the equipment.
- Putting the equipment into service.
- Providing ongoing maintenance.

It does the recipient country no good to receive equipment that it cannot maintain, either due to budgetary, personnel, or procurement reasons. In addition, there is the added challenge that equipment may come from various sources, resulting in unusual mixes of types. Additionally, lack of training may make it impossible for anesthesia care providers to know how to use the equipment. Health Partners International has created a, "How to Manage," series on all of the management issues involved in Healthcare Technology [80]. These guides cover the topics:

Guide 1: How to Organize a System of Healthcare Technology Management.
Guide 2: How to Plan and Budget for Healthcare Technology.
Guide 3: How to Procure and Commission your Healthcare Technology.
Guide 4: How to Operate your Healthcare Technology Effectively and Safely.
Guide 5: How to Organize the Maintenance of your Healthcare Technology.
Guide 6: How to Manage the Finances of your Healthcare Technology Management Team.

This group recognizes that human resources and management are essential in strengthening health systems, and also that the planning for and managing of assets are critical. Included also are health equipment, utilities, buildings, and other fixed assets.

Pulse Oximeters

Over 77,000 operating rooms worldwide operate without pulse oximeters, technology that is mandatory in HI countries. The number of operating theatres working without pulse oximetry ranges from 41 % in Latin America [81] to 49 % in south Asia, to 70 % in Sub-Saharan Africa. Lifebox, a registered charity founded in 2004 by WFSA, HSPH, and AAGBI, conducted studies that indicated that by closing the gap in pulse oximeter availability and use and by also increasing the use of the Surgical Safety Checklist worldwide, death rates could be lowered by 50 % [24].

Anesthesia Machines

As noted previously, significant amounts of equipment that have been donated to LMICs are hard to service, more complicated, and fragile than required, with parts that are difficult and costly to obtain. With the variety of material donated, even highly trained biomedical engineers in HI countries would be challenged to maintain all the machines.

Gradian Health Systems has confronted this problem and developed the Universal Anesthesia Machine. Dr. Paul Fenton had the initial concept and currently the machine has the following advantages for use in challenging environments [82]:

- Integrated oxygen concentrator delivers 10 l/min of 95 % O_2.
- Compatible with cylinder, pipeline, and portable oxygen as backup sources.
- Accepts all standard pediatric and adult breathing systems connections.
- Seamless transition to draw-over mode using room air during power outages and O_2 shortages.
- Accurate, low resistance draw-over vaporizers work without compressed gas.
- Calibrated delivery of isoflurane or halothane.
- Built-in oxygen monitor displays O_2 concentration of inspired gas and warns of hypoxic mixtures.
- Nitrous oxide can be used optionally and automatically shuts off if hypoxic mixture is detected.
- Hand-operated bellows allows ventilation without electric power or compressed gas.

Diamedica also produces a similar machine that is functional in extremely challenging environments [83]. This company produces a variety of portable anesthesia machines that can function with or without electricity. These examples illustrate the rethinking that is occurring in the development of medical equipment for LMICs.

While many of these innovations are significant individual achievements, the cost-effectiveness of these technologies has not been fully evaluated. In the end, much more infrastructural development will be required before healthcare centers in LMICs can fully use the available medical and surgical devices found in HICs.

Concluding Statement

The current status of anesthetic care in LMICs is truly representative of the conundrum of whether the glass is half empty or half full. As noted, there has been substantial progress in meeting many of the UN Millennium Development Goals. Now that the issues of the Global Burden of Surgical Disease are rising in the public consciousness and are starting to be addressed, there is cause for hope that resources required for improving anesthetic care worldwide can occur.

This will require increases in funding, equipment specifically developed for LMIC situations, anesthetic techniques appropriate to the practice settings, and increased training of personnel for the administration of these anesthetics. It may prove to be cost-prohibitive and even unnecessary to transplant HIC models of anesthetic administration into LMIC situations. Hybrid practice models may need to be developed to ensure that all patients are afforded anesthetic care in a timely manner, without cannibalizing needed personnel from the nursing or medical professions. In addition, strategies need to be created to induce practitioners to remain in their communities.

Appendix: How to Calculate a DALY

Definition: One DALY (disability adjusted life years) can be thought of as one lost year of "healthy" life. The sum of these DALYs across the population, or the burden of disease, can be thought of as a measurement of the gap between current health status and an ideal health situation where the entire population lives to an advanced age, free of disease and disability.

DALYs for a disease or health condition are calculated as the sum of the Years of Life Lost (YLL) due to premature mortality in the population and the Years Lost due to Disability (YLD) for people living with the health condition or its consequences:

Calculation:

$$\text{DALY} = \text{YLL} + \text{YLD}$$

The YLL basically correspond to the number of deaths multiplied by the standard life expectancy at the age at which death occurs. The basic formula for YLL (without yet including other social preferences discussed below) is the following for a given cause, age, and sex:

$$\text{YLL} = N \times L$$

where:
N = number of deaths.
L = standard life expectancy at age of death in years.

Because YLL measure the incident stream of lost years of life due to deaths, an incidence perspective has also been taken for the calculation of YLD in the original Global Burden of Disease Study for year 1990 and in subsequent WHO updates for years 2000–2004.

To estimate YLD for a particular cause in a particular time period, the number of incident cases in that period is multiplied by the average duration of the disease and a weight factor that reflects the severity of the disease on a scale from 0 (perfect health) to 1 (dead). The basic formula for YLD is the following (again, without applying social preferences):

$$\text{YLD} = I \times DW \times L$$

where:
I = number of incident cases.
DW = disability weight.
L = average duration of the case until remission or death (years).

Prevalence YLD.

The recent GBD 2010 study published by IHME in December 2012 used an updated life expectancy standard for the calculation of YLL and based the YLD calculation on prevalence rather than incidence:

$$\text{YLD} = P \times \text{DW}$$

where:
P = number of prevalent cases.
DW = disability weight.

From the World Health Organization:

http://www.who.int/healthinfo/global_burden_disease/metrics_daly/en/.

References

1. UN Millennium Summit (6–8 September 2000). http://www.un.org/en/events/pastevents/millennium_summit.shtml. Accessed Mar 20 2014.
2. Agency for Healthcare Research and Quality: "Addressing health disparities: a conversation with Thomas LaVeist, PhD, Director of the Hopkins Center for Health Disparities Solutions at the Johns Hopkins Bloomberg School of Public Health". 04–17 2013, Accessed 20 Mar 2014.
3. UN Millennium Development Goals Report 2013. http://www.un.org/millenniumgoals/pdf/report-2013/mdg-report-2013-english.pdf. Accessed 20 Mar 2014.
4. Jamison D, World Bank. Disease control priorities project. Disease control priorities in developing countries. Washington, DC: Oxford University Press/World Bank; 2006.
5. Farmer P, Kim JY. Surgery and global health: a view from beyond the OR. World J Surgery. 2008;32(4):533–6.
6. Abdullah F, Troedsson H, Cherian M. The World Health Organization Program for emergency surgical, obstetric and anesthetic care: from Mongolia to the future. Arch Surg. 2011;146:620–3.
7. WHO: Emergency and essential surgical care. http://www.who.int/surgery/globalinitiative/en/. Accessed 20 Mar 2014.
8. Médecins Sans Frontières: MSF Activities. http://www.msf.org/msf-activities. Accessed 20 Mar 2014.
9. Glenshaw M, Madzimbamuto FD. Anaesthesia associated mortality in a district hospital in Zimbabwe: 1994–2001. Cent Afr Med. 2005;51:39–44.
10. McCord C, Chowdhury Q. A cost effective small hospital in Bangladesh: what it can mean for emergency obstetric care. Int J Gynaecol Obstet. 2003;81:83–92.
11. Curci M. Task shifting overcomes the limitations of volunteerism in developing nations. Bull Am Coll of Surg. 2012;97(10):9–14.
12. Laleman G, Kegels G, Marchal B, Van der Roost D, Bogaert I, Van Damme W. The contribution of international health volunteers to the health workforce in sub-Saharan Africa. Hum Res Health. 2007;5:19–27.
13. World Bank. How we classify countries. http://data.worldbank.org/about/country-classifications. Accessed 20 Mar 2014.
14. CMS.GOV. National health expenditures 2012 highlights. http://www.cms.gov/Research-Statistics-Data-and-Systems/Statistics-Trends-and- Reports/NationalHealthExpendData/downloads/highlights.pdf. Accessed 20 Mar 2014.
15. World Bank. Health expenditure per capita (Current US$). http://data.worldbank.org/indicator/SH.XPD.PCAP Accessed 20 Mar 2014.
16. World Bank. GNI per capita ranking, Atlas method and PPP. http://data.worldbank.org/data-catalog/GNI-per-capita-Atlas-and-PPP-table. Accessed 20 Mar 2014.
17. Scheffler RM, Jiu JX, Kinfu Y, Dal Poz MR. Forecasting the global shortage of physicians: an economic-and needs-based approach. Bull World Health Organ. 2008;86:516–23.
18. Weiser TG, Regenbogen SE, Thompson KD, Haynes AB, Lipsitz SR, Berry WR, Gawande AA. An estimation of the global volume of surgery: a modeling strategy based on available data. Lancet. 2008;372:139–44.
19. CDC: Fast facts—inpatient surgery. http://www.cdc.gov/nchs/fastats/insurg.htm. Accessed 20 Mar 2014.
20. American society for Aesthetic Plastic Surgery 2012. http://www.surgery.org/media/statistics. Accessed 20 Mar 2014.
21. Braz LG, Braz DG, Braz JRC. Mortality in anesthesia: a systematic review. Clinics (Sao Paolo). 2009;64(10):999–1006.
22. Yii MK, Ng KJ. Risk-adjusted surgical audit with the POSSUM scoring system in a developing country. Br J Surg. 2002;89:110–3.
23. World Alliance for Patient Safety, WHO Guidelines for Safe Surgery (First Edition), 2008. 9–10.
24. Funk LM, Weiser TG, Berry WR, Lipsitz SR, Merry AF, Enright AC, Wilson IH, Dziekan G, Gwande AA. Global operating theatre distribution and pulse oximetry supply: an estimation from reported data. Lancet. 2010;376:1055–61.
25. Warner MW. Efforts Needed to Meet Anesthesiologist Demand. Physicians Weekly; 2011.
26. Walker I, Wilson I, Bogod D. Anaesthesia in developing countries. Anaesthesia. 2007;62 Suppl 1:2–3.
27. Hodges SC, Mijumbi C, Okello M, McCormick BA, Wlaker IA, Wilson IH. Anaesthesia services in developing countries: defining the problems. Anaesthesia. 2007;62:4–11.
28. Vo D, Cherian MN, Bianchi S, et al. Anesthesia capacity in 22 low and middle income countries. J Anesth Clin Res. 2012;3(4):207–11.
29. Conway MD, Gupta S, Prakash S. Building better partnerships for global health. McKinsey Quarterly; 2006, p. 1–8.
30. Mullan F. The metrics of the physician brain drain. NEJM. 2005;353:1810–8.
31. US Senate Committee on Foreign Relations, Testimony of Dr. Dr. Paul Farmer, July 15 2003.

32. Forum Libre I: Medecine, Sante et Democratie en Haiti. 1989, p. 11–20.
33. WHO, Maternal Mortality Fact Sheet, Fact sheet N°348, May 2012. http://www.who.int/mediacentre/factsheets/fs348/en/. Accessed 20 Mar 2014.
34. Notrica MR, et al. Rwandan surgical and anesthesia infrastructure: a survey of District Hospitals. World J Surg. 2011;35:1770–80.
35. World Health Organization, "Global Atlas of the Health Workforce". http://who.int/hrh/statistics/hwfstats/en/index.html. Accessed 20 Mar 2014.
36. Spiegel DA, Choo S, Cherian M, et al. Quantifying surgical and anesthetic availability at primary health facilities in Mongolia. World J Surg. 2011;35: 272–9.
37. Daugherty, et al. An analysis of the labor markets for anesthesiology. Santa Monica, CA: RAND Corporation; 2010.
38. Cristina Frangou, "Tensions Rise in Debate on Role of Europe's CRNAs". Anesthesiology News. 2007.
39. John Hayes, "Anesthesiologist-CRNA Teamwork Common, but Groups at Odds," Medscape Anesthesiology. 2012.
40. Tuffs A. German Hospital's use of trained nurse anaesthetists angers doctors. BMJ. 2007;334(7594): 607.
41. American Society of Anesthesiologists, "About the Profession". http://www.asahq.org/For-the-Public-and-Media/About-Profession.aspx. Accessed 20 Mar 2014.
42. American Association of Nurse Anesthetists, "Certified Registered Nurse Anesthetists at a Glance". http://www.aana.com/ceandeducation/becomeacrna/Pages/Nurse-Anesthetists-at-a-Glance.aspx. Accessed 20 Mar 2014.
43. British Anaesthetic and Recovery Nurses Association, "Becoming an Anaesthetic and Recovery Nurse". http://www.barna.co.uk/media/uploads/downloads/how-to-become-an-anaesthetic-and- recovery- nurse.pdf. Accessed 20 Mar 2014.
44. The Royal College of Anaesthetists, "Considering a Career in Anaesthesia". http://www.rcoa.ac.uk/careers-and-training/considering-career-anaesthesia. Accessed 20 Mar 2014.
45. Global Knowledge Exchange Network, An overview of education and training requirements for global healthcare professionals: nursing edition. 2009.
46. International Federation of Nurse Anesthetists, "About IFNA". http://ifna-int.org/ifna/page.php?16. Accessed 20 Mar 2014.
47. Australian and New Zealand College of Anaesthetists, "What is anaesthesia?" http://www.anzca.edu.au/patients/anaesthestist. Accessed 20 Mar 2014.
48. Global Knowledge Exchange Network, An overview of education and training requirements for global healthcare professionals: physician edition. 2009.
49. Newton M, Bird P. Impact of parallel anesthesia and surgical provider training in sub-Saharan Africa: a model for a resource-poor setting. World J Surg. 2010;34:445–52.
50. Ryan Greysen S, et al. Medical education in Sub-Saharan Africa: a literature review. Med Edu. 2011;45:973–86.
51. "Sweden Contributes $30m to 3MDG Fund," Mizzima. 2014.
52. WHO Country Office for Nepal, "Human Resource for Health (HRH)," WHO. 2008. http://www.nep.searo.who.int/EN/Section4/Section40.htm.
53. World Federation for Medical Education, "Standards". WFME. 2014. http://www.wfme.org/standards. Accessed 20 March 2014.
54. "European Diploma in Anaesthesiology and Intensive Care". European Society of Anaesthesiology. 2012. http://www.esahq.org/education/edaic/about.
55. World Health Organization: Guide to infrastructure and supplies at various levels of health care facilities—Emergency and Essential Surgical Care (EESC), Compiled from the WHO Manual Surgical Care at the District Hospital 2003. WHO/HPW/CPR 2005.
56. Rosseel P, Trelles M, Guilavogui S, Ford N, Chu K. Ten years of experience training non-physician anesthesia providers in Haiti. World J Surg; 2010; 34:453–8.
57. Shrestha BM, Rana NB. Training and development of anesthesia in Nepal: 1985 to 2005. Can J Anesth. 2006;53(4):339–43.
58. AMA International Health Database. http://www.ama-assn.org//ama/pub/about-ama/our- people/member-groups-sections/medical-student-section/opportunities/international-health- opportunities.page. Accessed 20 Mar 2014.
59. Curci M. Task shifting overcomes the limitations of volunteerism in developing nations. Bull Am Coll Surg. 2012;97(10):9–14.
60. Laleman G, Kegels G, Marchal B, Van der Roost D, Bogaert I, Van Damme W. The contribution of international health volunteers to the health workforce in sub-Saharan Africa. Human Resources for Health. 2007;5:19–27.
61. Mullan F. The metrics of the physician brain drain. New Eng J Med. 2005;353:1810–8.
62. Clemens MA, Pettersen G. New data on African health professionals abroad. Hum Res Health. 2007;6(1).
63. Hagopian A, et al. The migration of physicians from sub-Saharan Africa to the United States of America: measures of the African brain drain. Hum Res Health. 2004;2(17).
64. DeCamp M, Rodriguez J, Hecht S, Barry M, Sugarman J. An ethics curriculum for short term global health trainees. Global Health. 2013;9:5.
65. Goucke R, Morriss W. "Pain management in low and middle income countries—just put up with it?" Anaesthesia News. 2011. 293, p. 6.
66. Personal communication, Brett Gutsche.
67. Tobias JD, Columbia M, Kim Y, Davis J (2002) Anesthetic care in developing countries: equipment and techniques. South Med J. 95(2): 239–247.
68. Shinde G, Sharma N, Jadhav B, Jaisal P. Caesarean section under local anaesthesia: back to basics. Trop Doct. 2012;42:38–40.

69. Zafar A, Ahmad S, Ansari J. Office haemorrhoidectomy with local anaesthesia: a feasible day-case procedure. Trop Doct. 2009;39:69–70.
70. Munks DG, Alli MO, Abdel Goad EH. Optical urethrotomy under local anaesthesia is a feasible option in urethral stricture disease. Trop Doct. 2010;40:31–312.
71. Craven R. Ketamine. Anaesthesia. 2007;62 Suppl 1:48–53.
72. We Care Solar. http://wecaresolar.org/. Accessed 20 Mar 2014.
73. University of Utah, Technology venture development, P. 10–11. http://www.techventures.utah.edu/Documents/Student-Innovation-Report-2013.pdf. Accessed 20 Mar 2014.
74. National Academy of Sciences, The Global Health and Education Foundation. http://www.drinking-water.org/. Accessed 20 Mar 2014.
75. Congo Story. HEAL Africa Water Project. http://congostory.org/node/86?page=1. Accessed 20 Mar 2014.
76. Howie SR, Hill S, et al. Meeting oxygen needs in Africa: an options analysis from Gambia. Bull World Health Org. 2009;87:763–71. http://who.int/bulletin/volumes/87/10/08-058370/en/index.html. Accessed 20 Mar 2014.
77. Mavalankar D, et al. Managing equipment for emergency obstetric care in rural hospitals. Int J Gynaecol Obstet. 2004;87(1):88–97.
78. Howitt P, et al. The lancet and imperial college London (UK) commission: technologies for global health. Lancet. 2012;380(9840):507–35.
79. Health Partnership Scheme, Partnership for Global Health. http://www.thet.org/hps/. Accessed 20 Mar 2014.
80. Health Partners International. "How to Manage" series of health care technology guides. http://www.healthpartners-int.co.uk/our_expertise/how_to_manage_series.html. Accessed 20 Mar 2014.
81. Lifebox. http://www.lifebox.org/about-lifebox/the-pulse-oximetry-gap/. Accessed 20 Mar 2014.
82. Gradian Health Systems. http://www.gradianhealth.org/wp-content/uploads/2012/03/Gradian- Brochure-FULL-revised-4.23_reduced-size1.pdf. Accessed 20 Mar 2014.
83. Diamedica. http://www.diamedica.co.uk/english/product_details.cfm?id=208. Accessed 20 Mar 2014.
84. Buck N, Devlin HB, Lunn JN. The report of a confidential enquiry into perioperative deaths. London: Nuffield Provincial Hospitals Trust and the King's Fund; 1987.
85. Heywood AJ, Wilson IH, Sinclair JR. Perioperative mortality in Zambia. Ann R Coll Surg Eng. 1989;71:354–8.
86. Hansen D, Gausi SC, Merikebu M. Anaesthesia in Malawi: complication and deaths. Trop Doctor. 2008; 30:146–9.
87. Enohumah KO, Imarengiaye CO. Factors associated with anaesthesia-related maternal mortality in a tertiary hospital in Nigeria. Acta Anaesthesiol Scand. 2006;50:206–10.
88. Ouro-Gang'na Maman AF, Tomta K, Ahouangbevi S, Chobli M. Deaths associated with anaesthesia in Togo, West Africa. Trop Doct. 2005;35:220–2.
89. Debas HT, Gosselin R, McCord C, et al. Surgery. In: Jamison DT, Breman JG, Measham AR, et al., editors. Disease control priorities in developing countries. 2nd ed. Washington, DC: World Bank; 2006. Chapter 67Available from: http://www.ncbi.nlm.nih.gov/books/NBK11719/.
90. WHO Road Traffic Data. http://www.who.int/mediacentre/factsheets/fs358/en/. Accessed 25 Mar 2014.
91. WHO Data on Pregnancy-Related Complications and Death. http://www.who.int/mediacentre/factsheets/fs348/en/. Accessed 25 Mar 2014.
92. WHO Data on Club Feet. http://www.who.int/surgery/challenges/esc_congenital_nomalies/en/. Accessed 25 Mar 2014.
93. The World Bank. Knowledge in development note: international migration. 2009. http://econ.worldbank.org/WBSITE/EXTERNAL/EXTDEC/EXTRESEARCH/0,,content MDK:22451777~pagePK:64165401~piPK:64165026~theSitePK:469382~isCURL:Y,00. html. Accessed 25 Mar 2014.
94. Dubowitz G, Detlefs S, McQueen KA. Global anesthesia workforce crisis: a preliminary survey revealing shortages contributing to undesirable outcomes and unsafe practices. World J Surg. 2010;34(3): 438–44. doi:10.1007/s00268-009-0229-6.
95. Maki J, Qualls M, White B, Kleefield S, Crone R. Health impact assessment and short-term medical missions: a methods study to evaluate quality of care. BMC Health Ser Res. 2008;8:121. doi:10.1186/1472-6963-8-121.
96. Acherman LK. The ethics of short-term international health electives in developing countries. Ann Behav Sci Med Edu. 2010;16(2):40–3.
97. Perry L, Malkin R. Effectiveness of medical equipment donations to improve health systems: how much medical equipment is broken in the developing world? Med Biol Eng Comput. 2011;49:719–22. doi:10.1007/s11517-011-0786-3.

Planning a Mission, Fundraising, and Building a Team

5

Medge Owen and Helen Akinc

Introduction

Global health work can be many different things; exciting, frustrating, time-consuming, inspiring, life changing, however, one thing is certain, it is never boring. There are many important considerations when one goes about planning and executing a medical or surgical mission. Building the right relationships and executing a successful program can positively impact many lives, so getting it right is important. A poorly planned or executed program can negatively impact both participants as well as country hosts. The goal of this chapter is to lay the foundation for developing and executing a successful global health program through planning a mission, fundraising, and building a team.

M. Owen, M.D. (✉)
Wake Forest University, Winston-Salem, NC, USA

Kybele, Inc., Winston-Salem, NC, USA
e-mail: mowen@wakehealth.edu

H. Akinc, M.B.A.
NavyBrat LLC, Winston-Salem, NC, USA

Planning a Mission

Selecting and Assessing a Site

Selecting and assessing a site is an important initial consideration that highly influences the success of a program. Individuals or organizations must carefully ponder the political stability of the proposed country, priorities within the country, the state of the medical infrastructure, the presence of a local champion, language barriers, readiness for change among local practitioners, and overlap with work already under way by other organizations or individuals [1–3].

Site selection begins with a dialogue with a host country contact, usually a physician. Global health and medical meetings such as the World Congress of Anesthesiology (WCA) are excellent venues through which to meet and network with medical providers from other countries. The WCA is held every 4 years, and a schedule can be found on the website for the World Federation of Societies of Anaesthesiologists (www.anaesthesiologists.org). Many interesting panels and poster presentations highlight disparities and challenges that exist in providing anesthesia and surgical care across the world. When trying to understand the various needs that exist, it is important to start from the local host's perspective.

Once communication begins, if goals between the visiting and host organization are compatible and mutually beneficial, an invitation may be

R. Roth et al. (eds.), *The Role of Anesthesiology in Global Health: A Comprehensive Guide*,
DOI 10.1007/978-3-319-09423-6_5, © Springer International Publishing Switzerland 2015

extended for a site visit to the host country. Ideally, this should occur at least 9–12 months before arriving with a team. A site visit can involve a few individuals, identified as potential program organizers, who travel to the prospective country in order to build relationships with medical personnel and conduct a needs assessment [1]. It is helpful for the visiting physicians to closely align with the host physician to better understand his or her goals for partnership. It is also important to observe the conditions and medical practices that exist within several hospitals to develop a broader understanding of the medical landscape. Figure 5.1 provides an example of an assessment form developed and used by Kybele, Inc., a 501(c)(3) organization that promotes childbirth safety worldwide through educational partnerships (www.kybeleworldwide.org). While largely focused on obstetrics, obstetric anesthesia and newborn care, this assessment can be tailored to other surgical disciplines. Excellent considerations for pediatric-focused surgical programs have been summarized by Fisher et al. [4] and Schneider et al. [5]. Another screening tool has been developed by The WHO Global Initiative on Emergency and Essential Surgery Care (GIEESC), known as the Tool for Situational Analysis for Emergency and Essential Surgical Care [6].

During the site visit, one should assess and weigh the competence, influence, and leadership potential of the country host, otherwise deemed "the local champion." This individual will be pivotal to the overall success of the program and will assist with many elements of planning. A local champion paves the way for understanding local requirements, medical licensure, bureaucracy, legal issues, culture, and lays the groundwork for the program to be successful and well received. He or she must be hardworking and collaborative, with a positive demeanor, and capable of influencing change within their countries. A "local champion" is usually someone not too junior or senior. Young, junior colleagues lack clout within their healthcare systems and often can't influence change due to hierarchal barriers. Senior colleagues may not have the drive or interest to undertake a time-consuming collaboration due to administrative duties or upcoming retirement. It is very important, however, for senior colleagues to conceptually buy into the program, as they can become stumbling blocks if they are excluded.

One example of a local champion success story is that of Croatian anesthesiologist Dr. Dragica Kopic. One of the authors (MO) was speaking at a medical conference in Croatia and met Dr. Kopic. She was bright, energetic, and interested in learning about obstetric anesthesia but had little experience. Dr. Owen visited her local hospital and made numerous observations. Over the next few months, they continued to communicate via email. They conducted a survey of obstetric anesthesia practices in Croatia and found a limited use of regional anesthesia techniques. Dr. Owen invited her to present her findings at the Society for Obstetric Anesthesia and Perinatology's annual meeting [7] and sponsored her visit. Dr. Kopic also spent several weeks observing obstetric anesthesia patient care practices at Wake Forest and Duke Universities. Once inspired, her accomplishments were nothing short of remarkable. Within the year of her visit, she introduced into her university hospital the use of regional anesthesia techniques for labor and cesarean section. Prior to this, most patients either had no labor pain relief or general anesthesia for cesarean section. She initiated monthly childbirth education classes for prospective parents (Fig. 5.2). She raised funds to renovate and establish two special labor and delivery rooms—deemed "apartments" in Croatian—to allow a family member to attend the birth, which was previously not permitted. She organized a five-member obstetric anesthesia team among her colleagues and appeared on local television to discuss the merits of epidural analgesia for childbirth. Other hospitals in her region heard about her and started asking for help. To address the growing interest, Drs. Medge Owen and Margaret Sedensky, University of Washington, recruited a 14-member internationally based team of obstetric anesthesiologists, a midwife, and an obstetric internist to travel to Croatia in September 2005 to work within nine university hospitals throughout the country promoting the use of regional anesthesia for obstetric care (Fig. 5.3) [8].

Name of Institution ____

Leadership

Name of hospital administrator	phone # email
Enthusiasm for collaborative program	no interest 1 2 3 4 5 6 7 8 9 10 totally sold
Name of obstetrician	phone # email
Enthusiasm for collaborative program	no interest 1 2 3 4 5 6 7 8 9 10 totally sold
Name of anesthesia head	phone # email
Enthusiasm for collaborative program	no interest 1 2 3 4 5 6 7 8 9 10 totally sold
Name of nursing head	phone # email
Enthusiasm for collaborative program	no interest 1 2 3 4 5 6 7 8 9 10 totally sold
Name of labor ward head	phone # email
Enthusiasm for collaborative program	no interest 1 2 3 4 5 6 7 8 9 10 totally sold

Staffing

Number of obstetric attending	
Number of obstetric medical officers	
Number of obstetric residents	
Number of obstetric house officers	
Enthusiasm for collaborative program by team	none 1 2 3 4 5 6 7 8 9 10 totally sold
Number of anesthesia attending	
Number of anesthesia nurse anesthetists	
Number of anesthesia assistants	
Number of anesthesia students	
Enthusiasm for collaborative program	none 1 2 3 4 5 6 7 8 9 10 total
Number of labor ward midwives	
Number of assistants	
Enthusiasm for collaborative program	none 1 2 3 4 5 6 7 8 9 10 total

Morbidity and Mortality

What is the yearly total number of death for the past 3 years in hospital?
Number of still births for the past 3 years: fresh or macerated
In stillbirth numbers, can differentiate those who came in with fetal heart beats Yes No
Number of anesthesia related death in 3 years?
Any complications data collected?
Any other outcome collected of endpoint or process? Time

Obstetrics

Is there a hemorrhage protocol?
Is there a preeclampsia protocol?
Is magnesium available?
What drugs used to control blood pressure acutely? hydralazine labetalol nifedipine other
Are mothers allowed any fluids during labor?
The following are used to monitor baby in labor: Cardiotocography or fetal heart montor (FHM).
Doppler Hand held fetoscope
Is there a triage?
Is there a resuscitation area for mothers?
Is there preeclampsia or hemorrhage kit available?

Fig. 5.1 Site assessment form example. These document samples are the property of Kybele, Inc. If you use these or any part of these materials in publication, kindly reference that the materials were developed by Kybele, Inc

Is there oxygen available for mothers?
Is there emergency airway equipment available?
Is there an ICU or High dependency unit for ill patients?
Is there a manual for unit?
Is there an orientation schedule for new doctors
Is there overlap between new and old interns?
Is unit mainly run by residents or regular consultant rounds?
Are patients given any pain relief Yes No
Percentage getting pethidine?
Is regional labour analgesia given in the labor ward?
How many minutes before a patient is first seen by Ob staff? < 30min 30 – 60 min > 60min
Is blood easily available?
Do you operate an open door policy (patients not turned away for being full)?
Is there often delay to do c/s due to theatre issues?
Who transfers patient to theater?
Who transfers patients back to the ward?

Triage
Is there triage
Is there a time frame within which patient are seen
Is there a level system?
If level one, is there a process (cycle time of intervention)
Are there protocols?

Anesthesia
Is there a doctor anesthesia cover 24 hrs a day
How often are they summoned after hours?
How many anesthesia deaths in last 3 years? Both OB and non OB cases
Have you had deaths due to inability to intubate?
Death due to aspiration?
Do you have irregular supply of spinal needles bupivacaine ephedrine
Can you monitor blood pressure? EKG? O2 Saturation ? muscle relaxation?
Are these dugs always available propofol thiopentone succinylcholine vecuronium
Has anesthesia been involved in labor ward and how often?
No A few times Often All the time
Who is responsible for recovery room patients?
For past 3 years, yearly rate please-
How many deliveries
How many c/s
How many are done using spinals
How many are done using epidurals
How many are done using general anesthesia
Is there person in charge of anesthesia equipments?
Who is in charge of schedules for nurse anesthesia for doctors?
Is there shortage of anesthetists yes No
How many more is ideal?
Any regular anesthesia meeting?

Fig. 5.1 (continued)

Any anesthesia mortality log book?
Have anesthesia providers had neonatal resuscitation training?
Do you have pressure bags to deliver rapid fluids?
Do you have automated monitors?

Neonatology
Does the neonatal resuscitation area have oxygen bulb suction catheter suction clock ambubag neonatal mask drugs (naloxone, epinephrine)
Is NICU staff available for help in resuscitation?
Is the neonatal area in theater well stocked with bulb suction catheter suction clock oxygen ambu bag mask
Who is responsible for theater neonatal area stocking?
How often is training in neonatal resuscitation for midwives?

Nurses / Midwives
Number of midwives per shift?
Average decision to c/s time
Midwife or doctor led unit?
Do they go on courses for improvement?
Do the younger midwives go or the senior ones?
Relationship between midwives and obstetricians? Excellent Good Fair poor
What can improve patient care in the unit?
What are the major frustrations?

Theatre
How many theatres available for surgery?
How many ventilators available?
Is there defibrillator
Is there a dedicated OR for Obstetrics
Is there a dedicated team for OB
What volume per month?
Estimate of downtime per week/

Cesarean sections
Are patient left unattended on the corridor
Is there any fetal monitoring while waiting?
Are patients on their side?
Is oxygen available for them?
How long do mothers stay in recovery before transfer to ward
Do babies stay with mother?
What pain medicine is given postop?

Leadership
Any targets planned of death rates of time of processes of volume of work

Multidisciplinary
Any formal meeting in Labor ward about patients (daily)
Any formal review of adverse outcome or deaths

Fig. 5.1 (continued)

Any teaching meetings
Any meeting between Obstetric and anesthesia
Any meeting between nurses, obstetric, anesthesia and administration?

Administration
What incentives do staff have? Recognition awards lunch drinks bus pass ?
Any forum for staffs to give feedback on maternal care to administration?
Does administration visit the wards?
Is there a voluntary blood donation system?
Any specific targets or goals planned/

If a collaboration is wanted, what areas has potential for work collaboration and improvement?
Conclusion of visit

1. Nothing of significance can be achieved; best to continue to other causes
2. Suitable for a short interaction (course, lecture series, brief visitation)
3. Suitable for long term mission

Fig. 5.1 (continued)

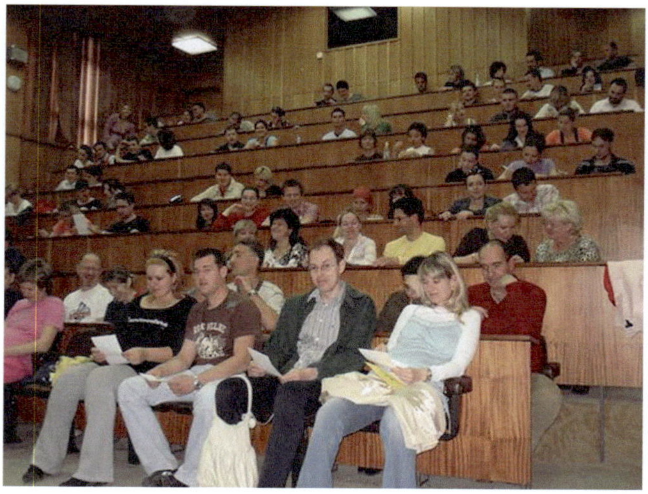

Fig. 5.2 Photo courtesy of Kybele, Inc. Dr. Dragica Kopic leads a family centered educational forum on options for labor pain relief in Split, Croatia

Focusing on countries with established anesthesiology training programs is cost-efficient and achieves broad impact because, upon graduation and job placement, young doctors can disseminate and promote new skills across a country [8]. Physicians in training are also quick learners and eager to perform new techniques. The sites selected should have an adequate healthcare infrastructure of supplies, even if there are limitations. Having to continuously bring equipment, medication, and supplies creates a culture of dependency, which cannot be sustained. It is far

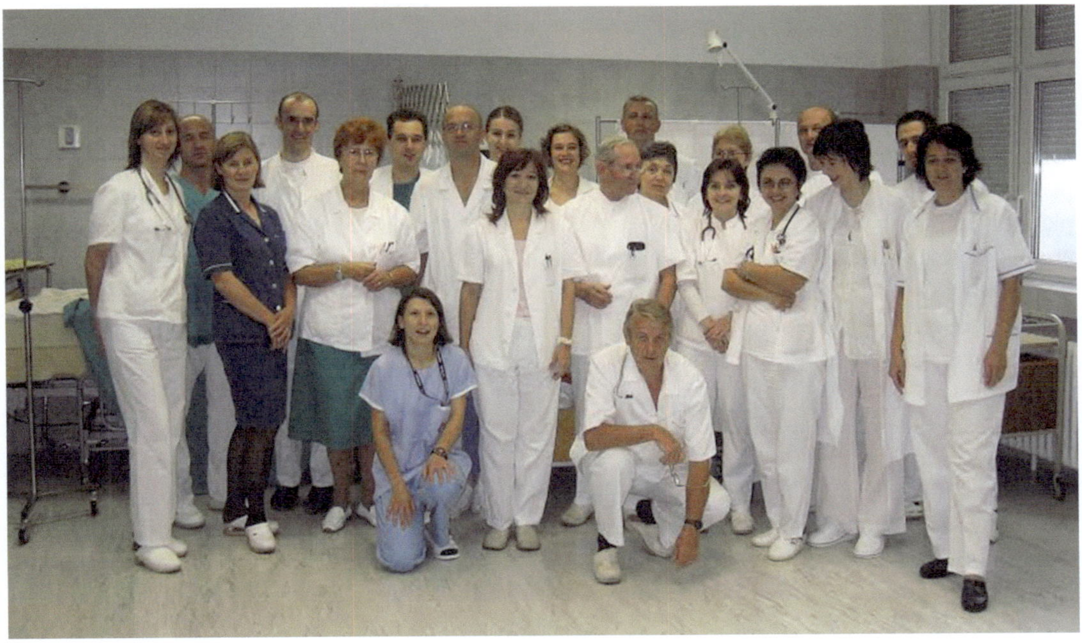

Fig. 5.3 Photo courtesy of Kybele, Inc. Australian anesthesiologist, Dr. Amanda Baric (kneeling front left), with colleagues at Sisak University Hospital, Croatia

more useful to provide education to better use the supplies already possessed and to develop internal supply chains through advocacy. This approach may limit projects in some of the poorest countries but unless a country has an established healthcare infrastructure it is unlikely that improvements can be sustained. To illustrate, Kybele conducted a program in the Republic of Georgia from 2006 to 2009 to encourage the use of regional anesthesia techniques for labor analgesia and cesarean section [9]. At the outset of the program, 10 % lidocaine was the only available local anesthetic and regional anesthesia was seldom used. Kybele sought permission from Ministry of Health officials initially to bring bupivacaine, ephedrine, and other supplies into the country for teaching demonstrations. Local physicians saw the immediate benefit of regional anesthesia techniques (Fig. 5.4) and joint advocacy persuaded the Health Ministry to include these medications on the national formulary. As a result, regional anesthesia techniques significantly increased, supply chains improved, and costs for epidural kits and spinal needles decreased across the country [9]. Had Kybele operatives continued to bring in supplies, the vast improvements may have never materialized.

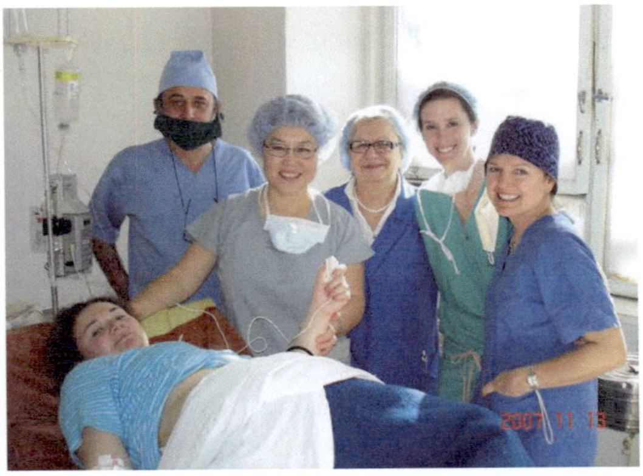

Fig. 5.4 Photo courtesy of Kybele, Inc. Grateful patient with labor analgesia in the Republic of Georgia with Kybele and local medical team

Pre-trip Planning

Once a site has been vetted and the decision to go has been made, pre-trip planning takes center stage. A project should be designed with input from the host physician to fit the specific needs of the country [1, 10]. Often, the host physician networks with other colleagues to determine interest within one or among multiple potential hospital sites. Goals of the trip, the number of participants, and required medical skill sets need to be planned in advance [11]. The local host can arrange housing, local transportation, and obtain permission for visitation and licensure for visitors. Figure 5.5 delineates the general responsibilities for a local host, team leader, and participants in advance of the trip.

Trips are often coordinated by one or two team leaders. These are individuals who have demonstrated leadership, flexibility, good judgment, intercultural competency, and strong interpersonal skills along with the requisite traits of superb clinical skills, strong work ethic, and honesty. The team leader or leaders build the team, make sure team members are prepared, and handle problems as they arise during the trip. An orientation packet should be sent to the trip participants approximately 3–4 months prior to departure. This should contain requirements regarding visas, immunizations, medications, and suggestions for travel, what to pack and much more. See Fig. 5.6 for the suggested contents of a pre-trip orientation packet.

Trip Execution

Once in-country, an introductory team meeting should be planned to outline the goals of the trip, roles of participants, and for team members to become acquainted. Orientation should be provided to the team that focuses on the host country culture, particularly as it relates to the practice of medicine, the role of doctors, nurses, and patients. Please see Fig. 5.7 for an example of an in-country orientation session that has been given by Kybele.

The actual trip itself will often present with unexpected glitches and surprises, both good and bad. It is appropriate to follow the "Traveler's 10 Commandments" (Fig. 5.8) and keep things lighthearted. No matter how much pre-trip research is done, how much vetting of participants, and how well prepared the team leader thinks the group is, there will always be surprises. Flexibility, calmness under pressure, and resourcefulness are important qualities of all participants. While on the trip, participants may need to be reminded that they are representatives of the coordinating organization or institution, and as such, need to exercise professionalism and cultural sensitivity. Particularly on a medical mission trip, the work can be intense and emotionally draining. It is important for trip leaders to assess the individual members participating and provide assistance when needed, to help someone understand a difficult situation. A common practice is to have a session in the evening where people can recount the events of the day and air any particular situations, concerns, or successes. This session also helps to more fully understand a participant, which is very useful for identifying future team leaders and assessing the fit of a particular individual for a specific role in possible future trips. Planning a sight-seeing outing at some point during the trip is fun, culturally enriching, and promotes team building (Fig. 5.9). While not to detract from the medical work at hand, this can give participants a needed break and a time to relax and reflect [1].

When entering a new hospital environment, participants are generally eager to jump right in and get started. Team members should be instructed to avoid this temptation, unless working with Operation Smile or other such organizations where this type of schedule is expected. Regardless of the sponsoring organization, it is important to take the time to observe and to build relationships with the local staff. In some cultures proper introductions to administration and hospital leadership are a prerequisite. Learn the names of colleagues and try to understand the local way of doing things. Western attitudes of superiority or "our way is the best way" should be avoided. It is important to realize that an approach from an institution abroad is not always the right one for the local environment and there can be negative ramifications. Think through situations carefully and make sure any technique

IN-COUNTRY HOST RESPONSIBILITIES:
1. Assist in the selection of host hospitals.
2. Provide names and contact information for host hospitals (name, email, cellphone, address).
3. Obtain obstetric related vital statistics from host hospitals (number of births, c/s rate, regional anesthesia usage, maternal and newborn mortality).
4. Help determine host hospital needs and equipment/supplies available, if possible.
5. Determine what credentialing will be required for Kybele teachers to do hands-on work.
6. Follow-up with local regulatory bodies regarding processing of credentials and issuing of temporary medical licenses.
7. Coordinate housing and transportation of the Kybele team in consultation/partnership with Kybele team leader. Kybele team should be housed together whenever possible.
8. Coordinate CME (in-country meeting) activities with team leader.

TEAM LEADER RESPONSIBILITIES BEFORE THE TRIP
1. Plan program details and dates with in-country host.
2. Determine trip budget in consultation with in-county host and Kybele administrative leadership.
3. Assemble team with skill sets/expertise requested by in-country host. Provide in-country host's and team participant's names and contact information to Kybele office administrator.
4. Prepare orientation packets in conjunction with Kybele office administrator. This will be mailed to participants approximately 3 months prior to trip (in collaboration with Kybele administration).
5. Assign team members lectures and hospitals assignments.
6. Learn if temporary medical licenses are required and ensure that these have been issued.
7. Organize team cultural orientation to occur within 1-2 days of arrival in-country.
8. Coordinate team pick up in coordination with in-country host.
9. Kybele office administrator will assist team leader with the following tasks:
-- Help ensure that team members complete Kybele application (with disclaimer) and provide CV and medical documentation to Kybele administration.
-- Prepare participant list and distribute to participants in coordination with team leader.
-- Collect participant documentation for team leader and supply a CD with relevant materials and emergency contacts.
-- Collect travel itineraries from participants.
-- Ensure evacuation insurance, visa requirements, vaccinations, medication, and disclaimers are collected from team members

DURING THE TRIP
1. Organize welcoming dinner for team member meet and greet. Additional instructions can be given.
2. Organize some cultural activities in conjunction with the cultural orientation
3. Help with SIM card purchase, money exchange, etc.
4. Team leaders must be present for entire Kybele program duration (does not include participant post trip sightseeing)
5. Organize closing dinner/debriefing at the end of the trip.
6. Collect participants' in-kind contribution sheets
7. Instruct on post-trip evaluation. All evaluations should stay within the team and not be distributed back to the host physicians.

AFTER THE TRIP
1. Gather participant reports and evaluations (for internal use only). Distribute to Kybele administration.
2. File FINAL trip executive report by one month following the trip that will be issued to Kybele

Fig. 5.5 Roles and responsibilities. These document samples are the property of Kybele, Inc. If you use these or any part of these materials in publication, kindly reference that the materials were developed by Kybele, Inc.

administration, participants and selected in-country contacts.
3. Gather photos and prepare a brief documentary for the Kybele website (or assign team member).
4. Help Kybele office administrator gather final participant in-kind contribution sheets.
5. Finalize budget and submit to Kybele administration with receipts.
6. Distribute evaluation to host-hospitals.
7. Consider research opportunities following the trip. Collect data for possible presentation at international society meeting. Ensure that review board guidelines are adhered to.
8. Consider sponsorship of in-country host to US/UK/Canada/Australia.
9. Determine if and when future Kybele involvement will occur.

Fig. 5.5 (continued)

being introduced won't introduce unnecessary expense or potential harm [1, 10]. Try to find creative solutions to local problems through partnership. Neither side has all the answers and mutual understanding can yield the best, innovative results [12, 13]. When building capacity, doing it the right way will undoubtedly take longer, but the outcomes are more likely to be sustained.

As such, teaching must be appropriately tailored to the setting [10]. Bring along a variety of handouts and power point presentations because visitors may be asked to make presentations without much advance notice (Fig. 5.10). Having a laptop is useful but be careful interchanging data across external memory devices as virus protection is often suboptimal. Bringing a textbook or two is also an appreciated gesture that can help for last minute lecture preparation and then be donated to the hospital. If doing clinical demonstrations, it is wise to bring familiar items such as epidural or spinal kits because one doesn't want to fumble around with unfamiliar supplies and local staff are interested in seeing what is commonly used back home (Fig. 5.11) [9]. Be sure that appropriate permission is granted by authorities to bring medication and supplies into the country, or contents may be seized at the border [1, 9]. Furthermore, it is nice to bring small gifts for those who make the stay special, as well as departmental leaders. It doesn't need to be expensive and can represent someone's hometown.

Media Opportunities

One needs to be prepared should the program become a focus of media attention. This came somewhat unexpectedly during Kybele's first team excursion to Turkey. Eight obstetric anesthesiologists visited ten teaching hospitals across the country and within 1 week; the program landed on the front page of a major national newspaper with a circulation in the millions. This led the first televised birth, a cesarean section with regional anesthesia, live on prime time national television (excerpts can be viewed at www.kybeleworldwide.org). This demonstrates that improving medical care and healthcare standards are important to the community at large, not just to those behind hospital walls. In fact, nearly every program Kybele has conducted has received print and television coverage (Fig. 5.12), so it is important to hone your message and be prepared [14].

Working with the media can help you spread an important message but there are a few things to remember when dealing with reporters. They are not medical experts and they have tight deadlines. With this in mind, present the most relevant information in simple terms and explain why it matters. Stick with two to three points and think about the best ways to present these points. Keep things easy to understand, interesting, and use vivid examples that will stick in people's minds. Practice out loud to make the message short and succinct. In conversation and storytelling, it is

Preparation for Kybele volunteers
Pre-departure orientation packet
Packets will be developed by team leaders and Kybele office administrator and will be sent to participants approximately 3 months before travel.

1. Materials will also be available for down load on the Kybele website (www.kybeleworldwide.org)
2. Orientation folders will include:
   a. Introductory cover letter (on Kybele letterhead)
   b. General country information
      i. Population and demographics handout
      ii. Photocopied cultural information
      iii. Guidebook
   c. General travel information
      i. What to take (clothes, prescription medication, money, mosquito spray, dietary concerns, small gifts for hosts, etc.)
      ii. Where to change money on arrival
      iii. Calling cards / cell phone information
      iv. www.travel.state.gov to register on-line prior to travel
      v. List of preferred airlines and travel routes
      vi. Contact information for preferred travel agents
      vii. Consular information (address and phone number)
      viii. Information about mandatory medical evacuation insurance (give websites or brochures)
      ix. Medical information: list required vaccinations or medications
   d. Travel disclaimer (Kybele letterhead) with return envelope
   e. Visa requirements: if visa required give instructions about how to get the visa. Provide application and consular and/or visa service contact information.
   f. Requirements for temporary medical license (photocopies of medical school diploma, residency certificate, letter of good standing, etc.)
   g. Speaker/Lecture assignments.
   h. Participant list to include
      i. Name and email address
      ii. Home address and home phone number
      iii. Institution and work title
      iv. Work number, fax and cell phone contact
      v. Notes (repeat participant, newcomer, past travel, etc.)
   i. Medical statistics
      i. Articles about maternal and newborn mortality in target country
   j. Traveler's 10 commandments
   k. Kybele brochure and business card
   l. Trip itinerary (if available, may need to be emailed 1 month prior to travel)
      i. Host hospital assignments and host contacts
      ii. Daily schedule (work and social schedule)
   m. Reminder checklist – dates by which items need to be received
      i. Credentials
      ii. Travel disclaimers
      iii. Flight information (flight information will be emailed to team

Fig. 5.6 Pre-trip orientation. These document samples are the property of Kybele, Inc. If you use these or any part of these materials in publication, kindly reference that the materials were developed by Kybele, Inc.

hosts and team prior to departure).

In-country cultural orientation

1. Orientation program will be developed by the in-country host and team leader.
2. Should be scheduled for teams prior to hospital work.
3. Orientation speakers may come from the US/Canadian consulates, USAID, local NGO's, Fulbright Association, Health Ministry representatives, hospital administrators.
4. Topics will include:
   i. Historical and cultural information
   ii. US/Canadian and host country relations
   iii. Safety and security issues
   iv. Medical system organization
   v. Maternal and newborn health issues

Fig. 5.6 (continued)

Cultural Orientation for Visiting Medical Team
Croatian Medical Association (Hrvatski liječnički zbor)
Šubićeva 9, 10 000 Zagreb, Croatia
tel: +385 1 46 93 300
+385 1 46 55 066

1500-1530: **Welcome and Opening remarks**
Minister of Science and Education for Croatia
President of Croatian Regional Anesthesia Association
Head of Anesthesia and Intensive Care Department, University of Split Medical School (organizing institution)

1530 -1600: **General Overview – U.S. Croatian Relations**
Political Affairs Officer, US Embassy, Zagreb

1600 -1630: **Cultural Overview – Croatia**
Cultural Affairs Officer, US Embassy, Zagreb

1630 -1700: **Women's Issues in Croatia**
Regional Director, STAR Network of World Learning

1700 -1730: **Coffee break**

17:30 -18:00: **Childbirth Organizational Structure in Croatia**
Local Obstetrician

18:00 -18:30: **Obstetric Anesthesia in Croatia**
Local Anesthesiologist

18:30 -19:00: **Kybele 2005 Croatia - Questions and Answers**
Kybele team leaders

19:00: Adjournment to dinner in a local restaurant

Fig. 5.7 In-country orientation. These document samples are the property of Kybele, Inc. If you use these or any part of these materials in publication, kindly reference that the materials were developed by Kybele, Inc.

1. Thou shalt not expect to find things as thou hast left them at home, for thou hast left home to find things different.
2. Thou shalt travel in a spirit of humility. The fact that others may think, speak, and act differently does not make them inferior.
3. Remember thy passport so that thou knowest where it is at all times, for a man without a passport is a man without a country.
4. Thou shalt not take anything, especially thyself, too seriously for a carefree mind is the beginning of fine travel.
5. Thou shalt not let thy traveling companions get on thy nerves, for thou art spending time and money to enjoy thyself.
6. Thou shalt not judge the people of a country by one person with whom thou has had trouble.
7. Thou shalt not worry, for he that worrieth hath no pleasure. And few things are ever fatal.
8. Blessed is the person who can say "thank you" in any language. Say it often.
9. Thou shalt when in Rome do somewhat as the Romans do, if in difficulty, thou shalt use common sense and friendliness.
10. Remember thou art a guest in every land and he that treateth his host with respect shalt indeed be treated as an honored guest.
    (Author unknown)

Fig. 5.8 Traveler's ten commandments

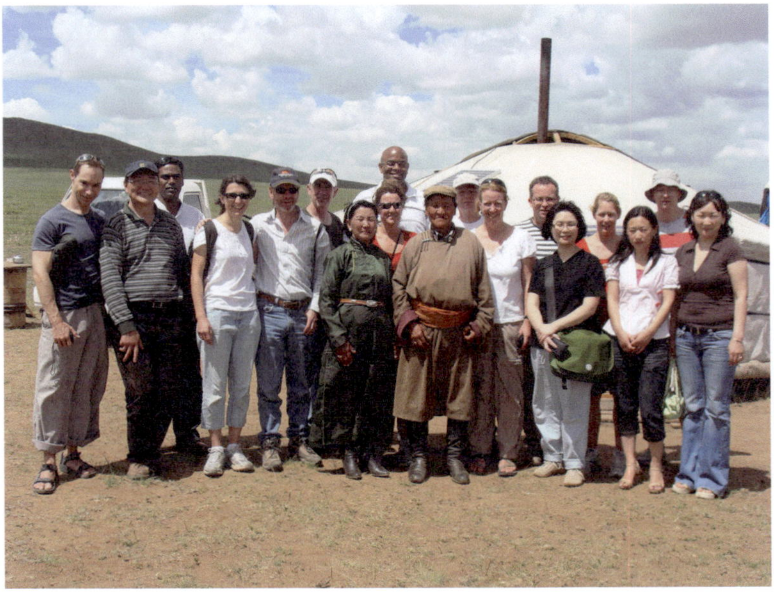

Fig. 5.9 Photo courtesy of Kybele, Inc. Kybele team visits a local gere in Mongolia

easy to let a story build to the climax, giving the most important information last. Reporters, however, want the impact first. It is important not to ramble as things can get off track. If that happens, one must steer the interview back around to the central message. Show passion and excitement, speak slowly and clearly, especially in dealing with language barriers. Finally, thank the interviewer for their interest in spreading a message that matters. Provide your contact information and

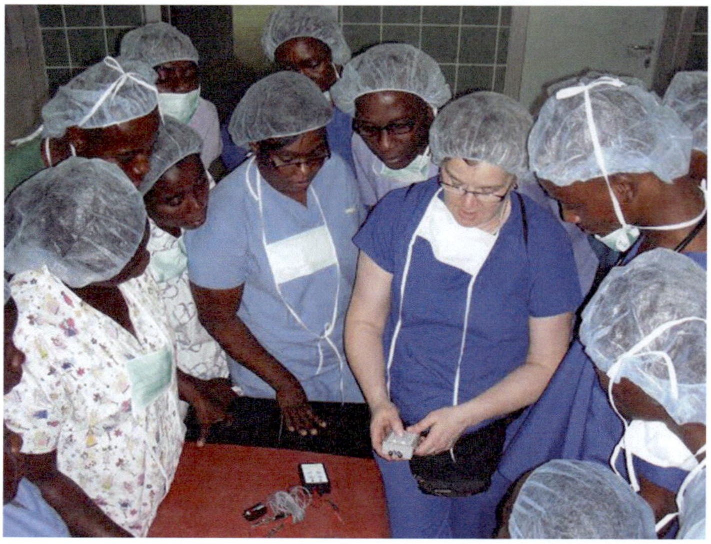

Fig. 5.10 Photo courtesy of Kybele, Inc. Dr. Holly Muir, Duke University Medical Center, engages in a small group tutorial in Ghana

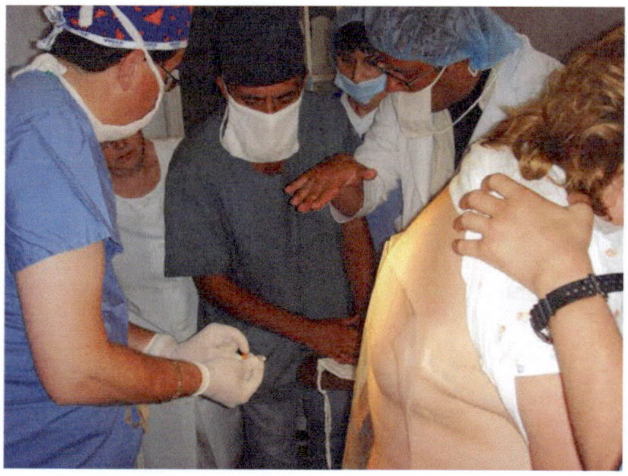

Fig. 5.11 Photo courtesy of Kybele, Inc. Dr. Virgil Manica, TUFTS University, conducts a bedside teaching demonstration in the Republic of Georgia

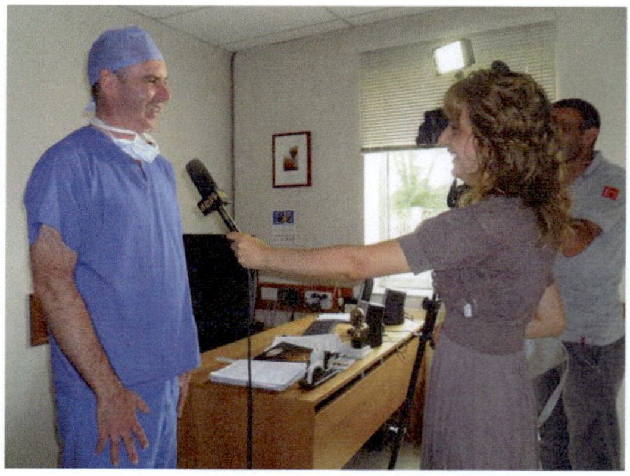

Fig. 5.12 Photo courtesy of Kybele, Inc. Dr. Simon Miller, British anesthesiologist, being interviewed by the press in Armenia

offer feedback and follow-up, if time allows. Ask where and when the interview will be released and try to get a copy of the news piece.

Post-trip Follow-Up and Evaluation

Following the trip, it is important for team members to communicate observations, impressions, and reflect back on the trip as a whole. Be careful with reports, however, to make sure that feedback is properly channeled to the trip leader for review and synthesis. Anything that is shared with the local host must be properly screened. It only takes one misplaced or well-intentioned but inaccurate comment from a participant in a trip report to threaten years of carefully developed relationships. It is common for participants to experience forms of culture shock when returning home. The experience abroad will have likely been emotionally stirring and meaningful, one that colleagues, friends, or family may have limited ability to understand. Written reports and presentations within home institutions are encouraged to help process what one has encountered. Assessments of the team members, both peer review and those of the trip leader, are informative and important (Fig. 5.13). The trip leader should gather all

Trip Country and Date:___________________________
Team Leader:____________________________________
In order to help strengthen our teams and help Kybele become even more effective in its mission, your feedback is really important and will be kept in confidence. Please take a few minutes to answer the following questions: Please answer the following questions using a 1-5 scale with one being strongly disagree and five being strongly agree.

1) The following qualities in a team member are important for this Kybele trip:

	1	2	3	4	5
a) Flexibility	__	__	__	__	__
b) Team Compatibility	__	__	__	__	__
c) Endurance/Stamina	__	__	__	__	__
d) Clinical Competency	__	__	__	__	__
e) Communication Skills	__	__	__	__	__
f) Cultural Sensitivity	__	__	__	__	__
g) Educational interaction	__	__	__	__	__
h) Adaptability	__	__	__	__	__
i) Timeliness	__	__	__	__	__

List the 3 qualities you feel are most important for team members to have:

__________________ __________________ __________________

	1	2	3	4	5
2) The trip was organized well	__	__	__	__	__
3) I knew what was expected of me daily	__	__	__	__	__
4) The accommodations were satisfactory	__	__	__	__	__
5) I felt safe while in the host country	__	__	__	__	__
6) Acceptable meals were provided	__	__	__	__	__
7) The hosts contributed to the experience	__	__	__	__	__
8) My teaching efforts were well received	__	__	__	__	__
9) Communication needs were met	__	__	__	__	__
10) I would participate on this team again	__	__	__	__	__

Please answer the following additional questions:
1) Is there a team member whose contribution to the Kybele work really stood out above the others? If yes, who, and describe their contribution?
2) If there were any team members who need to significantly improve in specific areas before participating in another Kybele trip, please identify the team member and explain.
3) What were your most important contributions to the team? Areas you would like to improve?
4) What were the strengths of your team leader? If there are areas you think the leader needs to improve, please describe.
5) What was the best part of this trip for you? The worst?
6) Any suggestions for him/her for future trips?
7) How will this trip impact your work in the future?
8) If there is a story or a memory you'd like to share from this trip, please do so in the space below.

Fig. 5.13 Team member assessment. These document samples are the property of Kybele, Inc. If you use these or any part of these materials in publication, kindly reference that the materials were developed by Kybele, Inc.

Name:

Country/Trip Date:

Question	Description
What was your intended role during this visit?	
What activities were you involved in during this trip?	
What did you accomplish? (i.e. lectures given, etc..)	
What barriers did you encounter in your work?	
What else remains to be done?	
What recommendations do you have about remaining priorities?	
What ideas do you have for future Kybele projects?	

Fig. 5.14 Team leader report. These document samples are the property of Kybele, Inc. If you use these or any part of these materials in publication, kindly reference that the materials were developed by Kybele, Inc.

information and generate a formal trip report that provides an overview of the entire program. Figure 5.14 is a template for the team leader report, which can be as short or as long as desired, as long as the questions are addressed. Host sites also need the opportunity to formally evaluate the quality of the program. An example of a host country assessment can be found in Fig. 5.15.

It is important to have ongoing, frequent communication with the host country physicians while the program is in place. Assuming that at some level, the goal of the program is to bring about change, to sustain that change requires attention, reinforcement, and maintaining the motivation to change. There are many ways to do this. At Kybele, team leaders and country hosts communicate frequently via email and Skype telecommunication. Kybele has found that including articles about host country leaders and others in electronic newsletters and news flashes generates pride and a sense of accomplishment within the host country. It is important to try to invite those identified as being strong host country leaders to visit the participant's hospitals to learn how the techniques they are being taught work in a different setting (Fig. 5.16). This creates a balanced sense of partnership and helps keep the communication lines open and strong. For lasting change to emerge, the motivation to change and to maintain that change must constantly be strengthened. The belief in self-directed change is highly cultural, and in some cases, the sponsoring organization is working against strongly held cultural beliefs that self-directed change is impossible. Seeing a system or technique work first hand solidifies the concept.

Ethical and Legal Considerations

It is important to manage the medical volunteers in such a way that the patient always comes first and that his/her personal information is protected. Determining who should be taught, and which skill sets and techniques should be taught, is a consideration, especially when working with individuals having less formal education and training than those performing the techniques back home (Fig. 5.17) [10, 15, 16]. Safety is the first and foremost priority. Informed consent

Hospital Name:______________________________

Date of Visit:________________________________

Your specialty: (circle one) Anesthesiologist
Obstetrician
Neonatologist
Other (please state specialty) _________________

Please mark either yes or no for your response to the following statements:

	Yes	No
We knew what to expect from the Kybele team.	____	____
The Kybele team was respectful to our culture	____	____
The Kybele team adapted to our needs.	____	____
The Kybele team members were knowledgeable about their specialties.	____	____
The Kybele team members made helpful suggestions.	____	____
The visit by the Kybele team met our expectations.	____	____
I plan to maintain contact with at least one Kybele team member.	____	____
I would like another Kybele team visit to our hospital in the future.	____	____
I would recommend a Kybele visit to other hospitals or facilities.	____	____

Please check the appropriate answer to finish the following statements:

	Excellent	Good	Fair	Poor	Terrible
The lecture(s) by the Kybele team members were:	____	____	____	____	____
The bedside teaching by the Kybele team members was:	____	____	____	____	____
The overall experience with the Kybele team was:	____	____	____	____	____

Please circle your response to the following statement:
The optimal duration for a Kybele team visit is: 1 week / 2 weeks / 3 weeks /4 weeks

Please answer the following questions to help us improve our program:

1) If you have a Kybele team visit again, what would you like to have the team accomplish?

2) Do you expect to change anything in your care of pregnant patients as a result of the Kybele program? If yes, please explain.

Fig. 5.15 Host country report. These document samples are the property of Kybele, Inc. If you use these or any part of these materials in publication, kindly reference that the materials were developed by Kybele, Inc.

3) What was the best part of the Kybele program?

4) Are there any Kybele team members who you consider outstanding in their performance during the Kybele program? If yes, please give their name and explain.

5) Are there any Kybele team members who were troublesome during the Kybele program? If yes, please give their name and explain.
6) What suggestions can you make for improving the program for the future?

Thank you very much for taking the time to complete this evaluation of the Kybele program at your hospital.

Fig. 5.15 (continued)

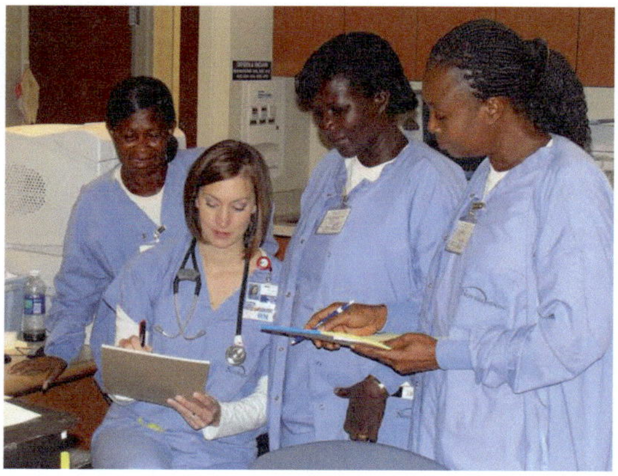

Fig. 5.16 Photo courtesy of Kybele, Inc. Midwives from Ghana observe obstetric care at Forsyth Medical Center, Winston-Salem, NC during an invited visit

from the patient is essential prior to any procedure and should be conducted in the patient's language and with respect to cultural and ethical beliefs [1]. Photographs at a bare minimum require permission of those being photographed and a recognition that standards of decorum vary greatly from culture to culture. As a general rule, participants should be advised to simply observe, listen, and build rapport during the initial phases of work. Photography is not the first priority and medical tourism should be avoided.

It is difficult to identify every single legal issue that could possibly arise while doing work overseas. Many cultures are not as litigious as the United States, but there can still be issues or medical complications. In the experience of the authors, getting liability insurance and malpractice insurance for all of the medical volunteers is usually not necessary or practical. Generally, with proper screening of participants, serious adverse events will be minimized. It is however advisable to obtain medical credentials of all participants, health and emergency contact information, and letters of recommendation. The local hosts should be made aware of any plans for resident physicians to be part of the visiting team (Fig. 5.18). They should only participate if it is mutually agreed to be beneficial and they must be accompanied by supervising credentialed physicians as per standards in developed countries [1].

To protect a nonprofit or other similar sponsoring organizations, insurance can be obtained to protect their officers and boards of directors. Some policies even provide ransom payments in the event a participant is kidnapped while working within the host country. In addition, many organizations require that volunteers sign a waiver, releasing the organization from any liability that arises from the volunteers' participation on a trip. If the individual refuses to sign the document, the person is denied a spot on the team. It is wise for sponsoring organizations to require that participants purchase supplemental emergency medical evacuation insurance. A simple internet search will reveal that there are many companies that provide this for a nominal fee. With so many ethical and cultural considerations, it is impossible to delineate policies that will govern every conceivable situation, but with care and common sense, risk can be minimized.

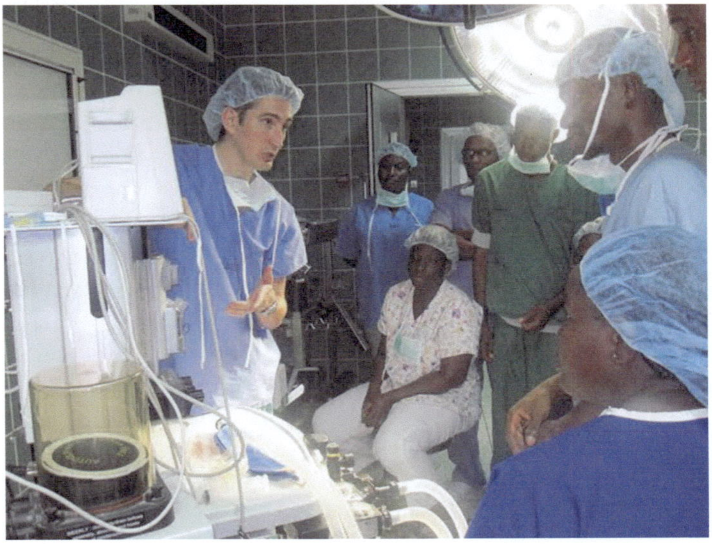

Fig. 5.17 Photo courtesy of Kybele, Inc. Dr. Michael Rieker, CRNA, instructs nurse anesthesia students at Ridge Regional Hospital, Accra, Ghana

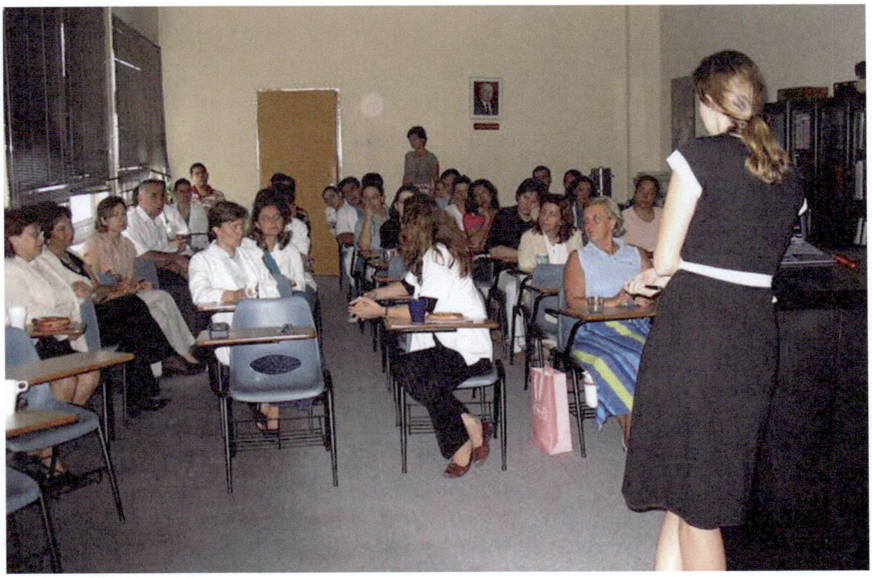

Fig. 5.18 Photo courtesy of Kybele, Inc. Dr. Brittany Clyne, obstetric anesthesia fellow, lectures at Uludag University, Bursa, Turkey

Research

Experimental procedures should not be performed on surgical missions [1]. Any research involving human subjects or record review needs institutional review board approval from both sponsoring institutions as well as host sites (Fig. 5.19). There is, by nature of this work, a grey area when it comes to who owns the data gathered during a trip. Normally data will be the property of the nonprofit or sponsoring organization. This may need to be explicitly stated in preparatory trip documents. Both the sponsoring organization and hosts should be aware of and approve anything presented or published in a public domain. It is preferable to involve the host country principals in collaborative research, presentations, and publications to improve their intellectual capital

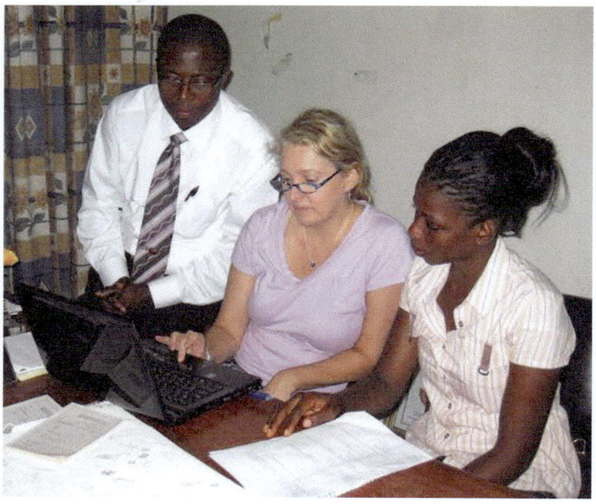

Fig. 5.19 Photo courtesy of Kybele, Inc. Dr. Medge Owen discusses research collaboration with Dr. Emmanuel Srofenyoh and Erica Ahiapokpor at Ridge Regional Hospital in Accra, Ghana

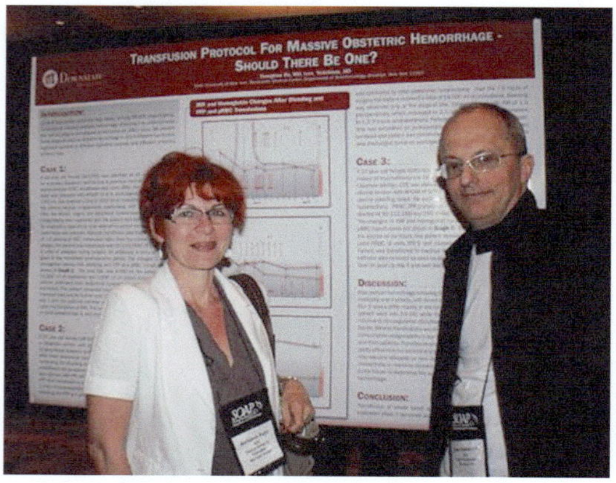
Transfusion Protocol For Massive Obstetric Hemorrhage -
Should There Be One?

Fig. 5.20 Photo courtesy of Kybele, Inc. Kybele team member Dr. Ivan Velickovic and Serbian host Dr. Boraslava Pujic present a poster of their work in Serbia at the annual meeting for the Society for Obstetric Anesthesiology and Perinatology

and visibility (Fig. 5.20). A useful discussion of research considerations in global health has been published by Stephen and Daibes [13].

Fundraising

There are a number of costs to consider when planning a global health program including passports, visas, immunizations, prescription medications, air fare, emergency evacuation insurance, meals, local housing, and local transportation. Over the years, Kybele has found that the average cost per person to make a 2-week medical mission trip is $2,000–$2,500. Costs can be covered in a variety of ways. Kybele uses a cost sharing approach whereby volunteers pay for their passport, visa, immunizations, and airfare with the remaining expenses divided between the organization and the local hosts. Having some financial ownership from the local hosts, even if it is small, creates buy-in, because some degree of cost generates a sense of value. There are a myriad of reasons for this; it facilitates acceptance of change, helps alleviate roadblocks, and invests the host in the whole process more completely. It also gives the organization leverage when asking for donations in the home country, as it is truthful to say that the local people are invested and materially contributing to the success of the mission.

An individual, or group of individuals, may want to start a nonprofit organization in order to bring about some type of change, support an ideal, or hope to help people, but quickly learn that raising money becomes the central task, at least for a while. In the beginning when one is starting up the nonprofit there will be expenses, such as getting registered and becoming incorporated. It takes significant time and expertise to complete the required forms and paperwork, which may vary from state to state. That is why it is important to get knowledgeable help and seek expert input from a lawyer and accountant who have experience in nonprofit work, to facilitate start-up, even though the process can still take months. Talk with people who are involved in other nonprofits. Collaboration is a good thing. See Fig. 5.21 for a quick run-down of frequently made mistakes to avoid.

Once a nonprofit is established, it is important to be judicious and a good steward of the funds received. The organization must be forthright regarding scope, quality, and quantity of the work they perform with honest evaluations available regarding how money is spent [1]. Many nonprofits struggle and eventually fail due to lack of funds, so it is not something to be taken lightly. Grants, corporate donations, individual donors, fund-raising special events, etc. are all ways to

1. **Cash flow crunch.** If fixed expenses are allowed to outpace cash flow, trouble lies ahead. If caught in time and measures can be taken to reduce expenses. This mistake will cost the organization financially and in terms of what projects can done.
2. **Conflict of interest.** Particularly with medical non-profits, the principals as well as many of the volunteers have other jobs and may be involved in research and data collection both in their jobs and in their volunteer work. It is easy to get tangled up in a messy conflict of interest situation. Working with an attorney to set up bylaws and take precautions through requiring signature on documents, memorandums of understanding among collaborating and supporting institutions will help prevent this mistake.
3. **Fuzzy boundaries.** This mistake relates to conflict of interest but is different. Institutions may want to benefit from the work the non-profit is doing, particularly if the organization is ahead of the curve in terms of where global healthcare is moving. If the boundaries between the non-profit and the larger institution are not clear, it may be very easy for the non-profit to be taken over by the larger institution.
4. **Unmonitored publications.** When an individual who participates in a medical mission trip writes an article, naming the non-profit, and makes insensitive comments about the host country infrastructure, people, state of medical technology, etc., that can go global and get back to the host country. In just a few taps of the keyboard, all the relationships that were built over time may be irreparably destroyed. Developing a policy and making participants aware of the need for great tact and sensitivity can help avoid this pitfall.
5. **Over-dependence on any one individual.** As in many aspects of life, allowing too many eggs to be in one basket is dangerous. If that volunteer, staff worker, head of the organization quits, is in an accident, or gets sick, and no one else knows how to do what the individual was doing, the organization will suffer and possibly die. Especially be wary of the volunteer who does everything. That person will burn out one day. It is important to build in redundancies.

Fig. 5.21 Fundraising mistakes to avoid. These document samples are the property of Kybele, Inc. If you use these or any part of these materials in publication, kindly reference that the materials were developed by Kybele, Inc.

build a cushion. In the authors' experience, to keep the fixed costs as low as possible, it is best to utilize volunteers as well as contract employees (who are essentially self-employed and work by the hour). Such a staff—some of whom are paid—can handle financial management, grant writing, event organization, correspondence, trip planning, and communications (newsletter, social media, etc.). The paid employees' hours may increase when needed, but the organization is not paying for time that is not being used. A reliable stream of monthly donors in the $10–$100 range will help cover the fixed costs. To maintain fiduciary responsibility and minimize risk, every nonprofit should have an accountant and a lawyer.

Developing a cushion of funds to enable the organization to provide services requires visibility, publicity, and asking for help. Having a sparkling, up-to-date website is essential. It must be updated on a continuous basis and there should be an easy way for the casual surfer to donate money if he/she is moved by the information provided on the site. Brochures are important, particularly when visiting potential donors. Speaking engagements, presenting at professional conferences, interviews on local television or for newspaper articles are all ways to get the word out (Fig. 5.22). The more people know about the organization, the more likely it is to lead to donations which ultimately improve success.

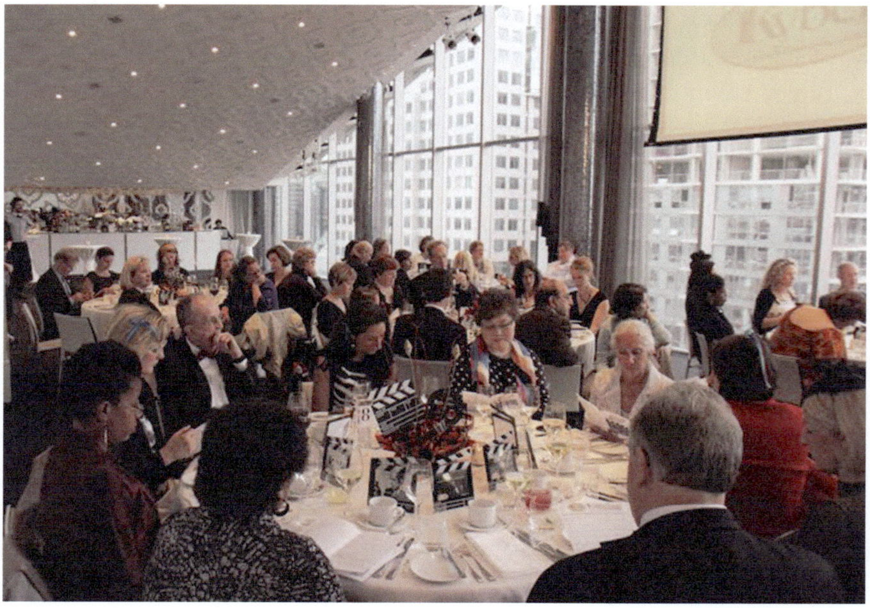

Fig. 5.22 Photo courtesy of Kybele, Inc. Kybele fundraising event at the Toronto International Film Festival Building in Toronto, Canada during the annual meeting for the Society for Obstetric Anesthesiology and Perinatology

Building a Team

For many participants on medical mission trips, the motivation to participate is multifaceted. The core human desire to help, to share expertise and gifts one has received, and to heal someone in need are at the center of many different types of medical volunteerism. Participating on a medical mission trip is also a way to enhance one's experience, as familiarization with global medicine is important in today's healthcare landscape and it can enhance one's resume. There are often significant research opportunities which are important in building an academic career. Others love travel and crave adventure. Still others have deep rooted religious convictions at the core. These are some of the motivations that typically lead individuals to participate, although there are undoubtedly other reasons.

How does one go about building a successful global health team when team members themselves may come from diverse medical backgrounds, institutions, and/or countries? The answer lies in finding individuals that are competent and experienced in their disciplines, yet flexible and adaptable [11]. It is not uncommon for very talented individuals to become unraveled or rigid when out of their comfort zone [17]. Depending upon the specific medical mission, a variety of medical skill sets will be needed (Fig. 5.23). Each has a different role and each has to be able to work together. It goes without saying that team members must be team players. Working in a different culture requires that team members have trust, patience, and good communication skills because in a medical setting, lives are at stake. Poor communication, ego, or power struggles should never be the root of adverse medical care. Cultures differ widely in how they express gratitude, criticism, respect, and power in ways that may not be easily understood by someone from another culture. Developing cultural competence results in an ability to understand, communicate with, and effectively interact with people across cultures [18]. While not everyone on the team will have equal cultural competence, everyone can and should be understanding and respectful of fellow team members and host country professionals. Never criticize individuals or medical practices openly or publically. When in doubt, ask questions. Also, never assume that everyone understands what is happening in a given encounter. If something doesn't make sense or seems off, that is the time to discretely ask questions and try to understand what is meant. When good preparation assures that everyone on the team is competent and skilled, then professionals should be allowed some leeway if using slightly different approaches.

Language barriers can pose problems in global contexts. It is important to have people on the team who are medically conversant in the target language or to make certain that there are skilled translators on hand. Undoubtedly some doctors in the host country will probably speak English; however, it is very important for visiting team members to speak slowly and use simple language to communicate. It also helps to write things down while speaking because many will read English but may miss the point during conversation. Another component to a successful team is to blend team members who have been on previous medical missions, particularly in the same host country, along with new, first-timers. The team members who have participated on prior trips to the same area will know the people, the way things work, and can help new team members adapt. Plus, the more experienced team members have a track record and the team leader will know their strengths and weaknesses, particularly if a formalized assessment tool is used to evaluate members at the end of the trip. It is important to bring new participants in order to get new insights, and to be on the lookout for new talent and leadership. An ongoing global health program should expand and grow and bringing new people is part of that process.

Building a diverse team is also a great way to strengthen home relationships with colleagues at work, acquaintances at other institutions, and even other NGOs. By broadening the base from where team members are recruited, it also gets the message out about a program or global health organization and increases its visibility. Building a team can also refer to the people who keep a

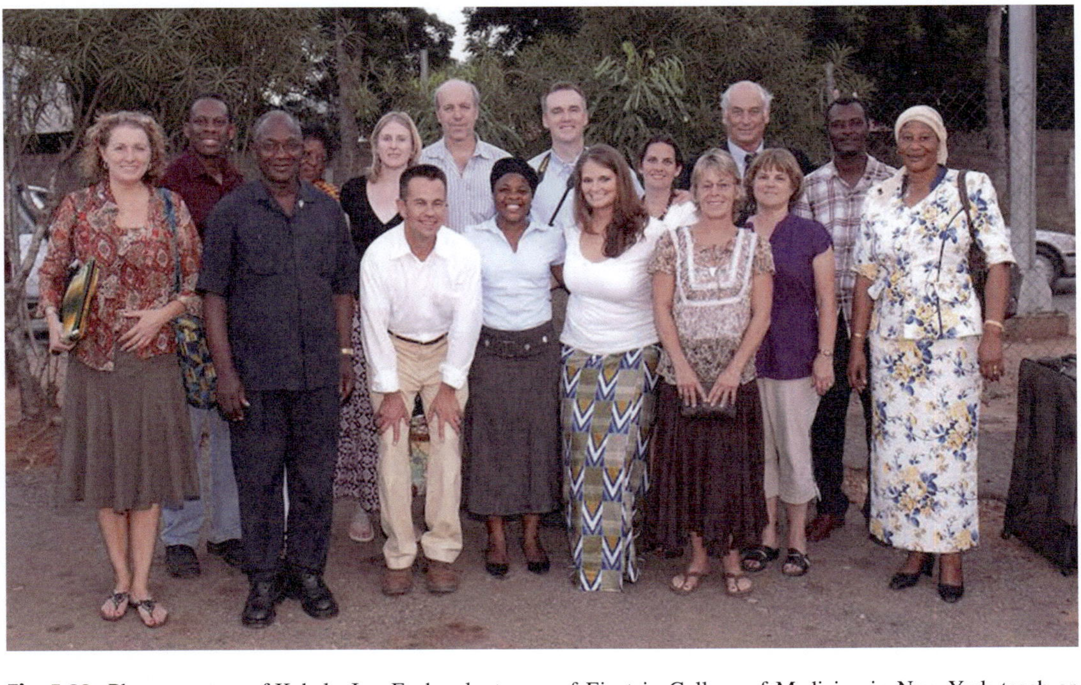

Fig. 5.23 Photo courtesy of Kybele, Inc. Each volunteer brings a particular skill set that can be used to achieve the mission's goals. (**a**) Dr. Mandisa Jones-Haywood of Wake Forest University teaches monitoring in Ghana. (**b**) Dr. Maria Small of Duke University and Dr. Kafui Demasio of Einstein College of Medicine in New York teach an ultrasound course on newly donated equipment in Ghana. (**c**) Dr. Mandisa Jones-Haywood of Wake Forest University teaches a course in CPR in Ghana

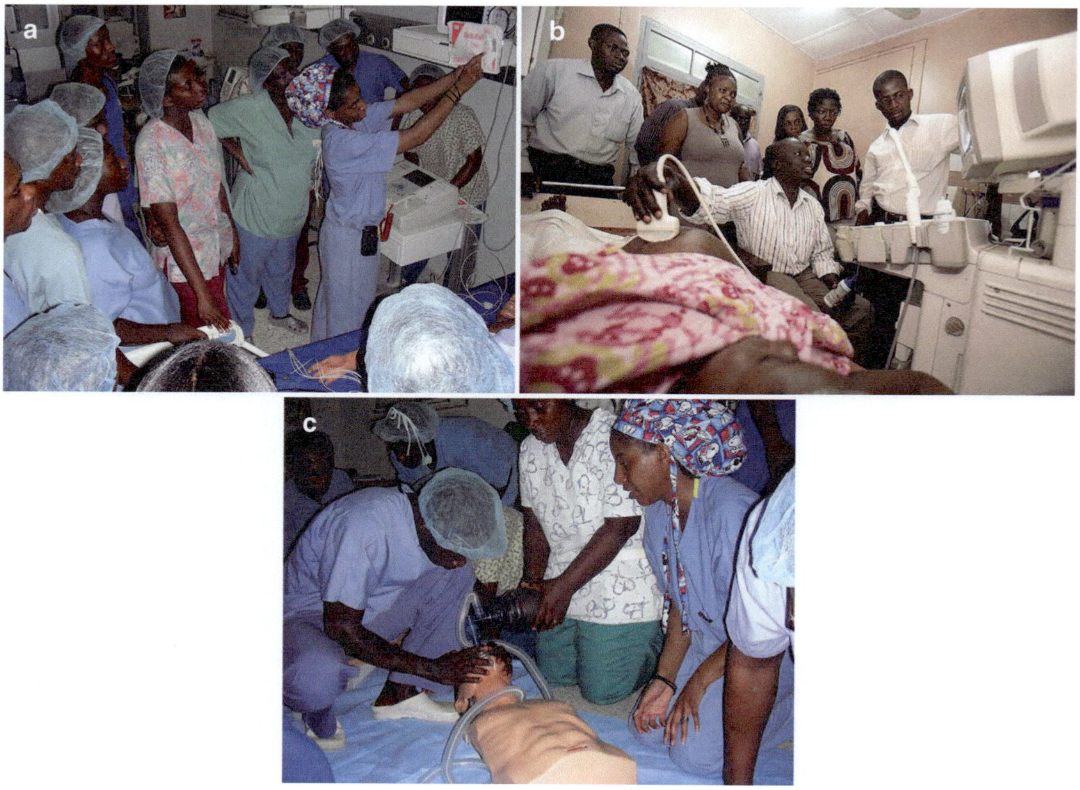

Fig. 5.23 (continued)

program or organization running on a daily basis. Typically, there will be employees, staff members, or volunteers who take care of daily operations. It takes special people and careful planning to assemble a global health team that works. The time and effort spent, however, can be immensely rewarding when a program is planned well and executed for success (Fig. 5.24).

Conclusion

In summary, planning and executing a successful global health mission can improve the lives of many, including patients, host country physicians, and participants. Simple expressions of gratitude as well as measured positive outcomes signal that a program has been well conducted. In the words of a grateful patient: "I didn't want to be alone. I was afraid that something may go wrong and nobody would notice. I was also afraid of the pain I am going to feel. After having the epidural, I am convinced that it helped me and eased my baby's way into this world. It helped me to live the most beautiful event of my life with enough strength to fully enjoy in it. Finally, I was lucky to have the competent and humane anesthesiologist who was there for me, and whom I felt was my sister to be with me and my son there." In the sentiment of a motivated host: "I'm in touch with my colleagues at the host hospitals almost every day. We are preparing epidural protocols which will be introduced in all hospitals. I think that is very important. It is the first time that anesthesiologists in my country are working together. Can you image that there are no guidelines about any field of anesthesia. I'm trying to change it." Finally, reflections of a changed participant: "Thank you so much for including me. The trip was very satisfying—personally and professionally—and has given me much momentum to make this type of development part of my

1. **Develop a great board of directors**. Ask people who are leaders in their fields. For a medical nonprofit, there should be approximately fifty percent who are in medical fields, and the remainder should be people from philanthropy, business, public relations, law, finance and other relevant fields. It is important that the board be a mix of people who will say what they think. Their expertise is important, not just their ability to write a big check.
2. **Grow slowly and deliberately**. Identify the keys to your particular brand of success and build on them. Rapid, unchecked growth may be appealing but it will not lead to success if growth outstrips cash flow.
3. **Keep at least six months operating expenses available in cash**. Grants and donors usually come through, but it may take significantly longer – on the order of months – than one expects or is promised. The letter may indicate that a $1 million grant has been awarded, but the money may arrive a year and a half later.
4. **Have fun and believe in what you are doing.** If it isn't fun and if you can no longer believe in what the organization is doing, it is time to walk away.
5. **Be flexible and open to change.**

Fig. 5.24 Nonprofit organization Keysto success. These document samples are the property of Kybele, Inc. If you use these or any part of these materials in publication, kindly reference that the materials were developed by Kybele, Inc.

career as well. Thank you for doing an amazing job setting up the support structures for this and making a difference."

Dare to dream. Strive to serve.

Acknowledgment The authors would like to acknowledge the hundreds of medical professionals who have volunteered with Kybele. We would like to thank Dr. Joe Tobin, chairman, and the department of anesthesiology at Wake Forest University for support.

References

1. Schneider WJ, Migliori MR, Gosain AK, Gregory G, Flick R. Volunteers in plastic surgery guidelines for providing surgical care for children in the less developed world: part II. Ethical considerations. Plast Reconstr Surg. 2011;128:216–22.
2. Buse K, Harmer AM. Seven habits of highly effective global public-private health partnerships: practice and potential. Soc Sci Med. 2007;64:259–71.
3. Petroze RT, Mody GN, Ntaganda E, Calland JF, Riviello R, Rwamasirabo E, Ntakiyiruta G, Kyamanywa P, Kayibanda E. Collaboration in surgical capacity development: a report of the inaugural meeting of the strengthening Rwanda surgery initiative. World J Surg. 2013;37:1500–5.
4. Fisher QA, Politis GD, Tobias JD, Proctor LT, Samandari-Stevenson R, Samuels P. Pediatric anesthesia for voluntary services abroad. Anesth Analg. 2002;95:336–50.
5. Schneider WJ, Politis GD, Gosain AK, Migliori MR, Cullington JR, Peterson EI, Corlew DS, Wexler AM, Flick R, Van Beek AL. Volunteers in plastic surgery guidelines for providing surgical care for children in the less developed world. Plast Reconstr Surg. 2011; 127:2477–86.
6. Reference for tool for situational analysis: http://www.who.int/surgery/publications/QuickSitAnalysisEESCsurvey.pdf.
7. Kopic D, Owen MD. Survey of obstetric anesthesia practices in Croatia. Anesthesiology. 2004;100 Suppl 1:A67.
8. Kopic D, Sedensky M, Owen M. The impact of a teaching program on obstetric anesthesia practices in Croatia. IJOA. 2009;18:4–9.
9. Ninidze N, Bodin S, Ivester T, Councilman L, Clyne B, Owen M. Advancing obstetric anesthesia practices in Georgia through clinical education and quality improvement methodologies. Int J Gynecol Obstet. 2013;120:296–300.
10. Peters JL, Boakye G, Harris M, Nsiah-Asare A, Antwi-Kusi A, Jabir AR, McAllister B, Hale D. Anesthesia teaching in Ghana: a 10-year experience. Int Anesthesiol Clin. 2010;48(2):23–37.
11. Wong EG, Trelles M, Dominguez L, Gupta S, Burnham G, Kushner AL. Surgical skills needed for

humanitarian missions in resource-limited settings: common operational procedures performed at Medecins Sans Frontieres facilities. Surgery. 2014;156:642–9. doi:10.1016/j.surg.2014.02.002.
12. Srofenyoh E, Ivester T, Engmann C, Olufolabi A, Bookman L, Owen M. Advancing obstetric and neonatal care in a regional hospital in Ghana via continuous quality improvement. Int J Gynaecol Obstet. 2012;116(1):17–21.
13. Stephen C, Daibes I. Defining features of the practice of global health research: an examination of 14 global health research teams. Glob Health Action. 2010; 3:1–9.
14. Kwok R. Two minutes to impress. Nature. 2013;494: 137–8.
15. Aliu O, Corlew SD, Heisler ME, Pannucci CJ, Chung KC. Building surgical capacity in low-resource countries: a qualitative analysis of task shifting from surgeon volunteers' perspectives. Ann Plast Surg. 2014;72:108–12.
16. Mellin-Olsen J. Varieties of teaching programs matched to country needs. Int Anesthesiol Clin. 2010; 48(2):9–21.
17. Fisher QA, Nichols D, Stewart FC, Finley GA, Magee WP, Nelson K. Assessing pediatric anesthesia practices for volunteer medical service abroad. Anesthesiology. 2001;95:1315–22.
18. Campbell A, Sullivan M, Sherman R, Magee WP. The medical mission and modern cultural competency training. J Am Coll Surg. 2011;212(1):124–9.

Developing Anesthesia Equipment for Low-Resource Environments

6

Angela Enright

Abbreviations

WFSA	World Federation of Societies of Anaesthesiologists
LMICs	Low- and middle-income countries
Hz	Hertz
HICs	High-income countries
UAM	Universal Anaesthesia Machine
UPS	Uninterruptible power supply
ISO	International Standards Organization
WHO	World Health Organization
AAGBI	Association of Anaesthetists of Great Britain and Ireland
HSPH	Harvard School of Public Health
NGOs	Nongovernmental organizations
V	Volt

Introduction

Anyone who has visited an operating room in a hospital in a resource-poor region will have seen anesthesia equipment sitting unused in corridors and store rooms, taking up space and serving as repository for assorted detritus (Fig. 6.1). The obvious question is why does good equipment remain unused and neglected when the anesthesia providers are frequently struggling to give anesthetics with minimal resources? This chapter will review and discuss issues involved in developing safe and appropriate anesthesia equipment for such environments.

A. Enright (✉)
Department of Anesthesia, University of British Columbia, Royal Jubilee Hospital, Victoria, BC, Canada
e-mail: ape@telus.net

Anesthesia Resources

Michael Dobson in his book Anaesthesia at the District Hospital says "good anaesthesia depends much more on the skills, training and standards of the anaesthetist than on the availability of expensive and complicated equipment." [1] All anesthesia providers wish to give safe anesthesia to their patients. However basic infrastructure, taken for granted in wealthy environments, is often not available in economically challenged areas. This means that special consideration has to be given to the suitability of anesthesia equipment for such regions.

In 2007, Hodges and colleagues studied the resources available in Uganda using a specially designed questionnaire given to 97 participants at a Ugandan anesthesia conference [2]. The response rate was 100 %. The survey requested information on equipment and drugs considered necessary to administer anesthesia to an adult for a laparotomy, to a child under 5 years for an appendectomy, and to a pregnant mother requiring anesthesia for cesarean section. Only the most basic equipment was included such as oxygen,

R. Roth et al. (eds.), *The Role of Anesthesiology in Global Health: A Comprehensive Guide*,
DOI 10.1007/978-3-319-09423-6_6, © Springer International Publishing Switzerland 2015

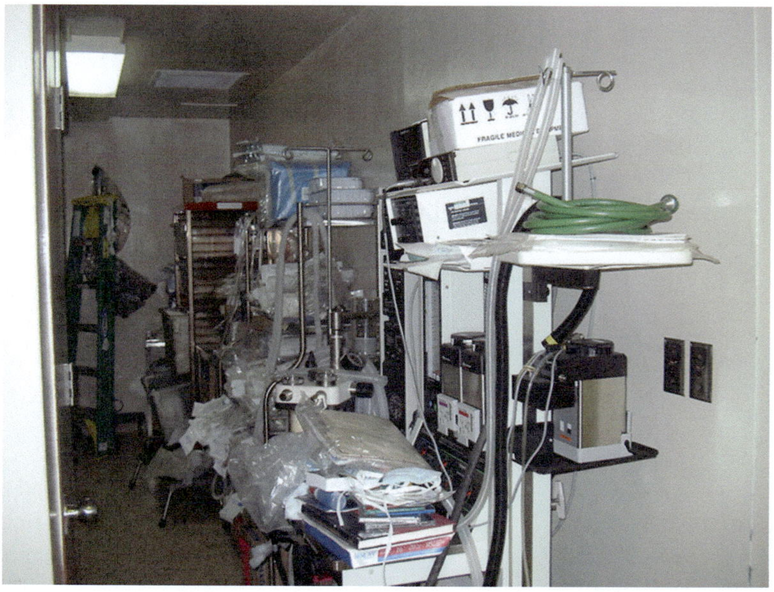

Fig. 6.1 Anesthesia machine used for storage

suction, pulse oximeter, blood pressure cuff, laryngoscope, endotracheal tube, and essential drugs. Twenty three (23 %) of the respondents had what they required to give safe anesthesia to an adult; 13 % could give safe anesthesia to the child and only 6 % could safely give general or spinal anesthesia for the cesarean section. This situation is not unique to Uganda but is reflected in studies from many other countries [3–6].

Looking at a basic element such as a reliable electricity supply, the World Bank developed some key performance indicators for Sub-Saharan Africa [7]. Factors such as number of outages per year and capacity of the system were included. Eastern and Southern Africa were doing better than Central and Western Africa in terms of capacity but the number of outages was highly variable from a low of 6 per annum in South Africa to a high of 407 in Guinea. These figures are borne out by information from published studies [3, 8] and particularly by a study done by Michael Dobson for the World Federation of Societies of Anaesthesiologists (personal communication). He contacted anesthesia providers in 122 countries requesting information on electrical supply and oxygen availability. Responses were obtained from 23 low- and middle-income countries (LMICs) which contained information from 52 hospitals. The results are contained in Tables 6.1 and 6.2.

Electrical problems occur not just due to power outages but also due to variations in voltage. A 240 volt (V) mains supply can come in as low as 180 V. Most western anesthesia equipment is designed to function with only a 5 % variation in voltage above or below the rated level. Dropping the voltage by this amount will cause most electrical and electronic equipment to stop working. Equipment that continues to function may overheat because the cooling fan runs more slowly. With microprocessors, a fall in mains voltage may cause the machine to reboot thus interrupting function for as long as the reboot takes, often several minutes. Higher incoming voltages may cause overheating or prompt fuses to blow.

Mains frequency presents a bigger problem than voltage irregularities. In North America a 110 V, 60 Hertz (Hz) system is used, which gives equivalent power to 240 V, 50 Hz but is safer in relationship to the risks of electric shocks. Many poorer countries use 110 V, 50 Hz systems. It is virtually impossible to convert 60 Hz equipment to run on 50 Hz mains. Transformers only work on voltage and not on

Table 6.1 Availability of electricity and oxygen in Africa

	Mains electricity			Oxygen piped			Oxygen cylinder		
Country	TH	RH	DH	TH	RH	DH	TH	DH	RH
Botswana	F	–	–	G	–	–	G	–	–
Cameroon	F	F	O	F	O	O	P	P	O
Egypt	F	F	P	G	G	O	G	G	G
Kenya	P	–	–	G	–	–	G	–	–
	G	P	P	G	O	O	G	F	P
	–	G	–	–	G	–	–	–	–
	F	F	P	G	–	–	G	G	F
	G	–	–	G	–	–	G	–	–
	G	–	–	G	–	–	G	–	–
Nigeria	F	–	–	F	–	–	F	–	–
	F	P	P	G	O	O	G	O	O
	P	–	–	O	–	–	G	–	–
	–	F	–	–	G	–	–	G	–
	P	–	–	G	–	–	–	–	–
Rwanda	F	–	–	O	–	–	G	–	–
South Africa	G	G	G	G	G	G	G	G	G
	G	G	F	G	G	F	–	–	G
	G	F	P	G	G	F	G	G	G
	G	–	–	G	–	–	–	–	–
	–	F	–	–	G	–	–	G	–
Tanzania	F	F	O	–	–	–	–	–	–
Tunisia	G	F	F	G	O	O	G	G	P
Uganda	F	–	–	–	–	–	–	–	–
	F	P	–	O	O	O	G	P	P

Key: *G* good availability, *F* fair (usually available), *P* poor (sometimes available), *O* unavailable, *Dash* no data received, *TH* tertiary hospital, *DH* district hospital, *RH* rural hospital

Table 6.2 Availability of electricity and oxygen in Asia

	Mains electricity			Oxygen piped			Oxygen cylinder		
Country	TH	DH	RH	TH	DH	RH	TH	DH	RH
India	F	F	P	G	O	O	–	G	F
Laos	G	F	P	G	O	O	G	G	P
Myanmar	F	–	–	G	–	–	G	–	–
Nepal	G	F	P	G	F	P	G	G	G
Philippines	G	–	–	G	–	–	–	–	–
	G	F	F	G	G	–	G	G	P
	F	–	–	G	–	–	–	–	–
	–	G	–	–	G	–	–	–	–
Sri Lanka	F	F	F	F	O	O	–	G	F
Vietnam	–	G	–	–	G	–	–	–	–

Key: *G* good availability, *F* fair (usually available), *P* poor (sometimes available), *O* unavailable, *Dash* no data received, *TH* tertiary hospital, *DH* district hospital, *RH* rural hospital

frequency. Therefore any equipment using an electric motor will not function for long and, after a few hours, the motor will be irreparably damaged. Generating companies with inadequate mains supply will often reduce the frequency which has the effect of reducing power to all appliances and can result in damage.

Oxygen shortages and cost problems are shared by both large and small hospitals in LMICs. It may not be possible to distribute cylinders because of poor road conditions which can deteriorate in rainy conditions. This is particularly likely in small, district hospitals. Costs vary from country to country but oxygen supplied in cylinders is much more expensive in LMICs than in industrialized countries, often by a factor of five to ten times more [9]. Nitrous oxide can be five to ten times more expensive per liter than oxygen. Because big hospitals use large amounts of oxygen, bills are often unpaid and the oxygen supply may be cut off. Some hospitals have been equipped with pipeline systems but many of these do not function because of the lack of trained people to maintain them. Using oxygen concentrators can reduce oxygen costs by about 60 % [10].

So what is the relevance of this information to anesthesia equipment? In high-income countries (HICs), anesthesia machines are high-tech workstations which require a stable electrical platform and compressed gases without which they cannot function. They contain sophisticated controls, monitoring, and alarm systems and can deliver a wide range of anesthetics to the patient. In addition, they have complex ventilators which can ventilate the lungs of even the sickest patient from intensive care. But this equipment needs highly trained and skilled biomedical technologists for service and maintenance. In the world where electricity is variable, and compressed gases are rare or nonexistent, these machines cannot function. Therefore the anesthesia provider must depend on a different type of anesthesia equipment to meet his needs. Unfortunately this fact is either unknown to, or ignored by, well-meaning donors or even purchasing agents in hospitals or ministries of health. Hence the common situation arises of good anesthesia equipment in one environment being totally useless in another.

How Do We Address This Issue?

In "Innovations," a quarterly journal published by the Massachusetts Institute of Technology [11], Timothy Prestero describes two approaches to solving design problems: the invention approach and the design approach. In the invention approach, the inventor sees a problem, designs technology to fix the problem, and then goes in search of a user who can and will use the technology. In the design approach, the inventor works with the end user to define the problem and the solution that will be usable in that context. Prestero notes; "a common failure of defining the technology before we have defined the user is that the approach puts the burden of adaptation on the user." Unfortunately, this is exactly how much anesthesia equipment has evolved. However there are exceptions to this where the designers have worked with the end users and have themselves experienced the environments where their equipment will be used. The Glostavent® anesthetic machine is one example; the Universal Anaesthesia Machine (UAM) is another.

Although both of these machines were designed by different anesthesiologists and engineers, and have some notable differences, they have much in common. Both are robust, easy to use, easy to service, and relatively low cost [12–14]. Oxygen is supplied by an oxygen concentrator which can produce oxygen concentrations over 90 %. An oxygen concentrator is a fairly simple apparatus that requires little servicing and maintenance, and produces oxygen from room air. Because voltage can vary greatly, the Glostavent® incorporates an uninterruptible power supply (UPS) unit that can work with voltage variations as high as 30 %. The UPS is a microprocessor-controlled battery backup unit, able to supply replacement alternating current automatically in the event of the mains power supply either being interrupted or being of inadequate quality. Following power failure, the UPS will supply approximately 20 min of reserve electricity. Different sized UPS units are available to suit budget and circumstances.

The UAM is designed to be able to deliver nitrous oxide or air as well as oxygen. It therefore has a safety mechanism that would prevent delivery of an hypoxic mixture of gases if the oxygen supply failed. Nitrous oxide cannot be delivered in the absence of the oxygen monitor. This monitor is electrically powered and has a rechargeable battery backup which should last for 2 h. Both UAM and Glostavent® only use cylinders as backup in the event of a power failure thus reducing costs for the provision of oxygen.

The major advantage of both of these machines is that they can be used for draw-over or continuous-flow anesthesia. A draw-over system is one where the patient breathes spontaneously through a circuit which enables him to "draw" the air through the circuit [1] (Fig. 6.2). The concentration of oxygen is never less than room air minus the fractional concentration of the inhaled agent.

The essential requirements of a draw-over system are a low-resistance vaporizer (a draw-over) and tubing which goes from the vaporizer to the patient. A one-way valve so that the patient does not breathe back into the vaporizer must be incorporated. Generally there are further additions to this basic circuit: reservoir tubing upstream of the vaporizer, with an inlet for oxygen, and a self-inflating bag or bellows, which must be placed downstream of the vaporizer to permit manual ventilation of the patient. This is the simplest and cheapest of anesthesia circuits. It is not perfect as it is a little cumbersome and may not be suitable for small infants although pediatric modifications are available. Nevertheless it is safe, reliable, and does not need compressed gases.

Both Glostavent® and UAM also permit use of a continuous flow system which is used in all high-tech anesthesia workstations. There is a continuous flow of carrier gas through the vaporizer. It requires compressed gases especially oxygen as there is the potential for hypoxia to occur. The ability to switch between one method and the other is a major feature of these two machines. If compressed oxygen is available, then a plenum system is very nice to use but, if oxygen supplies are low, then a draw-over system is safe and simple.

One of the differences between the Glostavent® and the UAM is the presence of a ventilator on

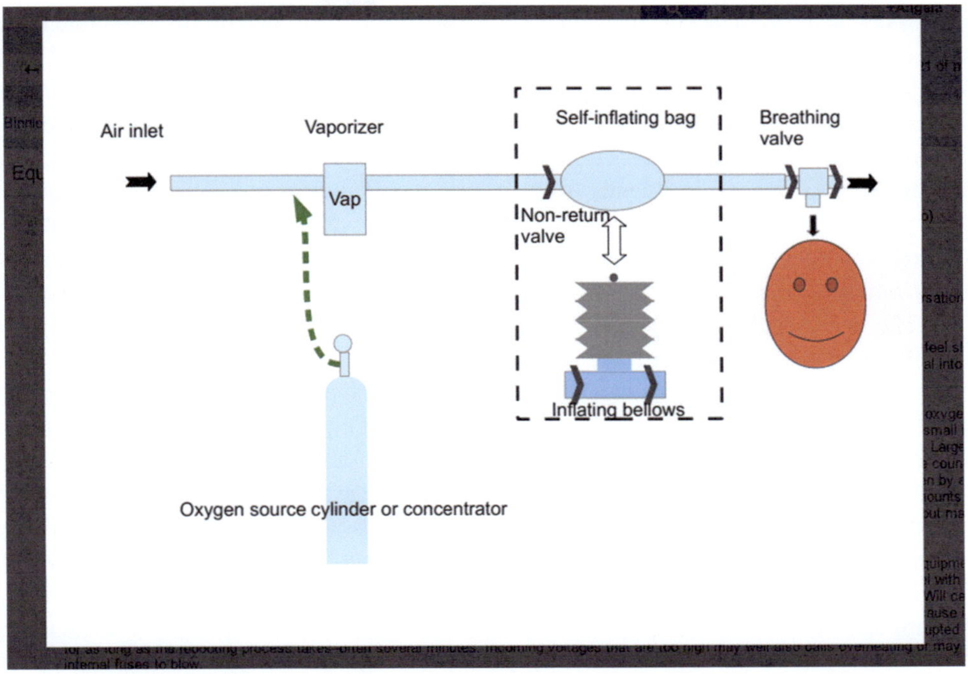

Fig. 6.2 Schematic of a draw-over circuit (M. Dobson)

the Glostavent® [12]. The Glostavent is gas-driven. It can run on compressed air produced by the oxygen concentrator, on oxygen from a cylinder, or from a central supply. The volume of driving gas necessary is just one sixth of the minute ventilation. The oxygen used to drive the ventilator is then returned to the breathing system thus increasing economy by using the same gas twice—once as a power source and then again as respired gas. For long cases, it can be tiring ventilating the patient by hand so the ventilator is very useful but not essential.

These two anesthesia machines meet the criteria of good design. They are efficient and effective in a low-resource setting. By using oxygen concentrators, they reduce the cost of providing oxygen and the organizational system required to provide it on a continuous basis. They can be used as draw-over or continuous flow systems depending on the patient and situational requirements. They need a minimum of maintenance which the local team can be readily trained to do. Finally both purchase and operating costs are significantly lower than the anesthesia workstations used in wealthy countries, making them much more affordable for hospitals with very limited budgets.

Standards

There are two types of standards that need to be addressed in terms of anesthesia provision anywhere in the world—standards for equipment and standards for anesthesia practice. In 2011 the International Standards Organization (ISO) issued well thought out standards for anesthetic machines suitable for low-income countries [15]. The importance of these principles is that manufacturers now have a value to which they should adhere when producing machines that can function without electricity or compressed gases. The ISO standard for high-tech anesthesia workstations [16] is not at all appropriate in these circumstances. ISO is also in process of producing a standard for a draw-over vaporizer (Mr. T. Longman personal communication ISO TR 18835). These highly technical documents are most easily understood by engineers. In order to assist anesthesia providers, the WFSA produced a document outlining essentials for anesthesia machines for LMICs that was approved by the General Assembly of the WFSA (122 countries) at the World Congress in Buenos Aires in 2012. An updated version of these recommendations is now available on the WFSA website.

The second type of standard is for anesthesia practice. The WFSA published its guidelines in 2010 [18] and includes recommendations for education, facilities, drugs, equipment and monitoring, and organization of the profession. Of particular interest here are the recommendations for monitoring of patients. There is universal agreement that the best monitor is the *full attention of a trained anesthesia provider* [18–20]. However all anesthesia providers need the assistance of appropriate monitoring equipment.

The WFSA categorizes such equipment into highly recommended, i.e., essential, recommended, and suggested. The authors note that highly recommended monitors are the minimum requirements for elective surgery even in resource-poor settings. In emergency cases, where life or limb is threatened, it may be acceptable to proceed without these monitors.

Oximetry

One of the highly recommended pieces of monitoring equipment is a pulse oximeter. This equipment came into general use in high-income countries in the early 1980s. The World Health Organization (WHO) Surgical Safety Checklist requires the presence of a functioning pulse oximeter on every patient [21]. However the cost of an oximeter is high and generally prohibitive for anesthesia providers in LMICs. Probes can cost over $100 each and have a use expectancy of only 6 months.

With this in mind, the WFSA, the Association of Anaesthetists of Great Britain and Ireland (AAGBI), the WHO, and the Harvard School of Public Health (HSPH) embarked on a project to develop a low-cost, full-service oximeter suitable for use in difficult circumstances. To this end, the Lifebox Foundation® was formed and specifications drawn up for a suitable oximeter. By the calculations of Funk et al. [22], 77,000 operating rooms in the world lack pulse oximeters. Anesthesia providers in low-income areas would like to have access to this technology. Lifebox Foundation® developed a full-service oximeter, suitable for use in difficult circumstances and meeting all international standards [23]. The oximeter will function on mains electricity, with rechargeable or disposable batteries.

Cost and education are the main factors reducing use of equipment in low-resource areas. The Lifebox Foundation® ensured that its oximeter was made available at a very reasonable cost and that it was accompanied by an education package. In fact, through the efforts of the Lifebox Foundation® more than 8,000 oximeters have been delivered to anesthesia providers in over 90 countries [24]. Education about oximetry and the surgical safety checklist has been provided by Lifebox volunteers in association with the local, regional, and national anesthesia societies thus making the program sustainable.

The project has been taken up enthusiastically by anesthesia societies, both receiving and donating, and nongovernmental organizations (NGOs) all over the world because knowledgeable people recognize that the oximeter is designed for use in difficult conditions, and will continue to function in spite of loss of electricity. Moreover it is available at low cost and thus fits Prestero's recommendations for design (i.e., it was designed and manufactured explicitly for the intended users). The Glostavent® and Universal Anesthesia Machines share the same design and cost benefits.

The Future

Slowly the need for anesthesia equipment suitable to low-resource areas is being recognized. New technology will bring improvement. The miniaturization and modernization of monitors will change the way things are done. Currently there are trials of a pulse oximeter using a smartphone [25]. Increasing use of capnography in the field will bring the development of less expensive capnographs. Perhaps increasing use of pumps for total intravenous anesthesia will bring about changes in the anesthesia machine as we know it. There will still be a need to provide oxygen-enriched air and to ventilate the lungs but vaporizers may become redundant.

The need for trained biomedical personnel who can maintain and service anesthesia equipment is recognized. As other areas of hospitals in low-income regions procure better equipment, that too will require maintenance and repair. Some suggest that fully trained biomedical engineers are not necessary [26] but that, given proper training, resources, and facilities, local technicians can provide most of the service required. With modern communication, it should be possible for a remote expert to lead a local technician through a repair. However manufacturers must recognize their obligation to provide training and follow-up for the products they sell. It may even be possible to design equipment without a service requirement. The development of this type of technology would go a long way toward solving the problems currently posed by the lack of trained technicians in LMICs.

Conclusions

There is a huge need for cost-effective, suitable equipment for anesthesia providers in low-resource areas. The challenges of variable electricity supply and quality, heat, cold, dust, and humidity need to be considered in design. Anesthesia equipment should be straightforward to operate and have safety features built in. Lack of biomedical technicians frequently necessitates that the anesthetist maintain and service the machine. Education of the end users is paramount. Without suitable education, even the best-designed equipment will not function well and will shortly be consigned to the equipment graveyard. It behooves manufacturers to realize that there is a huge market to be opened up if the cost and design of equipment, and the education and follow-up, are suitable for the locale in which it will be used.

Acknowledgement I would particularly like to thank Dr. Michael Dobson for his help in preparation of this chapter. His encyclopedic knowledge of anesthesia equipment and of working in low-resource areas were invaluable. He also created the schematic of the draw-over system.

References

1. Dobson MB. Anaesthesia at the district hospital. 2nd ed. Geneva: World Health Organization; 2000.
2. Hodges SC, Mijumbi C, Okello M, McCormick BA, Walker IA, Wilson IH. Anaesthesia services in developing countries: defining the problems. Anaesthesia. 2007;62:4–11.
3. Chao TE, Burdic M, Ganjawalla K, Derbew M, Keshian C, Meara J, McQueen K. Survey of surgery and anesthesia infrastructure in Ethiopia. World J Surg. 2012;36:2545–53.
4. LeBrun DG, Dhar D, Sarkar MIH, Imran TMTA, Kazi SN, McQueen K. Measuring global surgical disparities: a survey of surgical and anesthesia infrastructure in Bangladesh. World J Surg. 2013;37:24–31.
5. Knowlton LM, Chackungal S, Dahn B, LeBrun D, Nickereson J, McQueen K. Liberian surgical and anesthesia infrastructure: a survey of county hospitals. World J Surg. 2013;37:721–9.
6. Choo S, Perry H, Hessy AAJ, Abantanga F, Sory E, Osen H, et al. Assessment of capacity for surgery, obstetrics and anesthesia in 17 Ghanaian hospitals using a WHO assessment tool. Trop Med Int Health. 2010;15(9):1109–15.
7. Tallapragada V.S.N. P, Shkaratan M, Izaguirre AK, Helleranta J, Rahman S, Bergman S, 2009. Monitoring performance of electric utilities: indicators and benchmarking in Sub-Saharan Africa. World Bank, Washington, DC. © World Bank. https://openknowledge.worldbank.org/handle/10986/13030 License: CC BY 3.0 Unported. Accessed 19 Mar 2014.
8. Linden AF, Sekidde FS, Galukande M, Knowlton LM, Chackungal S, McQueen K. Challenges of surgery in developing countries: a survey of surgical and anesthesia capacity in Uganda's public hospitals. World J Surg. 2012;36:1056–65.
9. Howie S, Hill S, Ebonyi A, Krishnan G, Njie O, Sanneh M, et al. Meeting oxygen needs in Africa: an options analysis from the Gambia. Bull World Health Organ. 2009;87:763–71.
10. Friesen RM, Raber MB, Reimer DH. Oxygen concentrators: a primary oxygen supply source. Can J Anaesth. 1999;46:1185–90.
11. Prestero T. Better by design: how empathy can lead to more successful technologies and services for the poor. Innovations. 2010; 105–119.
12. Beringer RM, Eltringham RJ. The Glostavent: evolution of an anaesthetic machine for developing countries. Anaesth Intensive Care. 2008;36:442–8.
13. van Hasselt G, Barr KG. The first universal anaesthesia machine: an evaluation. JAP. 2011;4:128–34.

14. Rana RB, Agrawal JK, Manandhar ML, Shrestha N. An observational study of the Universal Anaesthesia Machine in Nepal. PMJN. 2011;11:36–41.
15. International standard 8835-7. Inhalational anaesthesia systems: part 7 anaesthetic systems for use in areas with limited logistical supplies of electricity and anaesthetic gases. Geneva: International Standards Organization; 2011.
16. International standard 80601-2-13-2011. Medical electrical equipment—part 2-13: particular requirements for basic safety and essential performance of an anaesthetic workstation. Geneva: International Standards Organization; 2010.
17. World Federation of Societies of Anaesthesiologists. Guidelines for tendering for anaesthesia machines. http://www.wfsahq.org/our-work/safety-quality. Accessed 20 Oct 2014.
18. Merry AF, Cooper JB, Soyannwo O, Wilson IH, Eichorn JH. International standards for a safe practice of anesthesia 2010. Can J Anaesth. 2010;57:1027–34.
19. Merchant R, Chartrand D, Dain S, Dobson G, Kurrek MM, Lagace A, Stacey S, Thiessen B. Guidelines to the practice of anesthesia—revised edition 2014. Can J Anaesth. 2014;61:47–71.
20. Association of Anaesthetists of Great Britain and Ireland. Recommendations for standards of monitoring during anaesthesia and recovery. 4th ed. 2007. p. 4. http://www.aagbi.org. Accessed 19 Mar 2014.
21. World Health Organization. Surgical safety checklist. Revised 1/2009. http://www.who.int/patientsafety/safesurgery. Accessed 19 Mar 2014.
22. Funk LM, Weiser TG, Berry WR, Lipsitz SR, Merry AF, Enright AC, et al. Global operating theatre distribution and pulse oximetry supply: an estimation from reported data. Lancet. 2010;376:1055–61.
23. Dubowitz G, Breyer K, Lipnick M, Sall JW, Feiner J, Ikeda K, et al. Accuracy of the Lifebox pulse oximeter during hypoxia in healthy volunteers. Anaesthesia. 2013;68:1220–3. doi:10.1111/anae 12382.
24. Lifebox. Saving lives through safer surgery. http://www.lifebox.org/projectupdates/. Accessed 20 Oct 2014.
25. Petersen CL, Chen TP, Ansermino JM, Dumont GA. Design and evaluation of a low-cost smartphone pulse oximeter. Sensors (Basel). 2013;13:16882–93.
26. Malkin R, Keane A. Evidence-based approach to the maintenance of laboratory and medical equipment in resource-poor settings. Med Biol Eng Comput. 2010;48(7):721–6.

7 Materials Management and Pollution Prevention

Jodi Sherman and Dorothy Gaal

Introduction

Medical progress has driven the development of new technologies and safer practices in health care. Ironically, modern industrialized medicine unintentionally contributes to environmental factors that threaten human health on individual, community, and worldwide scales. The healthcare sector in the United States (US) alone is responsible for 8 % of national greenhouse gas (GHG) production [1]. Anesthesiologists typically fail to consider the ecological implications of manufacturing, transporting, and disposing of drugs and devices employed in their practices. Hospitals, especially as regards perioperative care, are the leading energy consuming and waste-producing elements within the healthcare system. Only through understanding the interrelatedness and contribution of modern anesthesia practice to environmental issues can physicians work toward aligning commitment to patient care with community and ecological health [2].

J. Sherman, M.D. (✉) • D. Gaal, M.D.
Department of Anesthesiology, Yale University School of Medicine, New Haven, CT, USA
e-mail: jodi.sherman@yale.edu

Humanitarian medical service efforts in underserved areas in the last few decades have resulted in delivery of health care to hundreds of thousands of individuals who otherwise may not have been able to afford it. Facets of surgical mission efforts have been examined, such as the long- and short-term impact on the individual patient and healthcare system, quality assurance, and financial models. The well-meaning, altruistic anesthesia provider can contribute even more to the health of the host environment and the planet by weighing in on the ecological impact various elements of the humanitarian efforts make. Mission teams must be cautious not to abandon or export trash, nor to model wasteful behaviors to other parts of the world. In addition to humanitarian rewards, mission work affords an opportunity to learn how to import a conservation mindset back to the U.S.

Lead organizations and individuals recognize that success of these humanitarian efforts with regard to safety and quality requires some degree of standardization. Recent publications [3–6] endorsed by the American Society of Anesthesiology (ASA) and American Society of Plastic Surgery extensively describe fundamental components of service efforts. In this chapter, the focus of materials management is on aspects that impact the environment. Several stages are recognized when management and control of transported materials must be considered.

R. Roth et al. (eds.), *The Role of Anesthesiology in Global Health: A Comprehensive Guide*, DOI 10.1007/978-3-319-09423-6_7, © Springer International Publishing Switzerland 2015

Pre-trip Planning, Device Procurement, and Transportation

Planning

Who will participate in a mission and where the patient care will be delivered impact how much resources are consumed and pollution created by transportation. There is recognition that an individual nongovernment organization (NGO) cannot act in a silo and neglect the efforts of others. Potential services may be duplicated within a short time frame, with some teams having too few patients. Involving the local talent, rather than transporting an entire, self-sufficient, independently operating medical team, strengthens diplomatic efforts and local participants' confidence. This effort may include physicians, nurses, medical students, technicians, and translators.

Extremes of anesthesia supplies for missions range from a haphazardly filled duffle bag with assorted equipment to excessive numbers of boxes. Thoughtful teams recognize the need for a happy medium. Pre-trip planning with local hosts is essential to ensure availability of required equipment for safe and effective anesthesia care. It maximizes use of skilled human resources for provision of services to the greatest number of patients. Proper preparation also ensures prevention of shipment of unusable equipment and supplies that take up precious cargo space, waste fuel on transportation, and lead to exportation of unnecessary medical waste and pollution.

Site visit, trip evaluation forms from prior years, and close communication with host staff (physicians, nurses, hospital administrators, and operations support) are essential to shed light on facility conditions and equipment availability. Once on-site facilities are assessed, anesthesia teams can more easily establish the equipment and supplies that must be acquired. The sophistication, capabilities, and needs (education/physical) of the various sites are variable and evolving. The age and condition of anesthesia machines, defibrillators, autoclaves, and intensive care unit (ICU) ventilators, for example, are often below US standards. Calibration of vaporizers may be past due. Defibrillators may not be suited for infants. Suction may be nonexistent. Other times the equipment may be newer and well maintained. Some charitable organizations choose to be safe and bring all basic equipment; however these efforts can lead to increased shipping costs and transportation pollution.

Local, on-site anesthesia machines are frequently used by visiting anesthesiologists with great caution because they are often poorly maintained, and lack automation and modern safety features such as disconnect alarms, and oxygen proportioning systems. On one mission, for example, a near miss event occurred due to the accidental delivery of pure nitrous oxide (N_2O). The anesthesia machine predated standard positioning of the oxygen flow meter and the interlinking of the O_2-N_2O flow meter knobs. Additionally, an adult pulse oximeter was ill-fitting to the infant and functioned intermittently. Poor room lighting hindered physical examination of skin color. Fortunately, a free/facilitating anesthesiologist happened by and immediately diagnosed the problem prior to a hypoxia-induced cardiac arrest. Only after this near miss did the team appreciate the need for transportation of a portable defibrillator and appropriately sized probes. Transportation of a portable anesthesia machine might also have to be considered.

Anesthesia machines minimally have an oxygen source (often portable) or concentrating capability (as may be added to the portable Glostavent® (Fig. 7.1)), a vaporizer, and a variable fresh gas flow meter. It is not uncommon for the waste anesthetic gas (WAG) to be vented directly and passively out an operating room window. While the surgical team may be protected from the pharmacologic effects of these agents, the environment is not. Waste anesthetic gases are potent greenhouse gases (GHGs) [7], and an essential pollution prevention and cost saving strategy is through strict attention to use of lowest flow anesthesia [8]. Scavenging systems with carbon dioxide (CO_2) absorbents permit semi-closed circuits, reduce the total volatile agent used, and greatly reduce environmental impact; however, many host sites lack this technology. Portable machines may be brought on select trips

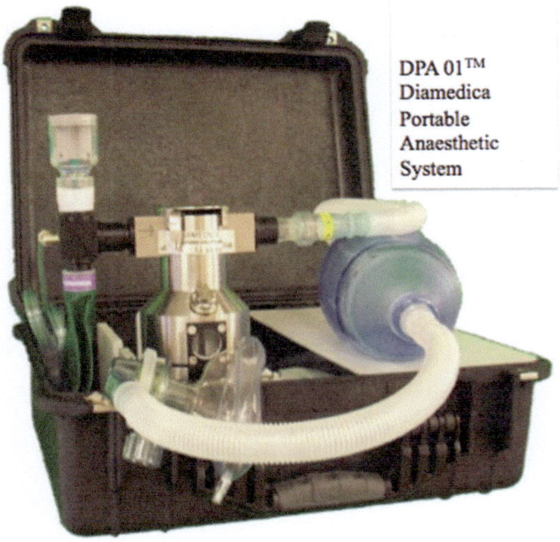

Fig. 7.1 Glostavent® portable anesthesia machine; oxygen concentrating capacity may be added on

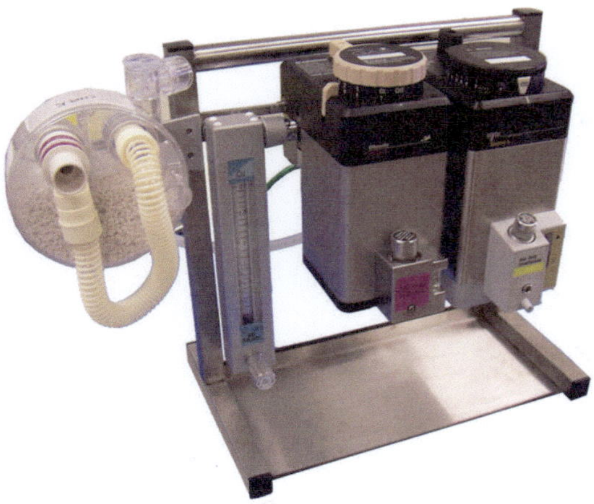

Fig. 7.2 G.A.S./U.V.S. portable anesthesia unit, with two vaporizers, variable flow meter, and CO_2 scavenging capability to permit semi-closed circuit

by the team (Fig. 7.2) and should be strongly considered if CO_2 absorbent capability is lacking in host countries. Regardless, backup non-rebreathing circuit systems must always be available although reliance on these systems wastes both oxygen and volatile anesthetics.

Similar to the anesthesia machine situation, local physiologic monitors may not be as contemporary as desired. Lacking capnography and pulse oximeter probes for small children, they may be unsuitable for general and especially pediatric use. NGO supplied monitors may permit team anesthesiologists to provide the same standard of monitoring that a patient at home receives.

The type of proposed surgeries, number of operating rooms (ORs) and operating days, patient population, and ages need to be known or carefully speculated to determine types and amounts of supplies. While purchasing local supplies can save shipment space and costs, or extend care when transported supplies run out, caution must be taken. Local safety control measures and oversight may be lacking, and labeling in a different language can be problematic. Teams should plan amounts of supplies as if single-use disposables will be used only once, though some devices may be safely reused.

Well-established organizations will have equipment and supply lists that include basic anesthesia equipment, as well as mission-specific lists that vary according to type of surgery and location. Specific types of missions may require all general anesthetics (GA) with breathing tubes (e.g., cleft lip/palate), while others may rely heavily on neuraxial techniques with GA backup (e.g., gynecologic surgery). Yet others may rely heavily on peripheral nerve blocks, such as is suitable for hand surgery. As much as possible, bringing individual procedure supply components instead of procedure kits can drastically cut down on the amount of waste [9]. Proper planning for type and number of anesthetics will ensure adequate supplies are on hand to maximize human resources, and prevent shipping of unnecessary supplies which may or may not be useful to the host team. Table 7.1 provides a sample basic anesthesia equipment list that may serve as a starting point for planning.

Device Procurement

Medical devices may be obtained for medical missions in a variety of ways, including pilfering from home institutions (not recommended), collecting opened but unused items from one's own hospital, appealing to manufacturers for donations of capital equipment and supplies, fundraising to purchase materials, and through

Table 7.1 Basic equipment recommended for a surgical mission[a] (adapted from Politis [6])

Type of equipment	Specific equipment
Anesthesia delivery	• Anesthesia machine with calibrated vaporizer • Machine circuits • CO_2 scavenging supplies • Gas analyzer • +/– continuous drug infusion pumps • +/– portable ultrasound machine
Monitors/lab	• Standard ASA: continuous pulse oximetry, end-tidal CO_2, automated noninvasive blood pressure, and multilead ECG (with lead pads); temperature monitoring and probes available • Twitch monitor • +/– invasive hemodynamic monitors • Point-of-care blood analyzer with adequate cartridges (caution: require refrigeration)
Airway management	• Facemasks, assorted sizes • Anesthesia circuits, appropriate size • Laryngoscope, blades, assorted sizes • Batteries, light bulbs • Video laryngoscope, blades, stylets assorted sizes • ETTs, stylets, assorted sizes • LMAs, assorted sizes • Bougies, assorted sizes • Ambu bag, appropriate size • $EtCO_2$ disposable detector • Suction tubing and instrument • Oral airways, nasal airways, assorted sizes • Nasal cannula, non-rebreather masks • Hydrogel
Vascular access	• IV catheters, assorted sizes • Tape and occlusive dressings • Tubing, appropriate type and size • Syringes, assorted sizes • Stop cocks • Alcohol swabs or alcohol solution and cotton swabs • +/– invasive
Emergency equipment	• Ambu/self-inflating bag • Cricothyrotomy kit • Intraosseous needle • Defibrillator, pads appropriate sizes • Portable oxygen tank • LMAs, assorted sizes • Bougie • Stat laboratory for point-of-care testing • Flashlights and batteries • Portable fiberoptic bronchoscope
Regional anesthesia supplies	• Ultrasound gel • Stimulatable needles, assorted sizes • Spinal and epidural needles, assorted sizes • Sterile drapes • Sterile prep • Sterile cotton • +/– spinal, epidural, PNB kits (Note: kits generate more waste than components)
Equipment/ maintenance	• Portable autoclave, indicator strips • Cleaning solutions, waste neutralizer • Bottle brushes • Tools • Repair kits

[a]Not intended as a comprehensive list

organizations that collect and manage larger scale medical equipment and supply donations to facilitate efficient and reliable distribution for those in need.

US hospitals generate more than 5.9 million tons of medical waste each year [10]. Much of that waste consists of unused medical supplies that are opened and unused but no longer sterile even if they have never contacted patients. Due to legal concerns and Food and Drug Administration (FDA) regulations, these supplies are not usable or resalable in the U.S. but may be enthusiastically accepted by many US-based charitable organizations for use in the developing world where they are so desperately needed. Supplies in opened packaging are re-sterilized and repackaged by donor institutions, then collected for distribution. R.E.M.E.D.Y. [11], Recovered Medical Equipment for the Developing World, founded by Dr. William Rosenblatt in 1991, was the first such not-for-profit organization dedicated to actively promoting the recovery of unused medical supplies for the purpose of global aid, pollution prevention, and cost-effectiveness. In addition to R.E.M.E.D.Y., many other not-for-profit medical equipment and supply organizations exist, including MedWish, MedShare, Procure, Afya Foundation, Intervol RUMS, IMEC International Medical Equipment Collaborative, and AWH Advocates for World Health. Some organizations focus on acquisition of supplies, and others on repurposed capital equipment [12].

The bulk of equipment and supplies for medical missions are procured through not-for-profit donation organizations. Institutions and manufacturers are often approached to fill supply gaps. It is possible to solicit donations of refurbished equipment from manufacturers, or borrow equipment from them for specific missions, such as portable ultrasound machines or echo machines. Mission groups typically house a central supply space from which all trips are stocked. Responsibility is with the mission organization to arrange and pay for shipment to final destinations.

Transportation of Supplies

Substantial advanced planning is required to ensure surgical and anesthesia supplies arrive intact and in a timely fashion. Supplies are gathered from donors, sorted, and then boxed. Historically, airlines used to be very generous with providing shipping. Boxes could be sent by general carrier with or without the team, free of charge. Gradually that largesse has disappeared. Some organizations have been able to piggyback supplies with the shipments of willing companies that regularly do business in the host country, allowing both economy and efficiency. In general, the bulk of supplies travel with mission team members, who must maximize opportunities to check supplies as personal luggage. Additional supplies are shipped separately, and overall thousands of dollars are now commonly spent on shipping of supplies for each mission. As a result of shipping expenses, fewer dollars exist for NGOs to fulfill their annual mission goals. Mission groups have been forced to reconsider their model for materials procurement, and to look hard for what can be safely and reliably sourced locally. Not only do these types of efforts save money, but they also reduce pollution by reducing shipping, as well as reducing manufacturing, use, and disposal of excess supplies. As noted, local procurement must proceed with caution.

For materials that will travel with the team, shipping arrangements should consider the timing, possible delays, and meticulous documentation for customs agents. Endorsement letters from government agencies or internationally recognized charities may facilitate transit through customs. Materials beyond their expiration dates should not be shipped, and open packages should be avoided because the discovery of even one may provoke confiscation of the entire shipment. Similarly, controlled substances should not be mixed with equipment supplies. Strict guidelines also exist regarding shipment of flammable and explosive substances, which must be sourced locally. If shipments are not timed appropriately, mission teams may be forced to scramble "on the ground" to purchase local materials at increased expense and waste of transportation and supplies that may not be usable without the mission team. Once the supplies arrive in the host country, with or without the team, they are brought to the hospital and stored. Advanced planning for secured transportation and storage locations is required to avoid theft, damage, loss, and waste.

Equipment Maintenance and Cleaning for Responsible Reuse

There is growing concern regarding the amount of waste generated in the ORs, which indirectly impacts public health and healthcare costs to society. Upwards of 1/3 of the 5.9 million tons of annual hospital waste in the U.S. originates in ORs [2, 9]. Strategies to reduce waste are critical to protect society from illness stemming from pollution, and to prevent the production of greenhouse gas formation through burning of fossil fuels for resource extraction, de novo manufacturing, and through waste incineration. Strategies that reduce waste save money directly in purchasing costs, and indirectly through prevention of illness and loss of productivity [2, 13–15].

Use of single-use disposable medical equipment is proliferating in the U.S., faster than anywhere else in the world. The reasons are multifactorial, and typically include cheaper purchase price though this neglects to consider that higher upfront costs of reusables are offset by numbers of reuse. Other reasons for selection of disposable devices include concern for infection prevention. For highly infectious patients, and for hard to clean items such as needles and IV tubing, disposables are warranted. However, indiscriminate broad use of disposables appears unwarranted as there is a paucity of evidence to support reduction of infection rates over properly cleaned reusables. The biggest reason for the trend toward disposables likely is due to the convenience of throwing used supplies away rather than cleaning them [16]. Upholding high standards of infection prevention during administration of anesthesia in underserved areas is critical; however caution must be taken to prevent the exportation of wasteful behaviors that are commonplace in the U.S.

Reduce

The primary resource conservation strategy both at home and abroad starts with opening and using less supplies whenever feasible. While humanitarian organizations noted above thrive on the excesses of the US health system as a source of medical supply donation and equipment refurbishment, waste reduction strategies in the U.S. must not be avoided to support their cause. When REMEDY was first instituted at Yale, OR nursing staff reported the program raised awareness of wasteful practices and staff consciously worked to open fewer materials while successfully collecting supplies. Over time, however, they anecdotally reported that they reverted to original wasteful habits and rationalized, "I'll just donate excess supplies so they won't go to waste." Unfortunately, only select supplies are desired by equipment donation organizations and so this attitude is misguided. Typically, medical missions provide an excellent opportunity to learn how to provide safe care with fewer supplies, and conservation practices ought to subsequently impact behaviors at home institutions.

In addition to clinical waste, another important opportunity for mission teams to reduce usage is through implementation of reusable food and beverage containers. One NGO provided each team member with a reusable coffee mug with the organization logo on it to help reduce waste, encourage conservation mindedness, and as a mission keepsake.

Reuse

Besides employing reusable devices when possible, an option that can lower environmental impacts is through the reprocessing of single-use devices (SUDs). Volunteers may be alarmed to discover that reuse of disposable items is commonplace in the developing world. Faced with financial restraints both in shipping and purchase, NGOs consider accepting these practices; however local standards of care must be honored as host regulations and customs may or may not permit reuse. There is precedent for SUD reuse practice in the U.S., and a growing industry around third-party reprocessing. The label "single use" is a manufacturer designation, and not an FDA designation. In 2000, the FDA issued a guidance document, "Enforcement Priorities for Single-Use Devices Reprocessed by Third Parties and Hospitals" to achieve standards and quality control [17, 18]. In addition to cost savings from waste stream diversion, third-party reprocessed devices in the U.S. may be sold to hospitals with as much as a 50 % discount [9, 13]. Substantial environmental savings can be achieved through reducing de novo manufacturing, transport of repeated quantities of single-use devices, and reducing disposal handling. While the same standards may be impossible to achieve in the developing world, reprocessing of simple SUDs such as supraglottic airways (SGA) and endotracheal tubes (ETT) on trips is routine, and efforts must be made by mission teams to attain high cleaning standards (Fig. 7.3). There is no limit to the number of times an airway device may be reused as long as it has been decontaminated and the cuff is in good working order. Many teams include an equipment decontamination and sterilization specialist, and travel with a portable autoclave.

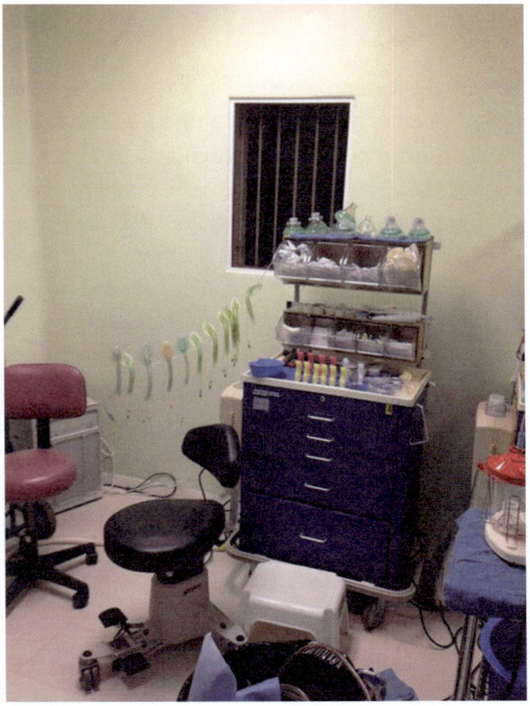

Fig. 7.3 Single-use disposable SGAs and Masks, drying after decontamination. Photo courtesy of Dr. Gabe Pitta

In the U.S., anesthesia breathing circuits are discarded after every use (and in some institutions, after any OR case even unused). In Europe and elsewhere, breathing circuits are routinely changed less frequently, ranging from once a day to once a week except in select cases of known or presumed infectious patients. Circuits are then often decontaminated for reuse, or discarded. To achieve safe reuse between cleanings, small microbial filters are placed in line with the circuit and discarded between patients, and condensate is routinely emptied after each use. McGain et al. found prolonging the interval between anesthesia breathing circuit decontaminations in this fashion results in financial, energy, and water savings, without any increase in significant microbial contamination rates [19]. Circuits are typically reused on missions, and it behooves the team to uphold these high standards of reuse.

Refurbished Equipment

US hospitals discard outdated equipment on a routine basis, as newer models and technology become available. Some will stipulate that vendors of new equipment take old equipment back to facilitate disposal; however few hospitals realize that it is indeed possible to contractually arrange for vendors to repurpose or responsibly recycle take-backs. Nonetheless, many vendors will try to salvage parts, and will donate refurbished or unused older models when asked, as part of organizational social responsibility. Some NGOs specialize in reclaimed equipment, though vendors also may be approached directly to satisfy mission needs and for permanent donation to hosts.

Cleaning

Infection prevention and control is of utmost priority, whether at home or abroad. Cleaning of medical devices can be particularly challenging in portable, foreign settings. Disinfectants have environmental impact themselves. All are intentionally toxic to destroy microorganisms, and while currently none is deemed "green," whenever possible, least harmful approaches must be employed [20, 21].

Classifying levels of infection risk must be matched with antimicrobial potency of disinfection materials and processes, to ensure care that is effective and safe for patients as well as limiting unnecessary exposure to staff, communities, and the environment through waste. Medical devices classified as critical (invasive, contacting sterile tissue) require sterilization. Semi-critical devices (contacting mucous membranes or non-intact skin) including laryngoscopes, ETTs, and SGAs require high-level disinfection (HLD). Noncritical devices (contacting intact skin) such as pulse oximeter probes and noninvasive blood pressure cuffs require low-level disinfection (LLD) [20].

Fisher et al. [2] describe at length several methods for HLD that are approved by the FDA [20]. These include glutaraldehyde 2–3.5 % (Cidex® and others), ortho-phthalaldehyde 0.55 % (Cidex-OPA® and others), and hydrogen peroxide 2.5 % with 2-furoic acid (Resert XL HLD). Always, devices intended for reuse must be checked for manufacturer recommendations for cleaning compatibility. Autoclaving can achieve either high-level disinfection or sterilization, depending on temperature, pressure, and time applied.

All cleaning starts with physical removal of excess bio-burden (body fluids and tissue) with detergent and water prior to disinfection and sterilization. For many anesthesia airway items, soaking in a bath of detergent and water and then scrubbing the lumen with a bottle brush can be effective in removing organic matter. Care should be taken to evacuate the accumulated condensate in breathing circuits between patients and before soaking; disposal is appropriately handled by sewage drain as with urine. After initial removal of bio-burden, items may then undergo the next steps to achieve disinfection or sterilization depending on their level of infection risk.

Autoclaving entails applying high pressures and heat to either sterilize or high-level disinfect equipment. Autoclaving at high temperatures is routinely employed to sterilize stainless surgical steel equipment. Autoclaving at lower temperatures and durations can be used for high-level disinfection [20], e.g., laryngoscopes and for classic reusable SGAs that are primarily silicone based. Device manufacturer guidelines should be carefully reviewed. Single-use disposable SGAs and ETTs may or may not be able to withstand HLD from autoclaving. All device cuffs must be fully deflated prior to treatment, and function must be tested prior to each use. Portable tabletop autoclaves are available in electrical or solar powered options, and some versions do not require water main hook up—helpful for mission work. Temperature sensitive test strips must be used to ensure quality control.

Glutaraldehyde is a HLD frequently used for heat-sensitive equipment, and therefore has broad application for missions. Glutaraldehyde is not a human carcinogen; however, several health effects have been reported amongst exposed healthcare workers including airway irritation and acute asthma exacerbation, eye irritation, nosebleeds, headaches, contact dermatitis, and staining of skin. Handling in a well-ventilated area is advised, and if that is not possible, a portable hood with charcoal filter is recommended. Ortho-phthalaldehyde (OPA) is a chemically related alternative that aerosolizes much less and is less irritating to the airway; however it can be difficult to rinse off of equipment and is a potent skin sensitizer. Further, OPA is considered toxic to aquatic life. Hydrogen peroxide is an oxidizer and suspected animal carcinogen with unknown human cancer potential. It can be a simple respiratory irritant but is not associated with any allergic response. In all cases, non-latex nitrile gloves and goggles are advised, and equipment must be rinsed prior to patient use. Proper disposal of sterilant and disinfectant waste includes binding with a neutralizer [20–24] (see below).

Waste Segregation, Disposal, and Minimization of Incineration

Waste Stream Segregation

Waste management by and large is a neglected issue, and ought to be of concern for responsible mission teams. It is essential to dispose of all waste safely, and in compliance with or exceeding country legislations. Proper waste management is an especially important area to educate hosts about. According to the WHO [25], a maximum of 20 % of hospital trash is comprised of biohazardous waste (regulated medical waste or RMW in the U.S.). In the OR setting, it is possible to achieve 10–15 % RMW in the U.S. and also abroad. The remaining 80 % of medical waste is nonhazardous, including paper, plastic, metal, glass, and food products, and is suitably handled as municipal solid waste (MSW) and ought to be landfilled. It is essential to keep hazardous waste out of the MSW stream to prevent occupational and community exposure. It is also important to avoid placing MSW into the hazardous waste stream since not only is hazardous waste significantly more expensive to dispose of, but its special treatment methods liberate potent toxins. Pollution prevention practices therefore emphasize proper waste stream segregation [10, 14, 15, 21–25].

Hazardous Waste

Incineration had been the most popular disposal method of hazardous waste in the U.S. in the past, and remains so in many developing countries. Dioxins, furans, and heavy metals are some of the most notorious toxicants liberated into the atmosphere through medical waste incineration, particularly through burning polyvinyl chloride (PVC) plastic that is ubiquitous in disposable medical devices, including IV tubing, ETTs, and LMAs. Dioxins, even in very small quantities, are potent carcinogens and up until recently, healthcare incineration was the single largest source of dioxins in the world. Newer emissions regulations in the 1990s led to the closure of thousands of medical incinerators in the U.S., as alternative safer treatment methods were enforced. Safer disposal methods include decontamination of biohazardous waste through autoclaving, then subsequent landfilling as MSW. Some blood products, chemicals, pharmaceuticals, and pathology specimens still do require incineration; however this should only amount to about 3 % of total hospital waste generated in the U.S. [13]. Many mission sites may lack autoclave capacity sufficient to handle treatment of the volume of OR waste, and sadly, incineration may be the principle method of disposal. Strict attention to waste minimization and proper segregation of trash is critical to minimize unnecessary burning, and hosts ought to be encouraged to set goals of increasing autoclaving capacity [2, 9, 10, 13–15, 21, 23–25].

Sharps Waste

Mission teams ought to carry disposable sharp bins from home to the destination site. It is dangerous and illegal to return this biohazardous waste back to the U.S., and so sharps bins are left behind for hosts to dispose of. Sharps disposal in the U.S. entails firstly heating at high temperatures to achieve disinfection, and then "rendering unrecognizable," e.g., through shredding or crushing; this waste is then safely destined for landfill [23]. Unfortunately, such high standards for sharps handling may be unachievable at host sites. Simple disposable containers may be easy to open, and sadly many stories of locals sorting through sharps waste for reuse exist. To avoid reuse, some locations rely on sealable drums and concrete pits. Mission teams must work with hosts to abide by local regulations and to consciously uphold the highest standards possible, while educating on best practices.

Pharmaceutical Waste

Pharmaceutical waste in the OR is handled either in a combined sharps/drug waste container or in a dedicated container for liquids with a binding and solidifying agent. The combined sharps/drug waste container ought to be handled as with any sharps waste, by high heating to decontaminate and then shredding or crushing to render unrecognizable. The container with solidified drug waste can be heat treated, or disposed of in landfill depending on the hazardous classification. In the U.S. many states require unused narcotics be wasted into sinks out of concern they might get extracted from solidifiers [26, 27].

Recycling

Within nonhazardous municipal solid waste, much could be diverted to recycling if facilities are present. Surprisingly, even in some developing countries there is a burgeoning market for recyclables. If the opportunity exists, it behooves mission staff to collect both clean, non-contaminated clinical waste such as simple cardboard and paper packaging, and high-quality plastic such as saline bottles, as well as personal waste such as beverage containers, and work with hosts to ensure recyclables make it to the appropriate facility. What is recyclable varies with location, technology advancements, and marketplace for materials and so communication is required with local facilities [9, 28]. Great care must be taken to avoid contamination of recyclables by hazardous materials. Not only is this responsible behavior for visitors, but it also sets an example for host facilities.

Disposal of Sterilant and Disinfectant Wastes

Unused disinfectant concentrates may be considered hazardous waste in the U.S., and the assumption in the mission setting is that sewage treatment facilities are incapable of handling these solutions. A simple and effective method of neutralizing OPA or glutaraldehyde is through addition of a glycine-based neutralizer (e.g., Glute-Out®) prior to dumping in sewage. Acid stabilized hydrogen peroxide solutions have a low pH and as such may need to be neutralized before drain disposal. These solutions are not toxic to aquatic life once the pH has been adjusted and may be disposed of to drain [20–23]. As always, all local regulations must be honored; however if standards are low it behooves the mission team to educate local staff about environmental concerns and uphold higher standards.

Lessons Abroad and at Home

Humanitarian medical service is incredibly rewarding work. Responsible mission work includes efforts to minimize wasteful practices and to prevent pollution, while providing safe and productive care. Several effective anesthesia equipment management strategies exist to minimize the environmental impact of care. Waste prevention begins with pre-trip planning in collaboration with hosts to determine required team members and equipment to minimize unnecessary transportation. Procurement is primarily through organizations specializing in reclaimed medical supplies and refurbished equipment. Waste anesthetic gases must be minimized; and CO_2 absorbent capacity is critical to permit low fresh gas flows. A decontamination and sterilization specialist is an essential team member for safe and responsible reuse of equipment. Proper waste disposal starts with strict attention to waste segregation. Care must be taken to avoid mixing of hazardous and nonhazardous waste, to keep sharps safe, to bind pharmaceutical waste, and to neutralize cleaning solutions prior to disposal. Special attention must be given to minimize incineration, and to support long-term autoclave capacity. Lessons learned not only benefit the local community, but they also can be employed at home to reduce the environmental impact of anesthesia practice on the global community.

References

1. Chung JW, Meltzer DO. Estimate of the carbon footprint of the US health care sector. JAMA. 2009; 302(18):1970.
2. Sherman J, Ryan S. Ecological responsibility in anesthesia practice. Int Anesthesiol Clin. 2010; 48(3):139–51. Lippincott Williams & Wilkins, Philadelphia, PA.

3. Fisher QA, Politis GD, Tobias JD, Proctor LT, Samandari-Stevenson R, Roth A, et al. Pediatric anesthesia for voluntary services abroad. Anesth Analg. 2002;95(2):336–50.
4. Schneider WJ, Politis GD, Gosain AK, Migliori MR, Cullington JR, Peterson EL, et al. Volunteers in plastic surgery guidelines for providing surgical care for children in the less developed world. Plast Reconstr Surg. 2011;127(6):2477–86.
5. Schneider WJ, Migliori MR, Gosain AK, Gregory G, Flick R, Committee of the American Society of Plastic Surgeons; Plastic Surgery Foundation. Volunteers in plastic surgery guidelines for providing surgical care for children in the less developed world: part II. Ethical considerations. Plast Reconstr Surg. 2011;128(3):216e–22.
6. Politis GD, Schneider WJ, Van Beek AL, Gosain A, Migliori MR, Gregory GA, et al. Guidelines for pediatric perioperative care during short-term plastic reconstructive surgical projects in less developed nations. Anesth Analg. 2011;112(1):183–90.
7. Sherman J, Le C, Lamers V, Eckelman M. Life cycle greenhouse gas emissions of anesthetic drugs. Anesth Analg. 2012;114(5):1086–90.
8. Feldman JM. Managing fresh gas flow to reduce environmental contamination. Anesth Analg. 2012;114(5):1093–101.
9. Practice Greenhealth. Greening the OR™. https://practicegreenhealth.org/initiatives/greening-operating-room. Accessed 6 June 2014.
10. Practice Greenhealth. Waste. https://practicegreenhealth.org/topics/waste. Accessed 6 June 2014.
11. R.E.M.E.D.Y.: Reclaimed Medical Equipment for the Developing World. http://www.remedyinc.org/. Accessed 6 June 2014.
12. American Medical Association. Medical supply recyclingprograms.http://www.ama-assn.org//ama/pub/about-ama/our-people/member-groups-sections/medical-student-section/community-service/medical-supply-recycling-programs.page. Accessed 6 June 2014.
13. Hunke TK, Ryan S, Hopf HW, Axelrod D, Feldman J, Torrillo T, et al. American Society of Anesthesiologists, Environmental Task Force. Greening the operating room manual. 2012. http://www.asahq.org/For-Members/Clinical-Information/Greening-the-Operating-Room.aspx. Accessed 6 June 2014.
14. World Health Organization. Health-care waste management. October 2011. http://www.who.int/mediacentre/factsheets/fs281/en/. Accessed 6 June 2014.
15. Health care without harm. https://noharm.org/. Accessed 6 June 2014.
16. Eckelman M, Mosher M, Gonzalez A, Sherman J. Comparative life cycle assessment of disposable and reusable laryngeal mask airways. Anesth Analg. 2012;114(5):1067–72.
17. FDA guidance document, "Enforcement Priorities for Single-Use Devices Reprocessed by Third Parties and Hospitals". August 14, 2000. http://www.fda.gov/MedicalDevices/DeviceRegulationandGuidance/GuidanceDocuments/ucm107164.htm. Accessed 6 June 2014.
18. United States Government Accountability Office. Report to the Committee on Oversight and Government Reform, House of Representatives. Reprocessed single-use medical devices: FDA oversight has increased, and available information does not indicate that use presents an elevated health risk. Washington, DC: United States Government Accountability Office; 2008. http://www.gao.gov/new.items/d08147.pdf. Accessed 6 June 2014.
19. McGain F, Algie CM, O'Toole J, Lim TF, Mohebbi M, Story DA, Leder K. The microbiological and sustainability effects of washing anaesthesia breathing circuits less frequently. Anaesthesia. 2014;69(4):337–42.
20. FDA issued a guidance document, Medical devices: sterility review guidance K90-1. August 30, 2002. http://www.fda.gov/MedicalDevices/DeviceRegulationandGuidance/GuidanceDocuments/ucm072783.htm. Accessed 6 June 2014.
21. Green Guide for Health Care. The Green Guide Version 2.2 operations section. 2008 revision. www.gghc.org. Accessed 6 June 2014.
22. Practice Greenhealth. Sterilants and disinfectants. https://practicegreenhealth.org/topics/chemicals/sterilants-disinfectants. Accessed 6 June 2014.
23. EPA medical waste. http://www.epa.gov/osw/nonhaz/industrial/medical/index.htm. Accessed 6 June 2014.
24. EPA hospital pollution prevention. http://www.epa.gov/region9/waste/p2/hospart.html. Accessed 6 June 2014.
25. World Health Organization. Waste from healthcare activities. November 2011. http://www.who.int/mediacentre/factsheets/fs253/en/.
26. Environmental Protection Agency, Management of Hazardous Waste Pharmaceuticals, 2014. http://www.epa.gov/osw/hazard/generation/pharmaceuticals.htm. Accessed June 6, 2014.
27. Managing pharmaceutical waste: a 10-step blueprint for healthcare facilities, Practice Greenhealth. August 2008. http://www.hercenter.org/hazmat/tenstepblueprint.pdf.
28. McGain E, Hendel SA, Story DA. An audit of potentially recyclable waste from anesthetic practice. Anaesth Intensive Care. 2009;37(5):820–3.

What Do Patients and Communities Expect of a Medical Mission?

8

V. Lekprasert, S. Pauswasdi, and B.M. Shrestha

Introduction

Every one wishes to live a healthy life. Many people worldwide are not so lucky. People become sick for many reasons and access to health care, which is a basic human right, may not be available. Those who can access these services may not be able to afford the cost. Any resources which they have might have been spent on basic primary needs like food, water, and shelter. There is nothing left for health care. This situation occurs more in less affluent countries.

International studies has shown that communities with low income, even those in affluent countries, have greater exposure to health damaging risk factors and thus have poorer health causing more illness and shorter life span.

Governments do plan to provide basic need and health care to their people but most of the time in developing countries, the plan is limited to paper only. Unstable and corrupt governments, lack of infrastructure, lack of understanding of priorities, and poor economy all play a part.

V. Lekprasert, M.D., M.S. (✉) • S. Pauswasdi, M.D.
Department of Anesthesiology, Ramathibodi Hospital, Mahidol University, Bangkok, Thailand
e-mail: varinee63@aol.com; varinee.lek@mahidol.ac.th

B.M. Shrestha, M.B.B.S., D.A., F.R.C.A.T.
Department of Anaesthesia and Intensive Care, Kathmandu Medical College Teaching Hospital, Sinamangal, Kathmandu, Nepal

The expectations and thus success of medical missions depend on many factors including quality and safety factors [1, 2], international collaboration, an understanding of the ethics and culture of the host region and establishment of a means to ensure sustainability and continuity. Recently, increasing public awareness of global health concept has led various organizations to create global collaborations in the form of medical missions [3]. The challenges of providing successful medical missions in underserved communities are multifactorial [4]. However, considering the principles of human rights, a conceptual framework can be summarized into three domains (quality, ethics and cultural relevance, collaboration) sharing the same goals of continuity and sustainability (Fig. 8.1).

Quality and Safety

Quality and safety are multifaceted issues. The Institute of Medicine (IOM) has identified six aims of quality medical care [5]:

- *Safety*: Providers must ensure that the medical care intended to benefit patients is not causing harm. This requirement is particularly applicable as many developing countries do not yet have safety standards built into their health care systems, and medical providers are often asked to practice outside of their expertise, which is both unsafe and unethical.

R. Roth et al. (eds.), *The Role of Anesthesiology in Global Health: A Comprehensive Guide*, DOI 10.1007/978-3-319-09423-6_8,

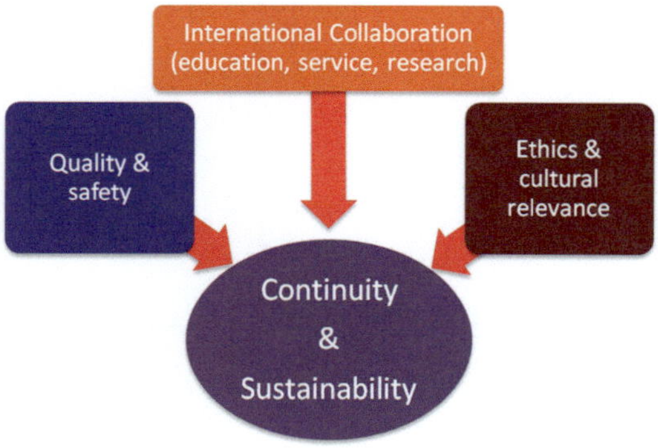

Fig. 8.1 A conceptual framework of the expectation of a medical mission (The pillars of successful medical missions)

- *Effectiveness*: Medical treatments must be based on scientific knowledge, and must produce beneficial, measurable results.
- *Patient-centered*: Care must be tailored to individual patient preferences, needs, and values. Patients should have authority over their own medical care, and their input must guide clinical decision-making.
- *Timeliness*: Patients requiring medical attention should have access to timely health care and follow-up care to avoid potentially harmful delays in treatment.
- *Efficiency*: Quality health care avoids wasting finances, time, equipment, and energy. Efficiency maximizes the impact of global health organizations.
- *Equitability*: The quality of medical care must be consistent across all patient types, irrespective of gender, ethnicity, socioeconomic status, and other personal characteristics. Similarly, visiting medical providers must hold themselves to the highest standards of quality care, as they would in their home countries.

Developing countries have poor economies and poor resources, which should not be a deterrent to providing quality care. Patients do wish to have quality care.

While low quality health care may be primarily a reflection of inadequate financial resources, there is evidence that quality can be enhanced in a number of ways even in the absence of additional resources [6].

Table 8.1 Types of resources needed for quality and safety in anesthesia

Human resources	Nonhuman resources
• Manpower	• Equipment/tools
• Education/knowledge	• Monitors
• Skills	• Drugs
• Experiences	• Blood supply

Ideally, people throughout the world should gain access to quality health care. However, there are considerable challenges in resources and organization to achieve all six key components. The World Federation of Societies of Anaesthesiologists (WFSA), which was founded in 1955 aims to make available the highest standard of anesthesia to all peoples throughout the world [7, 8]. The international standards recommended by the WFSA are aimed at anesthesia professionals everywhere to improve and maintain the quality and safety of anesthesia care. For some countries, these standards have already been implemented but for many countries or different areas in the same countries, these standards may represent a future goal. Nonetheless, the goal is always the best possible care and ongoing improvement for the safe practice of anesthesia [8].

Quality health care is about getting the right care to the right patient at the right time, and achieving the best possible outcome. Although it sounds simple, quality may vary for many reasons. Advanced technologies offer the promise of improving health, increasing life span, and reducing pain and suffering. However, working in multicultural areas requires knowledge of cultural differences and beliefs. What is considered the best care in one region may not be the best in many other, even adjacent, areas. The quality issue becomes even more complicated when facing a huge patient need and demand. In many areas worldwide, there is a problem of provider volume and density. When the ratio of patients to providers is overwhelming, the need is often determined by a combination of triage and weighing of risks and benefits for each patient.

Provision of quality anesthesia care requires both human and nonhuman resources (Table 8.1). Human resources include manpower, education, knowledge, skills, and experience of both physician

Table 8.2 Three phases in the WHO surgical safety checklist [9]

Sign in: Before starting anesthesia	*Time out*: Before starting surgery	*Sign out*: At the end of surgery
• Patient identification • Surgical marked site • Allergy • Difficult airway or aspiration risk • Bleeding risk and planned intravenous fluid therapy • Readiness of anesthesia machine, medications, pulse oximeter	• Confirmation of team members • Confirmation of the patient, procedure, and incision site • Antibiotic prophylaxis within the last 60 min • Anticipated critical events to surgeon, anesthesiologist, and nursing team • Availability of essential imaging	• Confirmation of the performed procedure • Complete counts of instrument, sponge, and needles • Correct specimen labeling • Addressing any equipment problems • Key concerns for patient recovery and management

and non-physician anesthesia providers. In addition, the multiple disciplines involve in the various components of safety must be considered. Therefore, multidisciplinary aspects of care through team training are vital. The World Health Organization (WHO) has introduced a surgical safety checklist in 2009, as a mean to improve surgical patient safety through multidisciplinary communication. The checklist was first launched in June 2008, and has been translated into at least six languages (Table 8.2). WHO 2009 surgical checklist comprises vital checks in three phases: sign in (before starting anesthesia), time out (before starting surgery), and sign out (at the end of surgery) [9]. The use of a checklist can be locally modified to suit the individual hospital setting. Recent studies show the benefits of operating room teamwork and communication, including reductions in morbidity and mortality among surgical patients in a diverse group of hospitals [9, 10].

Nonhuman resources include equipments, tools, monitors, anesthetic drugs, and blood supply. Provision of these resources is as important as medical logistics to support medical missions. The logistics of pharmaceuticals, medical and surgical supplies, devices and equipments are also essential for the continuity of care. In the resource-poor setting, this issue remains challenging.

A well-developed infrastructure is necessary to manage these resources for long-term use. Well-thought out strategic plans are required to make efficient use of limited resources. Considering the health of all as interconnected and closely linked to economic forces, resources must be used with the awareness of ongoing widespread poverty, world population growth, global warming, and depletion of limited natural resources. In other words, a "global mind-set" must be emphasized [11]. Although advanced anesthesia machines and equipments have provided better care for patients, overreliance on them may cause hidden problems and dangers. Evidence shows that many operating rooms in the developing world are littered with an accumulation of well-meaning mission donations in the form of unrepaired ventilators, and anesthesia machines, often labeled with the name and date of the mission [12]. Instead of modern and high-tech anesthesia machines, a simple medical ventilator such as the Bird respirator may be more practical in an area where electricity is not widely or consistently available (Fig. 8.2).

In addition simpler anesthesia machines and equipment may be easier for local staffs to maintain in working order. The literature reveals that short-term medical missions have improved the lives of patients in resource-limited area, but the ability to make a meaningful and lasting effect in the developing world is difficult [12].

Ethics and Cultural Relevance

Behavioral and cultural differences are significant barriers when working in different locations worldwide. Many models have been developed to cope with this problem. Rassiwala et al. reported two models of educational engagement: a 1-week program and a 4-week program for medical students [3]. Two physicians from the same university supervised the short program, while the longer program was coordinated by the nonprofit organization that worked with local health care

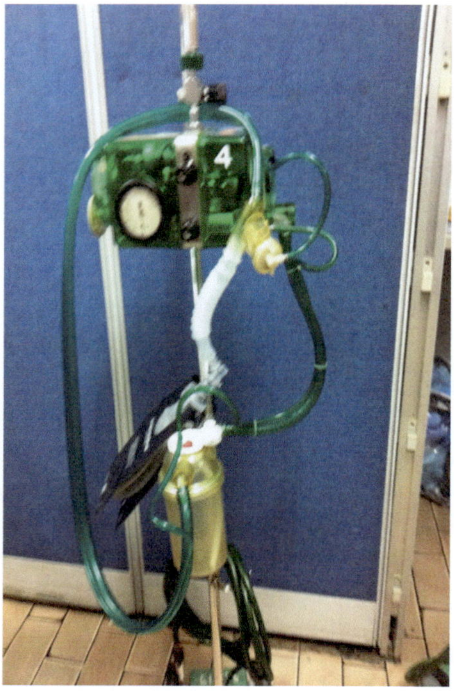

Fig. 8.2 Bird respirator at Ramathibodi hospital in Bangkok, kept in well-functioning condition for learning and teaching purposes

providers [3]. A longer duration program provided more time to develop good rapport, language and ethnic learning that bridges the cultural and ethical gaps between visiting medical students and the local population. The model of a longer duration of global health educational program helped medical students to incorporate their knowledge to better suit a resource-limited setting and also to build a better patient-provider bond. The same positive impact in terms of better collaboration and understanding of a cultural and social context was evident by senior physicians who may be able to stay in a place for long-term missions [13].

Despite good intentions, many international medical missions are unsuccessful. One of the major problems comes from cultural differences. Regardless of race or location, communication should proceed in a caring, and respectful manner to reduce culture-related communication problems, not only to the patients but also to local physicians on the basis of respect for their skills, knowledge, and traditions [13, 14]. Carrese et al. studied strategies for discussing negative information with Navajo patients in 34 Navajo informants [15]. There were three categories of informants: patients, traditional healers, and Western biomedical health care providers. The study suggested a four-stage approach to facilitate the bridging of cultural differences. The first stage is a patient assessment to assess the willingness and appropriate timing for any discussion. The next step is a preparation, which entails cultivating a trusting relationship, the involvement of family members, and facilitating the involvement of traditional healers if needed. The third stage is communication in a caring, kind, and respectful manner. Finally, the follow-through should be completed for the continuation of care.

International Collaboration and Sustainable Quality Health Care

Several issues are essential to maintain sustainable health care through international collaboration;

1. Education: in-country vs. oversea training programs;
2. Service: short-term vs. long-term and
3. Research: routine-to-research methodology

Education

In the developing world, education systems are poorly developed or nonexistent. Many peoples are uneducated and carry on with the traditional "cures" they received for generations when they were sick. To maintain good health free from many diseases, good hygiene is necessary—a concept that is also foreign to many in underdeveloped countries.

But even educated people in these countries often have very low expectations of the health care system—they experience cycles of health crises and do not maintain good health. An environment in health care must be created so that these people can also look for care when they need it, and not wait for the situation to become acute or critical. Most of the time these educated mass also do not trust the modern health care system and prefer to be treated by local medicine men. For example, Dhami Jhakri are the Nepalese words for shamans who are local healers and consulted by the local community. They are found in Nepal, parts of India, not only in remote villages but also in cities. Similar mediums, who practice often by spirit possession, are prevalent in other groups and tribes.

Poverty and lack of education, along with other social determinants, are proven barriers to health care. Various measures of health quality, including low life expectancies and high mortality rates, correlate to low levels of education [16]. People living in poverty usually have not been educated as to when, why, and where to access health care. Many mistakenly believe that their affliction is irreversible and permanent or the result of some wrongdoing on their part or the influences of evil spirits, and they are unaware of medical treatments that can treat or cure their condition. Additionally, general public health education is lacking, such as knowledge of proper hygiene and water treatment. It is the role of global health organizations to fill these educational gaps. By training health workers and community members to raise awareness about good health practices and opportunities to access medical care, global health organizations can produce far-reaching positive results.

The developed world needs to be educated and made more aware of poverty-induced health crises across the globe. Though general health education is readily available in affluent countries, education and advocacy about poverty-induced health crises throughout the world are necessary to spur developed nations to action.

Strasser described it well: "Despite the huge differences between developing and developed countries, access is the major issue in rural health around the world. Even in the countries where the majority of the population lives in rural areas, the resources are concentrated in the cities. All countries have difficulties with transport and communication, and they all face the challenge of shortages of doctors and other health professionals in rural and remote areas. Many rural people are caught in the poverty–ill health–low productivity downward spiral, particularly in developing countries." [17]

An earlier paper by Yancey reported "Health care providers are reminded at intervals that rich and poor, educated and illiterate people react similarly to excellent, considerate health services. Practice does not make for perfection in medicine; only excellent practice permits a close approximation to perfection. Poor people know of the presence and accessibility of the public teaching hospital in their community, yet they report to the hospital later than the higher income, private hospital individuals for care" [18]

And finally Clark reporting on volunteers in Ghana wrote: "Even though people are generally poor they still want to preserve their dignity. Valuable/expensive things offered on a silver platter tend to lose their value and have the tendency to be abused. Thus it is always advisable to let people bear some responsibility. This is why some communities have to pay a token fee for some of the services or medications. No matter how meager a fee paid, it is enough to let one value whatever is offered. If something very expensive is being offered for free, the notion is that it is meant to be thrown away; and that is why it is being given to them. They may even feel belittled by the totally free offer." [19]

Indeed, global health disparities and inequitable access to health care in developing countries should be an ongoing concern for many if not all physicians [20].

Thus evidence and research underscore that education is the key to sustainable changes in developing countries. Bidirectional education between low and high-resource countries can be beneficial to both sides. Low-resource countries gain knowledge, advanced clinical skills, and infrastructure organizing skill to meet their local needs. Students and faculty from high-resource countries also gain medical knowledge, clinical skills, cultural sensitivity, adaptability, flexibility and have more appreciation for public health and socioeconomic factors. The knowledge and experiences gained from working in low-resource countries can have long lasting beneficial effects on their career paths [7, 21, 22].

The World Federation of Societies of Anaesthesiologists (WFSA) has provided training opportunities in many areas around the world, both in-country training programs and overseas training programs. Candidates for oversea training must commit to return home to practice. The main advantage of overseas training program is the opportunity for the trainee to see the system and infrastructure support of anesthesia from the inside. The graduates can use knowledge and experience to organize infrastructures, improve anesthesia practice, and even become professional leaders in their homelands. However, local investments for infrastructure support and continuing education, as well as political commitments are essential to attract physicians and non-physician staff and retain those trained anesthesia providers in the areas of need. Studies reveal barriers to recruitment and retention of anesthesia providers that include poor working environment and limited appeal of health care jobs. These critical issues must be acknowledged and remedied in order to reduce the complex problem of "brain drain" [23]. In low-income and middle-income countries, well trained anesthesia providers, as well as other health care workers are very poorly paid. Thus, they either move to higher paying jobs locally or migrate to better-paid jobs abroad. In the past, the most commonly used strategy to retain those valuable health care personnel was compulsory rural service bonds and mandatory rural service for admission into postgraduate training programs. However, the new strategies including well-balanced workforce management policies, incentives, incremental improvement in public health facilities, better residential infrastructure, and local health care provider recruitment have shown promising impacts [23, 24].

At present the WFSA offers basic anesthesia training in two places: Bangkok Anesthesia Regional Training Centers (BARTC) in Thailand and Cluj-Napoca in Romania [7]. The center in Romania, which is supported by the WFSA and the European Society of Anaesthesiology's National Anesthesia Societies Committee (NASC) commenced in 2002. BARTC was established in 1996 with the collaboration of the Royal College of Anesthesiologists of Thailand (RCAT). RCAT feels the obligation to promote better global anesthetic care, apart from serving anesthesiologists in Thailand and cooperating with colleges/societies of anesthesiologists from various countries. Therefore, a 1-year WFSA-BARTC program was started in 1996, with Prof. Thara Tritrakarn (Thailand) as the first director and support from Prof. Mitsugu Fujimori (Japan), Dr. Kester Brown (Australia), and Dr. Haydn Plerndt (Australia). To date, WFSA-BARTC has 60 graduates from surrounding countries such as Laos PDR, Myanmar, Mongolia, Vietnam, Cambodia, and Bhutan. Feedback from the graduates emphasizes the great values of the program. In addition, WFSA-BARTC refresher courses have been conducted regularly in different countries where those graduates reside for continuing education as follows:

1991	Hanoi, Vietnam
1993	Ho Chi Minh City, Vietnam
1995	Ho Chi Minh City and Hue, Vietnam
1998	Vientiane, Laos PDR
1998	Haiphong, Vietnam
2004	Phnom Penh, Cambodia
2006	Ulaan Baatar, Mongolia
2007	Yangon, Myanmar
2010	Yangon, Myanmar
2011	Ulaan Baatar, Mongolia
2012	Ubonratchatani, Thailand
2013	Yangon, Myanmar

There are also short-term training programs sponsored by the WFSA in different countries as local health needs are identified, such as Romania, Israel, India, and South Africa. Many of these training courses have been extended to be of longer duration with additional subspecialty training [7].

At Ramathibodi Hospital in Bangkok, there is an additional a 1-year training program for Bhutan nurse anesthetists (Fig. 8.3). The program originally sponsored by the World Health Organization (WHO) was started in 2002 and continued for 5 consecutive years, with 21 graduates. After the graduates returned to Bhutan and practiced for sometimes, many requested to come back for additional short courses in areas such as

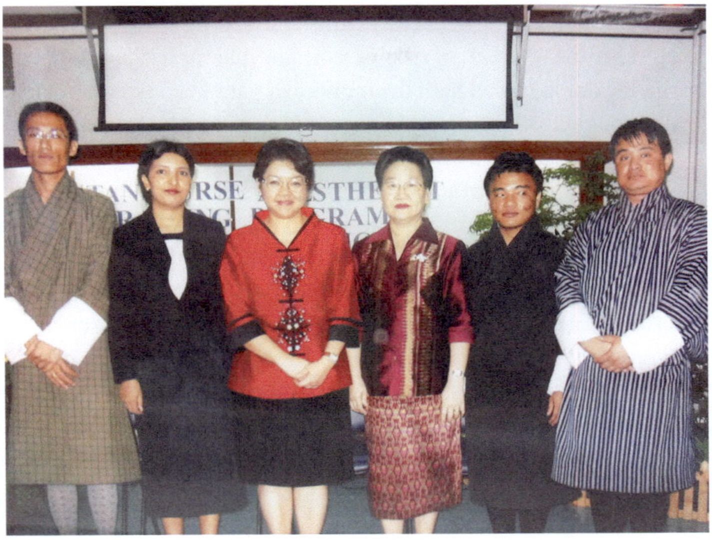

Fig. 8.3 A group of Bhutan nurse anesthetists graduated from Ramathibodi hospital, Mahidol University in 2003—Rinzin Dorji, Champa Sharma, Dr. Varinee Lekprasert, Dr. Surirat Sriswasdi, Dorji Gyeltshen, and Changlo

pain, intensive care, and cardiopulmonary resuscitation. WFSA-BARTC graduates also asked for the same courses, including anesthesia for special procedures such as kidney transplantation and laparoscopic surgery. Such actions clearly demonstrate the life-long learning mind and the great attitude of professional development in these alumnae to pursue quality health care in their homeland.

Every effort should also be done to recruit trainees into the specialty of anesthesia and to retain them locally. Thus, the continuity and sustainability of quality health care can be achieved.

Service

Ideally, long-term medical missions can alleviate the problems of short-term medical missions involving unfamiliarity with sociocultural differences, communication, and lack of follow-up care. It also can cultivate trusting relationship with patients and communities. However, long-term medical missions have higher costs, schedule constraints, and more complex logistics. Therefore, many global health activities use the form of short-term medical missions that could undermine the local health care system, by unfamiliarity with the local medical needs, diagnostic and management algorithm, and providing culturally irrelevant care. In addition, there are many lessons learned from various organizations, which have programs relying only on visiting volunteers to provide health care. For example, when the visiting surgeons leave the community and there is no surgeon to provide follow-up care or treat infections that may arise, serious complications may result. Such poor surgical outcomes can be avoidable if there is a continuity of care by local physicians. Thus, the impact on local medical systems could cause significant harm and hinder the success of the mission [25].

These global health activities use the form of short-term medical missions that may undermine the local health care system, and could cause significant harm and adversely affect the success of the mission [24]. Researchers have documented a number of reasons for these failures, including the economic situation of the country, hospital and national politics, personality conflicts, and continued lack of resources. In addition, language differences between the team and the host country add another challenge. Wolfberg emphasized the importance of developing strong relationships with local physicians with respect for their skills and traditions, so that follow-up care could be achieved when the visiting staff left the community [13]. Gorske discovered considerable risk for medical errors from short-term medical missions such as lack of understanding of the critical issue of the short-term medical mission setting itself and the increased risk of serious patient harm, lack of knowledge of the individual patient, and inadequate time for obtaining accurate and complete history [26].

Errors originated from lack of adequate health records, poor-setting infrastructure, and language barriers [25]. The nature of short stays in limited medical missions also causes complications due to insufficient patient screening, and lack of follow-up care. Extended medical missions clearly provide better outcomes, but the cost of such missions can be prohibitive. In addition, the current global burden of surgical disease is still high, and well-planned and organized short-term medical missions may be more cost-effective and cover a larger scope of world population health. Every possible means to bridge the gaps of cultural differences, ethical values and endemic barriers should be mobilized in order to achieve high quality in short-term medical missions. Without stable, collaborative partnerships with local physicians and community workers, it is difficult to enact sustainable improvements in health care quality from even well-intended missions.

Within Nepal, one of the authors (BMS) has helped organize surgical and medical camps in remote areas (Fig. 8.4). In these parts there is minimum equipment and drugs which sometimes have to be transported on the backs of donkeys. Oxygen cylinders are too heavy to be transported so most work is done with oxygen concentrators [27]. As there is no electrical power in remote areas generators are used. Other equipment such as portable halothane vaporizers, Ambu bags, foot suction (occasionally electrically powered), portable pulse oximeters, and other drugs and tubes is available. Esophageal stethoscopes are used as cardiac and respiratory monitors. Modified Bain circuits are available when an air–oxygen–halothane mixture is needed [28].

Research

In this twenty-first century, the health of people in the world is more closely linked than ever as we are all interconnected. Problems of limited resources, population growth, demographic changes, and environmental and biological dangers threaten us all. Research should be conducted even in underserved communities to improve quality health care and ascertain the effective use of limited resources.

In under-resourced locations, high technology research with surrogate outcome such as laboratory testing may not be relevant. However, research in these areas should involve various global health programs as a means to improve health care quality. It is also vital to create learning community services through continuing quality improvement projects or clinical research. Most international health service research is facing the problem of bringing research solutions into practice [29]. An effective way to get research into practice uses a different approach by formulating research questions from challenges in routine service or work. The so-called "Routine to Research" (R-2-R) has been described by Professor Vicharn Panich, director of the Knowledge Management Institute (KMI) in Thailand and has been shown to solve service/work problems while improving working quality at the same time (personal communication). Many models have been used to measure the success of R-2-R projects, such as quality, timeliness, and cost reduction. For example, a group of doctors and nurses from Siriraj hospital in Thailand noticed that after percutaneous coronary intervention (PCI), patients often experienced pain due to being immobile for up to 10 h after the procedure. To alleviate the pain, they described the "Siriraj Leg Lock" to confine the hip while allowing patients to freely move other parts of their body without compromising the postprocedural wound [30]. The study result showed significant less pain and more patient satisfaction without increasing wound complication.

Local communities tend to participate and cooperate well with research solutions since the working staffs that experience the problems conduct the research. The cycle of Continuous Quality Improvement (CQI) in communities can be sustained by the support of the program, on a national scale. In Thailand, four large organizations

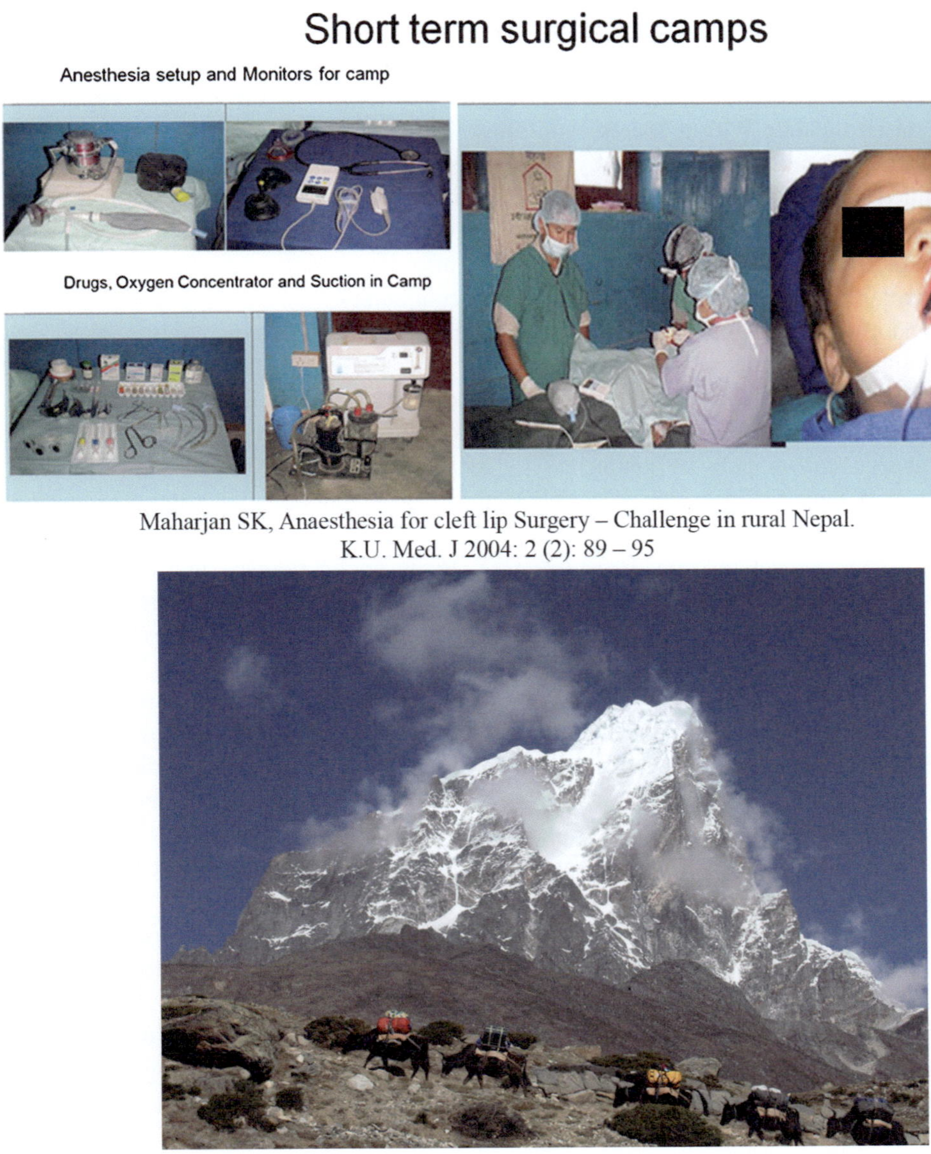

Fig. 8.4 Surgical camps in the Himalayas. Maharjan SK, Anaesthesia for cleft lip Surgery—Challenge in rural Nepal. K.U. Med. J. 2004: 2(2): 89–95

(Ministry of Health, Siriraj hospital, Thai Health Promotion Foundation, and the National Health Security Office) signed the Memorandum of Understanding (MoU) for the support of R-2-R in August 2008. Walley et al. suggested from their experience that these research and development programs should be linked and adapted for successful expansion [29].

Expectations from a Medical Mission

The Patients' Perspective

The first thing the patient expects from any medical team is that he/she will be well looked after and will be cured of his/her disease. While expecting these results, patients may have many other doubts about the team, perhaps related to previous experiences.

Questions raised include: Will he/she be listened to and heard properly and be seen by a properly qualified physician? Most of the time due to the large number of patients examined and treated and the short duration of stay of the medical team, there may be inadequate time to realize these ideals. Doubts may arise and with whatever sincerity the treatment was advised, the patient may not accept it. Patients believe that the team will respect his/her social and economic background. Any unnecessary remarks or comments from the team hurt their feelings and provoke resentment. Again, problems may occur for an otherwise successful medical mission. Patients who come for treatment are of different religious background. They may not like for any suggestion or misinterpretation of their religion from a visitor.

Similarly there are often local beliefs and customs in the society integral and even unique to them. To get away from unnatural beliefs and customs, it takes time and proper convincing. A medical team visiting for short periods, may find it very odd but these belief must be taken into account.

Now more and more patients based on past experiences know that they must be treated by qualified physicians and expect an ethical practice from them. They like to be given a proper explanation about their disease process, treatment, options and expected outcome. In more serious cases they may or may not want families to be involved in decision making for treatment and surgery. Patients do expect that the information about them will be confidential and protected.

Community Expectations

Community involvement plays a great role in achieving success or failure of medical missions. Normally the community has common denominators: a specific geographical area may have an organized government plan or be bound by social or cultural tradition. Usually with similar social and cultural attachments there is one voice which makes it easier for a medical team to function. But it is not always so. A community that is specified geographically will have many ethnic groups with a variety of social customs or beliefs. A politically demarcated community will have a party volunteer and work at the direction of the party affording benefit only for that particular party community.

Expectation differs across cultural, racial, and ethnic groups. Even then the community has many common expectations from a medical team.

- Good intention—Serve for the benefit of the local community without any self-interest.
- Qualified—Volunteers have appropriate medical training as well as accountability.
- There is no interference in religious views, social activities, and beliefs of the community.
- The ability to provide therapies that address the root causes exists.
- The team should not impose burdens on local health facilities: they should provide relevant care and not leaving behind medical waste.
- There should be no negligent care.
- Current standards of health care delivery or public health programs should be appropriately followed [31].
- Due permission and clearance should be obtained from the concerned authorities before initiating medical work.

Some medical missions believe that providing some care is better than providing none at all. Drs. Bishop and Litch, codirectors of the Kunde Hospital in Nepal, have explained why this philosophy is misguided:

- "It is inappropriate arrogance to assume that anything that a Western doctor has to offer his less developed neighbor is progress. These [Western physician] tourists are often working outside their trained specialty or have little concept of how that specialty applies to Nepal. They frequently don't understand local illness presentation, culture, or language. They often offer inappropriate treatment because they think they 'must give something.' The consultations are often one off, with little possibility for follow up and the local health providers are left to pick up the pieces with no record of the consultation. If an unregistered doctor on holiday in the United Kingdom offered general medical consultations in a shopping centre there would be a public and professional outcry." [32]

Conclusion

Countries should develop their own good health care system. International liaisons and support should be used to develop infrastructures, man power, and systems, until the countries become self-sufficient. Health care team should be able to provide total care to patients and satisfactory service to the community.

Patients and communities have high expectation of a medical mission, which should not be surprising since quality health care is a fundamental principle of human rights. Not only should the quality reach internationally accepted standards, but also continuity and sustainability should be available. Provision of safe anesthesia is difficult without appropriate human and non-human resources. International collaboration in education, service, and research with special consideration of ethics and cultural relevance are key success factors. Comprehensive health care policies and strategic plans from government are major challenges to retain trained anesthesia providers in the areas of need.

Severe shortages of trained health professionals plague developing countries, reflecting complex economic and political problems that will require decades for resolution. Until such time as surgical services are widely available and affordable in remote as well as urban areas of developing countries, anesthesiologists will continue to provide a valuable and personally rewarding contribution through short-term assistance [33].

Acknowledgement The authors would like to thank Professor Thara Tritrakarn of the department of anesthesiology, Siriraj hospital, Mahidol University for his kind help and valuable information regarding WFSA-BARTC program. Also Professor Vicharn Panich, the former director of the Knowledge Management Institute (KMI) in Thailand and Dr. Akarin Nimmannit from Siriraj hospital for the information of the Routine-to-Research (R-2-R) concept and practice in Thai health care. And finally Professor Babu Raja Shrestha, Professor of Anesthesia and Intensive Care, Kathmandu Medical College Teaching Hospital, Kathmandu, Nepal for his assistance in the preparation of this chapter.

References

1. Pierce EC. The 34th Rovenstine lecture. 40 years behind the mask: safety revisited. Anesthesiology. 1996;84:965–75.
2. McQueen KA. Anesthesia and the global burden of surgical disease. Int Anesthesiol Clin. 2010;48(2): 91–107.
3. Rassiwala J, Vaduganathan M, Kupershtok M, Castillo FM, Evert J. Global health educational engagement—a tale of two models. Acad Med. 2013;88:1651–7.
4. Enright A. Review article: safety aspects of anesthesia in under-resourced locations. Can J Anaesth. 2013; 60:152–8.
5. The IOM quality initiative: a progress report at year six. Institute of Medicine Newsletter. 1.1. Winter 2002. Accessed 24 Feb 2014—Through Global Health Course—High Quality Medical Care—UNITE for Sight—Module—6 ref. 1.
6. Skolnik R. Essentials of global health. Sudbury, MA: Jones and Bartlett; 2008. p. 147–66. Accessed 24 Feb 2014—Through Global Health Course—High Quality Medical Care—UNITE for Sight—Module—6 ref. 2.
7. Enright A, Wilson IH, Moyers JR. The World Federation of Societies of Anaesthesiologists: supporting education in the developing world. Anaesthesia. 2007;62 Suppl 1:67–71.
8. Merry AF, Cooper JB, Soyannwo O, Wilson IH, Eichhorn JH. International standards for a safe practice of anesthesia 2010. Can J Anaesth. 2010;57: 1027–34.
9. Haynes AB, Weiser TG, Berry WR, Lipsitz SR, Breizat A-HS, Dellinger EP, et al. A surgical safety checklist to reduce morbidity and mortality in global population. N Engl J Med. 2009;360:491–9.
10. Russ S, Rput S, Sevdalis N, Moorthy K, Darzi A, Vincent C. Do safety checklists improve teamwork and communication in the operating room? A systematic review. Ann Surg. 2013;258:856–71.
11. Benatar SR. Global health and justice: re-examining our values. Bioethics. 2013;27(6):297–304.
12. Farmer DL. The need for sustainability in contemporary global health efforts. Arch Surg. 2010;145(8): 752–3.
13. Wolfberg AJ. Volunteering overseas—lessons from surgical brigades. N Engl J Med. 2006;3564:443–5.
14. Schouten BC, Meeuwesen L. Cultural differences in medical communication: a review of the literature. Patient Educ Couns. 2006;64:21–34.
15. Carrese JA, Rhodes LA. Bridging cultural differences in medical practice. J Gen Intern Med. 2000;15: 92–6.

16. Marmot M. Social determinants of health inequalities. Lancet. 2005;365(9464):1099–104. Accessed 24 Feb 2014—Through Global Health Course—How to eliminate Patients barrier to Care—UNITE for Sight—Module—5 ref. 7.
17. Strasser R. Rural health around the world: challenges and solutions. Fam Pract. 2003;20:457–63. Accessed 18 Mar 2014.
18. Yancey AG. The challenge of providing health care for the poor: public hospital perspective. J Natl Med Assoc. 1987;79(1):107–11. Accessed 11 Mar 2014.
19. Clarke J. Cushioning cultural shocks: guidelines for volunteers in Ghana. Uniteforsight.org. Accessed 24 Feb 2014—Through Global Health Course—How to eliminate Patients barrier to Care—UNITE for Sight—Module—5 ref. 1.
20. Snyder J, Dharamsi S, Crooks VA. Fly-By medical care: conceptualizing the global and local social responsibilities of medical tourists and physician voluntourists. Global Health. 2011;7(6):1744–8603. Accessed 20 Mar 2014.
21. Dohlman LE. Anesthesia education across borders. Curr Opin Anaesthesiol. 2013;26:732–6.
22. Drain PK, Holmes KK, Skeff KM, Hall TL, Gardner P. Global health training and international clinical rotations during residency: current status, needs, and opportunities. Acad Med. 2009;84:320–5.
23. Sundararaman T, Gupta G. Indian approaches to retaining skilled health workers in rural areas. Bull World Health Organ. 2011;89:73–7.
24. Dubowitz G. Global health and global anesthesia. Int Anesthesiol Clin. 2010;48(2):39–46.
25. Pinto AD, Upshur REG. Global health ethics for students. Dev World Bioeth. 2009;9(1)1–10.
26. Gorske A. Harm from drugs in short-term missions. Review of the medical literature. The Center of the Study of Health in Missions; December 2009. http://www.csthmbestpractices.org/resources/Harm+From+Drugs+in+Short-term+Missions.pdf.
27. Shrestha BM, Singh BB, Gautam MP, Chand MB. The oxygen concentrator is a suitable alternative to oxygen cylinders in Nepal. Can J Anaesth. 2002;49(1):8–12.
28. Shrestha BM, Tweed WA, Basnyt NB, Lekhak BD. A modification of the Bain system for ambient air—oxygen inhalation. Anaesthesia. 1994;49:703–6.
29. Walley J, Khan MA, Shah SK, Witter S, Wei X. How to get research into practice: first get practice into research. Bull World Health Organ. 2007;85(6):424–5.
30. Pornratanarangsi S, Boonlert S, Duangprateep A, Wiratpintu P, Waree W, Tresukosol D, et al. The effectiveness of "Siriraj Leg Lock" brace on back pain after percutaneous coronary intervention:PCI. J Med Assoc Thai. 2010;93 Suppl 1:S35–42.
31. Suchdev P, Ahtrens K, Cllick E, Macklin L, Evangelista D, Grahm E. A model for sustainable short-term international medical trips. Ambul Pediatr. 2007;7:317–20. Accessed 10 Mar 2014.
32. Bishop RA, Litch JA. Medical tourism can do harm. BMJ. 2000;320(7240):1017.
33. Froese A. Anesthesia and the role of short-term service delivery in developing countries. Can J Anaesth. 2007;54(11):940–6.

Anesthesia in Resource-Poor Settings: The Médecins Sans Frontières Experience

9

Miguel Trelles, Patricia Kahn, Jason Cone, and Carrie Teicher

Introduction

Médecins Sans Frontières/Doctors Without Borders (MSF) is an independent medical humanitarian organization formed in 1971 by a small group of French doctors and journalists with the aim of providing emergency care to populations in danger. The underlying principle is that this assistance is offered based solely on need, irrespective of race, religion, gender or political affiliation. Surgical programs have been part of this response in some settings since the early 1980s [1]. With MSF now active in more than 70 countries, these surgical activities are undertaken in a wide array of contexts, ranging from conflict zones such as Afghanistan, Democratic Republic of Congo, and Syria, to natural disasters (e.g., the earthquake in Haiti and Typhoon Haiyan in the Philippines) to low-resource but more stable environments such as India and Burundi.

A key conclusion from this experience is that basic surgery should always be considered as an integral part of medical care, even in the most remote and impoverished settings, given its proven value in reducing mortality, morbidity and disability and improving quality of life [2, 3]. In working to translate this notion into practice, we and others have also learned that—contrary to a common view of surgery as unrealistically expensive and complex for difficult settings—basic surgical care provided at the low-cost district hospital level can be surprisingly cost-effective, and "might compare favorably with selected primary health interventions in terms of cost-effectiveness" [4–6].

What is also clear from our work in emergency/low-resource settings is that surgeons and anaesthetists need to discard preconceived notions of an inevitable link between the technical complexity of surgical and anesthesia techniques and the ability to reduce morbidity and mortality. On the contrary, we have found that keeping our interventions simple, accessible and sustainable within a given context is often the most effective way to best serve the needs of the many. In MSF-Belgium projects, the focus is on providing access to quality surgical and anesthetic management in programs that are well adapted to each context and to the needs of the local population.

Overview of Surgical and Anesthesia Activities

The countries and contexts where MSF-Belgium had surgical missions at the end of 2013 are shown in Table 9.1. All but two are in either

M. Trelles (✉)
MSF-Belgium, Brussels, Belgium
e-mail: Miguel.trelles@brussels.msf.org

P. Kahn • J. Cone
MSF-USA, New York, NY, USA

C. Teicher
Epicentre, New York, NY, USA

R. Roth et al. (eds.), *The Role of Anesthesiology in Global Health: A Comprehensive Guide*,
DOI 10.1007/978-3-319-09423-6_9, © Springer International Publishing Switzerland 2015

Table 9.1 Ongoing surgery projects, 2013

Country	Project	Context	Program description
Afghanistan	Kabul	Conflict	Obstetrics, general surgery
	Khost	Conflict	Obstetrics
	Kunduz	Conflict	Obstetrics, general surgery
Burundi	Gitega	Post-conflict	Obstetrics (fistula repair)
	Kabezi	Post-conflict	Obstetrics
DRC	Masisi	Conflict	Obstetrics, general surgery
	Niangara	Conflict	Obstetrics, general surgery
Haiti	Tabarre	Stable	Orthopaedics, general surgery
India	Mon	Stable	Obstetrics, general surgery
Mali	Douentza	Conflict	Obstetrics, general surgery
Mauritania	Bassikounou	Conflict	Obstetrics, general surgery
Pakistan	Timurgara	Conflict	Obstetrics, general surgery
Philippines	Guiuan	Natural disaster	Obstetrics, general surgery
Sierra Leone	Bo	Post-conflict	Obstetrics
South Sudan	Gogrial	Conflict	Obstetrics, general surgery
	Gumuruk	Conflict	General surgery
Somalia	Burao	Conflict	Obstetrics, general surgery
Syria	Jabal-Akkrad	Conflict	Obstetrics, general surgery

Table 9.2 Overview of surgical activities, 2010–2013

Indicator (#)	Total	2013	2012	2011	2010
Patients[a]	59,824	14,199	14,583	19,296	11,746
Cases[b]	77,048	19,395	19,145	22,964	15,544
Procedures[c]	83,004	21,774	20,865	24,101	16,264
Main surgical indicators					
Violent trauma[d]	4,767 (xx %)	1,445 (10.2 %)	1,277 (8.8 %)	1,086 (5.6 %)	959 (8.2 %)
Accidental trauma	10,283 (xx %)	3,808 (26.8 %)	3,075 (21.1 %)	1,927 (12 %)	1,473 (12.5 %)
Obstetrical[e]	25,719 (xx %)	6,337 (44.6 %)	6,785 (46.5 %)	7,644 (47.5 %)	4,953 (42.2 %)
Other pathologies	15,876 (xx %)	2,609 (18.4 %)	3,446 (23.6 %)	5,460 (34.0 %)	4,361 (37.1 %)
Total	56,605 CK 56,646	14,199	14,583	16,077	11,746
No. of projects[f]		18	22	21	19

[a]Number of new cases
[b]Number of Operating Room. visits
[c]Number of surgical procedures performed during an intervention. MSF data tools allow reporting up to three procedures. For data analysis, only the first entry is considered because not all projects reported multiple procedures in one surgical intervention
[d]Violent trauma cases as cause for intervention (only new cases)
[e]Percentage of Caesarean sections uses patient number (new cases) as the denominator
[f]Number of active projects during 2013

emergency settings (conflict or natural disaster) or post-conflict regions.

The core activity at these projects is the provision of lifesaving and essential surgery that requires only low technology and is based in district hospitals or in the subset of primary health centers with surgical capacity. Lifesaving surgery is defined as any procedure performed in response to an acute state in which the patient's life, organ, or limb is at stake and surgery must be done as soon as possible, usually within hours. Essential surgery addresses conditions that may not immediately affect health or life but will considerably impair the quality of life or present a serious future health threat, and that are amenable to a proven surgical treatment.

Table 9.2 gives an overview of the main surgical activities in these and 10 other (no longer

Table 9.3 Types of anesthesia used at surgical projects, 2013

	2013		2012		2011		2010	
Type of anesthesia	#	%	#	%	#	%	#	%
Spinal	7,208	37.2	7,294	38.1	7,797	39.7	5,224	33.6
General	7,945	41.0	7,971	41.6	7,961	40.5	7,033	45.2
Intubated	2,183	11.2	1,933	10.1	2,110	10.7	1,636	10.5
Local/regional	1,417	7.3	1,383	7.2	1,191	6.1	1,139	7.4
Combined/others	642	3.3	564	3.0	585	3.0	512	3.3
Total	19,395	100.0	19,145	100.0	19,644	100.0	15,544	100.0

Table 9.4 Ketamine doses and administration at MSF-Belgium surgical projects

Parameter	Anesthesia		Analgesia	
Route	IM/rectal	IV	IM	IV
Dose (mg/kg)	8–10	1–2	2–4	0.3–0.8
Onset (min)	5	1–2	5	1–2
Duration (min)	20–30	10–15	–	–
Maintenance (mg/kg)	5	0.5–1	–	–
Frequency (min)	20–30	15–20	–	–

active) surgery projects during the years 2010–2013 [7]. Focusing on the 14,199 patients treated in 2013, the most common indication for surgery was obstetrical (44.6 % of all patients), 79 % of which were Caesarean sections (data not shown). Accidental trauma was second (26.8 %), followed by violent trauma (10.2 %). At the same time, certain projects involved more complex, specialized types of surgery, for example, high-standard orthopedic procedures such as osteosynthesis and obstetric fistula repair.

In terms of anesthesia practice, around 90 % of all surgeries in 2010–2013 used either general or spinal anesthesia, as shown in Table 9.3. General anesthesia in most MSF contexts uses the intravenous agents ketamine and thiopental as well as the inhalation agent halothane. We consider ketamine an excellent choice for field settings due to its ease of use and safety profile and its widespread uptake throughout middle- and low-income countries (Table 9.4). (However, projects that use ketamine must have resuscitation material available, due to the known risk of respiratory arrest.) Drugs used for muscular relaxation and intubation include depolarizing agents (suxamethonium) and non-depolarizing agents (vecuronium, atracurium).

Spinal anesthesia (SA) is indicated for surgery below the umbilicus, i.e., lower limb surgery, surgery of the inguinal area and amputations; for Caesarean sections we use hyperbaric bupivacaine. Neither adrenaline nor opioids are added to our protocols, as we see no clear advantage.

Principles in MSF Field Anesthesia Practice

A key first principle in our surgical missions is that it is feasible, although challenging, to do safe anesthesia with basic tools and infrastructure: after all, millions of episodes of anesthetic administration are performed safely around the world every year in relatively low-technology settings. Clearly this requires anaesthetists with certain critical skills, but a trained anesthesiologist should know how to deal with the types of emergency situations (such as hemorrhagic shock or polytrauma), which happen everywhere. So in this sense there should be no essential difference between anesthetic practices in Western versus resource-poor settings; the difference is in practical implementation stemming from context-specific constraints.

The fundamental principles we apply to field anesthesia are:

- *Primum non nocere*—patient safety comes first. To achieve this,
- Simpler is often safer. We therefore keep protocols, equipment, etc. as basic as possible, which helps us implement
- The best practices for the majority of patients ("the best for most"). To achieve this,
- Flexibility is key to effectiveness.

On a practical level, MSF surgical/anesthesia activities follow these basic principles:

- Privacy and respect for the patient.
- Consent of the patient, or, if she/he is unable to consent, his or her representative must do so.
- Surgery is intrinsically linked to anesthesia, and vice versa.
- Surgical and anesthesia providers have a formal qualification or MSF validation.
- Surgery and anesthesia arsenals (techniques, equipment, and drugs) are safe, simple, and effective, allowing in most cases a low dependence on sophisticated technology.
- Tight collaboration between the surgical and anesthetic providers is assured.
- Before the start of new projects, a number of defined prerequisites must be in place.
- Surgery and anesthesia care encompass preoperative, intraoperative (perioperative), and postoperative care.
- Quality control is assured by following MSF policies, guidelines and protocols; and by appropriate record-keeping of patient files, including anesthesia/surgical information and other relevant clinical data.
- Emergency preparedness is essential, ensuring the maintenance of skills; the permanent availability of minimum materials, well-functioning sterilization facilities, and regular review; and updating of a Multiple Casualty Plan.

Key Challenges and How MSF Adapts

Adapting to the Local Cultural Context

Although perhaps not evident at first glance, cultural issues are essential to the way we work as field anesthesiologists. Informed consent provides a good example. Consent is important not only as an administrative procedure but, much more—especially in settings where many people cannot read—as a way of explaining to the patient (or family) what will happen during the surgery, what outcome(s) to expect and what difficulties and complications might arise. In many settings where we work, only males can provide consent, so for female patients we need approval from the husband or father. Sometimes the issues around obtaining consent delays surgery, and the medical team might sometimes consider going ahead in exceptional cases if there is urgent medical need but the family could not be briefed on the severity of the patient's condition. However, especially in contexts with high security constraints, it may be better not to proceed under these circumstances, because the reaction if a patient dies may be incomprehension, blame or even violence.

A situation we faced in one project after a natural disaster illustrates this problem. A 9-year-old girl arrived at a neighboring hospital (run by another international organization) that was treating pediatric patients. They called our surgeon to consult, and he determined that the child had acute abdominal pathology and urgently needed surgery. But when the anesthetist arrived and asked for the child's parents, he learned that they had gone to the market to buy milk for the child. The surgeon was in a quandary about whether to proceed, but after some discussion he accepted the need to wait. The medical team could not anticipate how the parents might react if they returned to find their child in the operating theatre; if the child died, they might think that the operation killed her. Since we were in a very violent neighborhood, it was conceivable that someone might have a weapon, or come back later to kill the surgical team. Fortunately the parents returned quickly and gave consent, and the surgery proceeded smoothly. But the story illustrates a risk that affects our decision-making.

Beyond informed consent, cultural norms related to modesty also affect our work. If an anesthetist wants to perform spinal anesthesia but the (female) patient arrives completely covered and refuses to even show her back, the medical team needs to be flexible, innovative and yet cautious. In our projects we work on the premise that everyone has the right to make decisions about their own body regardless of whether they are knowledgeable about medical issues or share our beliefs.

Table 9.5 Gender distribution of surgical patients, 2010–2013

	2013		2012		2011		2010	
Gender	#	%	#	%	#	%	#	%
Female	8,698	61.3	9,072	62.2	10,498	65.3	7,323	62.3
Male	5,501	38.7	5,511	37.8	5,579	34.7	4,423	37.7
Total	14,199	100.0	14,583	100.0	16,077	100.0	11,746	100.0

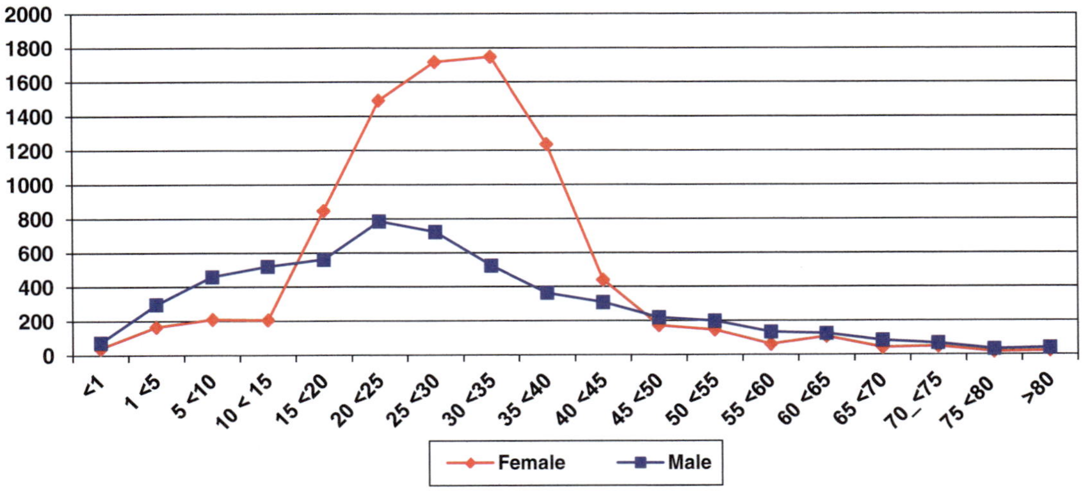

Fig. 9.1 Age distribution by gender at MSF-Belgium surgical projects, 2013

Adapting to the Patients' Profiles and Pathologies

Working in war-affected and underdeveloped countries with largely broken health systems means treating patients with very different profiles and pathologies than those in a typical Western hospital [8].

Although most of our surgical missions receive trauma patients, the majority of whom are male, overall more than 60 % of our surgical patients in 2010–2013 were women, as shown in Table 9.5. They were also overwhelmingly young (see 2013 data in Fig. 9.1), with a mean age of 28 years old for women and 27 for men. Another characteristic of the patients who reach our facilities is that they typically have an acute pathology, such as appendicitis, obstetric emergency, or strangulated hernia, since people with diseases like cancer or heart failure usually die in these settings due to lack of care. The decision to seek care is often difficult for our patients, because they may need money for the journey, or a means of transport. We therefore receive many patients who delayed leaving home when they became ill, or spent several days traveling to the hospital. Many have been treated by a traditional healer before coming to our hospital. Over the few days of these delays, an easily treatable pathology such as appendicitis can become life-threatening acute peritonitis.

The most common pathologies in our surgical patients are obstructed labor, acute abdomen and fractures (trauma), although this varies widely among projects. For obstetrical patients, a typical scenario is obstructed labor leading to a ruptured uterus, so the patient arrives in shock with the baby in her belly. We also see many cases of postpartum hemorrhage, as well as eclampsia and preeclampsia. Our general surgery projects frequently receive patients with visceral abdominal pathologies, such as peritonitis, often stemming from obstructed hernia. The number of trauma cases is highly dependent on the setting: for example, a project at a distant hospital in rural Congo may see fewer trauma cases because patients die before they reach the hospital. Most projects receive many patients with limb injuries, who tend to survive the initial trauma, as well as patients with blunt trauma of the liver or pancreas.

A common challenge these trauma cases present for anesthesiologists is the need to deal with hemorrhagic shock even when blood supplies are extremely limited. Under these circumstances it is sometimes necessary to use autologous hemotransfusion, a procedure that—while not well-known in Western countries—has saved many lives in MSF settings. Teams experienced with this procedure often perform autologous hemotransfusion from hemothorax and ectopic pregnancy. At the same time, the use of tourniquets, quick-clot gauzes, and intraosseus access with drill is common. Ketamine anesthesia has proven to be a good solution for this kind of pathology [9].

Despite this profile being heavily skewed towards acute pathologies, 95 % of our surgical patients in 2013 were considered to have a stable physical status prior to surgical intervention, since they received scores of ASA1 or ASA2 on the American Society of Anesthesiologists (ASA) scale. This scoring system subjectively categorizes patients into six subgroups based on preoperative physical fitness. It makes no adjustment for age, sex, weight, or pregnancy, nor does it reflect the nature of the planned surgery, the skill of the anesthetist or surgeon, the degree of preoperative preparation, or facilities for postoperative care, and thus may not provide the information best suited for our populations. At the same time, poor general health of our patients is another factor surgeons and anesthetists must often consider. For example, many patients in low-resource settings have chronic anemia, with levels of hemoglobin that are astonishingly low by Western standards and that potentially complicate any surgical intervention: we have seen cases of women arriving at our facilities with hemoglobin levels of 5 g/dl, well below the 12 g/dl which defines anemia in adult women, and even below MSF's threshold for proceeding to transfusion, i.e., 7 g/dl.

Clarity About Our Role and the Patient Population We Serve

Anesthetists working in Western countries usually rely heavily on technology for evaluating and monitoring patients, and typically want the same machinery to be available at our missions. However, this is often not feasible or wise, as the examples below illustrate. In practice, decisions on whether and what technology to transfer to the field, and what protocols to follow, go to the heart of understanding our role and how to best serve the most underserved patients—and have led MSF to the principles, mentioned earlier, of prioritizing simplicity and working towards sustainability [10].

For example, should we use an electrocardiograph in our surgeries? While the answer is obvious for Western settings, consider a rural hospital in a remote region of a low-resource country where we work with and train local staff. First, the nurse anesthetist must learn what an electrocardiogram is and in what situations we use it. Then she/he must learn about the different arrhythmias, how to distinguish them, and the drugs needed for each one—and, to be worth this considerable effort, all these drugs should be available locally. At the same time, intensive care facilities are scarce in these settings. Maintaining and repairing electrocardiograph equipment presents yet another set of problems. For these reasons, we have found it safer and more feasible in practice to rely on simpler monitoring protocols, which MSF developed based on the minimal standards for different levels of health care facilities as established by the World Health Organization (WHO) (2003). MSF standards call for the availability of equipment that is simple, safe, and easy to understand and maintain–at a minimum, oxygen (mainly with oxygen concentrators) and basic monitoring equipment (stethoscope, sphygmomanometer, pulse oximetry) must be on hand at all MSF missions with surgical activity. In addition, sites must have adult and pediatric resuscitation bags, suction device (which may be as simply as a foot sucker), laryngoscope set and intubation material, Magill forceps, anesthesia masks of different sizes, pressure infusion bag, and a standard list of drugs and consumables.

Another aspect of this basic-versus-high technology issue to consider is its potential impact on the patient population we serve. For example, our obstetrical surgery projects mainly prioritize Cesarean sections and other obstetrical emergencies. Expatriate medical personnel arriving at these projects sometimes suggest installing incubators for premature babies. But there are usually very few such facilities in the region—so having these incubators would transform our projects into the most advanced maternal centers far and wide, which in turn could end up drawing the country's elite as patients, rather than the local populations we came to serve and who otherwise have little access to care.

A related issue that influences our way of working, including the choice of equipment and protocols, is sustainability, given that MSF missions typically last from periods ranging from several months (e.g., after a natural disaster) to 4–5 years, and occasionally longer. For example, we could bring sophisticated anesthesia drugs used in the USA and elsewhere into our missions. But if we base protocols on these drugs, what happens when we leave? First, it will be difficult or impossible for the host country, institution or patients to access and afford these medicines. Second, there will be few staff trained in their use beyond those who worked with MSF. So instead we focus on medications that are commonly used in the region, that local staff know how to use, and that are affordable. When a project closes, we endeavor to leave behind a functional unit that can continue providing at least some basic care. Whether this is possible depends on many local factors, including security, availability of drugs and consumables, and the skill level and training of local staff (see following section). It also depends greatly on the circumstances of our departure, and is often impossible if we are forced to leave unexpectedly due to a host government withdrawing permission for us to work, or to increased security risks.

Managing Human Resources for Field Anesthesia

Anesthesia providers in MSF medical structures are drawn from a range of personnel that includes anesthesiologists, nurse anesthetists, other types of physicians or nurses, and anesthesia technicians. At the field level, the choice of anesthetist depends upon the human resources (HR) available, the type of project, whether or how much training is conducted, and the quality and quantity of surgical interventions. HR constraints, in turn, are shaped by both the quality and background of the anesthesia provider (anesthesiologist vs. nurse anesthetist; expatriate vs. national staff).

Expatriate anesthetists, especially those who are new to the field, are likely to face several challenges, starting with the fact that she/he may not be trained to work under adverse conditions or in very basic settings, or to use basic drugs such as ketamine [7].

The types and status of anesthesia equipment at surgical projects varies widely, but the standard equipment is usually very basic and high-standard biomedical devices are rare. Operating Theaters may lack monitors and/or defibrillator equipment, and anesthesia machines with ventilators are also uncommon (Ambu-type self-inflating bags offer one solution). Oxygen cylinders are not often available; in this case oxygen concentrators are a useful alternative. There must be a pulse oximeter that measures the saturation and pulse, as called for by the WHO-recommended standards and followed by MSF [9]. We do not use central venous catheters or central venous access due to the difficulty of assuring good-quality care of these devices in the field and to the need to avoid serious complications, especially infection, related to incorrect use.

This means that anesthesiologists at MSF projects usually have to rely mostly on clinical parameters, using their eyes, ears, and knowledge to make diagnoses without access to an arsenal of tools or tests, and to follow patients during surgery without advanced monitoring devices. She/he will probably need to take a blood pressure measurement with a cuff every 5 min during surgery, because typically no automatic machine is available. Without all the customary technology, the anesthesia provider's clinical skills are critical. Moreover, she/he is alone and fully in charge, and may even have to multitask—for example, functioning as a circulating nurse who hands supplies to the surgeon.

Such skills are not easy to find: surgeons and anesthesiologists are scarce, and those who function well in resource-limited settings are even rarer. For this reason, training is an important core activity of MSF-Belgium surgical missions. Different training schemes target different type of specialists, taking into consideration their skills and knowledge, as well as the skills and knowledge needed for implementing MSF's medical strategies and protocols.

Another important HR task is to train local staff. The need to do this may not be obvious, since some international organizations work by bringing in all essential personnel from outside—an approach that usually produces good outcomes from the project's beginning [11, 12]. However, it also means that the hospital usually closes at the end of the mission, since there is insufficient local capacity to continue its work. At MSF-Belgium we try to avoid this approach and instead to incorporate local staff development into our activities. A few years ago this often meant a "task shifting" model, especially in countries where there were simply not enough educated, highly trained people to meet the need for anesthesia services [13].

In practice, task shifting meant turning over anesthesia to someone without much education and who would work independently. This was MSF's approach in Somalia (e.g., in Guri'el, where we trained auxiliary nurses in safe anesthesia, which in this setting meant only ketamine and perhaps spinal anesthesia but not intubation [14]).

Where possible, we now look to "task sharing" —for example, by going into hospitals to coach and work alongside national staff for an extended period of time [15]. Sometimes we work with local staff who are certified nurse anesthetists but have not been trained to a high standard, sending doctors to work with them and improve their knowledge and skills. In other settings, we encounter staff with no training at all in anesthesia. So for example, at some projects in the Democratic Republic of Congo (e.g., Masisi), we worked alongside local staff for several years, teaching them the very basics at first and progressing all the way to intubation; now they are working independently.

Occasionally we do training in more advanced technologies for specific projects. One example is a peripherally inserted central catheter (PICC). These can only be used in selected projects, since in most settings they could do more harm than good. But we introduced them at two projects designated as trauma centers: Kunduz, in northern Afghanistan, which has an intensive care unit and where we trained local physicians on using PICC lines; and Tabarre, in Port-au-Prince, Haiti, where we trained nursing staff, who already have good training and strong skills.

Interacting with Local Staff

Expatriates usually account for only a small proportion of staff at our surgical projects, with national staff typically comprising up to 95 % of personnel. Our experience is that workplace interaction between these two groups often brings some predictable challenges, given the likelihood of a language gap and sometimes the very minimal skill level of local health workers. In some countries where we work, nurses study for only 6 months, and may not know how to perform basic arithmetic calculations or to correctly provide nursing care. Consequently, when an expatriate doctor asks a nurse to do something, the potential for misunderstanding and error is enormous. For example, in one of our projects, an anesthesiologist asked the nurse to give a patient "10 morphines" for postoperative pain. The order was then translated by a (non-medically specialized) translator; not long afterwards the patient went into respiratory depression. It emerged later that the nurse had understood the doctor's order to mean 10 ampules of morphine rather than 10 mg (i.e., one ampule), as the doctor had intended. So the patient got 10 times the intended dosage.

This unnecessary complication served as a reminder that our protocols should be designed with the lack of trained staff in mind, by returning to principles of operational simplicity and sustainability. Our protocols now call for giving as much medication as possible by mouth, and in the fewest possible doses.

It is also crucial for expatriates to remember that local staff are salaried workers with families and communities nearby, and often cannot match the intensive work schedule of outsiders present in the country for a short-term mission focused on doing humanitarian work.

Helping Patients Manage Pain

Pain management is especially challenging in MSF surgical projects for several reasons, starting with limitations on the types of medications available. Another factor is that patients may have a cultural expectation that pain is part of life, which can mean that that they do not complain about or even mention their pain. In our settings, we train the local staff that pain is also a vital sign. Therefore, patients should be systematically asked during ward rounds about the pain they are feeling, based on the use of scales. We mainly use the Face Rating Scale, where a range of different faces (from a big smile to a crying face) is showed to the patients.

Pain can be treated most effectively if it has been properly evaluated, although we recognize that the patient is the only person who can truly know his/her pain intensity. The use of an evaluation scale is mandatory in our projects, with results recorded as for other vital signs. Protocols for pain management are based on the following practices:

- The sooner treatment is initiated, the better.
- It is advisable to give medication before the pain becomes intense.
- Prescriptions should be systematic and taken regularly at fixed times.
- Oral dosing should be used as much as possible.
- Preference must go to multimodal analgesia.

In the MSF context, the analgesics available are WHO level 1, 2, and 3 drugs, including paracetamol, diclofenac, ibuprofen (Level 1), codeine, tramadol (Level 2), and morphine (Level 3). Morphine is the opioid of choice and is preferable to fentanyl (short duration) or pethidine/demerol (weak effect). However, it is difficult to use in the field because few of our staff members are trained to recognize morphine's complications. So we usually advise using and following WHO recommendations, which distinguish three level of pain management beginning with paracetamol and using morphine only at a last resort. Since the dosage requirement of individuals varies, the use of pain scores and clinical examination is mandatory.

Pragmatic Outcomes and Future Directions

In typical MSF field contexts, where the population's basic health needs are usually not being met, the issue of quality is often neglected. This neglect stems largely from the common misperceptions that placing priority on the expansion of coverage inevitably means less focus on quality, and that improving quality requires adoption of more expensive measures, leading to ever-escalating costs. In our experience, reality is much less black-and-white. Ensuring quality at our missions begins with the availability of clear institutional policies, relevant guidelines and strict protocols, all of which (as discussed throughout this chapter) should be well-adapted to the specific context. It also extends to providing the best possible work conditions for the surgical-anesthesia teams and requiring that they follow institutional practices to assure compliance and consistency in patient care.

In terms of monitoring quality, we use intraoperative mortality as a proxy for the delivery of safe anesthesia care. In 2013 MSF-Belgium reported 44 deaths related to its surgical interventions (cases = 19,395), an overall ratio of 0, 2 %—an outcome which demonstrates that it *is* possible to provide quality surgical-anesthesia care in field contexts. However, assessing certain other aspects of surgical care is more challenging, since the difficulty of following up with patients once they leave the hospital impedes the measurement of post-discharge outcomes. This issue is a well-recognized challenge in the field of global surgery; hopefully in the future, we and others will identify feasible ways to evaluate longer-term surgical outcomes and quality.

On a broader level, while it is widely recognized that there is an acute need for surgeons to deliver specialized services in low-income countries, the even greater need for anesthesia providers is often not highlighted [16]. In some humanitarian organizations, this gap is filled by expatriate anesthesia providers (specialized medical doctors and nurses), who make invaluable contributions to their programs and patients. However, it is also a reality that the growing gap between the so-called Western anesthesia practices and the requirements and limitations of field anesthesia make it increasingly difficult to find broadly trained anesthesia specialists with the capacity to be sufficiently adaptable and flexible, and to rely mostly on clinical skills rather than biomedical devices. A big challenge for the field of anesthesiology (and humanitarian organizations) over the coming years is therefore to improve the local anesthesia capacity in low-income countries and to train developed country specialists in the practice of field anesthesia.

References

1. Chu K, Rosseel P, Trelles M, et al. Surgeons without borders: a brief history of surgery at Médecins Sans Frontières. World J Surg. 2010;34(3):411–4.
2. Meara JG, Hagander L, Leather AJM. Surgery and global health: a Lancet Commission. Lancet. 2014; 383(9911):12–3.
3. Lavy C, Sauveen K, Mkandawine N, et al. State of surgery in tropical Africa: a review. World J Surg. 2011;35(2):262–71.
4. Grimes CE, Henry JA, Maraka J, et al. Cost-effectiveness of surgery in low- and middle-income countries: a systematic review. World J Surg. 2014; 38(1):252–63.
5. Gosselin RA, Maldonado A, Elder G. Comparative cost-effectiveness analysis of two MSF surgical trauma centers. World J Surg. 2010;34(3):415–9.
6. Spiegel D, Gosselin R. Surgical services in low-income and middle-income countries. Lancet. 2007; 370(9592):1013–5.
7. Wong EG, Trelles M, Dominguez L, et al. Surgical skills needed for humanitarian missions in resource-limited settings: common operative procedures performed at Médecins Sans Frontières facilities. Surgery. 2014;156(3):642–9.
8. Debas HT. Disease control priorities in developing countries. In: Jamison D et al., editors. Disease control priorities in developing countries. New York: Oxford University Press; 2006. p. 1245–60.
9. World Health Organization. Pulse oximetry training manual, Geneva. 2011. www.who.int/patientsafety/safesurgery/pulse_oximetry/tr_material/en/.
10. Luboga S, Mcfarlane SB, von Schreeb J, et al. Increasing access to surgical services in Sub-Saharan Africa; priorities for national and international agencies recommended by the Bellagio Essential Surgery Group. PLoS Med. 2009;6(12):1–5.
11. Chu KM, Ford NP, Trelles M. Providing surgical care in Somalia: a model of task shifting. Confl Health. 2010;5:12. doi:10.1186/1752-1505-5-12.
12. Ginzburg E, O'Neill WW, Goldschmidt-Clermont PL, et al. Rapid medical relief—Project Medishare and the Haitian earthquake. N Engl J Med. 2010;362:e31. doi:10.1056/NEJMp1002026.
13. Mavalankar D, Sriram V. Provision of anaesthesia services for emergency obstetric care through task shifting in South Asia. Reprod Health Matters. 2009; 17(33):21–31.
14. Chu KM, Trelles M, Ford NP. Quality of care in humanitarian surgery. World J Surg. 2011;35(6): 1169–73.
15. Dawson AJ, Buchan J, Duffield C, Homer CS, Wijewardena K. Task shifting and sharing in maternal and reproductive health in low-income countries: a narrative synthesis of current evidence. Health Policy Plan. 2014;29(3):396–408.
16. Marchbein D. Humanitarian surgery: a call to action for anesthesiologists. Anesthesiology. 2013;119(5): 1001–2.

Quality of Care: Maintaining Safety Through Minimum Standards

10

Kathryn Chu and Monique James

Introduction

One of the greatest challenges in executing effective surgical missions in low and middle resource countries (LMICs) is creating conditions that meet surgical and anesthetic standards of patient safety and quality care. When surgical teams from high income countries (HICs) perform operations in LMICs, they make use of existing hospitals or in emergency settings, sometimes establish makeshift clinical facilities [1]. Replicating HIC conditions would be impossible given technical and financial restraints. However, even with resource limitations and time constraints, establishing minimum standards of care is possible and necessary. Proper planning can maximize the quality of care in both elective and emergency surgical missions.

K. Chu, M.D., M.P.H. (✉)
Eerste River Hospital, Eerste River, South Africa
e-mail: Kathryn_chu@yahoo.com

M. James, M.D., M.P.H.
Icahn School of Medicine at Mount Sinai, Mount Sinai Hospital, New York, NY, USA

Safe Surgery and Quality of Surgical Care

"Surgical care is defined as any procedure that reduces physical disability and premature death by treatment of a surgical condition." [2] In recent years, the safety and quality of surgical care have gained much attention. With increased reporting of surgical outcomes, efforts have been made to minimize complications ranging from wrong-site surgery to preventable perioperative mortality. Patients also have a vested interest in provider-dependent outcomes when choosing a physician [3]. Safety in surgery includes minimizing adverse perioperative events such as 30-day mortality, surgical site infections, cardiac and respiratory complications. It also entails providing the conditions to improve quality of care. There are three pillars of quality of surgical care: structural inputs, processes of care, and direct outcomes measures [3]. Structural inputs include the availability and use of infrastructure and essential material or human resources. A safe structure, electricity, clean water, a blood bank, sterilization equipment, a post-anesthesia recovery unit, anesthetics and analgesics, and qualified surgical and anesthesia providers are the implements of care and the conditions in which the care is provided. Processes of care include protocols and surgical checklists, in other words, the way things get done in a health care system. Direct outcomes

R. Roth et al. (eds.), *The Role of Anesthesiology in Global Health: A Comprehensive Guide*,
DOI 10.1007/978-3-319-09423-6_10, © Springer International Publishing Switzerland 2015

measures include, at minimum, data on morbidity and mortality, which are ideally used in process and structural improvements [3].

Quality of Care in Resource-Rich Settings

In high income countries, multiple well-established systems are in place to measure and improve quality. For example in the USA, the Joint Commission is an organization that evaluates health care organizations and provides accreditation and certification [4]. As of 2010, all US hospitals were required to report compliance with 57 process measures [5]. In addition, various hospitals use the American College of Surgeons National Surgery Quality Improvement Program (ACS-NSQIP), a nationally validated, risk-adjusted, outcomes-based program that has been shown to decrease length of stay, complication rates, mortality, and health care costs [6–9]. The American Society of Anesthesiology's Anesthesia Quality Institute (AQI) maintains a database of perioperative outcomes and quality measures through the National Anesthesia Clinical Outcome Registry (NACOR) and regularly develops best practice guidelines for anesthesia practice through evidence-based medicine and consensus panels [10]. Adverse events are reported and available for later analysis through the Anesthesia Incident Reporting System (AIRS). Another program which uses incentive payments to encourage reporting is the Patient Quality Reporting System (PQRS) which evaluate adherence to process measures such as pre-incision prophylactic antibiotic administration and perioperative temperature monitoring [11].

In addition, patients themselves are invest time and money in finding hospitals and providers that give the best care available in the health care marketplace [3]—they seek the highest quality care through personal recommendations, national hospital rankings, and Internet rating sites such as Doximity. Patients have the ability to choose among providers because there is a high physician- and specialist-to-patient ratio and they have access to transportation and single- or third-party payment systems. In contrast, patients in LMIC have little choice where they receive surgical services; however, their providers should still strive to deliver high quality care.

Quality of Care in Resource-Limited Settings

The World Health Organization (WHO) estimates the frequency of worldwide perioperative events to be 3 % and surgical mortality to be 0.5 % with deaths and complications occurring disproportionately in LMICs [12]. Some countries in Sub-Saharan Africa (SSA) have reported perioperative mortality as high as 5–10 % [13, 14], and high anesthesia-related mortality rates have been reported in Malawi (1:500), Zimbabwe (1:500), and Togo (1:133) [15–17] which is significantly higher than in HIC (1:200,000) [18]. Most of these deaths are avoidable and due to lack of available blood products or inadequate or absent perioperative monitoring such as lack of pulse oximetry [15–17].

The quality of surgical care in LMICs is also difficult to measure. Human resources are limited and collecting routine outcome data is challenging. Longitudinal outcomes such as 30-day morbidity and mortality are particularly difficult to track when patients cannot return for follow-up and/or do not have contact information. Currently, most LMIC hospitals are not required by any regulatory body to report patient outcomes or implement quality process measures. National quality systems like NSQIP, AIRS, and PQRS and hospital accreditation organizations such as the Joint Commission do not usually exist.

International organizations such as the WHO and others that deliver surgical care in LMICs have begun to recognize this lack of oversight. In 2007, the World Health Organization (WHO) launched the Safe Surgery Saves Lives Project aimed at "improving the safety of surgical care around the world by ensuring adherence to proven standards of care in all states." [19] Acknowledging that anesthesia providers on medical missions will be practicing in areas with variable local quality standards, the remainder of this chapter focuses on the challenges of and strategies for providing safe and quality surgical care in LMICs including ways to implement minimum standards on location.

Minimum Standards for Surgical Missions

Pre-trip Assessment

Surgical missions in LMICs may be conducted in a variety of settings. Often, a team from a HIC is invited by a LMIC government hospital or a private organization to perform elective or semi-elective operations. In other instances, a humanitarian surgical team will set up surgical care in a post-disaster setting such as a hurricane or an earthquake, or during a conflict and perform emergency procedures where no preexisting structure or local partner is available [1]. In all instances, a pre-trip assessment is essential to quantify available resources. This can be done remotely but more ideally by a site visit prior to the start of the mission. In an emergency, the assessment can be done expeditiously before the entire surgical team is mobilized, and should be conducted by the team member(s) most experienced in surgical care for the specific setting.

This assessment refines mission objectives based on resources that are readily available or able to be mobilized. The specific role and capacity of local partners, surgical providers, nursing and support staff and the existing infrastructure, equipment, and supplies must be defined to meet the needs identified in the assessment. The types of procedures that can be safely performed must also be determined and team members briefed before the mission of these limitations. For example, if the LMIC setting does not have the postoperative monitoring or nursing ratio for cardiothoracic surgery, these procedures must not be allowed even if surgical providers have the skills to perform them. Recognizing when not to operate is as important in a low resource setting as knowing when to operate.

A useful assessment instrument is the Tool for Situational Analysis to Assess Emergency and Essential Surgical Care [20]. Developed in 2007 as part of The WHO Global Initiative on Emergency and Essential Surgery Care (GIEESC), the 152-item questionnaire evaluates infrastructure, human resources, procedures currently performed, and the availability of emergency equipment and supplies for resuscitation. It was developed for LMIC and can be used by local and international organizations alike.

Coordination with local health authorities must be clearly established prior to the mission. In elective missions, collaboration with a local partner organization and use of a preexisting hospital is likely. How the surgical mission will fit into the hospital's routine service delivery must be discussed with the appropriate management. Surgical missions can disrupt routine health care delivery but local staff may be reluctant to speak out because they do not want to seem unappreciative. In emergency missions, no functional hospital may exist. Obtaining permission from local health authorities, such as the Ministry of Health, to deliver care is important. Assuming that surgical intervention is welcome without an invitation from local health authorities is an arrogant attitude and can result in poor coordination and duplication of services, especially in large disasters with many humanitarian teams [21].

Minimum Intraoperative Standards and Quality Surgical Care in LMIC

In order to maintain safety and quality of care, surgical missions should strive to establish minimum standards. After large natural disasters, many humanitarian surgical mission teams are eager to provide care. However, the safety and quality of care of some of the teams have been questioned by the general public and other surgical teams. For example, after the 2010 earthquake in Port-au-Prince, many amputations were performed by surgical missions and criticism from other surgical teams arose regarding whether some of these were preventable if there had been higher quality of care or standardized protocols [22].

Structural Inputs

Médecins Sans Frontières (MSF), a medical humanitarian organization that has provided care in resource-limited settings for over 40 years, has established minimum criteria for structural inputs needed before humanitarian surgery can be delivered. These standards include a safe structure, electricity, clean water, a blood bank, sterilization equipment, a post-anesthesia recovery unit, anesthetics, analgesics, antibiotics, and qualified surgery and anesthesia providers [21]. Elective surgical missions should also adhere to these requirements [23]. While HIC resources such as intensive care units, invasive intraoperative arterial monitoring and computed tomography scan are not always available, basic structural, process, and outcome conditions should be established.

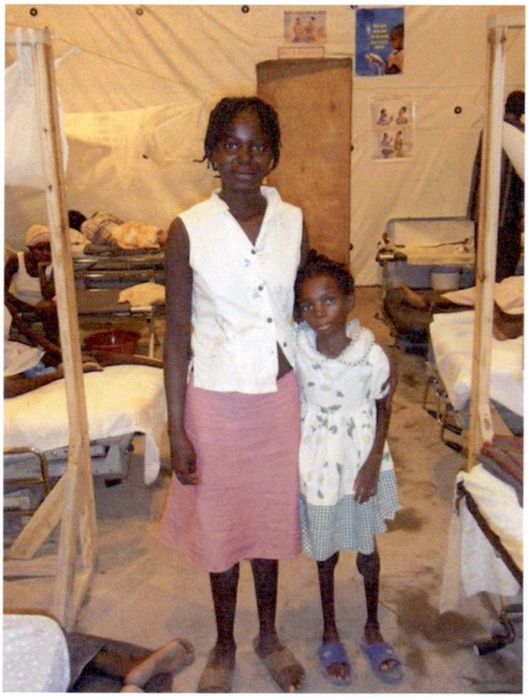

Fig. 10.1 In 2008, three hurricaines struck the island nation of Haiti. The Arbonite region was most severely afffected with the only hospital flooded and unusable. Medecins Sans Frontieres, a humanitarian organization, created a hospital in a warehouse in a few weeks. This hospital had an emergency department, inpatient wards, outpatient clinics and an operating theatre

Safe Structure

Surgical care must be delivered in a safe building. In 2008, extensive flooding ruined the local hospital in the Arbonite region of Haiti. During the pre-mission assessment MSF emergency coordinators determined the existing hospital could not be salvaged and a warehouse was converted into a temporary hospital with inpatient wards, an emergency department and an operating theater within a few weeks [1] (see (Fig. 10.1). After the 2010 earthquake in Port-au-Prince, over 200,000 persons died, thousands more were injured, and many buildings were structurally damaged including La Trinité, a MSF trauma hospital [24]. Alternative structures, including some government hospitals that were structurally safe but had not been providing surgical care, were identified and utilized. MSF also organized an inflatable tent hospital and eventually established a hospital in a container that included operating rooms and surgical wards [24] (see Fig. 10.2). These examples demonstrate that buildings that already in place, repurposed locations, or purpose-built portable structures can all serve as hospitals when required.

Electricity

Surgical care requires electricity to power anesthesia machines and surgical equipment such as operating room lighting, electrocautery, and suction. It is also helpful (but not necessary) to sterilize equipment using autoclaves, clean linens, and maintain refrigeration for the cold chain of medications and laboratory reagents. In LMICs, electricity is a precious commodity that is not readily available at all times. Some hospitals use back up generators during electricity shortages. Surgical missions must be prepared for these conditions by purchasing gasoline for host generators, bringing portable lighting, and using surgical and anesthesia equipment that are battery-operated. In response to the lack of reliable power sources in LMICs, many manufacturers have created medical technology that does not rely on electricity.

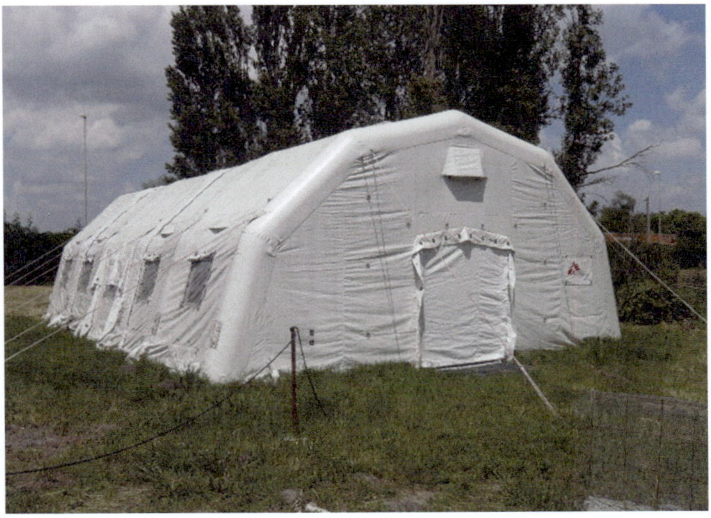

Fig. 10.2 A safe structure is needed for surgery. When a hospital or existing infrastructure is not available, alternatives are needed. Medecins Sans Frontieres has inflatable tents for emergencies which have several departments including emergency, inpatient wards, operating theatres, and even an intensive care unit. These tents have been recently used in the 2010 Haiti earthquake

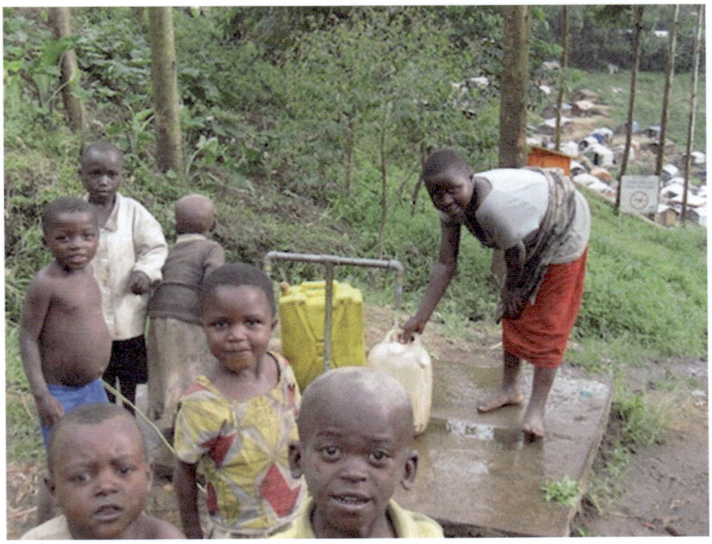

Fig. 10.3 Clean water is an essential right and access is a Millennium Development Goal. An estimated 15–20 L/person/day is needed for personal use and consumption but hospitals need up to 150–200/L/person/day for surgical procedures. Children collecting clean water at a common water point at an internally displaced camp, Masisi, Democratic Republic of Congo

Anesthesia machines with manual ventilators, oxygen compressors/concentrators with battery power capability and portable operating room lights, are just a few examples of equipment available for resource-limited settings [25]. For example, the Universal Anaesthesia Machine, manufactured by Gradian Health Systems, has a manual ventilator and oxygen concentrating mechanism that does not require compressed gases and can function in areas with unreliable power sources [26].

Clean Water

Clean water is needed to provide safe and quality surgical care. Routine hand washing by providers reduces wound infections and cross contamination and the spread of infection [27]. One of the Millennium Development Goals is to halve the number of persons living without drinking water and safe sanitation [28] (Fig. 10.3). The Sphere project, a volunteer initiative for humanitarian agencies has established minimum standards in humanitarian response and recommends 40–60 L of clean water/day/hospitalized patient [29]. For surgical care more is needed and used for cleaning and sterilizing surgical instruments and anesthesia machines, washing linens, and irrigating wounds. MSF recommends 100–300 L/patient/surgical procedure [30]. Sufficient water should be stored on the premises to ensure a steady and uninterrupted supply. If clean water is not available then water and sanitation experts should be a part of the surgical mission to supply or to chlorinate existing sources [31] (see Fig. 10.4).

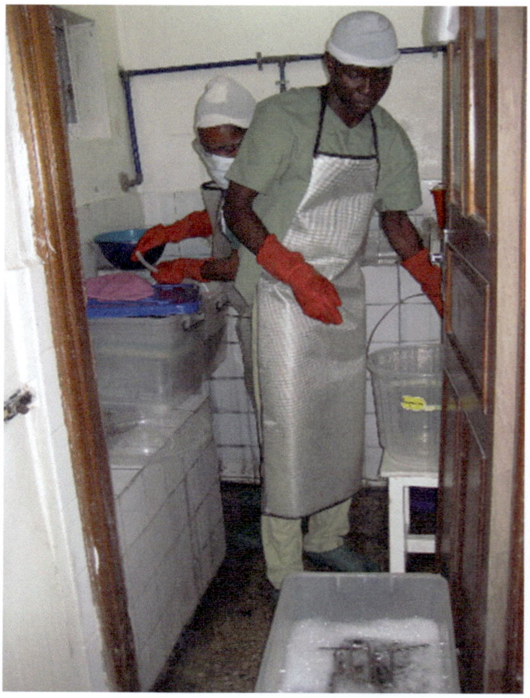

Fig. 10.4 Clean water is a minimum standard of care in humanitarian surgery because it is required for sanitation and sterilization. Photo by Pascale Choquenet

Blood Bank

Preoperative, intraoperative, and postoperative hemorrhage can be life threatening. The ability to transfuse a surgical patient with safe blood can save his or her life. In [29] LMICs, national transfusion services rarely exist and regional hospitals must rely on local blood banks with limited resources [32]. Each mission should have a transfusion protocol since blood is a precious commodity and should not be wasted. Elective surgical missions should identify the nearest blood bank. Emergency missions may have to set up their own system.

Organization should be aware that, at the minimum, blood banks must perform ABO typing and screening for human immunodeficiency virus (HIV), hepatitis B, hepatitis C, and syphilis [33]. Often the ability to store more than a few units of blood is limited by storage capacity and electricity. A list of prescreened potential donors with known blood types can be maintained especially for elective surgical procedures. If an effective blood cold chain does not exist, the transfusion of fresh, whole blood should be used [34]. More details on how to set up a blood bank can be found in the WHO manual, Blood Cold Chain [34].

Campaigns for voluntary unpaid donors are the ideal and safest way to maintain a blood bank; however, during short-term medical missions this can be both costly and time-consuming [33]. When relying on family replacement donors for whole blood during humanitarian surgical missions, the real risk of not transfusing must be weighed against the risk to the patient of contracting a transfusion transmitted illness (TTI) from an unscreened family member and the risk (or perceived risk) to the family member of contracting a TTI from the implements of blood collection [35]. Because of the complexities of providing safe banked or donated blood in a low resource setting, a protocol for blood conservation, intraoperative normothermia, and, if possible, pretreatment of existing anemia should also be in place for any surgical mission.

Sterilization Equipment

In order to safely perform surgery in any setting, sterilization equipment is needed. Simple autoclaves can be powered by wood burning, gas, or electricity and sterilize surgical equipment through high pressure steam at 121 °C for approximately 15–20 min. MSF uses several different models some pictured here (see Fig. 10.5).

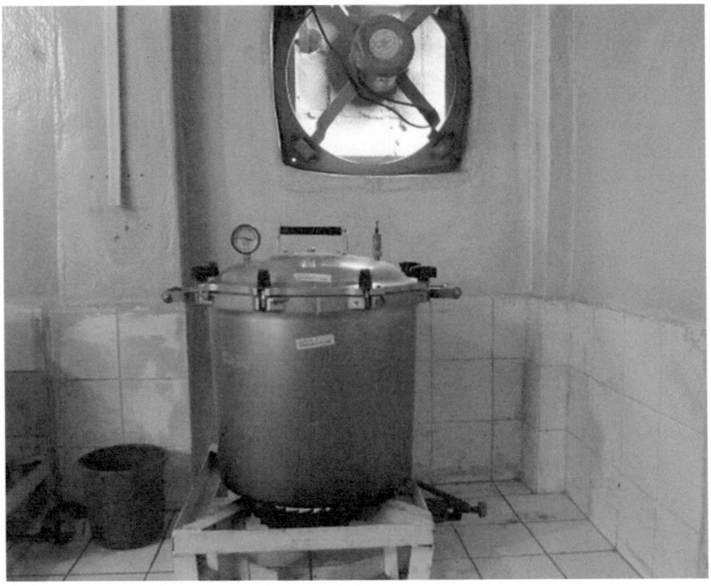

Fig. 10.5 Proper sterilization is a minimum standard for care for all surgical missions. Autoclaves can be small and basic like this 39 L wood burning one, which does not need electricity. Photo used with permission from Pascale Choquenet

Pharmaceutical Agents

Depending on the surgery general, regional, or local anesthetic agents and analgesics are required. For general anesthesia, inhaled anesthetics such as halothane, isoflurane, and sevoflurane may be used in functional anesthesia machines with vaporizers based on availability of agents and equipment. If these are not available, total intravenous anesthesia can be provided with anesthetics such as propofol, ketamine, thiopental, opioids, and benzodiazepenes [36]. In limited resource areas that do not have reliable oxygen supplies, regional and neuraxial anesthesia with local anesthetics may help to limit alterations in baseline patient physiology [37]. When providing any type of anesthesia care, access to resuscitation medications such as vasopressors, chronotropes, and ionotropes is imperative. Antibiotics covering a broad spectrum of gram-positive, gram-negative, and anaerobic organisms are needed for perioperative treatment and prophylaxis. If these basic medications are not available in the LMIC hospital where the surgical mission is to take place, then they must be brought in or sourced and managed on site (see Fig. 6). When considering medications needed for a medical mission, the WHO Model Lists of Essential Medicines are useful guides that can be tailored based on the clinical conditions and cases anticipated [38].

Anesthesia Monitoring and Equipment

The use of pulse oximetry for intraoperative monitoring saves lives. It is recommended as a minimum standard of monitoring by the WHO, yet over 70,000 operating rooms worldwide lack this essential equipment [39]. The WHO Patient Safety Pulse Oximetry Project aims to improve the safety of surgical care by training surgical providers how to use pulse oximeters [40] and works with organizations like Lifebox who donate pulse oximeters to LMIC hospitals that do not have them [41]. Although pulse oximetry fulfills the minimum standard for anesthesia monitoring, a noninvasive blood pressure cuff and thermometer can be helpful for preoperative assessment as well as intraoperative and postoperative monitoring. Anesthesia care should always be provided under the supervision and vigilance of a trained professional assigned to the care of each surgical patient [42].

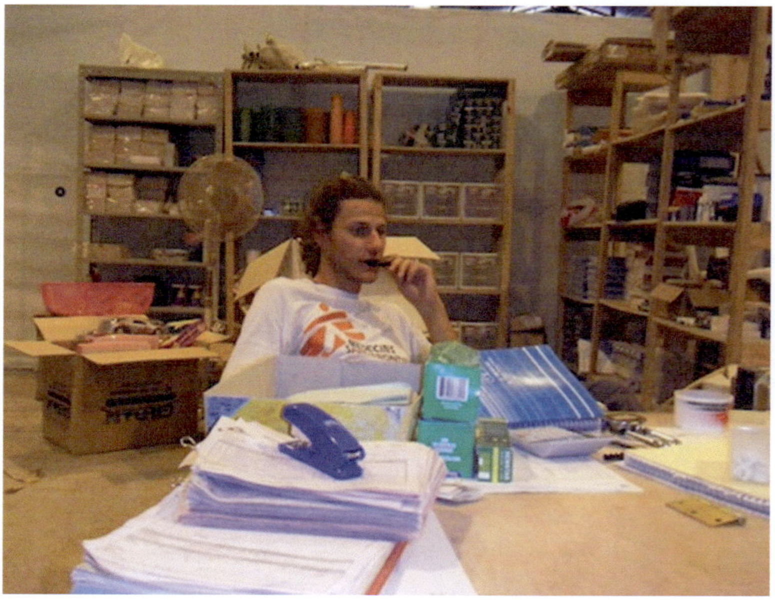

Fig. 10.6 A pharmacy that stocks essential medications such as anesthetic agents, antibiotics, and analgesics is needed in any surgical mission. If the local hospital does not have one, this must be created. Importing medications, even for humanitarian use, must be cleared with the appropriate authorities ahead of time

In emergency surgery, general anesthesia is often the appropriate anesthetic technique. Certain equipment and monitoring are needed to safely anesthetize patients. Airway management requires both oxygenation and ventilation. Oxygen sources include wall supplies, oxygen cylinders or oxygen compressors. Positive pressure ventilation can be applied with a bag valve mask with positive end expiratory pressure (PEEP) valve or with a ventilator. In preparation for medical missions, anesthesia providers should carry functional laryngoscopes and endotracheal tubes in a variety of sizes, supraglottic airways, oral airways, oro/nasogastric tubes and suction. These supplies allow for the adequate oxygenation and positive-pressure ventilation of a patient while decreasing the risk of aspiration.

In LMIC hospitals, regional and neuraxial anesthesia are invaluable anesthetic techniques. Routine use of regional and neuraxial anesthesia allows providers in low resource settings to avoid many of the economic and hemodynamic pitfalls and challenges that exist with routine use of general anesthesia [43, 44]. Spinal anesthesia can be used for a variety of lower extremity, pelvic, and abdominal surgeries particularly when oxygen is in limited supply. Regional anesthesia with the use of portable ultrasonography or nerve stimulation can provide adequate operative anesthesia, as well as postoperative analgesia for patients in hospitals with limited access to analgesic medications or limited postoperative patient monitoring [45, 46]. It is important to say that the rescue airway equipment mentioned above should always available in case of complications such as caudal spread of a neuraxial anesthetic or local anesthetic toxicity.

Postoperative Recovery Unit (PACU)

The immediate postoperative period can be a dangerous time if hypotension, hypoxia, hypercarbia, or ischemic events occur in unmonitored patients. If these life-threatening conditions are not accurately and quickly identified, they cannot be treated appropriately and death may follow quickly. Some LMIC hospitals do not have enough physical or human resources to have a dedicated PACU and patients are sent back to the postoperative surgical ward immediately after a procedure. This practice is especially risky after general anesthesia or in the face of respiratory or cardiac disease. Humanitarian surgeons should ensure a PACU exists at the hospital they are using, else one must be established. Experienced PACU nurses need to be part of the team if the pre-trip assessment shows a lack of qualified local personnel.

Qualified Surgical and Anesthesia Providers

One of the main reasons the unmet burden of surgical disease in LMICs is so great is the lack of surgical providers [47]. Surgical providers include all personnel involved in the delivery of surgical care including surgeons, anesthesiologists, PACU and surgical ward nurses. HIC surgical providers can play an important role in reducing the LMIC surgical burden through surgical missions. However, they should only provide care (including performing surgery and administering anesthesia) in LMIC for which they are qualified. If a surgeon cannot perform an amputation safely in the USA, then s/he should not be allowed to perform that operation other countries. If an anesthesia provider has not practiced pediatric cardiac anesthesiology since fellowship, s/he should not be allowed to do so during a mission.

Unfortunately, some surgical missions have given humanitarian surgery a bad reputation by adopting the attitude that LMIC patients can be "practiced upon" or that "any care is better than no care" [48, 49]. Surgical and anesthesia residents should not be allowed to operate or provide anesthesia without appropriate supervision regardless of the setting. Currently, no specific credentials are needed for HIC surgeons and anesthesiologists to work in surgical missions. Studies in high-income countries have shown that surgical quality is directly related to surgeon experience [50–53]. Surgeons and anesthesiologists planning to go on elective or emergency missions should receive special training to be better prepared for working in resource-limited settings. MSF and the International Committee for the Red Cross provide additional trauma training for their surgeons to work in war zones.

Processes of Care

The most important measure shown to improve quality of care is adherence to processes of care [3]. Basic protocols such as administration of perioperative antibiotics, the use of pulse oximetry for intraoperative monitoring, and checklists are processes than can be established on surgical missions. This might require pre-trip training of team members or on site training at the beginning of the mission with local staff.

Perioperative Antibiotic Protocols

Appropriate use of prophylactic antibiotics reduces postoperative infections [54]. Some patients will also need a course of postoperative antibiotics especially for contaminated conditions. Antibiotic protocols for common procedures, such as single dose prophylaxis for Cesarean sections can greatly reduce wound infections and endometritis [55]. Surgical missions should establish protocols for the procedures they perform. Antibiotic regimens may have to be adapted for the LMIC setting as there will be fewer choices of agents, but evidence based medicine should be practiced in humanitarian surgery just as pertains in HIC settings.

Checklists

Checklists save lives by standardizing basic safety checks and preparation for complex tasks. The airline industry has demonstrated this unequivocally with pre-flight checklists [56]. Checklists improve surgical quality by changing the culture of practice and ensuring that processes of care are followed [57]. In 2009, WHO published a 19-item surgical checklist that reduces morbidity and mortality in HIC and LMIC [58]. This checklist can be modified for each setting; its main purpose is to ensure that processes of care are adhered to for each individual patient. An adaptation of this surgical safety checklist for humanitarian surgery is shown in, Table 10.1 [1].

Table 10.1 Surgical checklist adapted for humanitarian surgery (adapted with permission from World Journal of Surgery, Chu [1])

1.	Perform anesthesia pre-operative evaluation
2.	Pulse oximetry is available and working
3.	Procedure explained to patient and written consent signed
4.	Confirm patient identification
5.	Mark operative site
6.	If significant fluid/blood loss expected, obtain appropriate intravenous access and ensure availability of fluid/blood products
7.	The appropriate surgical instruments are available to perform procedure
8.	Antibiotics have been given if wound is/expected to be contaminated
9.	Postanesthesia care is available
10.	Postoperative care protocol is established
11.	In a mass casualty, the procedure performed, date of dressing change or re-intervention are written on the bandage
12.	Patient and surgical data entered into a database

Checklists can greatly benefit surgical missions by improving communication between team members from different institutions and local and international providers who speak different primary languages.

Data Collection and Outcomes Assessment

Most surgical missions do not collect outcome data and therefore morbidity and mortality rates for humanitarian surgery are largely unknown. For example, numerous agencies performed thousands of procedures during the 2010 earthquake, but death and infection rates were not reported [59–62]. This resulted in undetected patient morbidity and mortality and an inability to improve the quality of care delivered. Some organizations collect patient demographic and procedural information and have conducted studies to determine morbidity and mortality. For example, MSF, using a standardized database containing nearly 20,000 procedures, reported an operative mortality rate of 0.2 %. Operation Smile, an organization which repairs cleft palates in LMICs, followed over 700 patients during a 4 week period in 19 countries giving individual surgeons feedback regarding complications and identifying areas of program improvement [63]. While these studies demonstrate the feasibility of data collection in resource limited settings, ongoing routine outcome data collection has not been reported by any humanitarian surgical agency. Moreover, since internationally standardized databases for humanitarian surgery do not exist, interpretation and comparison of data from various agencies are difficult [64].

Humanitarian surgery missions should be required to routinely collect data on structure, process, and outcome indicators. Local funding and human resources are often too scarce to conduct patient follow-up so surgical missions should ensure their budget allows the short-term employment of a local provider to track short and long term outcomes once the mission is over. Importantly, the surgical mission should analyze this data and give feedback to the host hospital or local agency. This information can be used to improve the quality of surgical care in future LMIC missions. When HIC providers carry out other public health interventions in LMIC such as maternal and neonatal care, HIV prevention, and vaccination programs, they are required by local ministries of health to submit data for routine monitoring and evaluation to improve program policy and protocols. There should be similar requirements for surgical missions. One proposed way to begin measuring surgical/anesthesia safety and increase awareness of avoidable perioperative complications in LMICs is the implementation and mandatory reporting of a postoperative mortality rate (POMR). POMR is defined as the number of perioperative deaths in ASA Classification I and II patients per 100,000 people [30]. This data is a basic part of any operating room log and can lead to further evaluation and comparison of surgical outcomes between countries. In addition, reporting of preventable mortality can help to stimulate action on the national and international levels.

Oversight and Regulation

As surgical missions become more commonplace, an international regulatory body should be created to provide oversight. While HIC standards cannot be completely translated to LMIC settings, as detailed above, minimum safe standards can be applied. Host LMIC or the HIC initiating the mission should require humanitarian surgeons and anesthesiologists to provide minimum standards through infrastructures such as appropriate medications and human resources, adherence to protocols, use of checklists, and simple databases to follow short and long term outcomes. An international regulatory body could maintain a central repository with standardized databases created for humanitarian surgery such as the clinical trials repository [65]. This regulatory body would receive post-mission reports from all humanitarian surgery missions and analyze complications in order to improve care. In the meantime, other resources exist. For example, the American College of Surgeons has a free online case log system and members who conduct humanitarian surgery can enter their cases [66].

Way Forward

Interest in global surgery is increasing exponentially [67]. It is estimated that surgical missions perform at least a quarter of a million procedures in LMIC; however, this is an underestimation since many missions do not publish their surgical activity [30]. Elective and emergency missions can help address the global burden of surgical disease. More importantly, they can improve the quality of care at LMIC host hospitals by introducing protocols, checklists, and a new culture of safety in global surgery. Such efforts demonstrate to local staff what can be achieved even in resource-limited settings.

Summary

The quality of surgical services in humanitarian settings is rarely assessed. Most LMIC countries are grateful for surgical care and do not have the resources to provide oversight. As HIC surgical and anesthesia providers increasingly become involved in surgical missions, the need to establish a framework for quality surgical delivery is more pressing.

Surgical missions must prepare for their trip in several ways. First, a pre-trip needs assessment must be conducted to assess existing resources and identify gaps in minimum standards in structural inputs, processes of care and outcome measures. A safe structure, electricity, clean water, sterilization equipment, a blood bank, a PACU, and appropriate medication and surgical providers are needed. Certain processes of care such as protocols and checklists should be decided upon ahead of time. A database should be established capturing patient demographics, procedural data, and outcomes. The mission and local administrators should decide which indicators can be realistically captured and how they will be collected especially longer-term outcomes. A well-defined mechanism for reporting data to local and international program directors and mission participants is needed; results should always translate into process or structural change. At the end of the surgical mission, local and international team members should give feedback and suggestions for improvements. All aspects of care, even structural inputs can be improved, especially if the project is a long term one. Humanitarian surgeons and anesthesiologists must strive to provide quality care and can be ambassadors for a new culture of safety in global surgery.

References

1. Chu KM, Trelles M, Ford NP. Quality of care in humanitarian surgery. World J Surg. 2011;35(6):1169–72. discussion 1173–1164.
2. Bickler S, Ozgediz D, Gosselin R, et al. Key concepts for estimating the burden of surgical conditions and the unmet need for surgical care. World J Surg. 2010;34(3):374–80.
3. Birkmeyer JD, Dimick JB, Birkmeyer NJ. Measuring the quality of surgical care: structure, process, or outcomes? J Am Coll Surg. 2004;198(4):626–32.
4. The Joint Commission. http://www.jointcommission.org. Accessed 1 May 2014.
5. Chassin MR, Loeb JM, Schmaltz SP, Wachter RM. Accountability measures—using measurement to promote quality improvement. N Engl J Med. 2010;363(7):683–8.

6. Hall BL, Hamilton BH, Richards K, Bilimoria KY, Cohen ME, Ko CY. Does surgical quality improve in the American College of Surgeons National Surgical Quality Improvement Program: an evaluation of all participating hospitals. Ann Surg. 2009;250(3):363–76.
7. Khuri SF. The NSQIP: a new frontier in surgery. Surgery. 2005;138(5):837–43.
8. Khuri SF, Daley J, Henderson W, et al. The Department of Veterans Affairs' NSQIP: the first national, validated, outcome-based, risk-adjusted, and peer-controlled program for the measurement and enhancement of the quality of surgical care. National VA Surgical Quality Improvement Program. Ann Surg. 1998;228(4):491–507.
9. Khuri SF, Henderson WG, Daley J, et al. Successful implementation of the Department of Veterans Affairs' National Surgical Quality Improvement Program in the private sector: the Patient Safety in Surgery study. Ann Surg. 2008;248(2):329–36.
10. Anesthesia Quality Institute. https://www.aqihq.org/index.aspx. Accessed 1 May 2014.
11. Physician Quality Reporting System. http://www.cms.gov/Medicare/Quality-Initiatives-Patient-Assessment-Instruments/pqrs/index.html. Accessed 1 May 2014.
12. Schlack WS, Boermeester MA. Patient safety during anaesthesia: incorporation of the WHO safe surgery guidelines into clinical practice. Curr Opin Anaesthesiol. 2010;23(6):754–8.
13. McConkey SJ. Case series of acute abdominal surgery in rural Sierra Leone. World J Surg. 2002;26(4):509–13.
14. Bickler SW, Sanno-Duanda B. Epidemiology of paediatric surgical admissions to a government referral hospital in the Gambia. Bull World Health Organ. 2000;78(11):1330–6.
15. Ouro-Bang'na Maman AF, Tomta K, Ahouangbevi S, Chobli M. Deaths associated with anaesthesia in Togo, West Africa. Trop Doct. 2005;35(4):220–2.
16. Hansen D, Gausi SC, Merikebu M. Anaesthesia in Malawi: complications and deaths. Trop Doct. 2000;30(3):146–9.
17. McKenzie AG. Mortality associated with anaesthesia at Zimbabwean teaching hospitals. S Afr Med J. 1996;86(4):338–42.
18. WHO guidelines for safe surgery 2009: safe surgery saves lives. Geneva; 2009.
19. Safe Surgery Saves Lives. http://www.who.int/patientsafety/safesurgery/en/. Accessed 10 May 2014.
20. Tool for Situational Analysis to Assess Emergency and Essential Surgical Care. http://www.who.int/surgery/publications/QuickSitAnalysisEESCsurvey.pdf. Accessed 7 May 2014.
21. Chu K, Stokes C, Trelles M, Ford N. Improving effective surgical delivery in humanitarian disasters: lessons from Haiti. PLoS Med. 2011;8(4):e1001025.
22. Unnecessary Amputations Performed in Haiti? http://limblossinformationcentre.com/2010/02/05/unnecessary-amputations-performed-in-haiti/. Accessed 7 May 2014.
23. Merry AF, Cooper JB, Soyannwo O, Wilson IH, Eichhorn JH. International Standards for a Safe Practice of Anesthesia 2010. Can J Anaesth. 2010;57(11):1027–34.
24. International Activity Report 2010-Haiti. http://www.msf.org/international-activity-report-2010-haiti. Accessed 7 May 2014.
25. Venticinque SG, Grathwohl KW. Critical care in the austere environment: providing exceptional care in unusual places. Crit Care Med. 2008;36(7 Suppl):S284–92.
26. The Universal Anesthesia Machine. http://www.gradianhealth.org/universal-anaesthesia-machine/. Accessed 16 May 2014.
27. Hand Hygeine in Healthcare Settings. http://www.cdc.gov/handhygiene/Basics.html. Accessed 12 May 2014.
28. UNICEF WASH strategies. http://www.unicef.org/wash/index_43084.html. Accessed 17 May 2014.
29. The Sphere Project. http://www.spherehandbook.org/en/appendix-2/. Accessed 27 May 2014.
30. McQueen KA, Parmar P, Kene M, et al. Burden of surgical disease: strategies to manage an existing public health emergency. Prehosp Disaster Med. 2009;24 Suppl 2:s228–31.
31. Water and Sanitation. http://www.msf.org/topics/water-and-sanitation. Accessed 17 May 2014.
32. Basavaraju SV, Mwangi J, Nyamongo J, et al. Reduced risk of transfusion-transmitted HIV in Kenya through centrally co-ordinated blood centres, stringent donor selection and effective p24 antigen-HIV antibody screening. Vox Sang. 2010;99(3):212–9.
33. Blood safety and availability. http://www.who.int/mediacentre/factsheets/fs279/en/. Accessed 17 May 2014.
34. The blood cold chain. http://www.who.int/mediacentre/factsheets/fs279/en/. Accessed 17 May 2014.
35. Erhabor O, Adias TC, Mainasara A. Provision of safe blood transfusion services in a low income setting in West Africa. Case study of Nigeria. In: Berhardt L, editor. Advances in medicine and biology, vol. 59. New York, USA: Nova Science Publishers; 2013. p. 1–58.
36. Mellor AJ. Anaesthesia in austere environments. J R Army Med Corps. 2005;151(4):272–6.
37. Morey TE, Rice MJ. Anesthesia in an austere setting: lessons learned from the Haiti relief operation. Anesthesiol Clin. 2013;31(1):107–15.
38. WHO model lists of essential medicines. http://www.who.int/medicines/publications/essentialmedicines/en/. Accessed 19 May 2014.
39. Walker IA, Newton M, Bosenberg AT. Improving surgical safety globally: pulse oximetry and the WHO Guidelines for Safe Surgery. Paediatr Anaesth. 2011;21(7):825–8.
40. WHO patient safety pulse oximetry project. http://www.who.int/patientsafety/safesurgery/pulse_oximetry/en/. Accessed 10 May 2014.
41. Lifebox. http://www.lifebox.org. Accessed 10 May 2014.

42. Chackungal S, Nickerson JW, Knowlton LM, et al. Best practice guidelines on surgical response in disasters and humanitarian emergencies: report of the 2011 Humanitarian Action Summit Working Group on Surgical Issues within the Humanitarian Space. Prehosp Disaster Med. 2011;26(6):429–37.
43. Inipavudu B, Mitterschiffthaler G, Hasibeder WR, Dunser MW. Spinal versus epidural anesthesia for vesicovaginal fistula repair surgery in a rural sub-Saharan African setting. J Clin Anesth. 2007;19(6):444–7.
44. Surgical care at the district hospital. http://www.who.int/surgery/publications/en/SCDH.pdf?ua=1. Accessed 27 May 2014.
45. Allcock E, Spencer E, Frazer R, Applegate G, Buckenmaier 3rd C. Continuous transversus abdominis plane (TAP) block catheters in a combat surgical environment. Pain Med. 2010;11(9):1426–9.
46. Buckenmaier 3rd CC, Lee EH, Shields CH, Sampson JB, Chiles JH. Regional anesthesia in austere environments. Reg Anesth Pain Med. 2003;28(4):321–7.
47. Ozgediz D, Hsia R, Weiser T, et al. Population health metrics for surgery: effective coverage of surgical services in low-income and middle-income countries. World J Surg. 2009;33(1):1–5.
48. Gilbert BJ, Miller C, Corrick F, Watson RA. Should trainee doctors use the developing world to gain clinical experience? The annual Varsity Medical Debate—London, Friday 20th January, 2012. Philos Ethics Humanit Med. 2013;8:1.
49. Ramsey KM, Weijer C. Ethics of surgical training in developing countries. World J Surg. 2007;31(11):2067–9. discussion 2070-2061.
50. Bilimoria KY, Phillips JD, Rock CE, Hayman A, Prystowsky JB, Bentrem DJ. Effect of surgeon training, specialization, and experience on outcomes for cancer surgery: a systematic review of the literature. Ann Surg Oncol. 2009;16(7):1799–808.
51. Dimick JB, Birkmeyer JD, Upchurch Jr GR. Measuring surgical quality: what's the role of provider volume? World J Surg. 2005;29(10):1217–21.
52. Rogo-Gupta LJ, Lewin SN, Kim JH, et al. The effect of surgeon volume on outcomes and resource use for vaginal hysterectomy. Obstet Gynecol. 2010;116(6):1341–7.
53. Wilt TJ, Shamliyan TA, Taylor BC, MacDonald R, Kane RL. Association between hospital and surgeon radical prostatectomy volume and patient outcomes: a systematic review. J Urol. 2008;180(3):820–8. discussion 828-829.
54. Bratzler DW, Houck PM. Antimicrobial prophylaxis for surgery: an advisory statement from the National Surgical Infection Prevention Project. Am J Surg. 2005;189(4):395–404.
55. Smaill F, Hofmeyr GJ. Antibiotic prophylaxis for cesarean section. Cochrane Database Syst Rev. 2002(3):CD000933.
56. Weiser TG, Haynes AB, Lashoher A, et al. Perspectives in quality: designing the WHO Surgical Safety Checklist. Int J Qual Health Care. 2010;22(5):365–70.
57. de Vries EN, Prins HA, Crolla RM, et al. Effect of a comprehensive surgical safety system on patient outcomes. N Engl J Med. 2010;363(20):1928–37.
58. Haynes AB, Weiser TG, Berry WR, et al. A surgical safety checklist to reduce morbidity and mortality in a global population. N Engl J Med. 2009;360(5):491–9.
59. Ginzburg E, O'Neill WW, Goldschmidt-Clermont PJ, Marchena E, Pust D, Green BA. Rapid medical relief—Project Medishare and the Haitian earthquake. N Engl J Med. 2010;362(10):e31.
60. MacIntyre NR, Jeffcoat DM, Chan DB, Lorich DG, Helfet DL. The experiences of a surgical response team in Haiti. Am J Orthop (Belle Mead NJ). 2010;39(4):172–201.
61. Merin O, Ash N, Levy G, Schwaber MJ, Kreiss Y. The Israeli field hospital in Haiti—ethical dilemmas in early disaster response. N Engl J Med. 2010;362(11):e38.
62. Peranteau WH, Havens JM, Harrington S, Gates JD. Re-establishing surgical care at Port-au-Prince General Hospital, Haiti. J Am Coll Surg. 2010;211(1):126–30.
63. Bermudez L, Carter V, Magee Jr W, Sherman R, Ayala R. Surgical outcomes auditing systems in humanitarian organizations. World J Surg. 2010;34(3):403–10.
64. Chu KM, Ford N, Trelles M. Operative mortality in resource-limited settings: the experience of Medecins Sans Frontieres in 13 countries. Arch Surg. 2010;145(8):721–5.
65. ClinicalTrials.gov. http://clinicaltrials.gov. Accessed 11 May 2014.
66. ACS Case Log System. http://www.efacs.org. Accessed 11 May 2014.
67. Wall AE. Ethics in global surgery. World J Surg. 2014;38(7):1574–80.

Legal and Ethical Issues in Global Health: A Trip Through the Vagaries of Truth and Culture

11

Jeffrey S. Freed

Introduction

Legal and ethical issues in global health should be considered a direct extension of those identical issues and principles we appreciate as an integral part of Western medicine and healthcare delivery. At no time should we consider the provision of healthcare or medical research in the developing world as outside the ethical and legal standards to which we adhere. This ideal often is at loggerheads with the practical realities of the developing world. However, as one who may well be or is an interloper in that world, one must take diligent care to preserve ethical and legal principles without trampling on established local cultural mores. Certain specific issues are unique to the developing and underdeveloped world. However, in no way will they, or should they, be addressed as deserving a lesser standard of ethical and legal observance. This, of course is a noble concept. But if one does not at least consider these principles prior to taking action, there will never be a coalescence of developed and developing world thought as well as behavior. It is not for us to impose our ethical and legal concepts on those in the developing world. Rather, it is for us to integrate lessons that have been learned at high cost into societies that have perhaps not yet identified the advantage of these principles to every individual, man and woman. These efforts are meant not to be paternalistic. They are meant to bring justice to those who may not have a voice, leveling the playing field no matter what the economic or social environment is in their world. Let us first examine the magnitude of the problem and the roots of these ethical and legal values in order to better understand how and why the medical community in the developed world has come to the beliefs and procedures to which we have agreed to adhere. This examination will also identify the complex issues that are faced when attempting to create ethical and legal guidelines in the healthcare structure of developing countries (Table 11.1).

The Problem

The problems encountered when delivering medical care in low- and middle-income countries (LMICs are myriad). They range from a lack of tangible resources (e.g., anesthesia machines) to the influence of local culture on the ability to deliver that same medical care (Figs. 11.1 and 11.2). When a 9-year-old presented to our hospital in Liberia with a gunshot wound to the abdomen, the obvious question was how it occurred. The mother, initially without much emotion, became irate when asked about the mechanism of

J.S. Freed, MD, MPH, FACS (✉)
Department of Surgery,
Icahn School of Medicine at Mount Sinai,
New York, NY, USA
e-mail: Jeffrey.Freed@mssm.edu

R. Roth et al. (eds.), *The Role of Anesthesiology in Global Health: A Comprehensive Guide*,
DOI 10.1007/978-3-319-09423-6_11, © Springer International Publishing Switzerland 2015

Table 11.1 Determinants for evaluation of problems in developing countries

Issues

- What is right? Depends on the definition
- What is best? Depends on the culture
- What can be done? Depends on the resources
- What is the law? Depends on the country

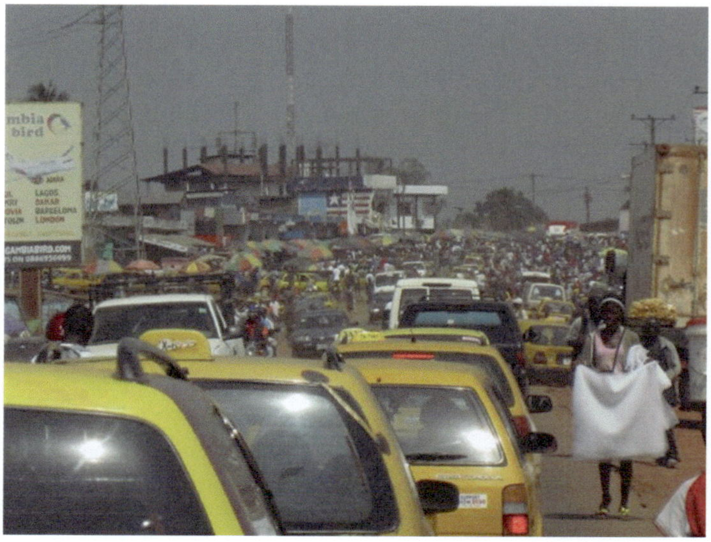

Fig. 11.1 Our home away from home

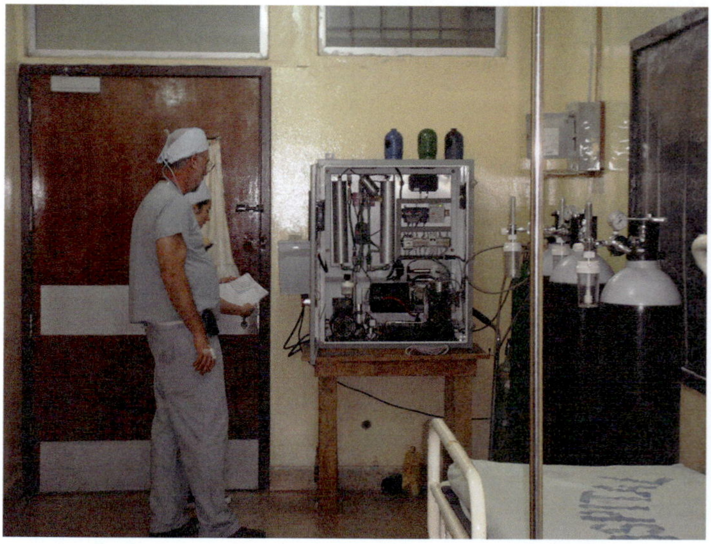

Fig. 11.2 Antiquated anesthesia equipment

the injury, specifically how a 9-year sustained a gunshot wound. This information was significant in diagnosis and planning of treatment for the injury. We were forced to proceed without the information when a local physician informed us that such questions were inappropriate. Apparently children were considered parental property and parents were not required to give explanations about their children's condition. It was a startling introduction to the local mores and an initiation into our understanding of ethical concepts in the developing world. These local mores are just another obstacle in the provision of adequate operative services in LMICs.

Surgery and anesthesia, referred to for practical purposes as operative services, are two of the most needed and most neglected areas of global health and two areas most often affected by legal and ethical issues. It has been estimated that operatively treatable diseases account for 11 % of the global burden of disease and more than 25 million disability-adjusted life-years [1]. This rough estimate includes injuries, malignancies, congenital anomalies, and complications of pregnancy, some of which may be cured if the affected populations had access to skilled surgical and anesthesia services. Unfortunately, the burden of these diseases disproportionately affects LMIC; overall it is estimated that only 3 % of the world's operations are performed in LMICs [2]. In many LMICs, operative services are concentrated in cities and only available to citizens who can afford them [3]. Several studies have shown that operative care can be delivered in a cost-effective manner in small hospitals [4]; however the current burden of disease in LMICs is not being adequately managed by the patchwork of surgical services supported by federal governments, international non-governmental organizations, and limited-resource surgical "mission trips." It is estimated that relief organizations perform nearly 250,000 operations in LMICs annually [5].

In 1996, Paul Farmer echoed in print what was known in the surgery/anesthesia community for some time; that surgery was the "stepchild" of global health [3]. Two billion people annually lack access to emergency or essential operative care and 175,000 anesthetics are delivered without even pulse oximetry, recognized as the standard of care in the developed world [6]. An estimated 500,000 mortalities per year in the developing world could be avoided were adequate surgical and anesthesia resources available. This is not just a medical problem. It is an ethical and moral problem that has not received the attention it should by developed countries that have the resources not only to deliver the necessary care, but also to educate and mentor surgeons and anesthesiologists in LMICs creating the skills to care for their own.

A major public misconception, primarily because of the universal emphasis on control of communicable disease (CD), is that those diseases are the principle cause of the significantly decreased life expectancy in the LMICs as compared to developed countries. Contrary to popular opinion, available data demonstrate that nearly 80 % of all non-communicable disease (NCD) deaths occur in low- and middle-income countries and these diseases are the major cause of mortality in these countries [7]. NCDs are the leading cause of death globally, killing more people each year than all other causes combined. The World Health Organization, explaining the reason for this, stated that the resources to prevent, diagnose, and treat these diseases are glaringly absent in LMICs. They further stated that NCDs are caused, to a large extent, by multiple behavioral risk factors that are pervasive aspects of economic transition, rapid urbanization and twenty-first-century lifestyles: tobacco use, unhealthy diet, insufficient physical activity, and the excessive use of alcohol and drugs, like khat chewing in Yemen [8]. The greatest deleterious effects of these risk factors are increasingly observed in LMICs, especially foisted upon poorer people within all these countries, mirroring the international underlying socioeconomic determinants. When examining these populations with great need, one identifies a repetitive cycle of poverty that exposes people to behavioral risk factors for NCDs while the resulting NCDs may become an important promoter for the downward spiral that leads families toward poverty [9].

At present, there is no universally accepted definition of "access to health services" [10]. For the purposes of this treatise, the definition by Peters et al. [11], which implies "the timely use of service according to need," will be operative. Utilization of healthcare is applied as an operational proxy for access to healthcare. Access has four dimensions: availability, geographic accessibility, affordability, and acceptability [12]. When considering ethical and legal issues in global health, acceptability becomes the most important barrier to successful deliverance of healthcare, as it must deal with local cultural issues, social issues, gender issues, and all the mystical and mythical issues observed and practiced in a society. This barrier is divided into tangible (e.g., monetary) or intangible (e.g., strongly held religious or spiritual beliefs).

It is often difficult to understand and always difficult to deal with the intangible. The tangible, in accessing health services, can stem from the demand and/or the supply side of the economic equation [13]. Demand-side determinants are factors influencing the ability to use health services at the individual, household or community level, while supply-side determinants are factors that interfere with the right of entry by individuals, households or the community. The need to identify the demand-side from the supply-side barrier is required to develop the necessary strategies to overcome the barrier. In fact, whether the barrier is tangible like money, or intangible like an immovable cultural mores, the application of ethical and legal principles should be the starting point for development of any solution.

Historical Background

We see a landscape of a significant portion of the world's population having experienced, and continuing to experience an inadequate access to what the United Nations declared in 1946 to be a "right to health." What has also been witnessed is the developed world community's multiple starts and reverses in an attempt to correct that phenomenon. The origins of these attempts date back millennia, as does the roots of the concepts of medical ethics and jurisprudence. A brief journey through the evolution of the development of medical ethics and jurisprudence focuses on how the questions of ethics and legal issues were identified in global health. Shortcomings in observance of those issues and failure to adhere to those rules and regulations enacted by multiple nations, countries, and agencies to enforce those principles are identified.

Historically, Western medical ethics, and the legal standards that evolved from these cultural principles, were inscribed by physicians in ancient documents like the Hippocratic Oath. The first recognized code of medical ethics, *Formula Comitis Archiatrorum*, was published in the fifth century AD, during the reign of King Theodoric the Great, the Visigoth ruler of Italy. As Middle Eastern influence increased in the medieval and early modern period, Islamic ethical medical doctrine was dispersed to the West. Writers like Ishaq ibn Ali al-Ruhawi, a Muslim physician, scribed the first complete book on the topic of medical ethics, entitled, *Conduct of a Physician*. Muhammad ibn Zakariya ar-Razi, Jewish thinkers like Maimonides, Roman Catholic scholastic thinkers including Thomas Aquinas, applied general rules and principles to questions of ethics and morals in order to resolve them, referred to as casuistry (that is, having the air of case law) in Catholic theology. These intellectual traditions continue in Catholic, Islamic and Jewish medical ethics to this day [14].

By the eighteenth and nineteenth centuries, medical ethics emerged as a more self-conscious discourse. In England, Thomas Percival, a physician and author, crafted the first modern code of medical ethics. He authored a pamphlet with the code in 1794 and wrote an expanded version in 1803, in which he coined the expressions "medical ethics" and "medical jurisprudence" [15]. In 1815, the Apothecaries Act was passed by the Parliament of the United Kingdom (UK). It introduced compulsory apprenticeship and formal qualifications for the apothecaries of the day under the license of the Society of Apothecaries. This was the beginning of regulation of the medical profession in the UK.

In 1847, the American Medical Association adopted its first code of ethics [16], based in large part upon Thomas Percival's work. While in the nineteenth century secularized medicine borrowed largely from Catholic ethics, in the twentieth century an approach articulated by thinkers such as Joseph Fletcher was distinctively liberal Protestant [17]. This liberalization led to the movement toward the appreciation of ethical and legal behavior throughout the developed world; however, it was the atrocities that occurred during the Second World War that focused humanity's attention on the need to deal with that type of heinous human experimentation, genocide and other crimes against humanity. The judgment by the war crimes tribunals at Nuremberg, in a new code that is now accepted worldwide, established ten standards by which physicians would have to conform when carrying out experiments on human subjects [18].

This code established a new standard of ethical medical behavior for the post-World War II human rights era. Among other requirements, this document enunciates the requirement of *voluntary informed consent* of the human subject. The principle of voluntary informed consent protects the right of the individual to control his own body. This code also recognizes that the risk must be weighed against the expected benefit, and that unnecessary pain and suffering must be avoided. Doctors should avoid actions that injure human patients. Also, the volunteer must be capable of understanding the nature of the research in which he or she partakes, including the risks and benefits. The principles established by this code for medical practice now have been extended into general codes of medical ethics [19]. It has also permeated the principles under which the medical and research community should function when working in the developing world.

Recent Developments

In the 1960s and 1970s, building upon liberal theory and procedural justice, much of the discourse of medical ethics went through a dramatic shift and largely reconfigured itself into what we now call bioethics [20]. Unfortunately, the legal discourse that followed progressed more slowly, with little teeth given to those codes and doctrine that were advocated and even enacted during the latter half of the twentieth century.

The goal of the memorialization of medical ethics and jurisprudence was to affect ethical behavior through cooperation among nations and by the creation of codified agreements, through the international law aspect of the human rights efforts. Examining the levels of interventions and how health officials can make use of it allowed for the passage of laws directing the behavior of individuals and nations. Such direction becomes a major undertaking when dealing with LMICs when they themselves have not necessarily set standards for ethical and legal action. Many of these countries have undergone social and political upheaval, being referred to as conflict or post-conflict nations (e.g., Congo, Liberia, and Nicaragua). The unrest sustained has often led to governments and nations being unable or unwilling to establish ethical and legal standards to which they would adhere when dealing with the health of their population.

Global health ethics and laws that nations have enacted have inadvertently created parallel legal systems. Specifically, each individual country must approve the international ethical principles, rights, and laws that have been created before those principles are instituted within the borders of their own country. Also, a treaty not recognized by a country results in that treaty having no force of law within that country. In view of the fact that international law is developed as a "bargaining evolution of theory," it often results in a simplified version of what was intended in order to be accepted by the multiple partners, both from developed and undeveloped worlds, participating in the process. In other words, laws and doctrine are created by compromise, often losing the initial intent and failing to accomplish hoped for goals.

Current Situations

Even though the Global Health community accepted the "right to health," especially in LMICs, it did not necessarily mean that the right to healthcare was accepted. In developing countries without the resources to provide adequate care, the desire to fulfill the goals of human rights in the healthcare arena is not often met. The intent of international laws and the quest for ethical deeds in providing the right to health (care) are based on ideas, but remains only an empty fantasy without the political and financial commitment of the global community. The creation of these humanitarian concepts is admirable. But very often something that should be progressively realized only reflects promoters' dreams by allowing the countries that most need these principles to escape any real pressure to enforce them. To bring sufficient pressure to correct this problem, human rights assessments would be necessary by unbiased observers and the results published so the facts would be universally appreciated. Anticipation of human rights violations by certain governments is required so steps can be taken to circumvent abuses [21].

The enforcement of global health laws and ethics requires an understanding of the societies that we are supposedly assisting. Developed nations must first establish that other societies are following the same rules and regulations that they have deemed appropriate. Developed nations must understand what the underlying right might be in any given society, and enforce the resolution utilizing that right. Mechanisms to accomplish this goal are available such as international tribunals that have been successful in documenting atrocities and calling to task those who have laid waste to established principles, laws, and ethics. Once the principles outlined above have been introduced, the clinical setting in which they will function starts to impact the deliverance of healthcare.

When one looks at the practical requirements of delivering "health" as established in the *Declaration of Human Rights* [22], the magnitude of that endeavor becomes clear. Perhaps even more than the need for surgical services in the LMCIs, is a worldwide anesthesia crisis. Most LMICs have less than 1 physician per 10,000 people and less than 1 anesthesiologist per 100,000 people, leaving an immense gap in the safe performance of operative services [23]. This void requires immediate attention to improve patient safety in low-income countries through education and support.

Measures to Improve Patient Safety

In order to address the marked disparity between the numbers of anesthesiologists in developed versus LCMIs (i.e., one anesthesiologist per 260 patients in the United States versus 1 anesthesiologist per 55,000 patients in Ghana) the American Society of Anesthesia Committee on Global Humanitarian Outreach is addressing this crisis in several ways:

1. Encouraging volunteerism.
2. Providing opportunities with reputable aid and mission organizations.
3. Supporting anesthesia education and training in LMICs.
4. Advocating for long term academic partnership with hospitals and universities in countries of need.
5. Providing for collaboration of organizations, institutions, and initiatives with common missions and philosophies.

Humanitarian efforts like these are essential in improving the state of health on a global stage.

Research

One area of scientific pursuit in the developing world that is significantly impacted by medical ethics is scientific research. Even more than other areas of healthcare in the LMICs, scientific research raises ethical issues, especially when funded by external sponsors from developed countries. Developing countries urgently need research to help address the enormous burden of disease. The disparities in resources previously described between developed and developing countries can promote exploitation in the case of externally sponsored research. Failure to understand that external sponsors may differ in their capability to appreciate different culture and educational status of the subjects in developing countries creates the need for significant internal and external oversight of research in LCMIs. Furthermore, in order to promote the ethical and legal climate for medical research, all countries should set national priorities related to their provision of healthcare. When externally sponsored research is proposed that does not address the national priorities of its host, the research must demonstrate its relevance and be justified to an appropriate independent research ethics committee. To enhance the capability of developing countries to conduct and oversee research that is in their best interest, the inclusion of a component to improve the local expertise in country should be a provision of any new healthcare and healthcare research. The most difficult part of the creation of this monitor would be to make it independent of both external and internal forces that often have their own agendas. An independent international organization without any direct interest in the results of the therapy or research could be established to provide services equivalent to an Independent Research Committee (IRB) at any North American academic institution. The committees would be comprised of similar members as Western IRBs including physician-scientists, ethicists, and lay people. The committee would function at arm's length from those issues on which it is evaluating and would be able to provide oversight while also performing an educational function for those in the host country. This IRB-type international committee would work hand-in-hand through every step of the process with a similar committee in the LMIC that had requested its services. The international community of developed nations would fund the program with the intent of its existence being self-limited until such time that any particular nation using it could afford its own independent organization.

Externally sponsored research often must cope with adverse and occasionally contradictory directions as to what may be ethically suitable. Finding an ethical framework for this situation requires application of the ethical and often legal principles that might be an anathema to the local authorities. In LMICs, Western ethical and legal conventions are occasionally seen as contradictory to acceptable local social and cultural behavior. An example of this is what we refer to in the West as female genital mutilation. In some countries on the African continent, this ritual is essential for a woman to be acceptable in her community and as a partner for marriage. Dealing with this type of cultural activity must be done with the utmost sensitivity. Providing such guidance and assisting in the education of those local professionals and citizens involved is part of the obligation of researchers and clinicians in establishing cohesive and mutually agreeable rules for the ethical review of research. The ethical framework for this process that has become the standard for global research is based on four principles:

1. The duty to alleviate suffering.
2. The duty to show respect for persons.
3. The duty to be sensitive to cultural differences.
4. The duty not to exploit the vulnerable.

> It is fundamental that these obligations are respected when research is planned and conducted. It is essential to ethical research that these principles be considered and that researchers take into account the context, social, cultural, and economic status of the study community. Institution of these principles will fulfill the minimum requirements to be considered ethical research [24].

An excellent example of research that has been effective and changed behavior in the developing world, especially India, dealt with adolescent health and development. The results of this research, presented as an analysis of data from six cross-national studies, representing 53 different countries, found that the success or the absence of parent–child relationships is an indicator of the likelihood of early sexual initiation, substance use, and depression among adolescents. The Child Development and Adolescent Health Center in New Delhi, India, has developed programs to better equip parents to manage behavioral problems and to recognize mental health problems among their adolescent children. Workshops were created to provide life skill education and promote mental health in secondary schools. They were designed to improve parents' communication with their children and enhance the capability of parents to prevent and identify common behavioral problems in adolescence. As a result of parent participation, several schools are now directly involving parents in mental health initiatives [25].

The difficulties of managing the multiple factors that compose what we term ethical research are often beyond the capability of LMICs and result in negative external oversight actions. The situation cited above could be considered one of "unethical ethics." The term unethical ethics is invoked when researchers, even with the best intentions, actions or policies that are believed to promote ethical research standards inadvertently cause serious damage to other important values, like the right to self-determination and the right to be compensated for damages incurred while participating in a study. In this case, the drive to promote the welfare of research participants unfortunately created a situation where it could be deemed difficult to conduct health related research, even if the research focused on important public health problems in that country. The preexisting Indian regulations protecting human participants involved in research were considered problematic enough to necessitate the US National Institutes of Health to cease all funding for biomedical research in India in 2013, and cautiously re-institute it in 2014 with severe restrictions and greater external oversight [26, 27].

The three core problems in the Indian study cited by the NIH were the following:

1. The research guidelines did not state how injuries suffered by research participants were to be compensated by research institutions and did not delineate how they were to be determined as "research related."
2. Protocol guidelines had an overly broad interpretation as to what counted as a research related harm, including for example use of placebo in a placebo controlled trial.
3. The Indian ethics review committees and licensing authorities had to help determine whether and to what extent compensation for harm was warranted, but was unclear as to what relevant skills and resources were available to do so.

The researchers conducting the study were making every effort to protect their study subjects. However, they failed to clearly define what were considered injuries to study subjects, the mechanism to identify those injuries and the methodologies to be used to determine compensation. As one cannot deduce the best efforts in this particular situation to create an ethical environment for the study resulting in harm to the study subjects, the researchers and the project they were conducting with their best efforts to work within the constraints of ethical research boundaries were deemed unsatisfactory. These results reflected the difficulty a scientist or scientific group unexpectedly faces even when the best efforts are effectuated.

The performance of ethical and legally acceptable research or clinical care in LMICs is often confounded when something unexpected is discovered. When a patient or subject undergoes a routine test at the doctor's office or is participating in a research study, a result that is surprising to the clinical personnel may be recognized. Regardless of the setting, test, or procedure, when it comes to incidental findings, President Barack Obama's Commission on Bioethics (referred to as the Bioethical Commission or just Commission) [28] has offered this recommendation: "anticipate and communicate." The Bioethics Commission recommended that all practitioners or research scientists anticipate and plan for incidental findings so that patients, research participants, and those involved in a patient or subject's care are informed before an intervention is undertaken. This recommendation holds true for all clinicians and researchers, including anesthesiologists.

Incidental findings have been conventionally defined as those results that originate from a test or procedure that have not been anticipated, producing an array of practical and ethical challenges for the subject or patient as well as the clinician or researcher. These "secondary findings" are not the primary objective of the test or the procedures performed, but are additional information to be considered and evaluated. These incidental and secondary findings may lead the physician/researcher to discoveries that were not previously considered, but may also result in uncertainty and grief if no equivalent benefit is derived and a condition for which no available treatment is found in that country.

The great majority of the present literature, that discusses incidental findings, relates to unforeseen genetic findings during clinical testing or research activities. In the developing world the majority of external humanitarian activities center round research and clinical care of infectious diseases. Recently, on a surgical mission to Phoebe, Liberia, a radiologist performed an ultrasound on a 5-year-old boy with massive splenomegaly thought to be secondary to malaria. The Liberian doctors believed that the child developed splenomegaly because of his refractory anemia. The sonogram revealed a massively enlarged heterogeneous spleen, multiple defects in the liver and extensive adenopathy in the abdomen and retroperitoneum compatible with lymphoma. The surgical team had not prepared the family for the possibility of a diagnosis that was untreatable and fatal in that setting. The lack of communication combined with the "incidental finding of

Table 11.2 ASA guidelines as to ethical behavior, based on AMA code of conduct

1. Patients' interests are foremost, including self-determination in decision making (includes minors in some situations)
2. Monitor themselves and others
3. Maintain confidentiality
4. Explain shared responsibility
5. No exploitive financial advantages
6. Provide care irrespective of ability to pay
7. Cooperative and respectful relationships with colleagues
8. Timely consultations
9. Strive to change laws and improve community of it betters patients
10. Secure controlled substances
11. Maintain skills

lymphoma" left the team emotionally disrupted and the family without hope for their child. This is a clear example of the need, especially in a setting where care is not available for "incidental or secondary findings," to think ahead before procedures are performed, and to prepare patients and their families for the chance of discovering an untreatable and possibly an incurable disease process. This is our ethical obligation.

The Bioethics Commission recommended that whether or not these incidental or secondary findings are identified, the clinician or researcher should proceed cautiously while following five recommendations considered basic guidelines no matter what the context of the finding. The guidelines are outlined in Table 11.2. The ultimate purpose of these guidelines is to ensure that the clinician or researcher, whether an anesthesiologist, other physician or non-physician scientist, fulfills the fundamental obligation to respect the subject's or patient's autonomy, beneficence, and right to informed decision making [29, 30].

The above tenets are an ideal. Commissions come and go but the principles that evolve remain unalterable. Yet there are times when the ideal cannot be met. On almost every mission to LMICs there is a moment when something is identified that challenges the principles. Whether the birth of a child with an omphalocoele (a large defect in the center of the baby's abdomen with intestines protruding) or an elderly emaciated woman with a cancer obstructing her bowel, there are times when an ethical decision must be made that is the opposite to the best medical care. The physician must decide *not* to treat the patient but to *allow* them to die. A lack of necessary resources for these cases would result in an inability to salvage these patients after the best operative intervention. Every instinct the physician has to try save a life must be tempered by the realities of functioning in these countries. And every effort must be made to transfer the reasons for your decision to the families and the local hospital staff who remain to care for these patients. Decisions based on long established bioethical canons may well appear as abandonment of the patient if those canons are not definitely expressed to the local caregivers invested in these patients. One has to have a strategy for dealing with these cases long before they appear in order to prevent animus among those who suffer the loss. This process must start before any specific case presents and is part of the obligation of any individual or team practicing or doing research in these settings.

These recommendations, extensively debated and reviewed have become the basis of an approach not only to care in the developed world but hopefully in the developing world in the future. The obligation of every physician, scientist or researcher approaching patient or subject intervention in LMICs is to understand and appreciate the significance of these guidelines and be willing and able to carry out his or her duties while maintaining these standards as best as possible in a different cultural and social environment. The operative team, often facing situations without authoritative solutions to complex medical problems based on experience in their developed country, must make decisions based on not only what is available in the field, but also on the ethical and legal issues addressed above. These guidelines that were developed by the Bioethics Commission apply not only to incidental and secondary findings, but also to all information about tests or procedures that might be sought or found in relationship to research study or clinical therapy or testing. This ideal is truly a goal to which we can aspire, both in ethical and legal arenas (Table 11.3).

Table 11.3 Guidelines of the bioethics commission

1. Individuals must be informed that incidental findings can occur
2. Professional groups develop unambiguous instructions for the categorization of these incidental and secondary findings
3. Directed research should occur to define the classes of and incidence of incidental and secondary findings including the costs, benefits, and harms these of these findings and preferences regarding the disclosure of the findings
4. Preparation of educational materials to inform all stakeholders (patients, practitioners, IRBs, etc.) about the ethical, practical, and legal implications of incidental and secondary findings
5. Affordable (and in some cases free) access to quality information must be available, both before and after testing

Ethical Guidelines of the ASA

The American Society of Anesthesiologists has developed guidelines for the ethical practice of anesthesiology that are applicable not only in the USA but also in any intervention with patients or subjects in LMICs [31].

To quote from the Preamble to Society's Guidelines for Ethical Practice, "Membership in the American Society of Anesthesiologists is a privilege of physicians who are dedicated to the ethical provision of health care." The Society has chosen to base these guidelines on the Principles of Medical Ethics of the American Medical Association (AMA) [32].

The AMA, as described in the historical discussion of ethics, was the first organization in the United States to codify the concept of ethical principles. Its beliefs were and still are that the medical profession has "long subscribed to a body of ethical statements developed primarily for the benefit of the patient." Any physician practicing under the aegis of the AMA is required to "recognize responsibility to patients first and foremost." While recognizing these principles, it must be remembered that they are not law but rather "standards of conduct that define the essentials of honorable behavior for the physician."

The AMA Principles are divided into nine specific sections. To summarize, a physician is encouraged to provide competent medical care with compassion and respect for human dignity and rights; professionalism must be maintained at all times and those not adhering must be reported; the law must be followed and efforts to improve those laws sought; the rights of patients and health professionals must be respected at all times including their privacy; a physician will continue his own education and encourage and support the education of others through interchange of knowledge; the physician maintains his independence as far as whom to treat (except in emergencies) and where to treat them; the betterment of the community shall be a constant goal of a physician; responsibility to the patient as paramount and: the physician shall support access to medical care for all people.

The practice of anesthesiology involves special problems relating to the quality and standards of patient care. Therefore, the ASA requires its members to adhere to the AMA Principles of Medical Ethics and any other specific ethical guidelines. It must be remembered that circumstances may arise when elements of the following guidelines may not apply and wherein individualized decisions may be appropriate. This is of special import when practicing or doing research in LMICs. The underlying principles, however, must never be ignored.

The ASA has created a document to outline the five areas in which an anesthesiologist must meet ethical responsibilities. These areas include responsibilities to patients, colleagues, facilities, communities, and themselves (Table 11.2). A brief summary will assist the reader to understand the goals of these individual tenets.

The patient–physician relationship involves special obligations for the physician that includes placing the patient's interests first and foremost, faithfully caring for the patient and always being truthful. This includes respect for the patient's self-determination; protection of all patients from disrespectful behavior and abuse from colleagues as well as themselves; maintenance of confidentiality; and guaranteeing of informed decision making and understanding of all parties involved in the anesthesia and post-anesthesia care. Also, anesthesiologists must not participate in exploitive financial relationships, always providing the same care for patients no matter their economic status.

The guidelines go on to speak of anesthesiologists maintaining professional interpersonal relationships with peers and non-physician staff and students, never taking advantage of those persons in their work roles or financially even while still monitoring the behavior and abilities of their peers. They must participate in their faculty's activities, including education, while maintaining a secure environment for the patient, staff, and the drugs they use. All anesthesiologists are required to appreciate their responsibility for improving the community and the society in which they participate, wherever their local facility exists in the developing world.

These guidelines issued by the AMA or ASA or any other agency or organization are meant to direct the healthcare provider, no matter what the rank or training, toward the consideration of the patient or subject as the most important member of any interaction. Any patient or subject is to be protected no matter what the circumstance. Ethical conundrums and legal conflicts will arise as a matter of course when treating or doing research or providing patient care. When the patient or subject is from an LMIC, the road is often fraught with bumps and potholes because of the inability of the patient to participate in the decision making process due to language or cultural differences.

The difficulties in patient participation for those residing in LMICs often are not just a matter of understanding language or technical terms, but rather, culturally being in a position to be part of the decision making process. Recently, a patient presented at the hospital in Niger where a fistula team was doing surgery. Previously, thinking that her bloody, foul-smelling vaginal discharge was secondary to a fistula, a medicine man in her village had given her herbs. These homeopathic medicants failed to resolve the problem and upon hearing of our fistula mission, she decided to seek our help. This was as much a medical decision as a cultural decision. Had she failed to resolve her problem, her husband would have abandoned her and the villagers would have ostracized her. In fact, on examination, she did not have a recto-vaginal fistula, but rather an extensive, fixed, ulcerated, necrotic cancer of her cervix, creating the offensive discharge. Unfortunately, in Niger, there is no treatment for this advanced gynecologic malignancy. This desperate woman was going to die from her disease. She should have been told that she had an untreatable problem to allow her to make arrangements for her multiple young children. In spite of our desire to inform her, we were unable to do so because her husband was not traveling with her. In the Niger culture only the husband could be told his wife's diagnosis. The husband could not come from the distant village where he lived, primarily because of financial issues. Therefore, our doomed patient was neither going to receive therapy nor be able to return home to prepare for her inevitable death. We were faced with an ethical issue without a satisfactory answer. After long discussions with the Niger hospital staff, we decided that it was more important to maintain the collegial relationship with the local community than it was to inform the woman of her diagnosis. This was done not only to respect the local tradition but just as importantly to protect the continuity of our mission for the sake of those not yet treated. This compromise, although not ideal, was the only way that many more women with a devastating condition could be returned to their normal lives. Long mores trumped our best efforts to be ethical, according to our own standards.

Global Health Law

As a consequence of rapid globalization, the need for a coherent system of global health law and governance has never been greater. Hazards are posed by contemporary globalization on human health and consequently there is an urgent need for global health law to facilitate effective multilateral cooperation in advancing the health of populations equitably. "Global health law" is an emerging field and there are many challenges to reaching its full potential to advance human health in just and effective ways [33].

Only recently have scholars engaged in a serious discussion of "public health law" [34], including a definition and theory of the field. The role of the state and civil society in health promotion and disease prevention within a country must be defined. Literature on the international dimensions of health is emerging but no similar systematic definition and exposition of a field we call "global health law" is apparent. This rapid and expanding globalization emphasizes the need for a coherent system of international health law and governance [35]. According to Taylor, a World Bank consultant and professor of public health law, "Although increasing global integration is not an entirely new phenomenon, contemporary globalization has had an unprecedented impact on global public health" [36] and is therefore responsible for the new challenges for international law and policy. It must be remembered that global health law is meant to facilitate effective cooperation between all nations for the purpose of advancing the health of populations equally.

Multinational corporations, in particular, have significant influence and power over global consumption of food, tobacco, pharmaceuticals, consumer and healthcare products and services. The production and delivery of these goods and services pose health hazards that span national borders, but often escape scrutiny under national laws. The global community, therefore, needs to develop effective ways to ensure the quality and safety of goods and services that are exchanged in international commerce. If this is not accomplished, unethical practices and the "push and pull" of market forces will pressure not only the business community but also doctors and nurses in LMICs to make critical choices about the welfare of their patients, often resulting in the forfeit of adequate resources needed for management of well-functioning healthcare systems [37].

Globalization is the driver of the considerably complex demand for effective mechanisms of global health governance. Today, the health of any population, especially one that is compromised, is not just determined by local facts, but rather is deeply affected by factors including the increasing integration and the internationalization of "the determinants of health." This complexity has contributed to the swift decrease in the actual ability of nation-states to protect the health of their populations by their own actions alone. The phenomenon has intensified the need for international cooperation among states [38], leading to the rapid increase in international organizations to try to establish legal codes to deal with these problems. A small sample of the most effective organizations include the UN system, organizations with significant involvement in health including the World Health Organization, the UN Children's Fund, the UN Food and Agricultural Organization, the UN Environment Program, the UN Population Fund, the International Labor Organization and the World Bank.

The need has also prompted non-governmental agencies to enter this arena including a wide variety of organizations coming at the problem from different perspectives such as religious groups, nongovernmental agencies and for-profit corporations like the pharmaceutical industry with a powerful and significant stake in international health policy. Also included are the more creative organizations like health research networks and, most significantly, public–private partnerships, an arrangement that is rapidly becoming commonplace. The need for more effective collective action among governments, businesses, civil society and other entities increases daily as the influences on health are more and more affected by external local international factors, including war or its many equivalents, trashing of the environment, trade or the lack thereof, investment both for internal and external sources and crime.

The seeds of the concept of global health law have developed from public international law. The law is ultimately designed only, to protect world health. The concepts are meant to protect the individual national sovereignty that is material in any international system. The subjects and the sources of international law, therefore, have been with specific intent, avoiding a "broad brush" approach to each issue. Global health law is a living entity continually attempting to be creative and non-intrusive in its attempts at global health governance. Academicians have emphasized global health governance, in contrast to prohibitory or regulatory products of "government" because it allows easy movement across public/private boundaries of the state, markets, civil society, and private lives [39]. Rather than a model of top-down social control, governance theory harnesses the creativity and channels the actions, ideas and resources of multiple actors that affect health.

The moral fiber of global health law is justice. This concept has been the consistent direction of the evolution of global health law and ethics. With this goal of greatly cherished social justice, the definition of global health law suggests that the state of affairs for healthy populations should be distributed fairly across social, racial, gender, economic, and geographic boundaries in all countries and regions. This is not to say that this justice must be rigidly equally allocated to every nation and region, but rather some equitable method of health protection for every human being must exist. Social justice must at least in part require reduction in socioeconomic disparities within and among countries. This demand for fair distribution has arisen out of the concept that every life has value. It should be the mission of the community of nations to alleviate poverty, the feeling of powerlessness and the needless suffering and death that harms everyone in the world's community by diminishing the public trust and discouraging social cooperation. The message delivered to those affected and to everyone in general should not be that the basic human needs of those less fortunate are of less concern than those who have the resources to attain their needs. "Social justice thus calls for policies that promote human dignity for all members of the international community equitably" (Fig. 11.3a,b) [33].

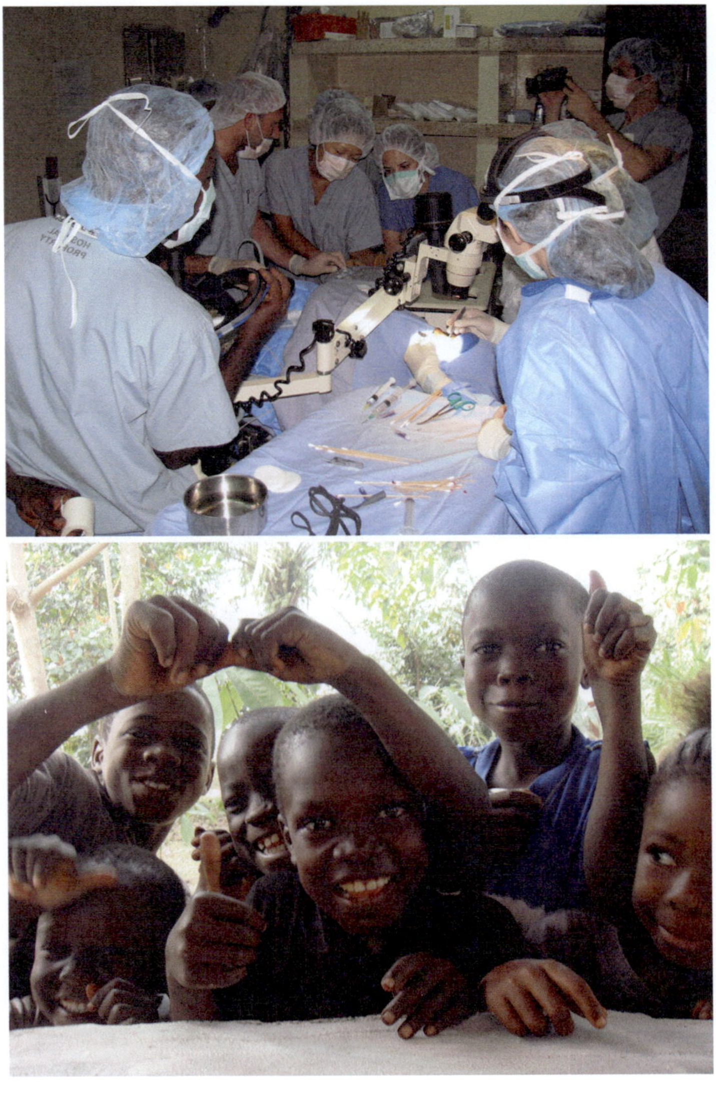

Fig. 11.3 (**a**) Doing what we do best. (**b**) The lives we hope to save

Conclusion

The information provided in this chapter should allow the reader to begin to understand the complexities of the ethical and legal issues that present themselves when one is involved in healthcare in the developing world. These issues are further complicated by the requirement of functioning within the same guidelines that control our activities while performing tasks in the developed world. This latter requirement is sacrosanct, and must be followed no matter what the context of the situation encountered in LMICs. The guidelines and codes that we are encouraged to follow present an expansive group of problems as different situations occur, while also providing an opportunity for reevaluation of the possibilities created by preexisting restraints. No two healthcare or medical decisions are generated by exactly the same circumstance, lending to the need for critical thinking when making decisions as to behavior in a particular setting.

No single chapter can describe all the ethical codes and legal systems that have been formulated to try to deal with healthcare issues in LMICs. However, this chapter is an introduction to those already in force, while also describing several of the contexts from which these answers to ethical and legal questions have evolved. In the process of this evolution, many individuals from Hippocrates to Hitler have influenced what is today considered ethical and legal. However, these present answers are fluid, with new problems and issues coming to the fore at a constant rate, and sometimes at a critical pace. No group of opinions or regulations can cover every possibility, especially since every issue encountered has a difference twist, in a different culture, in a different political atmosphere, and especially with different actors evaluating and acting on the certain variable conditions.

When a reader becomes part of the scenario and is faced with a set of circumstances not specifically covered by guidelines and rules, he or she must remember that LMICs are not test tubes in which to try a new and previously untried methodology. The people in LMICs have the same rights, privileges and needs that any person in any environment in the world has, and must be viewed with the same respect and justice that anyone anywhere is treated. Following this dictum will lead to the humane handling of any problem no matter what the ethical or legal issue.

References

1. Debas HT, Gosselin R, McCord C, Thind A. Surgery. In: Jamison DT, Breman JG, Measham AR, et al., editors. Disease control priorities in developing countries. 2nd ed. Washington, DC: World Bank; 2006. Chap 67.
2. Ozgediz D, Chu K, Ford N, et al. Surgery in global health delivery. Mt Sinai J Med. 2011;78(3): 327–41.
3. Farmer PE, Kim JY. Surgery and global health: a view from beyond the OR. World J Surg. 2008;32(4):533–6.
4. Ozgediz D, Jamison D, Cherian M, McQueen K. The burden of surgical conditions and access to surgical care in low- and middle-income countries. Bull World Health Organ. 2008;86(8):646–7.
5. McQueen KAK, Parmar P, Kene M, et al. Burden of surgical disease: strategies to manage an existing public health emergency. Prehosp Disaster Med. 2009;24 Suppl 2:S228–31.
6. Funk L, Weiser T, Berry W, Lipsitz S, Merry A, Enright A, et al. Global operating room distribution and pulse oximetry for surgical care. Lancet. 2010; 376:1055–61.
7. Miranda JJ, Casas JP, et al. Non-communicable diseases in low- and middle- income countries: context, determinants and health policy. Trop Med Int Health. 2008;13(10):1225–34.
8. Bulletin of the World Health Organization. Khat chewing in Yemen: turning over a new leaf. Bull World Health Organ. 2008;86(10):737–81.
9. Alwan A. Diseases and mental health. In: Global status report on noncommunicable diseases. World Health Organization. 2010, p. vii.
10. Penchansky R, Thomas JW. The concept of access: definition and relationship to consumer satisfaction. Med Care. 1981;19(2):127–40.
11. Peters DH, Garg A, Bloom G, et al. Poverty and access to health care in developing countries. Ann N Y Acad Sci. 2008;1136:161–71.
12. Gulliford M, Figueroa-Munoz J, Morgan M, Hughes D, Gibson B, et al. What does 'access to health care' mean? J Health Serv Res Policy. 2002;7(3):186–8.
13. Larson C, Williams J. Sociological context of TennCare: a public health perspective. J Ambul Care Manage. 2003;26(4):315–21.
14. Jonsen AR. Short history of medical ethics. New York, NY: Oxford University Press; 2000. p. 28–32.
15. Percival T. Medical ethics. Manchester: S. Russell; 1803.

16. American Medical Association [Internet]. Chicago: The Association; 2001. https://www.ama-assn.org/ama/pub/physicians/medical-ethics.page.
17. Fletcher J. Morals and medicine. Princeton, NJ: Princeton; 1954.
18. "Nuremberg Code" (PDF). U.S. National Institutes of Health. Retrieved 20 Jun 2012.
19. Kohler ED. The Nazi doctors and the Nuremburg code: human rights in human experimentation, and—cleansing the Fatherland—Nazi medicine and racial hygiene. Bull Hist Med. 1996;70(1):150–1.
20. Pellegrino ED. The origins and evolution of bioethics: some personal reflections Kennedy Institute of Ethics. Kennedy Inst Ethics J. 1999;9(1):73–88.
21. Kuszler P, Kochis B, Atkins D. Ethics, International Law and Human Rights, Sanford. depts.washington.edu/ihg/conference/ethicslawrights.doc.
22. United Nations General Assembly resolution 217 A (III). 1948.
23. Linden AF, Sekidde FS, Galukande M, Knowlton LM, Chackungal S, McQueen KA. Challenges of surgery in developing countries: a survey of surgical and capacity Uganda's public hospitals. World J Surg. 2012;36(5):1056–65.
24. Nuffield Council on Bioethics. The ethics of research related to healthcare in developing countries. http:/Nuffield bioethics.org. 2002, p. 126–34.
25. World Health Organization (WHO). Broadening the horizon: balancing protection and risk for adolescents. Geneva: WHO; 2001.
26. Shukla S. India's amended trials regulations spark research exodus. Lancet. 2013;382(9895):845–7.
27. Global bioethics BLOG: promoting reflections on and research issues in sub Saharan Africa. Research protections in India: a case of unethical ethics? 2001.
28. Presidential Commission for the Study of Bioethical Issues. Anticipate and communicate: ethical management of incidental and secondary findings in the clinical, research, and direct-to-consumer contexts. 2013.
29. Gutmann A. The bioethics commission on incidental findings. Science. 2013;342(6164):1321–3.
30. Ma M. Bioethicists issue guidance on handling incidental findings. JAMA. 2014;311(6):562–3.
31. American Society of Anesthesia Ethics Committee. Guidelines for the ethical practice of anesthesiology. (Approved by the ASA House of Delegates on October 15, 2003, last amended on October 19, 2011, and reaffirmed on October 16, 2013).
32. American Medical Association. Adopted June 1957; revised June 1980; revised June 2001.
33. Gostin LO, Taylor AL. Global health law: a definition and grand challenges. Public Health Ethics. 2008; 1(1):53–63.
34. Martin R, Johnson L. Law and the public dimension of health. London: Cavendish; 2006.
35. Fidler D, Gostin L. The new international health regulations: an historic development for international law and public health. J Law Med Ethics. 2006;33(4):85–94.
36. Taylor A. Encyclo of public health. International law and public health policy. Elsevier. 2008.
37. Lee K, Buse K, Fustukian S. Health policy in a globalising world. Cambridge: Cambridge University Press; 2002. p. 78–96.
38. Hunter ND. Risk governance and democracy in health care, Georgetown University Law Center. O'Neill Institute Working Paper Series. 2008, p. 1–60.
39. Gostin LO. Meeting basic survival needs of the world's least healthy people: toward a framework convention on global health. Georgetown Law J. 2008;96:331–92.

Part II

Specific Case-Related Implementation

Strategies for Patient Assessment and Scheduling

12

Laurent Jouffroy

Introduction

In many developing countries, especially in rural areas, lack of appropriate supplies and equipment create special challenges for the visiting anesthesiologist. Electricity may be unpredictable, oxygen and medical gas supplies and up-to-date monitoring systems may be nonexistent and the level of training of local health care providers can be variable [1, 2].

Furthermore, in many places, the practice of anesthesia focused primarily on the intraoperative care of the patient while limited attention is given to comprehensive medical assessment prior to surgery. When visiting areas where medical care is scarce, the anesthesiologist must be especially prepared to manage a range of conditions normally handled by a multispecialty team. By paying careful attention to the preoperative process, many potential serious complications related to anesthesia can be averted.

L. Jouffroy, M.D. (✉)
French Society of Anesthesia and Intensive Care, Anesthesiology and Critical Care, Ambulatory Surgery Unit, Clinique du Diaconat, Strasbourg, France
e-mail: laurent.jouffroy67@gmail.com

General Considerations

The preoperative assessment of patient should begin by taking the following into consideration:

1. Many patients have never had medical care previously, and therefore a thorough history and physical examination are necessary to rule out preexisting medical conditions. Unidentified medical conditions such as congenital heart disease may affect anesthesia care, especially in environments with limited facilities for dealing with perioperative complications [3].
2. Familiarity with locally endemic diseases and conditions is necessary to understand perioperative risk factors (e.g., parasitic infections: malaria, dengue fever, HIV/AIDS) [4].
3. Some anesthetic risks are unappreciated or unknown (e.g., difficult airway, natural rubber latex allergy). Every attempt should be made to identify them ahead of time.
4. Depending on the hospital and the country, access to certain routine medications may be limited.
5. A language barrier may exist resulting in potential confusion and misunderstanding.
6. Access to preoperative laboratory work-up and imaging may be limited.
7. Where knowledge and technical means to deliver regional anesthesia are limited, general anesthesia may be a more appropriate option [5].

R. Roth et al. (eds.), *The Role of Anesthesiology in Global Health: A Comprehensive Guide*, DOI 10.1007/978-3-319-09423-6_12, © Springer International Publishing Switzerland 2015

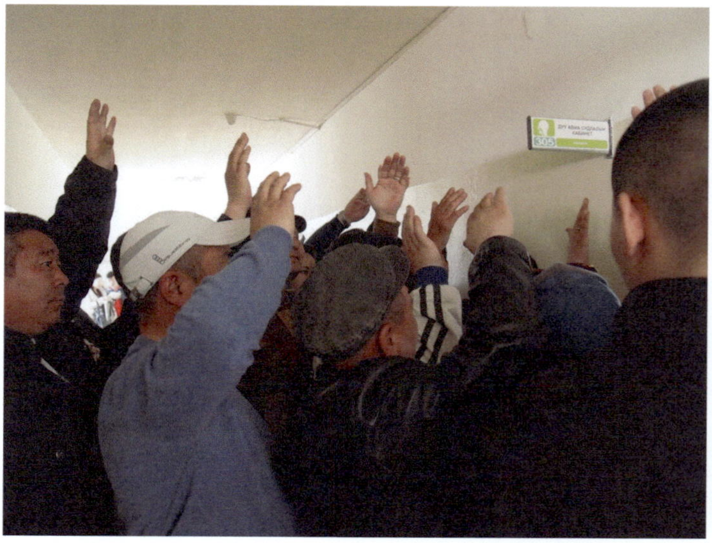

Fig. 12.1 Waiting for pre-operative evaluation

Patient Assessment

The *American Society of Anesthesiologists Task Force on Preanesthesia Evaluation* defines preanesthesia as the process of clinical assessment that precedes the delivery of anesthesia care for surgery and for nonsurgical procedures [6].

Preanesthesia evaluation includes the review of medical records (laboratory and imaging) as well as a compressive history and physical examination (Table 12.1).

Most patients should be assessed prior to the day of surgery, to allow adequate time for interventions such as preoperative testing or changes in medical regimen. For patients with low severity of disease or medium- or low-risk surgical procedures, the preanesthesia assessment may be performed on the day of surgery. But in some cases, especially in regions where access to a medical facility is limited, it can be difficult to arrange a pertinent assessment prior to the day of surgery.

While the preoperative assessment should ideally be completed by an anesthesiologist, in many cases a non-physician provider (e.g., trained nurse or anesthesia trainee) may be the most qualified individual to provide anesthesia care.

Table 12.1 Basic standards for preanesthesia care

Committee of origin: standards and practice parameters (approved by the ASA house of delegates on October 14, 1987, and last affirmed on October 20, 2010)
These standards apply to all patients who receive anesthesia care. Under exceptional circumstances, these standards may be modified. When this is the case, the circumstances shall be documented in the patient's record
An anesthesiologist shall be responsible for determining the medical status of the patient and developing a plan of anesthesia care
The anesthesiologist, before the delivery of anesthesia care, is responsible for:
1. Reviewing the available medical record
2. Interviewing and performing a focused examination of the patient to:
2.1 Discuss the medical history, including previous anesthetic experiences and medical therapy
2.2 Assess those aspects of the patient's physical condition that might affect decisions regarding perioperative risk and management
3. Ordering and reviewing pertinent available tests and consultations as necessary for the delivery of anesthesia care
4. Ordering appropriate preoperative medications
5. Ensuring that consent has been obtained for the anesthesia care
6. Documenting in the chart that the above has been performed

Table 12.2 American Society of Anesthesiologists physical classification [7, 8]

ASA physical status classification system
ASA Physical Status 1—a normal healthy patient
ASA Physical Status 2—a patient with mild systemic disease
ASA Physical Status 3—a patient with severe systemic disease
ASA Physical Status 4—a patient with severe systemic disease that is a constant threat to life
ASA Physical Status 5—a moribund patient who is not expected to survive without the operation
ASA Physical Status 6—a declared brain-dead patient whose organs are being removed for donor purposes

Preoperative Testing

Preoperative testing, as a component of the preanesthesia evaluation, may be indicated for various purposes, including but not limited to: discovery or identification of a disease or disorder that may affect the perioperative course, verification or assessment of an already known disease, disorder, medical or alternative therapy that may affect perioperative anesthetic care, and formulation of specific plans and alternatives for perioperative anesthetic care.

After obtaining the patient history, performing the physical examination and reviewing preoperative testing, the patient's ASA status should be noted (Table 12.2). The ASA classification identifies patients according to the level of systemic illness.

A patient's poor medical conditions and inappropriate selection for surgery when matching risk to procedure benefit, and inadequate preoperative preparation are factors associated with increased mortality in developing countries [9, 10].

Specific Clinical Considerations

Cardiac Risk

In general, cardiac risk factors are determined by the patient's condition prior to surgery, the prevalence of co-morbidities (as it relates to functional capacity), and the magnitude and duration of the planned surgical procedure. In rural environments a number of factors can contribute to an increased risk of cardiac complications during surgery. Examples include insufficient knowledge of the patient's prior medical conditions (especially as it may relate to endemic disease), inadequate airway control, lack of appropriate monitoring equipment, undetected hypoxia, and lack of resuscitation drugs and colloids and other fluids [11–13].

A thorough assessment provides the clinician an opportunity to initiate medical therapy, coronary interventions, and specific surgical and anesthetic techniques tailored to each individual. Active or unstable cardiac conditions include unstable coronary artery disease, decompensated heart failure, significant arrhythmias, and severe valvular disease.

The Lee index is one of the most accurate indices for predicting cardiac risk in non-cardiac surgery [14]. It emphasizes the value of clinical data in perioperative risk stratification. The Lee index contains five independent clinical determinants of major perioperative cardiac events: a history of ischemic heart disease, a history of cerebrovascular disease, heart failure, insulin-dependent diabetes mellitus, and impaired renal function. High-risk type of surgery is the sixth factor. All factors are equally weighted with one point given to each.

The incidence of major cardiac complications is estimated at 0.4, 0.9, 7, and 11 % in patients with an index of 0, 1, 2, and 3 or more points, respectively (Table 12.3).

Cardiac complications after non-cardiac surgery depend not only on medical risk factors but also on the type of surgery being performed, the urgency, magnitude, type, and duration of the procedure, as well as changes in body core temperature, blood loss, and fluid shifts [15].

With regard to cardiac risk, surgical interventions can be divided into low-risk, intermediate-risk, and high-risk groups with estimated 30-day cardiac event rates (cardiac death and MI) less than 1 %, 1–5 %, and superior to 5 %, respectively (Table 12.4). Although only a rough estimation, this risk stratification provides a good indication of the need for cardiac evaluation, drug treatment, and assessment of risk for cardiac events [16]. Evaluation of functional capacity is considered to be another essential component in preoperative cardiac risk assessment [17, 18]. Functional capacity is measured in metabolic equivalents (METs). One MET equals the basal metabolic rate. Exercise testing provides an objective assessment of functional capacity. Without testing, functional capacity can be estimated by the ability to perform a number of activities of daily living (Table 12.5).

When functional capacity is high, the prognosis is excellent, even in the presence of stable ischemic heart disease or risk factors (>4 metabolic equivalents). On the other hand, when functional capacity is poor or unknown (<4 metabolic equivalents), consideration of other risk factors is required to determine the patient's risk for perioperative morbidity.

Table 12.3 LEE cardiac risk index [16]

Classical LEE risk index	Clinical risk determinants	Clinical LEE risk index
1 Point	*High-risk surgical procedures* • Intraperitoneal • Intrathoracic • Suprainguinal vascular	Not applicable
1 Point	*History of ischemic heart disease* • History of myocardial infarction • History of positive exercise test • Current complaint of chest pain considered secondary to myocardial ischemia • Use of nitrate therapy • ECG with pathological Q waves	1 Point
1 Point	*History of congestive heart failure* • History of congestive heart failure • Pulmonary edema • Paroxysmal nocturnal dyspnea • Bilateral rales or S3 gallop • Chest radiograph showing pulmonary vascular redistribution	1 Point
1 Point	*History of cerebrovascular disease* • History of transient ischemic attack or stroke	1 Point
1 Point	*Preoperative treatment with insulin*	1 Point
1 Point	*Preoperative serum creatinine* >2.0 mg/dL	1 Point

Pulmonary Disease

Preoperative pulmonary care involves identifying patients at high risk for postoperative pulmonary complications and optimizing respiratory function for those with preexistent pulmonary disease [19, 20]. Postoperative pulmonary complications include atelectasis, bronchospasm, pneumonia, respiratory failure, and exacerbation of chronic lung disease.

Table 12.6 indicates conditions and risk factors that significantly increase the risk of such complications.

Smoking cessation before surgery should be initiated as soon as possible (at least 6–8 weeks prior to surgery, 4 weeks at a minimum) [21, 22].

Table 12.4 Surgical risk estimate: risk of myocardial infarction and cardiac death within 30 days after surgery

Low risk <1 %	Intermediate risk 1–5 %	High risk >5 %
Breast	Uncomplicated abdominal	Aortic and major vascular surgery
Dental	Carotid	Peripheral vascular surgery
Endocrine	Peripheral arterial angioplasty	Surgeries with major blood loss or fluids shifts involving the chest or abdomen
Eye (cataract)	Endovascular aneurysm repair	
Gynecology	Head and neck surgery	
Dermatologic procedures and Reconstructive	Neurological/orthopedic—major (hip and spine surgery)	
Orthopedic—minor (knee surgery)	Thoracic, renal/liver transplant	
Urologic—minor	Urologic—major (radical prostatectomy)	

Table 12.5 Estimated energy requirements for various activities

Functional capacity	METs	Physical activity without symptom	Estimated surgical risk
High	>10	Can participate to strenuous sport like swimming, singles tennis, basketball, or skiing?	
Good to very good	7–10	Can do heavy work around the house like scrubbing floors or lifting or moving heavy furniture Can participate in moderate recreational activities like golf, dancing, doubles tennis, football, bicycling at a regular pace Can walk uphill? Can walk on level ground at 4 mph (6.5 kph)? Run a short distance?	Low
Moderate	4–7	Can climb two flights of stairs? Can do light works around the house (dusting, washing dishes)?	
Low	<4	Can take care of yourself? Can eat, dress, or use the toilet? Can walk indoors around the house? Can walk a block or two on level ground at 2–3 mph (3–5 kph)?	Moderate to High
Not assessable	?		

kph indicates kilometers per hour, *MET* metabolic equivalent, *mph* miles per hour

Adapted from Fletcher et al. [18]

Preoperative Assessment of Respiratory Disease

The most commonly encountered preexisting respiratory conditions of clinical relevance to the anesthesiologist include chronic obstructive pulmonary disease (COPD), asthma, and obstructive sleep apnea syndrome (OSAS).

- For COPD, clinical findings of obstruction (wheezing, increased dyspnea), or a history of recent upper respiratory infection (coughing, sputum production) require particular attention and consideration. Major risk factors include type of surgery, type and duration of anesthesia, general health status, and smoking history, rather than specific lung function parameters [23].

Table 12.6 Surgical risk estimate: good evidence for postoperative pulmonary complications

Patient-related risk factor	Procedure-related risk factor	Laboratory test
Advanced age	Aortic aneurysm repair	Albumin level <30 g/L
ASA class = or > II	Vascular surgery	
Chronic heart failure	Thoracic surgery	
Functionally dependent	Abdominal surgery	
Chronic obstructive disease	Neurosurgery	
Obesity smoking	Head and neck surgery Emergency surgery	
Alcohol abuse	General anesthesia	

Modified from Smetana et al. [19]

- Asthma [24]: Preoperative assessment of the patient with asthma should focus on the patient's pulmonary status to determine the level of respiratory dysfunction and to assess the effectiveness of current therapy. A review of baseline exercise tolerance, hospital visits due to asthma (including whether endotracheal intubation or IV infusions were required), allergies, and previous surgical/anesthetic history is essential. The patient's medication regimen should be reviewed providing important clues as to the level of disease severity.

  Asthma can be divided into four categories:

1. Mild intermittent disease (use of short-acting bronchodilators on an as-needed basis).
2. Mild persistent disease (daily controller medication such as low-dose inhaled corticosteroid (ICS) leukotriene modifier, or theophylline).
3. Moderate persistent disease (low- or medium-dose ICS with a long-acting bronchodilator).
4. Severe persistent disease (daily symptoms, multiple medications such as high-dose ICSs, oral steroids, bronchodilators).

This classification should help to identify patients at risk for pulmonary complications and prepare the anesthesiologist to initiate therapy for potential bronchoconstriction and to plan perioperative care to minimize the risk of acute exacerbations.

- Obstructive sleep apnea syndrome [25, 26]: OSAS poses a high risk factor for encountering a difficult airway and post operative respiratory obstruction. In addition to a through history and physical examination prior to surgery, a standardized questionnaire can be helpful in assessing OSAS (e.g., Berlin questionnaire).

Pulmonary Function Tests

Preoperative spirometry and chest radiography are not predictive of postoperative pulmonary complications and cannot be recommended on a routine basis [27]. Clinical findings remain the most accurate predictor of postoperative pulmonary complications. Aggressive treatment based on the use of bronchodilators, antibiotics, corticosteroids, physical therapy, smoking cessation, and correction of malnutrition may be beneficial in reducing postoperative pulmonary complications.

Renal Disease

The patient with preexisting renal disease poses a particular challenge to the safe delivery of anesthesia. Renal complications are more likely to occur in:

1. Patients with preexisting renal dysfunction.
2. Patients with chronic heart disease, chronic obstructive lung disease, peripheral occlusive vascular disease, obesity.
3. Patients undergoing vascular procedures with aortic cross clamping, cardiopulmonary bypass.
4. Lengthy surgical procedures and/or procedure with major blood loss and major fluids shifts.

In non-cardiac surgery, the Kheterpal score is useful for the identification of patient at risk for postoperative renal impairment [28]. For patient without preexisting renal dysfunction seven identified preoperative predictors of acute renal failure include age, emergency surgery, liver disease, elevated body mass index, high-risk surgery, peripheral vascular occlusive disease, and chronic obstructive pulmonary disease necessitating chronic bronchodilator therapy. The score is applied as follows:

- Class I (0–2 risk factors) is not related to a relative risk of acute kidney injury (AKI).
- Class II (3 risk factors) is related to a relative risk of AKI from 4 %.
- Class III (4 risk factors) is related to a relative risk of AKI from 8.8 %.
- Class IV (5 risk factors) is related to a relative risk of AKI from 16.1 %.
- Class V (6 and more risk factors) is related to a relative risk of AKI from 46.3 %.

While a number of strategies have been suggested to minimize nephrotoxic insults, there is limited evidence to support the value of prophylactic and therapeutic interventions in patients at high risk for developing perioperative renal failure [29].

Obesity

The Overseas Development Institute (ODI) currently puts the number of overweight and obese adults in developing countries at more than 900 million. Moreover, the number of overweight and obese adults has risen from 250 million to nearly a billion in the last 30 years [30]. The body mass index (BMI) is the most widely used classification. Patients are considered overweight with a BMI between 25 and 29.9 kg/m^2 and obese with a BMI between 30 and 49.9 kg/m^2. Patients with a BMI of 50 kg/m^2 or greater are considered superobese.

Obesity is accompanied by co-morbidities such as coronary artery disease, hypertension, OSAS and/or diabetes mellitus. Perioperative risk assessment should, therefore, focus on cardiac and pulmonary dysfunction as well as nutritional status [31].

Preoperative assessment of risk factors and clinical evaluation as well as ECG examination is essential in obese patients. To identify patients at risk for difficult airway, a neck circumferences of at least 43 cm as well as a high Mallampati score and male gender are predictors for difficult laryngoscopy and hence intubation [32]. Preoperative testing is indicated in obese patients in order to detect abnormal glucose/HbA1C levels and/or anemia [27].

Diabetes Mellitus

Diabetes mellitus is a growing public health issue affecting people both in developing and developed countries [33]: approximately 150 million people have diabetes mellitus worldwide, and this number may very well double by 2025. Much of this increase will likely occur in developing countries. By 2025, while most people with diabetes in developed countries will be aged 65 years or more, in developing countries the age range is in the 45–64-year bracket during some of their most productive years.

Patients with diabetes are more likely to require surgery [34]. Elevated blood glucose in the perioperative period is a risk factor for surgical site infection [35] and diabetic patients are at greater risk for postoperative heart failure [36]. Both type I and II diabetic patients have a higher rate of difficult laryngoscopy than non-diabetic patients [37].

It is not necessary to test blood sugars routinely on all patients during the preoperative assessment. Screening for diabetes/risk of hyperglycemia can be based on history and examination or investigations of glycemic control. Risk factors include age, sex, family history of diabetes, low exercise level, and obesity [38, 27].

Anemia

Anemia is an especially important public health concern in developing countries and is responsible for significant morbidity and mortality. About two billion people worldwide are estimated to suffer from anemia and it is reported to account for more than 700,000 deaths per year in Africa and Southeast Asia. The highest prevalence of anemia is in preschool-age children (47 %) although nonpregnant women constitute the largest group (468 million) [39]. Underlying causes for anemia are multi-factorial and largely preventable and include nutritional deficiencies, infections, multiple pregnancies, and hemoglobin disorders.

Low preoperative hemoglobin levels and a high level of surgical intervention can predict the need for intraoperative blood transfusion and potentially poor postoperative outcome. Low hemoglobin levels are associated with increased perioperative morbidity in surgical patients, longer recovery from procedures that involve blood loss, and a higher likelihood of postoperative infection. Depending on the hospital, and the lack of availability of routine blood tests, it may be beneficial to bring the equipment required to measure hematocrit (a small portable device), especially if procedures involving blood loss are anticipated. Given the risks and costs associated with allogeneic blood transfusion and the low availability of blood for transfusion, strategies have been developed for preoperative correction of anemia and prevention of perioperative blood transfusion needs as preoperative iron supplementation which may be considered to correct preoperative anemia [40].

Substance Abuse and Addiction

In many developing countries, alcohol and cigarette use is rising rapidly and often at an earlier age. Intravenous drug use, involving heroin, amphetamine, and opiates, is on the rise [41].

Alcohol use disorders (AUDs) are associated with alcohol-related postoperative complications such as higher rates of wound infection, acute withdrawal and organ failure. For the preoperative detection of AUDs, the combined use of a standardized questionnaire (e.g., CAGE questionnaire) together with laboratory testing such as GGT (g-glutaryl transferase) and carbohydrate-deficient transferrin (CDT) is superior to either one alone [42, 43]. Alcohol abstinence for at least 1 month has been shown to reduce perioperative complications from 74 to 31 % [44].

HIV/AIDS

According to the 2007 WHO/UNAIDS estimates, at the end of 2007, more than 95 % of HIV infections worldwide occur in developing countries with two-thirds occurring in sub-Saharan Africa where over 28 million people are living with HIV. Infection rates are lower in Asia and the Pacific, where over seven million are infected. However, since this syndrome is not specific, it is rarely recognized, even when clinically apparent.

Preoperative Evaluation for HIV-Infected Patients [45]

Preoperative evaluation of the HIV-infected patient is similar to that of the general population; however, comorbidities, active substance use, and the presence of methicillin-resistant Staphylococcus aureus may be more prevalent in the HIV-infected population (see Table 12.7).

In most developing countries, heterosexual transmission is the dominant mode of spread, and mother to child transmission of HIV is much

Table 12.7 Surgical management considerations for HIV-infected patients with comorbidities and other conditions

Comorbidity risks	Pre- and perioperative recommendations
Hepatic dysfunction • *Increased prevalence of hepatic dysfunction from ART or from preexisting liver disease* *Surgical risk* • Co-infection with HBV or HCV may predispose to increased bleeding risk due to coagulopathy or thrombocytopenia	*Recommendation* • Assess for hepatic dysfunction preoperatively because of the possible impact on dosing or selection of anesthetics, perioperative antibiotics, and other medications
Renal dysfunction • *Increased prevalence of renal dysfunction from HIV-associated nephropathy (HIVAN) and other causes*	*Recommendations* • Assess for renal dysfunction preoperatively because of the possible impact on dosing or selection of anesthetics, perioperative antibiotics, and other medications • If there are renal function changes in the perioperative period, review ART regimen for agents that may require renal dose adjustment
Coronary artery disease and cardiac abnormalities • *Increased prevalence of CAD from metabolic dysfunction due to HIV infection and/or ART* • *QT prolongation or other cardiac abnormalities may occur in advanced HIV infection or in patients receiving certain medications*[a]	*Recommendations* • Assess for coronary artery disease preoperatively. Perform careful review of preoperative EKG results
Respiratory complications • *Prevalence of underlying pulmonary disease is increased due to the increased risk for bacterial pneumonia and high prevalence of smoking in HIV-infected patients* *Surgical risk* • Risk for postoperative pneumonia is increased in HIV-infected patients	*Recommendation* Carefully evaluate for respiratory complications in the perioperative period
Thrombocytopenia and neutropenia • *Idiopathic thrombocytopenic purpura may occur at any stage of HIV infection* *Neutropenia is common in HIV-infected individuals with severe immunosuppression*[b]	*Recommendations* • Consult with hematologist prior to surgical procedure when platelet counts approach 50,000 per μL • Routine use of G-CSF not recommended but in perioperative period may consider G-CSF[c] use to maintain absolute neutrophil count >1,000 cells/mm
Hemophilia	*Recommendation* • Coordination between surgical team and hematologist is recommended for transfusion of factor replacement in anticipation of surgery

(continued)

Table 12.7 (continued)

Comorbidity risks	Pre- and perioperative recommendations
Substance use (SU) • *SU disorders are more prevalent in HIV-infected individuals than in the general population* *Surgical risks* • Increased risk for complications from surgery and anesthesia, notably cardiac complications associated with cocaine use • Increased risk for withdrawal symptoms in the postoperative period for unrecognized alcohold, benzodiazepine, or heroin use	*Recommendations* • Obtain detailed history of substance use • Consider obtaining urine toxicology screen, with patient consent • For elective surgery, observe appropriate period of abstinence with the use of substitute medications such as methadone or benzodiazepines as appropriate
Methicillin Resistant Staphylococcus aureus (MRSA) • *Community-acquired MRSA infection is more common in MSM than in the general population*	*Recommendations* • Assess for a history of previous MRSA infection/colonization, particularly in MSMs • Use vancomycin instead of cefazolin for prophylaxis when indicated in patients with positive history of MRSA
Drug allergies • *HIV-infection is associated with a higher incidence of medication allergies*	*Recommendation* • Obtain a careful history of allergies

HBV hepatitis B virus, *HCV* hepatitis C virus, *MSM* men who have sex with men, *PI* protease inhibitor, *ZDV* zidovudine

[a]Anti-arrhythmics, methadone, PIs, antipsychotics, or macrolide antibiotics can cause QT prolongation or other cardiac abnormalities, especially if more than one such agent is administered concurrently

[b]Neutropenia may be caused by medications (e.g., ZDV, TMP-SMX), HIV infection itself, bone marrow infiltration from malignancy or systemic infection

[c]G-CSF is recommended over GM-CSF due to theoretical concerns regarding potential stimulation of HIV replication by the latter, although the possible mechanism by which GM-CSF might affect HIV-1 replication remains unclear

[d]Alcohol withdrawal may be life-threatening if symptoms are not recognized early

more common. Transmission associated with injecting drug use is particularly frequent in parts of South and South East Asia and Central and South America. Acquisition of infection from contaminated blood remains a problem, especially in parts of sub-Saharan Africa and South Asia. Women and children are at especially high risk for transfusion transmitted HIV infection, the former because of the high incidence of anemia and hemorrhage associated with pregnancy and childbirth, and the latter because of malarial anemia [46].

Perioperative Medication Management of HIV-Infected Patients

Clinicians should continue antiretroviral therapy (ART) in the perioperative period with as little interruption as possible, particularly for patients co-infected with hepatitis B virus (HBV) who are receiving an ART regimen that also has activity against HBV.

Specific Considerations

Difficult Airway

Airway assessment is paramount when assessing anesthesia-related morbidity. Many unnecessary deaths are a result of airway problems in healthy young patient in developing countries [47].

The American Society of Anesthesiologists defines a difficult airway as the clinical situation in which a conventionally trained anesthesiologist experiences difficulty with facemask ventilation of the upper airway, difficulty with tracheal intubation, or both [48] (Table 12.8).

No single predictive sign for difficult airway management is sufficient by itself and the preanesthesia assessment needs to combine a number of validated evaluation criteria (Table 12.9).

Systematic multimodal screening for difficult intubation should include the Mallampati classification (Fig. 12.2), the thyromental distance (<3 finger breaths), the mouth opening or interincisor distance (<3 cm), and the upper lip bite test (ULBT).

- The Mallampati classification [49–51].
- The ULBT [52] consists of three classes: class I, the lower incisors can bite the upper lip, making the mucosa of the upper lip totally invisible; class II, the same biting maneuver reveals a partially visible upper lip mucosa; and class III, the lower incisors fail to bite the upper lip.

Table 12.8 Current recommendations from the ASA for airway assessment preoperatively

Recommendations for evaluation of the airway
History. An airway history should be conducted, whenever feasible, before the initiation of anesthetic care and airway management in all patients. The intent of the airway history is to detect medical, surgical, and anesthetic factors that may indicate the presence of a difficult airway. Examination of previous anesthetic records, if available in a timely manner, may yield useful information about airway management
Physical examination. An airway physical examination should be conducted, whenever feasible, before the initiation of anesthetic care and airway management in all patients. The intent of this examination is to detect physical characteristics that may indicate the presence of a difficult airway
Multiple airway features should be assessed
Additional evaluation. Additional evaluation may be indicated in some patients to characterize the likelihood or nature of the anticipated airway difficulty. The findings of the airway history and physical examination may be useful in guiding the selection of specific diagnostic tests and consultation

Particular attention to the evaluation for possible difficult intubation should be paid in certain medical conditions such as obesity, large

Table 12.9 Components of the preoperative airway physical examination

Airway examination component	Nonreassuring findings
Length of upper incisors	Relatively long
Relation of maxillary and mandibular incisors during normal jaw closure	Prominent "overbite" (maxillary incisors anterior to mandibular incisors)
Relation of maxillary and mandibular incisors during voluntary protrusion of the lower jaw	Patient cannot bring mandibular incisors anterior to (in front of) maxillary incisors
Interincisor distance	Less than 3 cm
Visibility of uvula	Not visible when tongue is protruded with patient in sitting position (e.g., Mallampati class greater than II)
Shape of palate	Highly arched or very narrow
Compliance of mandibular space	Stiff, indurated, occupied by mass, or nonresilient
Thyromental distance	Less than three ordinary finger breadths
Length of neck	Short
Thickness of neck	Thick
Range of motion of head and neck	Patient cannot touch tip of chin to chest or cannot extend neck

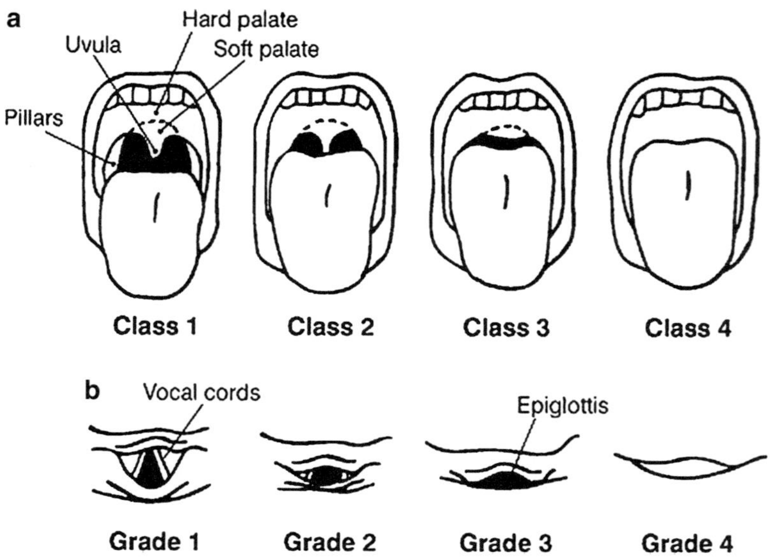

Fig. 12.2 (**a**) Mallampati classification modified by Samsoon and young: Class 1—visualization of the soft palate, Class 2—complete visualization of uvula, Class 3—visualization of the base of the uvula, Class 4—soft palate is not visible at all; (**b**) Laryngoscopy according to the classification of Cormack and Lehane: Grade I—most of the glottis visible, Grade II—only the posterior extremity of the glottis visible, Grade IV—not even the epiglottis visible [6]

neck circumference (more than 45 cm), OSAS, diabetes, fixed cervical spine, ENT pathologies, and preeclampsia.

Pulmonary Aspiration

Perioperative pulmonary aspiration is defined as aspiration of gastric contents (Practice Guidelines for Preoperative Fasting) occurring after induction of anesthesia, during a procedure or in the immediate period after surgery [53]. Aspiration is a known risk of anesthesia and it is avoidable with proper management strategies. Preoperative assessment and identification of patients at risk for aspiration allow the clinician to initiate fasting, medication administration, and appropriate anesthetic techniques to minimize the risk of pulmonary aspiration. In developing countries, higher risk of aspiration is related to inadequate airway management, lack of awareness, and understanding of the anesthesia providers.

Predisposing factors for increasing incidence of aspiration include:

1. Coexisting diseases or conditions that can affect gastric emptying or fluid volume: e.g. obesity, diabetes, hiatal hernia, gastroesophageal reflux, neurological deficit, emergency surgery (particularly in a trauma patient), bowel obstruction, or opioid medication taken by the patient.
2. Patients in whom airway management might be difficult, inadequate (light) anesthesia, or the supine position.

The primary method for reducing the risk of aspiration is to ensure that the patient has an empty stomach before induction of anesthesia, particularly for elective surgical procedures. The routine request to fast patients prior to surgery has evolved with time to emptying the stomach prior to induction of anesthesia so that nowadays several anesthesia societies suggest shorter fasting times with regards to liquids in fit healthy patients. Fasting is the recommended approach to reducing the quantity of gastric contents. According to the ASA definition, preoperative fasting is defined as a prescribed period of time before a procedure when patients should restrict the oral intake of liquids or solids.

A number of recommendations have been proposed related to the duration of fasting and the type of foods that should be avoided. For Preoperative Fasting Status, the ASA guidelines suggest:

1. Adults: Clear liquids at least 2 h (e.g., water, fruit juices without pulp, carbonated beverages, clear tea, black coffee).
2. Children: Clear liquids at least 2 h; breast milk at least 4 h; infant formula at least 6 h.
3. Solids or nonhuman milk at least 6 h.
4. Fried or fatty foods or meat, additional fasting time: at least 8 h or more.

The European Society of Anesthesiology guidelines suggest clinicians [54]:

- Increase the emphasis on encouraging patients not to avoid fluids for any longer than is necessary:
  "Adults and children should be encouraged to drink clear fluids (including water, pulp-free juice and tea or coffee without milk) up to 2 h before elective surgery (including caesarean section)".
- Offer practical, pragmatic advice on chewing gum, smoking and drinks containing milk:
  "Patients should not have their operation cancelled or delayed just because they are chewing gum, sucking a boiled sweet or smoking immediately prior to induction of anesthesia".
- Consider the safety and possible benefits of preoperative carbohydrates:
  "It is safe for patients (including diabetics) to drink carbohydrate-rich drinks up to 2 h before elective surgery".
  "Drinking carbohydrate-rich fluids before elective surgery improves subjective well-being, reduces thirst and hunger and reduces postoperative insulin resistance".
- Fasting in obstetric patients:
  "Women should be allowed clear fluids (as defined above) as they desire in labor".
  But "Solid food should be discouraged during active labor".

These recommendations are of particular importance in warmer climates where dehydration

Table 12.10 Several therapeutic strategies have been applied to decrease the risk of aspiration

Preoperative pharmacologic interventions
1. Gastrointestinal stimulants (e.g., metoclopramide, cisapride)
2. Blockage of gastric acid secretion
a. Histamine-2 receptor antagonists (e.g., cimetidine, ranitidine, famotidine)
b. Proton pump inhibitors (e.g., omeprazole, lansoprazole)
3. Antacids (e.g., sodium citrate, magnesium trisilicate)
4. Antiemetics (e.g., ondansetron, droperidol)
5. Anticholinergics (e.g., atropine, glycopyrrolate)
6. Multiple agents/drugs *versus* single agents/drugs

can post a significant risk to the patient's health prior to surgery.

Patients should be informed of fasting requirements sufficiently in advance of their procedures. Verification of patient compliance with fasting requirements should be assessed prior to the procedure. Nevertheless for patients at risk for aspiration, some preoperative pharmacologic interventions have been proposed (ASA 2011) (Table 12.10.)

Allergy [55]

Substances most responsible for immediate allergic reactions during anesthesia are neuromuscular blockers (63 % of reactions), latex (14 %), hypnotics (7 %), antibiotics (6 %), plasma substitutes (3 %), and morphine-like substances (2 %). Allergic reactions to local anesthetics are very rare, especially when one considers how often they are used. To date no anaphylactic reaction to halogenated anesthetic agents has been published.

The preanesthesia evaluation has to include a systematic search for potential hypersensitivity reactions, taking into account the great number of drugs and devices to which the patient may be exposed during the perioperative period.

Patients at risk for anaphylactic/anaphylactoid reaction are the following:

- Patients with a documented allergy to one of the drugs or products likely to be used.
- Patients with a history of possible allergic reaction during a previous anesthesia.
- Patients with a history of possible latex allergy.
- Children having had multiple surgeries, particularly those with spina bifida and myelomeningocoele.
- Patients with a history suggesting allergy to vegetables, fruits or cereals known to have frequent cross-reactivity with latex (such as kiwi, banana, papaya, avocado, chestnut, buckwheat).

Knowledge of any previous allergic reactions to medications and the nature of the reaction are critical information for the anesthesiologist as well as the other members of the perioperative team to obtain. For patients with hypersensitivity to latex, exposure to even low amounts of latex-containing particles is sufficient to induce a severe anaphylactic reaction. A latex-free operating environment, in which no latex gloves or accessories are used should be established.

Malignant Hyperthermia [56, 57]

Malignant hyperthermia (MH) is serious condition characterized by acute hyperpyrexia developing during or immediately after general anesthesia.

Exposure of patients with mutations predisposing them to MH following exposure to volatile anesthetics, including halothane, isoflurane, enflurane, desflurane, and sevoflurane, or to a depolarizing muscle relaxant such as succinylcholine, can precipitate life-threatening muscle contractures, increases in heart rate and body temperature, rhabdomyolysis, myoglobinuria, and metabolic acidosis. The mortality rate for MH is 80 % in untreated patients but about 5 % with timely treatment.

If malignant hyperthermia is suspected from a family history of adverse events with the administration of anesthetics or when a patient has a reaction suspicious for malignant hyperthermia, a muscle biopsy is indicated but usually not available. No physical findings identify MHS patients.

Local or regional anesthetic techniques are good choices where possible. If general anesthesia has to be used, avoidance of triggering agents is advised and preparation of the anesthesia machine includes removing vaporizers, flushing through the machine with 100 % oxygen and using a new breathing circuit. An anesthesiologist on a medical mission needs to be prepared for malignant hyperthermia and must carry dantrolene or make sure that it is available.

Drug Interactions

Routinely prescribed medications have many potential interactions with drugs used during surgery, but few situations prohibit concurrent administration. The perioperative medical regimen should be reassessed in view of the nature and half-life of the medications. Many medications are continued through the perioperative period, with the last dose taken with a sip of clear liquid up to 2 h prior to the procedure, and quickly resumed during recovery (Table 12.11).

Medical Records

It is imperative that the anesthesiologist documents all findings related to the perioperative interaction in the patient's record and insures its accessibility to both the patient and the local

Table 12.11 Medications and their use or discontinuation during the perioperative period [58, 59]

	Should be continued	Should be discontinued
Cardiovascular [60]		
Beta blockers [61] (e.g., metoprolol, atenolol, nebivolol)	Until and including the day of operation	/
Ace inhibitors (*ACEI*) (e.g., captopril, lisinopril) *Angiotensin receptor blockers* (*ARB*) (e.g., losartan, candesartan)	Until the day before of operation	On the day of the operation (general anesthesia)
Calcium channel blockers [62] (e.g., nifedipine, diltiazem)	Until and including the day of operation	/
Nitrates (e.g., nitroglycerin, isosorbide)	Until and including the day of operation	/
Alpha-2 agonists (e.g., clonidine)	Until and including the day of operation	/
Aspirin [63, 64]	Unless noted otherwise	STOP at least 5 days prior to surgery in high risk of bleeding procedures
Clopidogrel	Unless noted otherwise	STOP at least 1 week prior to surgery
Oral anticoagulants	Unless noted otherwise	STOP at least 5 days prior to surgery
	In patients undergoing surgery with a low risk of serious bleeding, such as cataract or minor soft tissue surgery (carpal tunnel, dermatologic procedures), continuation should be considered instead of instituting bridging therapy	*In high-risk patients or in case of surgical procedures with a high risk of serious bleeding, discontinuation of medications and bridging therapy with LMWH are highly recommended for the perioperative period*
LMWH – Prophylactic dose – Half or full therapeutic dose	Until the day before of operation	STOP 12 h before surgery STOP 24 h before surgery
Diuretics (e.g., furosemide, hydrochlorothiazide)		On the day of the operation
Cardiac rhythm management medications (e.g., digoxin, beta-blockers, quinidine, amiodarone)	Until and including the day of operation	/

(continued)

Table 12.11 (continued)

	Should be continued	Should be discontinued
Statins (e.g., atorvastatin, simvastatin)	Until and including the day of operation	/
Cholesterol lowering medications	Until the day before of operation	On the day of the operation.
CNS medications		
Anticonvulsants (e.g., phenytoin, tegretol)	Until and including the day of operation	/
Antidepressants (e.g., imipramine, sertraline)	Until and including the day of operation	/
Monoamine oxidase inhibitors		STOP at least 2 weeks prior to surgery
Antianxiety medications (e.g., diazepam, lorazepam)	Until and including the day of operation	/
Antipsychotics (e.g., haloperidol, risperdal)	Until and including the day of operation	/
Lithium	Until and including the day of operation	/
Antiparkinson drugs (e.g., sinemet)	Until and including the day of operation	/
Vitamins/nutritional supplements		
"Over-the-counter" *vitamins*		STOP at least 10–14 days prior to surgery
Herbal/alternative preparations [65, 66] (e.g., Ginseng, Garlic, Ginko, Echinacea, Ephedra)		STOP at least 1 week prior surgery, and 1 week after
Pulmonary medications		
Asthma medications (e.g., theophylline, inhaled steroids)	Until and including the day of operation	/
COPD medications (e.g., theophylline, ipratropium, inhaled steroids)	Until and including the day of operation	/
Pulmonary hypertension medications (e.g., sildenafil, prostacyclin, others)	Until and including the day of operation	/
Endocrine		
Insulin	– Type 1 should take 1/3 the day of surgery – Insulin pump continued at the lowest basal rate	– Type 2 take none
Oral diabetic medications metformine	Until the day before of operation	On the day of the operation STOP 24–48 h before surgery
Thyroid medications (e.g., synthroid, dessicated thyroid, propylthiouracil)	Until and including the day of operation	/
Steroids (*oral and inhaled*) (e.g., prednisone, cortef)	Until and including the day of operation	/
Oral contraceptives	Until and including the day of operation	/
Renal		
Phosphate binders, renal vitamins, iron, erythropoietin, others	Until the day before of operation	On the day of the operation.
Gynecology/urology		
Prostate medications (e.g., terazosin, tamsulozsin)	Until and including the day of operation	/
Hormonal medications	Until and including the day of operation	/
Oral contraceptives	Until and including the day of operation	/

(continued)

Table 12.11 (continued)

	Should be continued	Should be discontinued
Analgesics		
Opiate containing analgesics (e.g., vicodin, tylox, methadone)	Until and including the day of the operation, without exception	/
Nonsteroidal anti-inflammatory compounds (e.g., ibuprofen, naproxen)		STOP at least 5 days prior surgery
Gastrointestinal		
Gastroesophageal reflux (GERD) medications (e.g., ranitidine, omeprazole)	Until and including the day of operation	/
Antiemetics (e.g., ondansetron, metoclopramide)	Until and including the day of operation	/
Autoimmune medications		
Methotrexate	Until and including the day of operation Unless risk of acute renal failure	/
Etanercept (Enbral)		STOP 2 weeks prior to surgery
Infliximab (Remicade)		STOP 6 weeks prior to surgery
Adalimumab (Humira)		STOP 8 weeks prior to surgery

Table 12.12 Statement on documentation of anesthesia care

Committee of origin: quality management and departmental administration (approved by the ASA house of delegates on October 15, 2003, and last amended on October 16, 2013)
Documentation is a factor in the provision of quality care and is the responsibility of an anesthesiologist. While anesthesia care is a continuum, it is usually viewed as consisting of preanesthesia, intraoperative/procedural anesthesia and postanesthesia components. Anesthesia care should be documented to reflect these components and to facilitate review. Documentation may be through a paper record, an electronic system, or a combination, as specified by the practice and the facility where patient care is provided. CMS has separate detailed requirements for the contents of peri-anesthesia care documentation that should be addressed, if pertinent
The record should include documentation of:
I. Preanesthesia Evaluation
A. Patient interview to assess:
1. Patient and procedure identification
2. Verification of admission status (inpatient, outpatient, "short stay", etc.)
3. Medical history
4. Anesthetic history
5. Medication/Allergy history
6. NPO status
B. Appropriate physical examination, including vital signs and documentation of airway assessment
C. Review of objective diagnostic data (e.g., laboratory, ECG, X-ray) and medical records
D. Medical consultations when applicable
E. Assignment of ASA physical status, including emergent status when applicable
F. Formulation of the anesthetic plan and discussion of the risks and benefits of the plan (including discharge issues when indicated) with the patient or the patient's legal representative and/or escort.2
G. Documentation of appropriate informed consent(s)
H. Appropriate premedication and prophylactic antibiotic administrations (if indicated)

medical facility (Table 12.12). These records help to discuss the best anesthetic strategies. At every stage of the process, appropriate coordination between anesthesiologist, anesthesia providers, surgeons and operating-room staff is achieved. But in many countries, hospitals do not maintain individual medical records and it is the responsibility of each patient to carry his or her own record. If this is the case, it is highly recommended that the perioperative anesthesia record be created in the local language. In addition, a copy or photograph of the anesthesia record should be kept with the visiting medical team in the event paper records are permanently lost.

Information and Consent

Obtaining medical consent for anesthesia during outreach missions can be a significant challenge as a result of cultural and linguistic and logistical barriers. Very often, the high volume of patients and the logistics of the screening process can be such that the first interaction with a patient occurs in the operating room. Whenever possible, every effort should be made to arrange for a preanesthesia consultation prior to the day of surgery. This meeting can be done concomitantly with the surgeon(s) in a parallel fashion or separately. Anesthesiologists must insist on having adequate time to evaluate and discuss surgical risks with patients and their family members even if this assessment reduces the number of potential surgical cases performed. The anesthesiologist must ensure that patients—or in the case of minors, their family members—fully appreciate the risks specific to the delivery of anesthesia and have an opportunity to address their concerns prior to the operation. Arrangements must be made to communicate and obtain written consent in a language that is accessible to patients and their family members.

Patient Identification

In many developing countries, patient identification is often more difficult because of the language barrier, of the *other race effect* (difficulty to recognize faces from other race), of the close similarity of names, or because of lack of familiarity with local names (Fig. 12.3). Here, as elsewhere in the process, assistance by an interpreter is very helpful. In the author's experience a useful method is to obtain Polaroid photography of the patient with his or her name, date of birth, diagnosis, and treatment plan. The patient is then asked to present this identification card upon entering the operating room for verification. Standard time-out checklists are absolutely paramount to avoid serious medical errors or oversights.

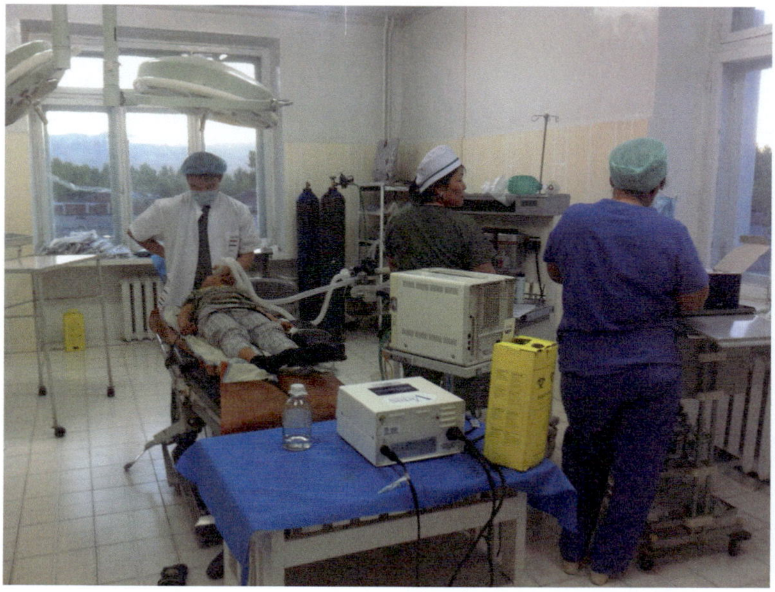

Fig. 12.3 At induction

Scheduling

In scheduling cases, the anesthesiologist must take into account a number of important elements including the nature and urgency of the operation to be performed, the age and medical condition of the patient, the availability of postoperative care (monitoring and intensive care), the limitation of drugs and life sustaining equipment. It is recommended that the team including the surgeon, nursing staff, and anesthesiologist discuss the order and priority of the cases on a daily basis to avoid any miscommunications that could result in unnecessary cancelations, medical errors, or prolonged fasting for patients.

Individual Considerations

As mentioned above, particular attention should be paid to certain anesthetic risks:

- Difficult airway: A portable storage kit should be adapted to the specific skills of the local practitioner and healthcare facility. In developing countries, the minimum content includes: rigid laryngoscope blades, tracheal tubes of assorted sizes, tracheal tube guides, supraglottic airway. More advanced equipment such as videolaryngoscopes, flexible fiber-optic intubation equipment or exhaled carbon dioxide detectors are rarely available unless brought along by the anesthesiologist.
- Risk of anaphylaxis: Patients sensitized to latex must be scheduled at the beginning of the day and in a latex free environment.
- Malignant hyperthermia: A patient with predisposition to malignant hyperthermia must be scheduled at the beginning of the day in order to avoid perioperative exposures to potential gas contamination.

Conclusion

While great strides in technology and technique have greatly improved the overall safety of anesthesia delivery worldwide, incomplete or improper preoperative assessment of the patient continues to be the one the most significant sources of morbidity and mortality. The visiting anesthesiologist must not only be well prepared for unexpected clinical challenges, but also strive to advance the education and training of local providers. It is only can short-term medical interventions can result in long-term sustainable change.

References

1. Capello CS, Gainer VG, Adkisson GH. The safe practice of anesthesia in developing countries. CRNA. 1995;6:91–5.
2. Walker IA, Wilson IH. Anesthesia in developing countries: a risk for patients. Lancet. 2008;371: 968–9.
3. Tobias JD, Kim Y, Davies J. Anesthetic care in developing countries: equipment and techniques. South Med J. 2002;95:239–47.
4. Misra S, Koshy T. Anesthesia in developing countries: one-way traffic? Anesth Analg. 2009;108:674–5.
5. Jochberger S, Lederer W, Mayr VD, Luckner G, Wenzel V, Ismailova F, Ulmer H, Hasibeder WR, Dünser MW, Helfen Berührt Study Team. Anesthesia in developing countries: one-way traffic? Anesth Analg. 2009;108:675.
6. American Society of Anesthesiologists Task Force on Preanesthesia Evaluation. Practice advisory for preanesthesia evaluation: an updated report by the American society of anesthesiologists task force on preanesthesia evaluation. Anesthesiology. 2012; 116:522–38.
7. Cullen DJ, Apolone G, Greenfield S, Guadagnoli E, Cleary P. ASA physical status and age predict morbidity after three surgical procedures. Ann Surg. 1994;220:3–9.
8. Owens WD. American society of anesthesiologists physical status classification system is not a risk classification system. Anesthesiology. 2001;94:378.
9. Bainbridge D, Martin J, Arango M, Cheng D, Evidence-based Peri-operative Clinical Outcomes Research (EPiCOR) Group. Perioperative and anaesthetic-related mortality in developed and developing countries: a systematic review and meta-analysis. Lancet. 2012;380:1075–81.
10. Khan M, Khan FA. Anesthetic deaths in a developing country. Middle East J Anesthesiol. 2007;19:159–72.
11. Jochberger S, Ismailova F, Lederer W, Mayr VD, Luckner G, Wenzel V, Ulmer H, Hasibeder WR, Dünser MW, Helfen Berührt Study Team. Anesthesia and its allied disciplines in the developing world: a nationwide survey of the Republic of Zambia. Anesth Analg. 2008;106:942–8.

12. The Task Force for Preoperative Cardiac Risk Assessment and Perioperative Cardiac Management in Non-cardiac Surgery of the European Society of Cardiology (ESC) and endorsed by the European Society of Anaesthesiology. Guidelines for pre-operative cardiac risk assessment and perioperative cardiac management in non-cardiac surgery. Eur J Anaesth. 2010;27:92–137.
13. Fleisher LA, Beckman JA, Brown KA, Calkins H, Chaikof E, Fleischmann KE, Freeman WK, Froehlich JB, Kasper EK, Kersten JR, Riegel B, Robb JF. ACC/AHA 2007 guidelines on perioperative cardiovascular evaluation and care for noncardiac surgery: executive summary—a report of the American College of Cardiology/American Heart Association Task Force on Practice Guidelines (writing committee to revise the 2002 guidelines on perioperative cardiovascular evaluation for noncardiac surgery)—developed in collaboration with the American Society of Echocardiography, American Society of Nuclear Cardiology, Heart Rhythm Society, Society of Cardiovascular Anesthesiologists, Society for Cardiovascular Angiography and Interventions, Society for Vascular Medicine and Biology, and Society for Vascular Surgery. J Am Coll Cardiol. 2007;50:1707–32.
14. Lee TH, Marcantonio ER, Mangione CM, Thomas EJ, Polanczyk CA, Cook EF, et al. Derivation and prospective validation of a simple index for prediction of cardiac risk of major noncardiac surgery. Circulation. 1999;100:1043–9.
15. Mangano DT. Perioperative medicine: NHLBI working group deliberations and recommendations. J Cardiothorac Vasc Anesth. 2004;18:1–6.
16. Boersma E, Kertai MD, Schouten O, Bax JJ, Noordzij P, Steyerberg EW, Schinkel AF, van Santen M, Simoons ML, Thomson IR, Klein J, van Urk H, Poldermans D. Perioperative cardiovascular mortality in noncardiac surgery: validation of the Lee cardiac risk index. Am J Med. 2005;118:1134–41.
17. Hlatky MA, Boineau RE, Higginbotham MB, Lee KL, Mark DB, Califf RM, Cobb FR, Pryor DB. A brief self-administered questionnaire to determine functional capacity (the Duke activity status index). Am J Cardiol. 1989;64:651–4.
18. Fletcher GF, Balady GJ, Amsterdam EA, Chaitman B, Eckel R, Fleg J, Froelicher VF, Leon AS, Pina IL, Rodney R, Simons-Morton DA, Williams MA, Bazzarre T. Exercise standards for testing and training: a statement for health-care professionals from the American Heart Association. Circulation. 2001;104:1694–740.
19. Smetana GW, Lawrence VA, Cornell JE. Preoperative pulmonary risk stratification for noncardiothoracic surgery: systematic review for the American College of Physicians. Ann Intern Med. 2006;144:581–95.
20. Arozullah AM, Daley J, Henderson WG, Khuri SF. Multifactorial risk index for predicting postoperative respiratory failure in men after major noncardiac surgery. The National Veterans Administration Surgical Quality Improvement Program. Ann Surg. 2000; 232:242–53.
21. Theadom A, Cropley M. Effects of preoperative smoking cessation on the incidence and risk of intraoperative and postoperative complications in adult smokers: a systematic review. Tob Control. 2006;15:352–8.
22. Thomsen T, Tønnesen H, Møller AM. Effect of preoperative smoking cessation interventions on postoperative complication and smoking cessation. Br J Surg. 2009;96:451–61.
23. Henzler D, Dembinski R, Kuhlen R, Rossaint R. Anesthetic considerations in patients with chronic pulmonary disease. Minerva Anesthesiol. 2004;70: 279–84.
24. Applegate R, Lauer R, Lenart J, Jason Gatling J, Vadi M. The perioperative management of Asthma. J Aller Ther. 2013;S11.
25. Gali B, Whalen FX, Schroeder DR, et al. Identification of patients at risk for postoperative respiratory complications using a preoperative obstructive sleep apnea screening tool and postanesthesia care assessment. Anesthesiology. 2009;110:869–77.
26. Gross JB, Bachenberg KL, Benumof JL, et al. Practice guidelines for the perioperative management of patients with obstructive sleep apnea: a report by the American Society of Anesthesiologists Task Force on Perioperative Management of patients with obstructive sleep apnea. Anesthesiology. 2006;104:1081–93.
27. Idem 6.
28. Kheterpal S, Tremper KK, Englesbe MJ, et al. Predictors of postoperative acute renal failure after noncardiac surgery in patients with previously normal renal function. Anesthesiology. 2007;107:892–902.
29. Zacharias M, Gilmore IC, Herbison GP, et al. Interventions for protecting renal function in the perioperative period. Cochrane Database Syst Rev. 2005;9, CD003590.
30. Keats S, Wiggins S. Future diets: implications for agriculture and food prices. London: Overseas Development Institute Report; 2014.
31. Coe AJ, Saleh T, Samuel T, Edwards R. The management of patients with morbid obesity in the anaesthetic assessment clinic. Anaesthesia. 2004;59: 570–3.
32. Brodsky JB, Lemmens HJ, Brock-Utne JG, et al. Morbid obesity and tracheal intubation. Anesth Analg. 2002;94:732–6.
33. World Health Organization 2003. Diabetes mellitus. Fact sheet N°138. Available online: http://www.who.int/mediacentre/factsheets/fs138/en/.
34. Clement S, Braithwaite SS, Magee MF, et al. Management of diabetes and hyperglycaemia in hospitals. Diabetes Care. 2004;27:553–91.
35. Ata A, Lee J, Bestle SL, et al. Postoperative hyperglycemia and surgical site infection in general surgery patients. Arch Surg. 2010;145:858–64.
36. Charlson ME, MacKenzie CR, Gold JP, et al. Risk for postoperative congestive heart failure. Surg Gynecol Obstet. 1991;172:95–104.
37. Mashour GA, George A, Kheterpal S, et al. The extended Mallampati score and a diagnosis of diabetes

mellitus are predictors of difficult laryngoscopy in the morbidly obese. Anesth Analg. 2008;107:1919–23.

38. Idem 4.
39. De Benoist B, McLean E, Egli I, Cogswell M. Worldwide prevalence of Anaemia 1993–2005: WHO Global Database of Anaemia. World Health Organization, 2008. Available online: http://www.who.int/vmnis/anaemia/en/.
40. Hodges SC, Mijumbi C, Okello M, McCormick BA, Walker IA, Wilson IH. Anaesthesia services in developing countries: defining the problems. Anaesthesia. 2007;62:4–11.
41. Uchtenhagen A. Substance use problems in developing countries. Bull World Health Organ. 2004; 82:639–718.
42. Ewing JA. Detecting alcoholism. The CAGE questionnaire. JAMA. 1984;252:1905–7.
43. Martin MJ, Heymann C, Neumann T, et al. Preoperative evaluation of chronic alcoholics assessed for surgery of the upper digestive tract. Alcohol Clin Exp Res. 2002;26:836–40.
44. Tonnesen H, Rosenberg J, Nielsen HJ, et al. Effect of preoperative abstinence on poor postoperative outcome in alcohol misusers: randomized controlled trial. BMJ. 1999;318:1311–6.
45. New York State Department of Health AIDS Institute. Perioperative management of HIV-infected patients. 2012. Clinical Guidelines. Available at: www.hivguidelines.org.
46. Grant AD, De Cock KM. HIV infection and AIDS in the developing world. BMJ. 2001;322:1475–8.
47. Cherian M, Choo S, Wilson I, Noel L, Sheikh M, Dayrit M, Groth S. Building and retaining the neglected anaesthesia health workforce: is it crucial for health systems strengthening through primary health care? Bull World Health Organ. 2010;88: 637–9.
48. American Society of Anesthesiologists Task Force on Management of the Difficult Airway. Practice guidelines for management of the difficult airway. Anesthesiology. 2013;118:251–70.
49. Mallampati SR. Clinical assessment of airway. Anesthesiol Cl N Am. 1995;13(2):301–6.
50. Samsoon GLT, Young JRB. Difficult tracheal intubation: a retrospective study. Anaesthesia. 1987;42: 487–90.
51. Cormack RS, Lehane J. Difficult tracheal intubation in obstetrics. Anaesthesia. 1984;39:1105–11.
52. Khan ZH, Mohammadi M, Rasouli MR, et al. The diagnostic value of the upper lip bite test combined with sternomental distance, thyromental distance, and interincisor distance for prediction of easy laryngoscopy and intubation: a prospective study. Anesth Analg. 2009;109:822–4.
53. American Society of Anesthesiologists Committee. Practice guidelines for preoperative fasting and the use of pharmacologic agents to reduce the risk of pulmonary aspiration: application to healthy patients undergoing elective procedures—an updated report by the American Society of Anesthesiologists Committee on Standards and Practice Parameters. Anesthesiology. 2011;114:495–511.
54. Smith I, Kranke P, Murat I, Smith A, O'Sullivan G, Søreide E, Spies C, Bas in't Veld. Perioperative fasting in adults and children: guidelines from the European Society of Anaesthesiology. Eur J Anaesth. 2011;28:556–69.
55. Mertes PM, Malinovsky JM, Jouffroy L, Working Group of the SFAR and SFA, Aberer W, Terreehorst I, Brockow K, Demoly P, ENDA and the EAACI Interest Group on Drug Allergy. Reducing the risk of anaphylaxis during anesthesia: 2011 updated guidelines for clinical practice. J Investig Allergol Clin Immunol. 2011;21:442–53.
56. Hopkins PM. Malignant hyperthermia: advances in clinical management and diagnosis. Br J Anaesth. 2000;85:118–28. Malignant hyperthermia.
57. Hopkins PM. Malignant hyperthermia. Curr Anaesthesia Crit Care. 2008;19:22–33.
58. Hollevoet I, Herregods S, Vereecke H, Vandermeulen E, Herregods L. Medication in the perioperative period: stop or continue ? A review. Acta Anaesth Belg. 2011;62:193–201.
59. Mercado DL, Petty BG. Perioperative medication management. Med Clin N Am. 2003;87:41–57.
60. Wolf A, McGoldrick KE. Cardiovascular pharmacotherapeutic considerations in patients undergoing anesthesia. Cardiol Rev. 2011;19:12–6.
61. Fleischmann KE, Beckman JA, Buller CE, Calkins H, Fleisher LA, Freeman WK, Froehlich JB, Kasper EK, Kersten JR, Robb JF, Valentine RJ. American college of cardiology foundation/American Heart Association task force on Practice guidelines; American Society of echocardiography; American Society of nuclear cardiology; Heart rhythm Society; Society of cardiovascular Anesthesiologists; Society for cardiovascular Angiography and Interventions; Society for vascular Medicine; Society for vascular Surgery. J Am Coll Cardiol. 2009;54:2102–28.
62. Wijensundera DN, Beattie WS. Calcium channel blockers for reducing cardiac morbidity after noncardiac surgery: a meta-analysis. Anesth Analg. 2003; 97:634–41.
63. Douketis JD. Perioperative management of antithrombotic therapy: antithrombotic therapy and prevention of thrombosis, 9th ed: American College of Chest Physicians Evidence-Based Clinical Practice Guidelines. Chest. 2012;141(2 Suppl):e326S–50.
64. Oscarsson A, Gupta A, Fredrikson M, et al. To continue or discontinue aspirin in the perioperative period: a randomized, controlled clinical trial. Br J Anaesth. 2010;104:305–12.
65. Baillard C, Bianchi A, Gehan G, et al. Anaesthetic preoperative assessment of chronic medications and herbal medicine use: a multicenter survey. Ann Fr Anesth Reanim. 2007;26:132–5.
66. Ang-Lee MK, Moss J, Yuan CS. Herbal medicines and perioperative care. JAMA. 2001;286:208–16.

13 Perioperative Follow-Up and Quality Maintenance

Curtis L. Baysinger, Ivan Velickovic, and K.A. Kelly McQueen

Introduction

The overall burden of surgical disease has a significant impact on global health. In 2013 a World Bank independent commission estimated the magnitude to be 28 % of the total global burden of disease and that the burden of surgical disease is likely to eclipse that due to infectious diseases by year 2016 [1, 2]. In those countries in which some data collection has been possible, preventable anesthesia deaths are very high and aggravate the burden of surgical disease [3–5]. Postoperative complications are rarely followed in low and middle income countries (LMICs) once the patient leaves the operating theater. This missing information impedes accurate conclusions on the role of anesthesia and surgical intervention in averting surgical disease burden. The extent to which postoperative complications contribute to these problems is currently not known.

A lack of trained personnel, inadequate supplies, poor and not enough equipment, constrained pharmaceutical access, and a woefully inadequate infrastructure have all been touted as the major barriers for improving anesthesia care in low income countries (LICs); however, in both low and middle income countries, the core problem may well be a failure of implementation of medical knowledge. Implementation requires bridging the gap between knowing what to do and actual application of the knowledge within a system robust enough to deliver care. Changing the systems by which care is delivered by process improvement should be the major focus for quality improvement in anesthesia in LMICs [6, 7]. Improving the processes by which postoperative care is delivered is critical to improving postoperative quality and outcome.

Quality improvement is a moving target—once achieved, effort is required to maintain improvement. Successful quality maintenance following short term surgical interventions requires a long term commitment from both visitor and the host facility beyond that associated with the visit itself. This long term commitment should include a calendar of repeat short visits and ongoing interaction between the intervention team and the host facility in between visits. When short term visits have been used to provide only proper training of health care workers, this alone has been insufficient in most situations to effect

C.L. Baysinger, M.D. (✉)
K.A.K. McQueen, M.D., M.P.H.
Department of Anesthesiology, Vanderbilt University Medical Center, 1211 Medical Center Dr., Nashville, TN 37232, USA
e-mail: curtis.l.baysinger@vanderbilt.edu; kelly.mcqueen@vanderbilt.edu

I. Velickovic, M.D.
Department of Anesthesiology, State University of New York Downstate Medical Center, University Hospital of Brooklyn, 450 Clarkson Ave., Brooklyn, NY 11203, USA
e-mail: ivan.velickovic@downstate.edu

R. Roth et al. (eds.), *The Role of Anesthesiology in Global Health: A Comprehensive Guide*, DOI 10.1007/978-3-319-09423-6_13, © Springer International Publishing Switzerland 2015

meaningful improvement in LMICs. Waldemar et al. in a review of targeted training program for providers of neonatal resuscitation noted no effect on neonatal mortality rates after training of health workers who performed the resuscitation [8]. Heitmann et al. noted a similar lack of skill retention in providers following Advanced Cardiac Life Support training in Haiti [9]. Thus, if outcomes in LMICs are to improve and if quality improvement occurring during short term visits is to be maintained, it is insufficient to improve only the training of a group of health care workers or to increase the resources that are available in a system. Processes of care have to be improved [7]. Targeted data collection continued by the host health care providers after a short term intervention team departs is the first step. Distribution of this data to all members of a health care system to allow appropriate decision making is required for change to be successful [7].

Maintenance of quality improvement initiatives has the potential for great success at low cost. Since resource scarcity is one of the most daunting aspects of providing health care in LMICs, reduction in systems waste is essential for expanding essential surgical services. Quality improvement processes and changes in systems procedures are proven to reduce in waste of valuable materials, and scarce resources can then be allocated more appropriately [7, 10]. The changes in behavior from these improvements can be accomplished at minimal cost and do not rely on the use of advanced technologies [10]. An emphasis on vigilance in physical diagnosis by providers of anesthesia care without use of advanced technologies may be the most efficacious approach [11]. These and other successful quality maintenance initiatives following short term interventions require modified use of implementation science techniques that have found success in high income countries.

The Need for Adequate Data Collection

Quality improvement in surgery and anesthesiology requires data collection and analysis so that steps to improve care can be outlined and implemented because "that which cannot be measured cannot be improved" [12]. Data on perioperative morbidity and mortality is lacking in most LICs and some MICs. In those countries in which it is collected, the data almost never includes events outside of the immediate intraoperative period [13]. In many LICs there is no written patient record of surgical care beyond the ubiquitous surgical case log in each institution, and accurate statistics are not recorded [14]. In most institutions, deaths occurring within a 30 day period are not recorded either. This makes the tracking of outcomes and mortality within a country nearly impossible (Fig. 13.1). Even if a system to collect health information exists, the data are often incomplete and many times the outcomes are so discouraging to the governing bodies having health care responsibility that they go unutilized [13]. This situation is difficult for most visiting practitioners in high income nations to comprehend.

Underreporting could be changed if the capture of both intraoperative and postoperative surgical and anesthesia mortality rates became a global health priority [1, 13, 15]. As an example where recognition of a specific disease burden and its measurement lead to focused action and improvement, maternal mortality was shown to be a significant contributor to overall world disease in the 1980s. The adoption of mandatory reporting of maternal mortality ratios (MMRs) by the World Health Organization's (WHO) focused world attention on the unacceptable high rates of maternal mortality [16] and galvanized action to reduce it. The tracking of MMR allowed monitoring of quality improvement programs aimed at its reduction and each country was then able to track and compare its results with another country [13]. Tracking of the MMR also led to the inclusion of the reduction of maternal mortality in the United Nations' Millennium Declaration Goals (MDGs). As a result significant progress has been made [17]. A similar worldwide initiative to focus on one easily measured surgical and anesthetic outcome might spur many initiatives to improve anesthetic and surgical quality much like the MDGs did for maternal and child health.

Adoption of a perioperative mortality rate (POMR) defined as the number of American Society of Anesthesiologist (ASA) classification

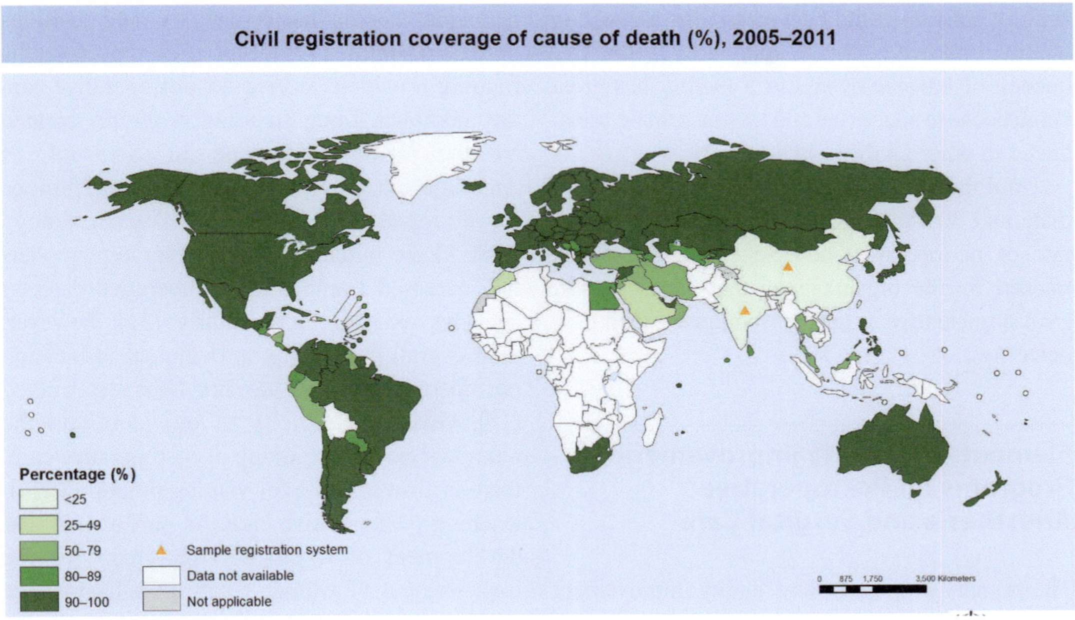

Fig. 13.1 Countries registering cause of death by percentage of total deaths captured. Adpated with permission from World Health Organization Statistics 2013, World Health Organization Global Health Observatory Map Gallery. http://gamapserver.who.int/mapLibrary/app/searchResults.aspx. Accessed 14 April 2014

I and II deaths per 100,000 population or as the fraction of deaths divided by the total number of operations recorded, could serve as the metric which could galvanize the world's efforts to improve surgical outcomes. Separate ratios for deaths within the immediate operative period and those occurring within 30 days should be recorded [18]. These ratios should be stratified for ASA status focusing only on ASA I and II patients. Although surgical procedures in LICs are often performed on ASA I and II patients who are trauma victims, many of whom would die in the field without care, ASA I and II patients should not die in the perioperative period in a system with reasonable surgical skill and anesthetic delivery [13]. Although either of the above suggested ratios is not specific to anesthetic related death, both can be easily measured, are not reliant upon interpretation, and represent the overall quality of surgical care.

Since most operating rooms in LICs record intraoperative death, most often in a paper log of operative procedures, governmental agencies could be incentivized to collect and report the data if funding of surgical improvement projects were contingent upon their collection. In many MICs whose health care systems have significant centralized control, data collection by subordinate hospitals occurs only if required by a central health agency. Furthermore, the current surgical log books found in virtually all low and middle income countries could be easily altered to collect in-hospital postoperative data in addition to that recorded in the immediate surgical period with minimal increase in effort on the part of health care providers. The WHO could report immediate and postoperative mortality ratios for each of its members along with the other data it currently reports. It could become an important measure of a country's public health and patient safety and spur the adoption of future MDGs aimed at improving surgical care.

In the absence of centralized data collection, the most available measure in the majority of LMICs is the frequency of adverse events in a given health delivery facility following surgical and anesthetic care, which is a rough measure of whether patients are helped or harmed. Although the argument is made above that expanded, centralized reporting of mortality rates among healthy patients is the best metric for measuring quality improvement, the reduction in the frequency of adverse events in a facility has great value because successes and lessons can be transferred to other facilities in a country.

Until there is an international mandate, immediate and 30-day perioperative mortality and the rate of perioperative adverse events should be tracked by the organizations that sponsor short term surgical trips as they try to improve their own outcomes.

Elements of Quality Improvement Programs for Postoperative Anesthesia and Surgical Care

The primary purpose of any quality improvement program is to improve patient care [12]. The current model for improving health care quality in general follows the Donabedian framework in which the physical and human structure of the system, the process by which care is delivered, and outcomes of care delivered are assessed [19].

System Structure

The Need for Adequate Numbers of Trained Personnel

The prevention of postoperative adverse events requires trained individuals. Many LICs and some middle income countries (MICs), have an extraordinary lack thereof, the magnitude of which is not well understood due to lack of data on numbers of providers within many LICs [1, 5, 15]. In Uganda, one of the few LICs from which data has been collected, reports in 2008 noted that there were only 14 anesthesiologists for a population of 30 million, giving a ratio of 1 provider per 2.1 million population [1, 20, 21]. In neighboring Kenya there are only 13 anesthesiologists that work in public hospitals serving a population of 32 million [15]. While joint education projects between facilities within a LIC and outside education organizations are ongoing in some areas to improve the lack of trained providers [22], the high cost of training relative to per capita income means many training positions in LICs go unfilled [15]. Moreover, reports on the training providers receive for postoperative care are unknown. Long standing programs created by the World Federation of Societies of Anaesthesiologists (WSFA) and the Committee for European Education in Anaesthesiology (CEEA) are initiatives that can serve as models for increased training in perioperative care by agencies external to a country [23]; however, their overall impact in improving anesthesia and postoperative quality has not been determined [15]. Given the scarcity of providers and the unknown extent of training in postoperative care, there is always a role for visiting practitioners in teaching postoperative care. As part of a 2 year development of a process road map for the improvement of women's care in a health care facility by the Kybele organization and Ridge Hospital in Ghana (Fig. 13.2) [24, 25], post-cesarean section care was identified as a process for improvement and the visiting team developed a program of education for post-cesarean care.

In many MICs resources exist to support training of an adequate number of providers, but standards to insure the quality of the training are often lacking. One focus for short term visit teams to MICs should be not only to provide education, but to partner with interested host facility personnel in creating training standards. During a recent Kybele team visit to Serbia by two of the authors (CB and IV), the local host was engaged in outlining a strategy for education of practitioners outside of the host facility. A curriculum that could be standardized for wide spread use is being created.

In addition to production of trained individuals, the retention of trained practitioners is difficult because the rate of pay for health care practitioners is very low. Once trained in their home country, many anesthesia providers have the qualifications to work elsewhere and thus migrate to better paid positions outside their home country. A "brain-drain" is thus created [15, 20] and the scarce resources used to train in-country providers are exported to more developed nations when those persons leave. The detrimental effect on postoperative care is probably

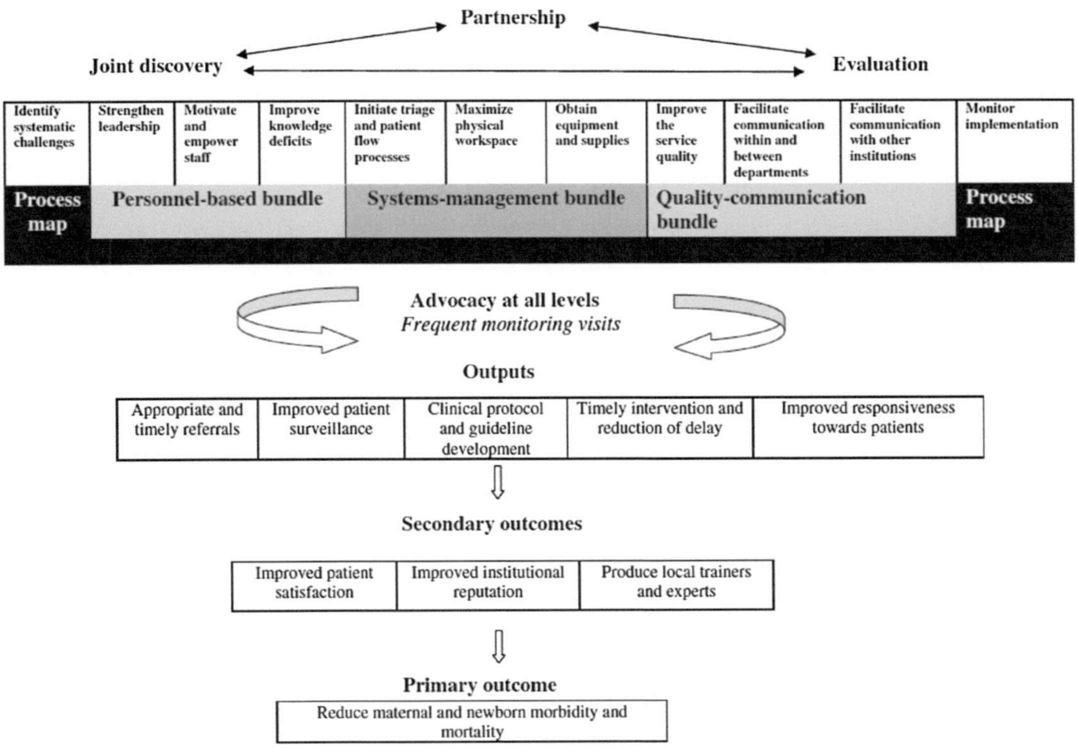

Fig. 13.2 Kybele-Ghana Health Services/Ridge Hospital, Accra process improvement map. Adapted with permission from Srofenyoh et al. Advancing obstetric and neonatal care in a regional hospital in Ghana via continuous quality improvement. Int J Gynaecol Obstet. 2012; 116:17–21 [25]

significant, but currently not quantified. As a process improvement, visiting teams could use morale improving measures to encourage and bolster local practitioners; examples are noted below in the section entitled "Workforce Morale."

The Need for Adequate Infrastructure and Supplies

The prevention of adverse events requires adequate infrastructure and supplies. The lack of transportation for supplies and inadequate support staffing compound the inability to provide essential materials for safe anesthesia care of reasonable quality. Hodges et al., in their report of anesthesia services in Uganda in 2007 using a standardized survey tool, noted that only 23 % of hospitals surveyed could provide a safe general anesthetic for an adult, 13 % could so do so for a child, 28 % could do spinal anesthesia safely, and that resources to provide safe anesthesia for cesarean delivery were available in only 6 % of facilities [3]. Equally dismal percentages for adequate equipment maintenance and drug availability were noted. Although adequate resources do not translate into quality anesthesia provision, provision of necessary resources is required. Donated equipment can be a useful means of improving physical resources, but it must meet the need of the host facility otherwise it will be discarded and can then become a significant environmental hazard to an individual facility as waste disposal is almost non-existent in most LICs. The troubleshooting and subsequent disposal of inappropriate equipment further drains scarce resources and degrades quality care [26]. The WHO has published guidelines that charitable organizations could use for equipment donations [27].

In contrast to surgical facilities in most wealthy western countries, virtually all facilities in LICs and most in MICs do not have a post-anesthesia care unit (PACU) attached to the operating room.

Patients are most often returned to the regular wards or sent to areas little different from them following an operative procedure. Recently reported evidence from France reinforces that establishment of PACUs significantly reduce postoperative adverse events [28]. Unfortunately, resources in most LMICs will likely not be available to provide such a specialized area in facilities in which it currently does not exist. Resources in LICs would probably be better spent on higher priorities. In MICs, extensive facilities were often constructed with operating areas near patient rooms dispersed throughout a facility without dedicated PACUs. The creation of centralized PACUs is unlikely in these settings as the cost of changing this infrastructure would be substantial. Quality improvement could focus on more extensive preanesthetic assessment and preparation and alterations of intraoperative anesthetic techniques to reduce the possibility of anesthesia related post-anesthesia complications. Since airway obstruction and respiratory complications are among the most frequent causes of postoperative morbidity [29], the use of regional anesthesia as a strategy to reduce adverse events could be encouraged as a measure to improve quality. For example, in a recent report of a Kybele sponsored trip to Georgia, Ninidze et al. reported an increase in the use of regional anesthesia for cesarean delivery [30]. While specific effects on postoperative adverse events were not noted, the report was done in the context of improving total perioperative care in which increased use of regional anesthesia was thought to improve maternal outcomes.

Although the only randomized controlled trial examining the effects of pulse oximetry introduction failed to show a reduction in adverse effects postoperatively [29], its widespread use to improve patient outcomes during the immediate operative period is now part of the *International standards for a safe practice of anaesthesia* [31]. Best practice guidelines vary considerably among organizations in all health systems, but virtually all guidelines demand use of pulse oximetry and compliance among practitioners for its use is nearly 100 % when made available [31]. Currently The Global Oximetry project promotes the widespread adoption of pulse oximetry during the operative period [32]. As an initiative, visiting teams could promote pulse oximetry use into the postoperative period regardless of patient location and, with their host facility, adopt processes to implement immediate care when hypoxemia is detected.

Process Improvement Systems

In many LMICs, systems for care delivery have typically evolved slowly and the reasons for processes used are often not know by the current workers within the system. This leads to difficulty in introducing new ideas quickly. In many LMICs the problem being addressed has often existed for so long that it has survived attempts in the past to solve it, has been cast off as a result of resource lack, and is approached by the workers in the system as being unsolvable [7]. Improving workplace morale, changing workplace behavior and culture, and change implementation are required for process improvement.

Workforce Morale

Improving process to prevent of adverse events requires good workforce morale. The poor infrastructure and lack of medical supplies noted above are commonly found in LICs and some MICs and lead to poor workforce morale [15]. Provider psychological reaction to the organizational structure in which the provider works has an almost equal effect. A recent systematic review of studies examining factors contributing to poor health care worker morale in LICs, noted that while financial constraints and poor resource availability ranked near the top of factors associated with poor morale (90 % and 80 % respectively), lack of career development and lack of recognition by the organization for worker contributions ranked nearly as high (85 % and 70 %, respectively) [33]. In contrast, poor infrastructure was reported by only 45 % of workers as contributing to low morale. As part of their ongoing improvement, the above mentioned Kybele–Ghana partnership began a program recognizing individual nurse suggestions, implemented a monthly nurse recognition award, and sponsored an out of country educational trip to the United States for those nurses who were recognized as team leaders. Although the effects on overall morale were not measured, other improvements in work performance measures (decreased work tardiness for example) were noted.

Workforce Behavior and Culture

The prevention of adverse events is likely to be incentivized by changes in behavior and culture. As an example, the attitudes and practice habits of anesthesiologists and other anesthesia providers in LMICs regarding vigilance have not been evaluated or studied. However, the behavior of local anesthesia providers has been anecdotally noted by humanitarians, visiting physicians, and surgical teams providing care through nonprofit organizations. Often anesthesia providers will leave a patient under anesthesia for a variety of reasons, including caring for another patient, being called to an emergency, and in the most shocking of situations, for a lunch break leaving no one else in attendance. The process of providing a thorough hand-off of care to persons who will care for a patient in the postoperative period is not often performed. These practices were common place in developed countries prior to 1950, but a culture of vigilance and the availability of safety monitors which demand continuous assessment has forever changed the standard of care for an anesthesia provider in the immediate and postsurgical period. However, for providers who have rendered pre- and post-anesthetic and surgical care for years and decades without monitors, and often with minimal resources, an emphasis on vigilance may have waned. Vigilance in many LICs needs to be reintroduced, and postoperative hand offs to other health personnel need to be mandatory.

Vigilance may be enhanced by the simple measure of identifying the sicker vs. the healthiest postoperative patient. The good success in reducing maternal mortality reported by the Kybele-Ghana experience may lie in separating the sick from the less sick by screening for preeclampsia and post-delivery hemorrhage. This action allowed scarce and overworked care givers to focus their attention on those patients who needed it most. Similarly an index of patient risk for postoperative difficulty could be generated using a combination of unstable intraoperative hemodynamics, excessive surgical blood loss, and complexity of preoperative medical conditions. Postoperative care givers could identify those patients with increased risk vs. those with less and thus focus their scarce time preferentially.

Team building will help change workplace behavior. Team building encourages participation by all stakeholders in perioperative care. Regular meetings ensure all persons have a say in the change process that affects them. Ensuring that everyone can speak during meetings and using power elevating techniques allow individuals, including those who are low in the organizational structure to feel that that they have input [7]. Shortly after The Kybele-Ghana project began, both the visiting team and the facility hosts agreed that monthly morbidity and mortality conferences and monthly service meetings would occur. All stakeholders at the host facility participated, and everyone were encouraged to have input.

Implementation of Process Change

Prevention of adverse events requires change to the processes and ways of doing work; "all change will not result in improvement, but any improvement will need to result in change" [7]. Although the application of implementation science to LIMC health care systems is in its infancy, Ramaswamy and Barker [7] and Berwick [10] (based on his review of successful project implementation in an LIC [Peru] and an MIC [Russia]) suggest common factors that can lead to successful implementation and maintenance of quality improvement (Tables 13.1 and 13.2). These authors state that successful implantation will often lead to higher quality with consumption of fewer resources and better quality care that often costs less compared to the provision of defective care [7, 10]. The challenge of improving postoperative care relies upon consuming fewer resources. Implementation of better processes needs to be the focus in LICs in particular that often waste many of the scarce resources that they can ill afford to lose [7].

Table 13.1 Factors for successful quality improvement implementation

• Clear improvement goals
• Participation by all stakeholders
• Defining measures to achieve goals
• All providers help build infrastructure and data collection means
• All participate in generating change ideas
• Education of learned successes to those outside a facility

Table 13.2 Team behaviors for successful quality improvement

• Specify defined goals, understood by all stakeholders
• Use team building during project development
• Build infrastructure, especially data collection
• Empower local leadership to move forward despite a larger changing policy environment
• Spread new improvements in stages

Table 13.3 Common reasons for resistance to change by organizations

• Lack of buy-in to need for change
• Uncertainty about future career effects, position qualifications
• Fear of learning new ways of doing things
• Lack of trust in external suggestions
• No participation in planning by stakeholders
• Perceived lack of communication by leadership
• Fear of failure

One core principle is how changes are introduced to the stakeholders who they will affect; either resistance will be encountered, or providers will accept them and the implementation will more likely be successful [7]. Travis et al. and Ramaswamy and Barker et al. have outlined common reasons for resistance to change among stakeholders within a system (Table 13.3) [7, 34]. During the early evolution of the Kybele–Ghana partnership, need for the routine involvement of an organizational systems consultant who had worked with organizations in overcoming resistance to adoption of change by stakeholders was identified. Thus a non-medical person who fulfilled this role was made a routine part of the visiting team and met with small groups of health providers during external team visits to facilitate acceptance of agreed measures to process development.

Formulating clear aims to improve perioperative anesthetic and surgical care upon which all stakeholders agree can be difficult because not all will accept that a problem is everyone's to solve and or even whether solving a given problem is necessary. Group meetings may require participation of large groups of people from the entire organization. Leadership has to emphasize the importance of the project and show unwavering commitment to it. The aims should be couched in terms of measurable results that are easily operationalized and understood to all who are participating in the change [7, 10]. For example, since adoption of pulse oximetry in the postoperative period will likely improve outcome, the number of patients who had low oxygen saturation readings and the number of interventions might be used as a metrics to monitor post-anesthetic care.

Work flow charts, which contain all participants in the system, have not often been used in LMICs to diagram work processes; however, their use in other settings has often led to personal insights that create individual ownership for improvement [10]. Trade-offs between accurate recording of those measures vs. ease in producing relevant data is often necessary [7]. Display of the data to all stakeholders will keep interest in the quality improvement high and will lead to acceptance of change when progress is shown [7, 10]. While advanced technology to collect data, such as use of mobile phone devices which are common in LMICs is possible, it is important to focus on simplicity of data gathering and presentation [7]. During the development of the process map used by the Kybele–Ghana partnership, individual intermediate improvement goals were identified and progress toward each goal was measured by a "colored smiley face" (from a red frowning face meaning no progress to a green smiling face meaning total implementation). This chart was updated by the visiting team and host partners at each repeat visit and displayed where all stakeholders could easily see it. Although the effect of the device was not quantified, progress could be easily determined by all in the facility.

Spreading Local Successes

Transferring change to other parts of the health care system outside of a local system that has had success requires spread to other parts of a country. Many times that spread will be impeded as it occurs in a country's political climate where overall health care policy changes are frequent due to frequent political leadership changes [10]. Because virtually all LICs and most MICs have not had much experience with large scale quality improvement programs, the most effective approach to disseminate a successful project would be use of a deliberate timetable in which a program is implemented in a health care district, followed by ramping up through successive regions of a country [7]. Workshops conducted every 3–6 months, first within a district involving stakeholders from a health care facility, and then among stakeholders within a region would identify reasons for success and help remove barriers [7]. Recent success has been reported by the Institute for Healthcare Improvement (IHI) and by Berwick who used this approach in improving care to patients with hypertension over large regions in Russia [10, 35]. In many MICs, where a health care delivery system may be under significant centralized control, change to an established procedure may require permission by a higher level governmental organization. Centralized health ministries may view change to a long-standing policy as unnecessary and thus impede the dissemination of local innovation.

Maintaining Outcomes

Few reports of success from LMICs in areas of anesthesia related quality improvement exist Reports from other areas of health care delivery, primarily aimed at reduction in the burden of infectious disease, are few as well, but show that implementation and maintenance of quality improvement programs using the tools outlined above can be effective [6, 10, 36–39].

What is very clear is that those programs that have been successful had ongoing visiting program-host interaction during times when the visiting team is not on site. The necessary systems changes to effect meaning full quality improvement will not come from sporadic visits from either internal or external well-meaning health care organizations. Narrowly focused quality improvement projects without building wide focused systems for monitoring and response will most likely fail [7, 40]. External organizations interested in helping should thus be ready to commit to a long term relationship with the facility or health system with which they interact. Trust between the leadership of the visiting team and the host and a good working relationship is critical for overall success.

With modern communication technology, and the availability of internet and wireless communication in most LMICs, host team members can communicate easily with their external counterparts at almost no expense. The benefit for monitoring progress between team visits and the ability to better plan visits in greater detail is obvious.

An ongoing relationship between visitor and host is one of the main reasons why the above mentioned Kybele–Ghana partnership reported success in reducing maternal mortality and the rate of stillbirths through partnership with a health care facility in Accra, Ghana. After initial site visits over a 2 year period of time by the Kybele organization and establishment of their process improvement map, results in the major outcome variables were impressive: maternal mortality declined 34 %, case fatality rates from preeclampsia and hemorrhage decreased from 3.1 % to 1.1 % and from 14.8 % to 1.9 % respectively, and stillbirths declined by 36 %. All of this occurred despite a 36 % increase in patient admissions and a substantial increase in patient acuity. Success was attributed to use of many of the implementation strategies mentioned above, including a long term commitment by all parties to process improvement, formal support from by the country's senior health leadership, training by staff in quality improvement processes, participation by all parties involved at the health care facility, identification of local persons who take ownership of the process, and identification of a measure of outcome that was easily obtained and made known to all [24, 25].

Surgical Safety Checklist

World Health Organization | Patient Safety
A World Alliance for Safer Health Care

Before induction of anaesthesia → **Before skin incision** → **Before patient leaves operating room**

Before induction of anaesthesia

(with at least nurse and anaesthetist)

Has the patient confirmed his/her identity, site, procedure, and consent?
- ☐ Yes

Is the site marked?
- ☐ Yes
- ☐ Not applicable

Is the anaesthesia machine and medication check complete?
- ☐ Yes

Is the pulse oximeter on the patient and functioning?
- ☐ Yes

Does the patient have a:

Known allergy?
- ☐ No
- ☐ Yes

Difficult airway or aspiration risk?
- ☐ No
- ☐ Yes, and equipment/assistance available

Risk of >500ml blood loss (7ml/kg in children)?
- ☐ No
- ☐ Yes, and two IVs/central access and fluids planned

Before skin incision

(with nurse, anaesthetist and surgeon)

- ☐ **Confirm all team members have introduced themselves by name and role.**
- ☐ **Confirm the patient's name, procedure, and where the incision will be made.**

Has antibiotic prophylaxis been given within the last 60 minutes?
- ☐ Yes
- ☐ Not applicable

Anticipated Critical Events

To Surgeon:
- ☐ What are the critical or non-routine steps?
- ☐ How long will the case take?
- ☐ What is the anticipated blood loss?

To Anaesthetist:
- ☐ Are there any patient-specific concerns?

To Nursing Team:
- ☐ Has sterility (including indicator results) been confirmed?
- ☐ Are there equipment issues or any concerns?

Is essential imaging displayed?
- ☐ Yes
- ☐ Not applicable

Before patient leaves operating room

(with nurse, anaesthetist and surgeon)

Nurse Verbally Confirms:
- ☐ The name of the procedure
- ☐ Completion of instrument, sponge and needle counts
- ☐ Specimen labelling (read specimen labels aloud, including patient name)
- ☐ Whether there are any equipment problems to be addressed

To Surgeon, Anaesthetist and Nurse:
- ☐ What are the key concerns for recovery and management of this patient?

This checklist is not intended to be comprehensive. Additions and modifications to fit local practice are encouraged. Revised 1 / 2009 © WHO, 2009

Fig. 13.3 World Health Organization Surgical Safety Checklist. Adapted with permission from WHO Surgical Safety Checklist and Implementation Manual WHO Surgical Safety Checklist. http://www.who.int/patientsafety/safesurgery/tools_resources/SSSL_Checklist_finalJun08.pdf. Accessed 14 April 2014

Similar success has been reported by another Kybele sponsored health care team in an MIC. Ninidze et al. recently reported on the success of a similar collaborative quality improvement project to increase the use of regional anesthesia for labor and for cesarean section in the nation of Georgia [30]. Over 3 years, four visits were made by an outside consulting group who provided education in the use of regional anesthesia and introduced quality improvement processes and measurement tools. The use of general anesthesia for cesarean delivery declined from approximately 80–30 % overall at participating hospitals and the use of epidural analgesia for labor increased from 20 % to approximately 45 %; no changes were noted at control hospital within the country. Reasons cited by the authors for success were similar to that noted by the Ghana–Kybele partnership.

An example where quality improvement has not been uniformly successful is in adoption of the WHO Surgical Safety Checklist (SSCL) in LMICs (Fig. 13.3) [41]. When successfully implemented, the WHO SSCL has led to significant reduction in anesthetic and surgical complications. Bergs et al. in a recent systematic analysis of seven studies evaluating the implementation of the WHO SSCL in hospitals in developed countries and LMICs noted an approximate 40 % reduction in any complication (30-day mortality, surgical site infection, excessive blood loss, unplanned emergency surgery, pneumonia), a 23 % reduction in mortality, and a 43 % reduction in surgical site infection [42]. Weiser et al. in a prospective study of the WHO SSC introduction in four hospitals in developed countries, two hospitals in MICs and one hospital in a LIC, noted a one-third reduction in complications a drop in overall surgery associated death from 3.7 to 1.7 %, and increased compliance with six essential safety measures (airway evaluation, use of pulse oximetry, IV access, prophylactic antibiotic administration, confirmation of surgical site, and sponge count verification) from 19 to 51 % [43]. However, the authors of this second study were unable to determine if the use of the checklist had been retained after the study period. Indeed, although Borchard et al. reported a 70 % overall compliance with elements in a recent systematic review of SSCL adoption in developed countries [44], other studies have noted barriers to their adoption. One study from France noted wide variation in their adoption attributable to organizational and cultural factors [45].

Widespread implementation in LMICs may be unsuccessful. Alitoor et al. evaluated the implementation of the SSCL in hospitals in Pakistan and noted a lack of surgical site identification in 13 % of the surveyed procedures, no antibiotic prophylaxis in 38 %, and no recording of patient allergies and instrument counts in 54 % and 21 % of the procedures, respectively [46]. SSCL adoption may be more critical in LMICs than in more developed countries as the largest decrease in complications (74 % in one study) occurred in LMICs as compared to high income countries (HICs) [41]. Levy et al. emphasized that effective adoption of checklist elements in a hospital in a developed country required the use of the elements of implementation science noted in the discussion above [47]. Vivekanantham et al. noted that barriers to adoption in LICs are cultural in nature, and require education efforts and compliance monitoring in that setting [48].

For the SSCL to be most effective in improving care, it is essential that safety equipment, rescue medications and blood, which are emphasized in the list, be available in the setting where implementation is desired. While the WHO and Safe Surgery Saves Lives researchers have recognized that the SSCL will require modification based on local infrastructure, the outcomes related to the check list have not been compared nor stratified related to these local modifications. For instance, when the SSCL was initially evaluated, pulse oximetry was not routinely available in a majority of operating theaters in LICs [49]. Of even greater concern is that oxygen is often not available in many operating theaters of LICs, and that blood banking and the availability of non-banked blood is infrequently planned for and rarely available outside hospitals providing the highest level of care in LICs. In fact, oxygen has only been recently added to the WHO Essential Medicine list [27]. These realities anecdotally contribute to a sense of futility in the poorest settings when the list is modified for the resource reality on the ground.

Conclusions

For the past two decades, the pressing needs of the global HIV epidemic have shifted the focus of LMIC health care systems away from surgical and anesthesia infrastructure, and, by extension, away from outcomes analysis and improvement interventions. As LMICs build and improve surgical infrastructure to meet the growing surgical needs related to chronic disease, maternal and child health, and trauma, it is essential to include processes for tracking, reporting, and benchmarking anesthesia and surgical outcomes. Recent advocacy for the perioperative mortality ratio including reporting of a separate ratio for postoperative mortality presents a realistic opportunity to evaluate and track patient safety and outcomes related to anesthesia and surgery. Systems-wide, infrastructure and cultural changes will be required for the much needed quality improvement in the postsurgical period in most LMICs and even as infrastructure lags behind. LMICs should be encouraged that early implementation of these processes will decrease postoperative morbidity and mortality.

References

1. Dubowitz G, Detlefs S, McQueen KA. Global anesthesia workforce crisis: a preliminary survey revealing shortages contributing to undesirable outcomes and unsafe practices. World J Surg. 2010;34: 438–44.
2. Jamison D, World Bank, Disease Control Priorities Project. Disease control priorities in developing countries. New York: Oxford University Press, World Bank; 2006.
3. Hodges SC, Mijumbi C, Okello M, McCormick BA, Walker IA, Wilson IH. Anaesthesia services in

developing countries: defining the problems. Anaesthesia. 2007;62:4–11.

4. Khan MU, Khan FA. Anaesthesia-related mortality in developing countries. Anaesth Intensive Care. 2006; 34:523–4.
5. Hansen D, Gausi SC, Merikebu M. Anaesthesia in Malawi: complications and deaths. Trop Doct. 2000; 30:146–9.
6. Barker PM, Mphatswe W, Rollins N. Antiretroviral drugs in the cupboard are not enough: the impact of health system's performance on mother-to-child transmission of HIV. J Acquir Immune Defic Syndr. 2011;56:e45–8.
7. Ramaswamy R, Barker PM. Quality Improvements in Resource-Poor Countries. In: Sollecito WA, Johnson JK, editors. McLaughlin and Kaluzny's Continuous Quality Improvement in Health Care. Burlington, MA: Jones and Bartlett Learning; 2013.
8. Waldemar AC. Newborn-care training and perinatal mortality in developing countries. N Engl J Med. 2010;362:614–23.
9. Heitmann D, Whittaker P, Goedecke E, Goptz I. Teaching advanced cardiac life support in a developing country: pitfalls and potential solutions. Ann Emerg Med. 2008;51:505.
10. Berwick DM. Lessons from developing nations on improving health care. BMJ. 2004;328:1124–9.
11. McIntyre JWR. A unified approach to providing general anaesthesia monitoring with special reference to developing countries. Int J Clin Monit Comput. 1990;7:147–55.
12. Dutton RP. Why have a quality management program? Int Anesthesiol Clin. 2013;51:1–9.
13. McQueen KA. Global anesthesia crisis and quality improvement. Int Anesthesiol Clin. 2014;52:109–19.
14. Mathers CD, Fat DM, Inoue MF, Rao C, Lopez AD. Counting the dead and what they died from: an assessment of the global status of cause of death data. Bull World Health Organ. 2005;83:171–7. 52:109–19.
15. Dubowitz G. Global health and global anesthesia. Int Anesthesiol Clin. 2010;48:39–46.
16. Mahler H. The safe motherhood initiative: a call to action. Lancet. 1987;1:668–70.
17. Peterson HB, Haidar J, Merialdi M, Say L, Gülmezoglu AM, Fajans PJ, et al. Preventing maternal and newborn deaths globally. Obstet Gynecol. 2012;120:636–42.
18. World Health Organization. WHO Guidelines for Safe Surgery. http://whqlibdoc.who.int/publications/2009/9789241598552_eng.pdf. Accessed 24 Apr 2014.
19. Donabedian A. The quality of care: how can it be assessed? JAMA. 1988;260:1743–8.
20. Ozgediz D, Jamison D, Cherian M, McQueen K. The burden of surgical conditions and access to surgical care in low-and middle-income countries. Bull World Health Organ. 2008;86:646–7.
21. Ozgediz D, Galukande M, Mabweijano J, Kijjambu S, Mijumbi C, Dubowitz G, et al. The neglect of the global surgical workforce: experience and evidence from Uganda. World J Surg. 2008;32:1208–15.
22. Ozgediz D, Wang J, Jayaraman S, Ayzengart A, Jamshidi R, Lipnick M, et al. Surgical training and global health: initial results of a 5-year partnership with a surgical training program in a low-income country. Arch Surg. 2008;143:860–5.
23. Mellin-Olsen J. Varieties of teaching programs matched to country needs. Int Anesthesiol Clin. 2010;48:9–21.
24. Engmann C, Olufolabi A, Srofenoyh E, Owen M. Multidisciplinary team partnerships to improve maternal and neonatal outcomes: the Kybele experience. Int Anesthesiol Clin. 2010;48:109–22.
25. Srofenyoh E, Ivester T, Engmann C, Olufolabi A, Bookman L, Owen M. Advancing obstetric and neonatal care in a regional hospital in Ghana via continuous quality improvement. Int J Gynaecol Obstet. 2012;116:17–21.
26. Howie SR, Hill SE, Peel D, Sanneh M, Njie M, Hill PC, et al. Beyond good intentions: lessons on equipment donation from an African hospital. Bull World Health Organ. 2008;86:52–6.
27. World Health Organization. WHO model list of essential medicines. http://www.who.int/selection_medicines/list/en/. Accessed 7 Apr 2014.
28. Tiret L, Desmonts JM, Hatton F, et al. Complications associated with anaesthesia—a prospective survey in France. Can Anaesth Soc J. 1986;33(3 Pt 1):336–44.
29. Moller JT, et al. Randomized evaluation of pulse oximetry in 20,802 patients: II Perioperative events and postoperative complications. Anesthesiology. 1993;78:445–53.
30. Ninidze N, Bodin S, Ivester T, Councilman L, Clyne B, Owen M. Advancing obstetric anesthesia practices in Georgia through clinical education and quality improvement methodologies. Int J Gynaecol Obstet. 2013;120:296–300.
31. Merry AF, Cooper JB, Soyannwo O, Wilson IH, Eichhorn JH. International Standards for a Safe Practice of Anesthesia. Can J Anesth. 2010;57:1027–34.
32. Thomas GM, McHugh GA, O'Sullivan E. The global oximetry initiative. Anaesthesia. 2007;62 Suppl 1:75–7.
33. Willis-Shattuck M, Bidwell P, Thomas S, Wyness L, Blaauw D, Ditlopo P. Motivation and retention of health workers in developing countries: a systematic review. BMC Health Serv Res. 2008;8:247–55.
34. Travis P, Bennett S, Haines A, Pang T, Bhutta Z, Hyder AA, et al. Overcoming health-systems constraints to achieve the Millennium Development Goals. Lancet. 2004;364:900–6.
35. Institute for Healthcare Improvement. The Breakthrough Series: IHI's Collaborative Model for Achieving Breakthrough Improvement. IHI Innovation Series. 2003. http://www.ihi.org/resources/pages/ihiwhitepapers/thebreakthroughseriesihiscollaborativemodelforachievingbreakthroughimprovement.aspx. Accessed 14 Apr 2014.
36. Agyepong IA, Adjei S. Public social policy development and implementation: a case study of the Ghana

National Health Insurance Scheme. Health Policy Plan. 2008;23:150–60.
37. Agyepong IA, Sollecito WA, Adjei S, Veney JE. Continuous quality improvement in public health in Ghana: CQI as a model for primary health care management and delivery. Qual Manag Health Care. 2001;9:1–10.
38. Bukonda N, Tavrow P, Abdallah H, Hoffner K, Tembo J. Implementing a national hospital accreditation program: the Zambian experience. Int J Qual Health Care. 2002;14 Suppl 1:7–16.
39. Legros S, Massoud R, Urroz O. The Chilean legacies in health care quality. Int J Qual Health Care. 2002;14 Suppl 1:83–98.
40. Durand MA. Quality improvement and the hierarchy of needs in low resource settings: perspectives of a district health officer. Int J Qual Health Care. 2009;22:70–2.
41. Haynes AB, Weiser TG, Berry WR, Lipsitz SR, Breizat AH, Dellinger EP, et al. A surgical safety checklist to reduce morbidity and mortality in a global population. N Engl J Med. 2009;360:491–9.
42. Bergs J, Hellings J, Cleemput I, Zurel Ö, De Troyer V, Van Hiel M, et al. Systematic review and meta-analysis of the effect of the World Health Organization surgical safety checklist on postoperative complications. Br J Surg. 2014;101:150–8.
43. Weiser TG, Haynes AB, Dziekan G, Berry WR, Lipsitz SR, Gawande AA, Safe Surgery Saves Lives Investigators and Study Group. Effect of a 19-item surgical safety checklist during urgent operations in a global patient population. Ann Surg. 2010;251:976–80.
44. Borchard A, Schwappach DL, Barbir A, Bezzola P. A systematic review of the effectiveness, compliance, and critical factors for implementation of safety checklists in surgery. Ann Surg. 2012;256:925–33.
45. Fourcade A, Blache JL, Grenier C, Bourgain JL, Minvielle E. Barriers to staff adoption of a surgical safety checklist. BM J Qual Saf. 2012;21:191–7.
46. Alitoor A, Nigah-e-Mumtaz S, Syed R, Yousuf M, Syeda A. Surgical safety practices in Pakistan. J Pak Med Assoc. 2013;63:76–80.
47. Levy SM, Senter CE, Hawkins RB, Zhao JY, Doody K, Kao LS, et al. Implementing a surgical checklist: more than checking a box. Surgery. 2012;152:331–6.
48. Vivekanantham S, Ravindran RP, Shanmugarajah K, Maruthappu M, Shalhoub J. Surgical safety checklists in developing countries. Int J Surg. 2014;12:2–6.
49. Funk LM, Weiser TG, Berry WR, Lipsitz SR, Merry AF, Enright AC, et al. Global operating theatre distribution and pulse oximetry supply: an estimation from reported data. Lancet. 2010;376:1055–61.

14 Women's Rights to Pain Relief After Surgery and Labor Analgesia

Fiona Turpie and Ronald B. George

Introduction

The health and socioeconomic development of any country is dependent on the well-being of women. However, women are still dying in childbirth and from treatable conditions because they don't have access to the most basic surgeries and perioperative care, including analgesia. Safe anesthesia for cesarean delivery saves lives during obstructed births but, when not available, can lead to mortality for the mother and fetus. Whether it is a cesarean, childbirth, or any number of surgical procedures, they are immeasurable painful components of women's lives.

Access to pain management is a human right. However, less than 50 % of all patients with acute postoperative, chronic, or cancer pain are adequately managed [1]. Unfortunately in low and middle income countries (LMIC) the incidence of pain is significantly higher [2]. Following surgery or childbirth, acute pain may limit the recovery and function of women in the postoperative period as these women fight to reduce poverty, hunger, and threats to their environmental on a daily basis. In contrast, pain associated with labor and delivery is the most important anesthetic-related concern for expectant mothers in high income countries [3]. Young girls and women in LMIC suffer the greatest ill-health consequences from low status, poverty, and denial of basic human rights [4].

Human Rights and Inhuman Pain

Pain is, in part, a learned experience. It does not necessarily only reflect the presence of a noxious stimulus but reflects interactions with a person's internal and external environment and her/his learned behaviors from cultural experiences. Pain is a complex milieu of physiology, psychology, and sociological factors. When managed poorly, pain also has major physiological, psychological, economic, and social ramifications for patients, their families, and society [5]. Given the wide variety of cultural environments, countless variations in the experience and manifestations of pain are to be expected. Regardless of its definition, source, or influence from environmental factors, the management of pain is a public health emergency on a global scale.

Pain is defined as a physical suffering or discomfort caused by illness or injury [6]. The International Association for the Study of Pain defines pain as an unpleasant sensory and emotional experience

F. Turpie, M.D., F.R.C.P.C., D.T.M.H.
Department of Anesthesiology, Pain Management, and Perioperative Medicine, Dalhousie University, Halifax, NS, Canada

R.B. George, M.D., F.R.C.P.C. (✉)
Department of Women's & Obstetric Anesthesia, IWK Health Centre, 5850 University Ave., Halifax, NS, Canada, B3P 0B7
e-mail: rbgeorge@dal.ca

R. Roth et al. (eds.), *The Role of Anesthesiology in Global Health: A Comprehensive Guide*, DOI 10.1007/978-3-319-09423-6_14,

associated with actual or potential tissue damage, or described in terms of such damage [7].

Advocates for pain management have pointed out repeatedly that inadequate pain management is a violation of human rights. Less than 50 % of patients with acute, chronic, or cancer pain are adequately managed [1, 8]. It was demonstrated that pain impacts the quality of life for 20 % of adults and 50 % of the elderly [1, 5, 8]. Pain related to untreated cancer effects more than 70 % of those 10 million diagnosed annually and the number of diagnosed cases is expected to exceed 20 million by 2020 [8]. In 2012 there were more than 35 million people living with Human Immunodeficiency Virus (HIV), creating a large burden of pain related morbidity as pain affects more than 60 % of those during their illness with HIV [8]. HIV has a particularly dramatic prevalence in developing countries, with more than 70 % of diagnosed cases living in sub-Saharan Africa; 12 million are women over the age of 15 [9]. Not only is pain a physiologic response but also a pathological response which increases both morbidity and mortality. It has an impact on individuals' quality of life.

In LMIC, health care delivery is focused on high-level objective goals such as treating prevalent cancers and developing vaccinations and treatments effective against HIV and malaria. While working towards these necessary goals to improve lives in developing countries we should not lose focus on analgesia management, the pain suffered by women, and the impact of pain on quality of life indicators.

In the past 30 years there has been expansive growth in our knowledge of the physiology and psychology of pain. We now have numerous pharmaceutical and non-pharmaceutical interventions to aid our patients. However, the gap between our understanding of the biology of pain and our pervasive failure to implement effective pain management strategies continues to grow. In LMIC, this gap is, for the most part, ignored despite pandemic suffering from HIV and Acquired Immune Deficiency Syndrome (AIDS), poverty, oppression and violence, and war and its aftermath [5].

Untreated pain after surgery increases heart rate, systemic vascular resistance, and circulating catecholamines, placing patients at risk of myocardial ischemia, stroke, bleeding, and other complications. Unrelieved acute pain commonly elicits pathophysiologic neural alterations, including peripheral and central neuronal sensitization, that evolve into chronic pain syndromes [10]. Physically, these responses include reduced mobility and consequent loss of strength, disturbed sleep, an increased susceptibility to disease, dependence on medication, and codependence on family members and other caregivers [5]. The psychological and likely societal ramifications of chronic pain are profound. The WHO has revealed that mental illness is four times more likely to afflict those with chronic pain issues compared to those without pain [5].

Declaration of Montreal, 2010

At the conclusion of the 2010 World Congress on Pain, the International Association for the Study of Pain hosted delegates to the International Pain Summit, comprised of representatives from 130 countries who gathered to address the tragedy of unrelieved pain globally. At the conclusion of the Summit, the delegates adopted the Declaration of Montreal, which states that access to pain management is a fundamental human right. Within this declaration, it is stated that there is 'inadequate access to the treatment of acute pain caused by trauma, disease and terminal illness and failure to recognize chronic pain is a serious chronic health problem akin to other chronic diseases such as diabetes or chronic heart disease' [11]. Reasons for this failing including: major deficits in knowledge of health care professionals regarding the mechanisms and management of pain, lack of national policies declaring pain management as a public health problem, inadequate levels of research funding, and severe restrictions on the availability of opioids and other essential medications critical to the management of pain [11]. The World Health Organization (WHO) estimates that five billion people have limited or no access to controlled medicines to treat moderate to severe pain [8]. Supporting this statement, experts demonstrated that "every country in the world is now party to at least one human rights treaty that addresses health related rights as well as other rights that relate to the conditions necessary for health" [1] (Table 14.1).

Pain is a ubiquitous throughout our lives and throughout our practice as anesthesiologists. The mandate of the World Federation of Societies of Anaesthesiologists (WFSA) is to maintain the highest standards of anesthesia, pain medicine, trauma management, resuscitation, and preoperative/critical care medicine to all peoples of the world and advocate for improved pain management [12]. They have acknowledged that pain has been both poorly managed and over looked both in developed and developing countries [13]. The WFSA have adopted the three steps of the WHO analgesic treatment ladder starting with non-opioid adjuncts, secondly stepping up to low potency opioids, and then if necessary the addition of a high potency opioid to manage moderate to severe pain (Fig. 14.1).

Table 14.1 The Declaration of Montreal

The Declaration of Montreal [11]
Article 1. The right of all people to have access to pain management without discrimination
Article 2. The right of people in pain to acknowledgment of their pain and to be informed about how it can be assessed and managed
Article 3. The right of all people with pain to have access to appropriate assessment and treatment of the pain by adequately

The 2010 Declaration of Montreal formalized the position of the World Federation of Societies of Anesthesiologists (WSFA) on acute and chronic pain. Future global health anesthesiology research and policy will be guided by the Declaration

Each of the medications on the ladder, acetaminophen, ibuprofen, and morphine are found on the WHO List of Essential Medications updated every 2 years and directed at the primary health care requirements of a population [1]. They are selected with regard to disease prevalence, safety, efficacy, and comparative cost-effectiveness [14]. The *Essential List* advocating the pharmaceutical needs of individuals allows each nation to expand on the list according to national health goals and individual needs. The goal of the *Essential List* is to establish standards of health care supplies and to improve national standards of care.

The Realities of Pain Management Among Women in LMIC

Women experience more severe pain, more recurrent pain, and longer duration of pain than men [15]. Moreover, pain affects a higher proportion of women than men and they are less likely to receive treatment compared to men [16, 17]. Upwards of 20 % of women may suffer from continued severe acute pain after labor and delivery of their children [18]. Since acute pain is a risk factor for chronic pain, it can be postulated that the experiencing the pain of childbirth may shape a woman's "pain future," having a profound effect on her life.

Access to pain management is poor for all people in LMIC, gender inequalities contribute to the pain suffered women globally. This can be due to various cultural, economic and political barriers. Pain from menstruation and/or childbirth is diminished by caregivers and deemed 'natural'.

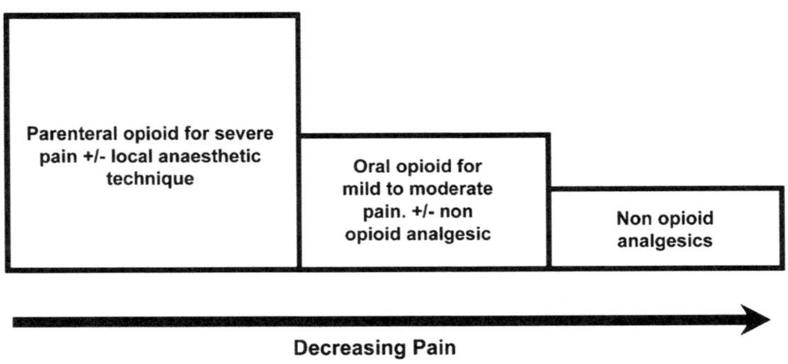

Fig. 14.1 World Federation of Societies of Anaesthesiologists modified analgesic ladder for acute pain [13]

Women are among the most commonly cited vulnerable groups along with children, the elderly, patients living with HIV/AIDS or other chronic diseases, those with mental or physical disabilities, ethnic minorities, and socioeconomically disadvantaged groups [19, 20]. A large percent of the female population are potential mothers, and the detrimental effect of maternal death on household income, household productivity, and household disintegration has been widely described [21]. During and after a disaster, women have to assume the role of head of household. This may include management of household finances and food supply, in addition to childcare and other responsibilities [20].

Pregnancy may be the defining period of a women's life. In most parts of the world pregnancy can also be a life threatening condition. Access to safe and pain free surgical care during pregnancy is a critical prerogative for all women. The ability to provide quality analgesia is likely an indicator of the level quality of care facility can deliver. In the opinion of the authors, the rate of death of women in LMIC could be improved by providing them with access to quality health services such as analgesia. However, in reality, most women experience serious barriers to accessing services. Even if they do reach them, the services themselves are often of insufficient quality or effectiveness. The main components are the health professionals within their 'enabling environment' that comprise a functioning health care system including effective transportation, drugs, equipment and supplies [21]. A lack of trained surgical providers is among the most significant barriers to essential surgical and postsurgical care. LMIC have a crisis of human resources where the workforce of surgeons, obstetricians, and anesthesiologists is severely depleted [22]. This scarcity is due in part to a paucity of education, training, and economic opportunities for physicians and other health care workers.

Pain and Childbirth

In the advocacy of pain management as a human right, the Declaration of Montreal states that it is the right of all people to have access to pain management for acute pain caused by trauma, disease, or terminal illness without discrimination. The pain of pregnancy is not caused by any of these injuries described but by the physiological preparation of the uterus and cervix to expel the fetus through the vagina. Labor causes severe pain for most women. The pain of labor for nulliparous women was similar to the trauma of having a digit amputated [23]. There is no other circumstance where it is considered acceptable for an individual to experience untreated severe pain, amenable to safe intervention, while under a physician's care [24]. The American College of Obstetricians and Gynecologists together with the American Society of Anesthesiologists have stipulated that in the absence of a medical contraindication, a women's request is a sufficient medical indication for pain relief during labor [24].

In China, most women in labor are primigravidas whose fear of labor pain leads them to request cesarean deliveries rather than risk labor without effective analgesia; their fears may be justified as less than 1 % of women in labor are given analgesia [25]. As a result, the rate of cesarean deliveries is as high as 50 % in many hospitals in China. In these situations, more available labor analgesia may reduce the rate of cesarean deliveries and resulting morbidity and mortality by reducing fear of labor pain.

The logistics of pain management during labor are complex. There is the physiology of both mother and fetal circulation to consider and the choice of drug and delivery may have impact one or both parties. Some methods of pain management, such as labor analgesia, can be costly and labor intensive. Neuraxial labor analgesia is the primary modality in high-income countries. However, epidural analgesia uses numerous disposables and large volumes of medications. The ability to supply the medications and disposable equipment must be considered when planning to provide a labor analgesia service. All classes of drugs used traditionally on labor units for pain management of labor are listed in the WHO List of Essential Medicines. This includes opioids, naloxone, local anesthetics, and nitrous oxide [26]. Providing pain relief during labor is both necessary and feasible in developing countries.

Neuraxial analgesia is a highly effective method of providing pain relief during labor [27, 28]. Regardless of economic situation, some women in labor wish to have analgesia for childbirth. Unfortunately, access to epidural analgesia during labor is limited in LMIC [29]. In a survey of women in LMIC, 85 % of respondents indicated they would request labor analgesia if available but only 40 % received any form of analgesia during childbirth [30]. Costs of staffing and supplies associated with providing neuraxial analgesia can be prohibitive in LMIC [13, 31]. With limited resources for epidural analgesia, spinal analgesia may be a useful alternative for relief of labor pain [32, 33].

Pain management during labor permits a calm and stable environment for the infant's delivery. It will offer the workers the ability to demonstrate compassion and empathy instead frustration. Perhaps the learned behavior of pain and its needed endurance will be recognized as unnecessary and bring these women to a supervised skilled setting for delivery. Skilled delivery would offer the women greater chances of survival and perhaps even reduce the complications affecting the neonate leading to longer-term survival of both mother and child.

To truly promote women's rights and the right to pain relief, a greater investment in education and health, including reproductive health and family planning must be made [4]. Beyond difficult accessibility, women have limited access to health care in LMIC because of traditional beliefs surrounding religion and ethnicity into which modern medical care does not fit [34]. The authors postulate that exposure and education of women may have women ignore traditional beliefs and choose safe labor pain relief over cesarean delivery. The next section describes in more detail the international efforts to advance the health of women in the context of the Millennium Development Goals.

Table 14.2 The United Nations Millennium Goals

The United Nations Millennium Goals
Goal 1. Eradicate extreme poverty and hunger
• Reduce extreme poverty by half
• Productive and decent employment
• Reduce hunger by half
Goal 2. Achieve universal primary education
• Universal primary schooling
Goal 3. Promote gender equality and empower women
• Equal girls' enrollment in primary school
• Women's share of paid employment
• Women's equal representation in national parliaments
Goal 4. Reduce child mortality
• Reduce mortality of children under 5 years of age by two-thirds
Goal 5. Improve maternal health
• Reduce maternal mortality by three-quarters
• Access to reproductive health
Goal 6. Combat HIV/AIDS, malaria, and other diseases
• Halt and begin to reverse the spread HIV/AIDS
• Halt and reverse the spread of tuberculosis
Goal 7. Ensure environmental sustainability
• Have proportion of population without improved drinking water
• Halve proportion of population without sanitation
• Improve the lives of slum-dwellers
Goal 8. Develop a global partnership for development
• Internet use

As discussed above, the Millennium Development Goals were created to help focus resources for the achievement of several universal human rights and global priorities by the year 2015

The Millennium Development Goals and Pain

When women are treated as objects and not as fully human, they have few or no rights and their health suffers. Basic human rights generally include a right to: (a) respect as a person of value or worth, (b) security of person (safety), (c) privacy/confidentiality, (d) food, nutrition, and housing, (e) freedom from any form of discrimination, (f) information and education, (g) benefits of scientific progress, (h) freely informed consent, (i) reproductive choices, and (j) equitable access to health services of good quality [4].

To galvanize purpose and organize efforts toward the achievement of basic human rights for all people, at the turn of the twenty-first century, the United Nations (UN) created an ambitious set of eight goals to be achieved by 2015 (see Table 14.2).

Although there have been great strides made to improve conditions for the marginalized minorities, for women and children under five in developing countries, the objective deadlines of the MDGs will not be met. Still more than 1 billion people live in extreme poverty, with a total of 385 million still living on less than 1.25 dollars a day. There is still a huge gender gap for those employed, with the gender-employment ratio resting at almost 30 % in Africa [35]. Women still fill positions of lesser employment [36]. Primary school education in developing countries has reached 90 % [37]. A child under five is twice as likely to die if her mother has not had a primary school education [36]. For this reason, the UN is in the process of setting a post-2105 agenda for continued work [38].

The survival of children under five (MDG 4) and the reduction in maternal mortality (MDG 5) may be key pain related goals. Reducing by almost half, the child mortality incidence has fallen 12.4 million in 1990 to 6.6 million in 2012 [39]. Despite this fall in the child mortality rate, the rate of neonatal deaths is increasing [39]. Asphyxia is the cause of 9 % of the neonatal deaths. In dealing with the pain of the laboring woman, a reduction in some of the complications of labor can result in successful instrumental delivery allowing those infants to be delivered without serious morbidity or complications which would result in lower infant mortality rate [39, 40].

MDG 5 addresses a woman's right to maternal health care. The original goal, to reduce the maternal mortality ratio by two-thirds has had some success with a reduction in maternal deaths of 47 % from 1990 to 2010 [40]. Even though there has been great progress, 50 million babies are still born without skilled attendants present [40]. Postpartum hemorrhage is still a large contributing factor to maternal mortality in much of the developing world.

MDG 4 and 5 are unified by the need to empower women both in poverty and in developing countries, include objective measures of their success. The goals include the need for education on reducing the mortality of children under five by measuring mortality reduced by mortality rates and the reduction in the maternal mortality ratio. Currently there is no consideration of a woman's suffering and pain and how that may affect work towards the achievement of the MDGs.

The MDG each has gender biases directed towards the improvement of marginalized women and the children under their care in impoverished and developing countries. Potential examples of these biases in LMIC include the preference for male children, which may result in lower investment of resources for female children. This leads to women being disadvantaged in the battle to combat hunger. As women are responsible for most work in the home, pregnant women perform heavy physical labor far into their pregnancies. This significant workload may contribute to preterm delivery and fetal growth restriction, which leads to decreased under-five survival. Another example: Women's lives can be improved by ensuring environmental sustainability and access to clean water near where people live. Since the daily task of collecting water mostly falls to female members of the household, clean accessible water could mean more time to concentrate on their own and their children's health. Thus, bringing an improved water supply to somewhere near residential concentrations can both improve the health of a population and reduce the burden of a particularly taxing and time-consuming form of labor.

The Three Delays of Maternal Mortality: Pain Delay

The conceptual details first described by Thaddeus and Wade of the three delays relating to maternal mortality in the developing world are applicable to all aspects of women's health care in the developing world [41]. The woman must first recognize that pain may be key to an underlying pathophysiologic condition or simply to childbirth itself. It may require consultation with other women in the village including a traditional birth attendant prior to the recognition of a problem. If no problem is identified when there is one present, the obstruction to skilled assistance is postponed. Women, the earth over, place their children and their commitments before their own well-being (Fig. 14.2).

In rural communities, where the women have both limited education and access to information

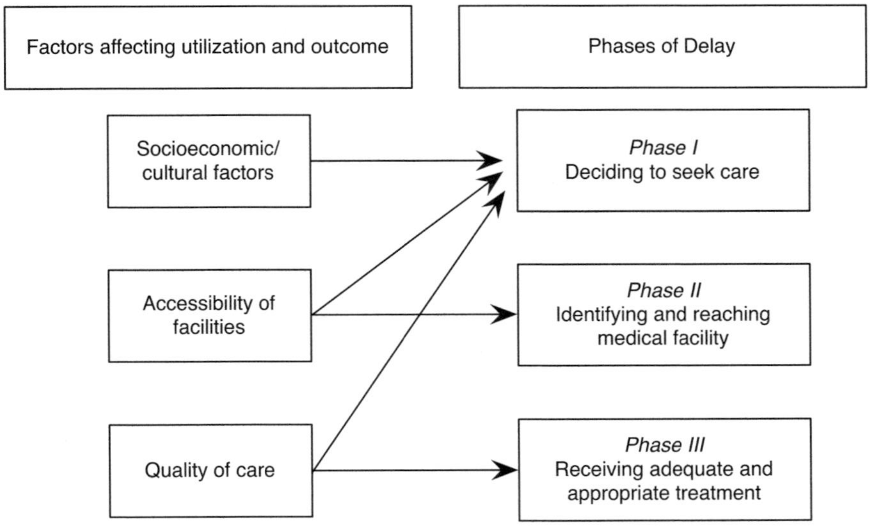

Fig. 14.2 The Thadeus and Maine delay model [41]. Thadeus and Maine describe the complex care seeking behavior of women in low resource settings as having three phases; the decision to seek care, gaining access to a medical facility, and receiving the services needed. Each of these phases is influenced by a web of social and cultural issues, transportation and geography of the local health care landscape, and the quality of personnel and services in-country

because of cultural and sociological constraints they often must seek approval from a head of household to seek treatment. It is often that the male holds both the pecuniary support and social approval needed to seek transport to that health care facility and more importantly the money to provide the care. If the male head has moved to an urban center to support his family, seeking assistance may delay a woman's search for care.

If both financial support and permission are given, the next issue will be for the woman to find transport to the clinic or center, which may be able to help her. She may need to walk, but with severely incapacitating pain that may not be possible. She may need to find public transport, which has an unpredictable schedule. When the need is urgent she may need to exercise the option of hiring a motor or a bicycle. The limited accessibility may delay a woman from the needed care, immaterial of the source of her pain. Finally when she does arrive at the health care facility, the doctor or other health care professional may be unavailable to either assess her pain but perhaps more importantly manage her pain. Each step in the delay model prolongs the pain and its impact on quality of life.

Availability of analgesics. Almost at the same time as the Montreal Declaration, there was another summit in the Netherlands, sponsored by the International Federation of Health and Human Rights of which the British Medical Association and the Amnesty International observing [42]. A resolution was passed by the World Medical Association General Assembly stating that individuals in pain had the right to pain management. The WMA also declared that drug control policies should be reviewed. The goal of this review was to ensure that drugs such as morphine were available in countries where there may be unnecessary mechanisms of restriction in place.

The woman herself. Traditional beliefs religion and ethnic origin were identified as reasons that the women would avoid hospital [34]. Birth was perceived as a test of endurance. In Uganda women are expected to deliver without fear but a multitude of traditional therapies are offered, including back massages, sitting submerged in water mixed with forms of herbal medicine to clean, disinfect and 'widen the birth canal', spreading topical herbs inside the vagina and herbal elixirs to deliver the placenta [43].

System issues. Once access to the drugs is secured, the patient needs access to an individual who will treat her pain. The closest medical care may be a clinic staffed only by nurses or other health care workers without the knowledge or the training to assess and treat her pain. Either by systematic or self-referral she must seek out a physician who must then set aside their own beliefs to treat the pain. There are many biases of health care professional including concern about the patient's needs for pain management and the balance of dependence and addiction. A broader education amongst all health care professionals to teach empathy and compassion with appropriate and necessary management of pain, which may take on many forms during one's life, is required globally [44].

Mismanaged and under recognized pain has huge implications on physiological, social economic, and social cultural levels irrespective of women's pain. Pain can have significant, pervasive repercussions if not managed properly. It is associated with lost time of work, slower return to activities of daily living, and reduced physical recovery after the injury, be it surgical or otherwise. Improved relationships once pain is under control have been documented, including in the postpartum period after the delivery that improves mother–infant bonding.

Conclusion

Pain becomes a life-defining event for many women in developing countries; be it the untreated and often ignored pain of child birth, acute surgical pain, or even the disregarded palliative pain of end of life pathology. As health care professionals, we must seek out strategies and interventions to change this cycle. Acknowledgement of pain and recognition of its further impacts is only the first step. Both our increased acknowledgement and awareness of pain in women must be utilized for advocacy of pain management in women. The Declarations of Human Rights, the Millennium Development Goals and the Declaration of Montreal are inching us forward towards a future where pain management is a human right. But more will be needed. Addressing the pain of women and their right to appropriate management in developing countries will take great effort by supporting the education of those who are to manage the pain as health care professionals and those who must ensure the supply of the drugs. These skills must be shared with the emphasis on both empathy and compassion. Education is key.

References

1. Cousins MJ, Brennan F, Carr DB. Pain relief: a universal human right. Pain. 2004;112(1–2):1–4.
2. Adams V, Worldwide Palliative Care Alliance. Access to pain relief: an essential human right. A report for World Hospice and Palliative Care Day 2007. Help the hospices for the Worldwide Palliative Care Alliance. J Pain Palliat Care Pharmacother. 2008; 22(2):101–29.
3. Carvalho B, Cohen SE, Lipman SS, Fuller A, Mathusamy AD, Macario A. Patient preferences for anesthesia outcomes associated with cesarean delivery. Anesth Analg. 2005;101(4):1182–7.
4. Thompson JE. Poverty, development, and women: why should we care? J Obstet Gynecol Neonatal Nurs. 2007;36(6):523–30.
5. Brennan F, Carr DB, Cousins M. Pain management: a fundamental human right. Anesth Analg. 2007; 105(1):205–21.
6. The Oxford English Dictionary. 2nd ed. Oxford: Oxford University Press; 1989.
7. IASP Taxonomy: International Association for the Study of Pain; 2014 [cited 2014]. Available from: http://www.iasp-pain.org/Education/Content.aspx?ItemNumber=1698&navItemNumber=576 - Pain.
8. Lipman AG. Pain as a human right: the 2004 Global Day Against Pain. J Pain Palliat Care Pharmacother. 2005;19(3):85–100.
9. Global Health Observatory—Number of Women Living with HIV: World Health Organization; 2014. Available from: http://www.who.int/gho/hiv/epidemic_status/cases_adults_women_children/en/.
10. Siddall PJ, Cousins MJ. Persistent pain as a disease entity: implications for clinical management. Anesth Analg. 2004;99(2):510–20. table of contents.
11. International Pain Summit Of The International Association For The Study Of Pain. Declaration of Montreal: declaration that access to pain management is a fundamental human right. J Pain Palliat Care Pharmacother. 2011;25(1):29–31.
12. World Federation of Anaesthesiologists, WFSA Constitution: World Federation of Anaesthesiologists; 2013. Available from: http://www.anaesthesiologists.org/guidelines/wfsa-constitution.

13. Size M, Soyannwo OA, Justins DM. Pain management in developing countries. Anaesthesia. 2007;62 Suppl 1:38–43.
14. Manikandan S, Gitanjali B. National list of essential medicines of India: the way forward. J Postgrad Med. 2012;58(1):68–72.
15. Alabas OA, Tashani OA, Tabasam G, Johnson MI. Gender role affects experimental pain responses: a systematic review with meta-analysis. Eur J Pain. 2012;16(9):1211–23.
16. Bartley EJ, Fillingim RB. Sex differences in pain: a brief review of clinical and experimental findings. Br J Anaesth. 2013;111(1):52–8.
17. Fillingim RB, King CD, Ribeiro-Dasilva MC, Rahim-Williams B, Riley III JL. Sex, gender, and pain: a review of recent clinical and experimental findings. J Pain. 2009;10(5):447–85.
18. Eisenach JC, Pan PH, Smiley R, Lavand'homme P, Landau R, Houle TT. Severity of acute pain after childbirth, but not type of delivery, predicts persistent pain and postpartum depression. Pain. 2008;140(1):87–94.
19. Miller AC, Arquilla B. Disasters, women's health, and conservative society: working in Pakistan with the Turkish Red Crescent following the South Asian Earthquake. Prehosp Disaster Med. 2007;22(4):269–73.
20. Bloem CM, Miller AC. Disasters and women's health: reflections from the 2010 earthquake in Haiti. Prehosp Disaster Med. 2013;28(2):150–4.
21. D'Ambruoso L, Abbey M, Hussein J. Please understand when I cry out in pain: women's accounts of maternity services during labour and delivery in Ghana. BMC Public Health. 2005;5:140.
22. Hoyler M, Finlayson SR, McClain CD, Meara JG, Hagander L. Shortage of doctors, shortage of data: a review of the global surgery, obstetrics, and anesthesia workforce literature. World J Surg. 2014;38(2):269–80.
23. Chestnut DH, Polley LS, Wong CA, Tsen LC, Ebooks Corporation. Chestnut's obstetric anesthesia. London: Elsevier Health Sciences; 2009. Available from: http://msvu.eblib.com/patron/FullRecord.aspx?p=1429863.
24. ACOG Committee Opinion #295: pain relief during labor. Obstet Gynecol. 2004;104(1):213.
25. Fan ZT, Gao XL, Yang HX. Popularizing labor analgesia in China. Int J Gynaecol Obstet. 2007;98(3):205–7.
26. WHO Model list of essential medicines: World Health Organization; 2013. Available from: http://www.who.int/medicines/publications/essentialmedicines/en/.
27. Anim-Somuah M, Smyth R, Howell C. Epidural versus non-epidural or no analgesia in labour. Cochrane Database Syst Rev. 2005;4, CD000331.
28. Stewart A, Fernando R. Maternal ambulation during labor. Curr Opin Anaesthesiol. 2011;24(3):268–73.
29. Schnittger T. Regional anaesthesia in developing countries. Anaesthesia. 2007;62 Suppl 1:44–7.
30. Imarengiaye CO, Ande AB. Demand and utilisation of labour analgesia service by Nigerian women. J Obstet Gynaecol. 2006;26(2):130–2.
31. Viitanen H, Viitanen M, Heikkila M. Single-shot spinal block for labour analgesia in multiparous parturients*. Acta Anaesthesiol Scand. 2005;49(7):1023–9.
32. Dyer RA, Reed AR, James MF. Obstetric anaesthesia in low-resource settings. Best Pract Res Clin Obstet Gynaecol. 2010;24(3):401–12.
33. Anabah T, Olufolabi A, Boyd JC, George RB. Low-dose spinal anaesthesia provides effective labour analgesia and does not limit ambulation. South Afr J Anesth Analg. 2014(In Press).
34. Gabrysch S, Campbell OM. Still too far to walk: literature review of the determinants of delivery service use. BMC Pregnancy Childbirth. 2009;9:34.
35. The United Nations we can end poverty millenium development goals and beyond fact sheet: Goal 1 eradicate extreme poverty and hunger.: United Nations; 2013. Available from: http://www.un.org/millenniumgoals/poverty.shtml.
36. The United Nations we can end poverty millenium development goals and beyond fact sheet: Goal 3 promote gender equality and empower women.: United Nations; 2013. Available from: http://www.un.org/millenniumgoals/gender.shtml.
37. The United Nations we can end poverty millenium development goals and beyond fact sheet: Goal 2, achieve universal primary education.: United Nations; 2013. Available from: http://www.un.org/millenniumgoals/education.shtml.
38. Beyond 2015: United Nations; 2015. Available from: http://www.un.org/millenniumgoals/beyond2015.shtml.
39. The United Nations we can end poverty millenium development goals and beyond fact sheet: Goal 4, reduce child mortality: United Nations; 2013. Available from: http://www.un.org/millenniumgoals/childhealth.shtml.
40. The United Nations we can end poverty millenium development goals and beyond fact sheet: Goal 5, reduce maternal mortality: United Nations; 2013. Available from: http://www.un.org/millenniumgoals/maternal.shtml.
41. Thaddeus S, Maine D. Too far to walk: maternal mortality in context. Soc Sci Med. 1994;38(8):1091–110.
42. Lema MJ. World medical leaders declare that pain treatment is a human right … and it couldn't come at a worse time. Pain Med. 2012;13(12):1531–2.
43. Kyomuhendo GB. Low use of rural maternity services in Uganda: impact of women's status, traditional beliefs and limited resources. Reprod Health Matters. 2003;11(21):16–26.
44. Lohman D. Pain care as a human right. Pain Pract. 2014;14(3):199–203.

Saving Sight in Developing Countries

15

Ebby Elahi and Natalie F. Holt

General Considerations

While many basic ophthalmic procedures may be performed under topical or local anesthesia provided by the ophthalmologist, others require deeper sedation or anesthesia administered by an anesthesiologist. During intraocular surgery, for instance, relaxation of the extraocular muscles and control of intraocular pressure (IOP) can be quite critical. Many anesthetic agents and maneuvers have influences on IOP and therefore affect surgical conditions (Table 15.1). In orbital surgery, the oculocardiac reflex, secondary to pressure on the optic nerve, may lead to significant bradycardia and hemodynamic instability. Finally, because microsurgical maneuvers require immobility of the patient, intravenous sedation must be carefully titrated to reduce head movement while maintaining adequate oxygenation.

E. Elahi, M.D. (✉)
The Icahn School of Medicine at Mount Sinai, 1034 Fifth Avenue, New York, NY 10028, USA
e-mail: Drelahi@FAeye.com

N.F. Holt, M.D.
Yale School of Medicine, 333 Cedar Street, TMP 3, P.O. Box 208051, New Haven, CT 06520, USA

Patient Evaluation

Ophthalmic surgeries are usually low-risk procedures associated with little morbidity or mortality. They are most often performed on patients at the extremes of age—the elderly and very young—both of whom merit unique considerations in the context of anesthesia. Medical history is best addressed using a systems-based approach, with a focus on the cardiovascular, pulmonary, and neurologic systems. A useful way to screen for occult cardiovascular disease is to inquire about the patient's ability to exercise at 4 metabolic equivalents (METs) without dyspnea, chest pain, or lightheadedness. An example of an activity that uses about 4 METs is climbing one to two flights of stairs. Pulmonary evaluation should take into account recent upper respiratory infections, smoking history, and signs and symptoms suggestive of obstructive sleep apnea (e.g., snoring, obesity). The neurologic evaluation should note any preexisting deficits of the central or peripheral nervous system. The patient should also be screened for aspiration risk factors. For pediatric patients, preoperative evaluation should also include information about birth history (e.g., prematurity) and developmental history (e.g., difficulty/failure reaching developmental milestones), asthma or other respiratory problems, and recent infections. The patient's mental status and ability to communicate adequately with the medical team is of critical importance, especially during conscious

R. Roth et al. (eds.), *The Role of Anesthesiology in Global Health: A Comprehensive Guide*,
DOI 10.1007/978-3-319-09423-6_15, © Springer International Publishing Switzerland 2015

Table 15.1 Effect of anesthetic drugs and maneuvers on intraocular pressure (IOP)

Agent	Effect
Ventilation pattern	Hypoventilation increases IOP, hyperventilation decreases IOP
Intravenous induction and inhaled agents	All decrease IOP except possibly ketamine; etomidate decreases IOP but myoclonus upon injection may be dangerous in setting of ruptured globe
Narcotics	Decrease IOP
Succinylcholine (Suxamethonium)	Increase IOP
Nondepolarizing neuromuscular blocking agents	Decrease IOP
Hypertonic solutions (dextran, mannitol)	Decrease IOP
Acetazolamide	Decrease IOP

sedation cases in which the patient's ability to remain motionless can be critical. Finally, it is important to elicit any personal or family history of complications related to anesthesia.

Laboratory testing prior to ophthalmic surgery is not usually necessary. However, hemoglobin and bleeding time may be sought for more extensive interventions such as oculofacial procedures in which blood loss is expected or in patients on medications that might affect blood clotting. Recent evidence suggests that antiplatelet and anticoagulant medications do not increase the occurrence of significant bleeding complications during cataract surgeries, even when regional blocks are performed; therefore, these medications should be continued in patients who use them chronically for cardiovascular conditions [3]. Patients with type II diabetes should be counseled to hold insulin and oral hypoglycemic agents on the day of surgery. For patients with type I diabetes, a basal infusion of insulin should be continued once nil per os (NPO), and a glucose-containing solution should be infused during surgery. A recent analysis by Operation Smile International demonstrated that the majority of children treated during its medical mission had an age–weight ratio at or below the Centers for Disease Control and Prevention's (CDC) 50th percentile; however, the majority had near-normal hemoglobin levels. This underscores the fact that mild-to-moderate malnutrition is relatively common in developing countries. Therefore, it is best to use weight-based drug and fluid calculations [4].

Management of Anesthesia

General Principles

In developed countries, safety standards, monitoring requirements, the availability of drugs and supplies, as well as an adequate supply of well-trained anesthesia providers are such that anesthesia-related mortality is extremely low—less than 1 in 100,000 in the USA [5]. By contrast, in developing countries, deaths attributable to anesthesia in the range of 1 in 133 [6], 1 in 144 [7], and 1 in 504 [8] have been reported. To maintain a safe level of care, basic intraoperative monitoring should include means to assess oxygenation, ventilation, and circulation. Since 2007, the WHO, together with the World Federation of Societies of Anaesthesiologists (WFSA), the Association of Anaesthetists of Great Britain and Ireland (AAGBI), and others have supported the Global Oximetry Initiative to advocate the provision of pulse oximetry as a minimum monitoring standard during the provision of anesthesia [9]. Pulse oximetry offers the benefit of establishing a basic measure of adequacy of tissue perfusion and oxygenation as well as providing a continuous display of heart rate. When general anesthesia is administered, continuous capnography is the gold standard for ensuring correct placement of the airway and adequacy of ventilation. An esophageal or precordial stethoscope provides an alternative means of assessing adequacy of ventilation when capnography is not available. The WFSA has published recommendations on international standards for the safe practice of anesthesia based on available levels of infrastructure (basic, intermediate, optimal) [10]. This includes suggested minimum drug requirements (Table 15.2). The WHO also has a Model List of Essential Medicines [11].

For ophthalmic procedures, maximizing the use of local and regional anesthesia offers the benefit of minimizing equipment and monitoring needs. It is therefore an ideal approach for the majority of

Table 15.2 Recommended supplies and anesthesia drugs based on level of health care facility

Rural hospital or health center (sparse operating room or minor procedure room only)	District or provincial hospital (100–300 beds)	Referral hospital with intensive care facilities (300–1,000 beds)
Supplies		
Equipment: Capital		
	Complete anesthesia, resuscitation and airway management systems including:	Same as Level 2 with these additions per operating room and ICU bed:
Adult and pediatric self-inflating breathing bags with masks	Reliable oxygen source	ECG monitor
Foot-powered suction	Vaporizer	Anesthesia ventilator, reliable electric power source with manual override
Stethoscope, sphygmomanometer, thermometer	Hoses and valves	Infusion pumps
Pulse oximeter	Bellows or bags to inflate lungs	Pressure bag with IV infusion
Oxygen concentrator or tank oxygen and draw-over vaporizer with hoses[a]	Face masks (size 00–5)	Electric or pneumatic suction
Laryngoscopes, bougies	Pediatric anesthesia system	Oxygen analyzer
	Oxygen supply failure alarm, oxygen analyzer	Thermometer or temperature probe
	Adult and pediatric resuscitator sets	Electric warming blanket
	Pulse oximeter, spare probes, adult and pediatric	Electric overhead heater
	Capnograph	Infant incubator
	Defibrillator (one per OR suite/ICU)	Laryngeal mask airways (sizes 2–4)
	ECG monitor	Intubating bougies, adult and child
	Larygnoscope, Macintosh blades (1–4)	Anesthetic agent (gas and vapour analyzer)
	Oxygen concentrator[s] cylinder	
	Foot or electric suction	
	IV pressure infusor bag	
	Adult and pediatric resuscitator sets	
	Magill forceps and/or bougie	
	Spinal needles (25G)	
	Nerve stimulator	
	Automatic noninvasive blood pressure monitor	
Equipment: Disposable		
Examination gloves	ECG electrodes	Same as Level 2 plus:
IV infusion/drug injection equipment	IV equipment and fluids (normal saline, Ringer's lactate, dextrose 5 %)	Ventilator circuits
Suction catheter size 16F	Pediatric giving sets	Yankauer circuits and suckers
Airway support equipment, including airways and tracheal tubes	Suction catheter size 16F	IV infusion tubing
Oral and nasal airways	Sterile gloves sizes 6–8	Disposable suction machines
	Nasogastric tubes 10–16F	Disposables for capnography, oxygen analyzer

(continued)

Table 15.2 (continued)

Rural hospital or health center (sparse operating room or minor procedure room only)	District or provincial hospital (100–300 beds)	Referral hospital with intensive care facilities (300–1,000 beds)
	Oral airway size 000–4	Sampling lines
	Tracheal tube size 3–8.5 mm	Water traps
	Spinal needle size 22G and 25G	Connectors
	Battery size C	Filters—Fuel cells
Drugs		
Ketamine 50 mg/mL	*Same as Level 1 but also*:	*Same as Level 2 but also*:
Lidocaine 1 or 2 %	Thiopental 500 mg/1 g powder or Propofol	Propofol
Diazepam 5 mg/mL or Midazolam 1 mg/mL	Suxamethonium bromide 500 mg powder	Nitrous oxide
Morphine 10 mg/mL	Pancuronium	Various modern neuromuscular blocking agents
Pethidine (Meperidine) 50 mg/mL	Neostigmine 2.5 mg injection	Various modern inhalation agents
Epinephrine 1 mg	Ether, halothane, other inhalation agents	Various inotropic agents
Atropine 0.6 mg/mL	Lidocaine 5 %, heavy spinal	Various antiarrhythmic agents
	Bupivacaine 0.5 %, heavy or plain	Nitroglycerine for infusion
	Hydralazine 20 mg injection	Calcium chloride 10 % 10 for injection
	Furosemide 20 mg injection	Potassium chloride 20 % 10 mL injection for infusion
	Dextrose 50 % 20 mL injection	
	Aminophylline 250 mg injection	
	Ephedrine 30/50 mg ampule	
	Hydrocortisone	
	±Nitrous oxide	

Modified from Merry AF, Cooper JB, Soyannwo O, Wilson IH, Eichhorn JH. International Standards for a Safe Practice of Anesthesia 2010. *Canadian journal of anaesthesia = Journal canadien d'anesthesie*. 2010;57(11):1027–34. Table 1
[a]Oxygen stored in cylinders is common in outlying hospitals. Tanks of various sizes are available, with difference capacities of oxygen storage. Type E cylinders hold 625 L oxygen; Type G hold 5,300 L oxygen; and Type H hold 6,900 L oxygen. While in the USA oxygen tanks are green, the WHO specifies that oxygen cylinders are white

cases. It should be recognized that although it is possible for a visiting medical mission group to transport disposable supplies and drugs, the team will often be dependent on the host nation for daily sterilization of equipment. Therefore, the quality of this sterilization equipment may be a limiting factor in terms of case turnover. It is advisable to provision supplies for at least a full day of surgical procedures without needing to re-sterilize equipment. Carrying disposable back-up instruments can also provide a safety net in the event reusable instruments become unavailable.

In some countries, traditional NPO guidelines are circumvented, especially for those patients who are only expected to receive regional ophthalmic blocks or "minimal" sedation [12]; however, this practice is controversial, and following the ASA Practice Guidelines on Preoperative Fasting is the safest approach (Table 15.3) [13].

As with any anesthetic, it is useful to utilize a pre-anesthetic checklist to ensure that basic preoperative patient information and the necessary anesthesia equipment is available prior to the start of each case (Table 15.4 and Fig. 15.1).

Regional Blocks

Topical local anesthesia and regional orbital blocks may be employed for most intraocular and

Table 15.3 Summary of fasting guidelines to prevent pulmonary aspiration

Ingested substance	Minimum fasting period (h)
Clear liquids (water, carbonated beverages, tea, black coffee)	2
Breast milk	4
Infant formula	6
Nonhuman milk	6
Light meal (toast, clear liquids)	6
Heavy meal (fatty foods)	8

Adapted from Practice guidelines for preoperative fasting and the use of pharmacologic agents to reduce the risk of pulmonary aspiration: application to healthy patients undergoing elective procedures. Anesthesiology 2011;114:495

Table 15.4 Pre-anesthetic checklist

Patient's Name: Date of Birth: Weight:		Procedure:	
ASA Physical Status	1 2 3 4 5 E	Anesthetic resources	
Mallampati Class	I II III IV	Airway – Masks – LMAs, Tubes – Working laryngoscopes – Bougies	☐ ☐ ☐ ☐
Aspiration Risk?	Yes No	Breathing – Circuit, leak-tested – Soda lime, no color change	☐ ☐
Allergies?	Yes No	Suction	☐
Important Medications (e.g., insulin, seizure drugs)		Drugs and Devices – Oxygen cylinder, full and off – Vaporizers – Monitors, alarms on – Based drugs labeled – Fluids available – Thermometer, temperature probe	☐ ☐ ☐ ☐ ☐ ☐
Relevant Medical Problems (e.g., diabetes, asthma)		Emergency – Epinephrine – Self-inflating bag – Tilting table – Succinylcholine	☐ ☐ ☐ ☐
History of anesthesia-related problems			

Modified from Merry AF, Cooper JB, Soyannwo O, Wilson IH, Eichhorn JH. International Standards for a Safe Practice of Anesthesia 2010. *Canadian journal of anaesthesia = Journal canadien d'anesthesie.* 2010;57(11):1027–34

periorbital procedures. The increased use of phacoemulsification for cataract extraction has led to a greater use of topical anesthesia for cataract surgery, while most vitreoretinal procedures require a denser anesthesia provided by regional blocks [14]. Among the regional techniques available are the retrobulbar, peribulbar, and sub-Tenon's block. Relative contraindications to regional ophthalmic block include blindness in the contralateral eye, significant myopia, elevated IOP, and trauma or perforation of the globe [15]. Whether these blocks are performed by an anesthesiologist or ophthalmologist varies by institution and experience of the provider. Regardless, it is the responsibility of the anesthesiologist to monitor the patient's vital signs during the performance of any regional anesthetic.

Retrobulbar and Peribulbar Blocks

Traditionally, the four rectus muscles of the eyes were thought to form a distinct cone around the globe whose apex was at the optic foramen. Retrobulbar blocks are performed such that local anesthetic is injected directly into the intraconal space, allowing for profound and rapid anesthesia and akinesia (globe immobility) of the rectus muscles with a low volume of anesthetic. Subsequently, it has been recognized that the connective tissue around the rectus muscles is incomplete. Therefore, local anesthetic injected outside the orbital cone may diffuse into the intraconal space and produce results similar to those achieved from a retrobulbar block with relatively less risk. This is the principle behind the peribulbar block, which is theoretically safer owing to the position of the needle on injection more removed from the optic nerve and other critical brainstem structures.

The retrobulbar block is performed by directing a needle toward the apex such that local anesthetic is injected into the intraconal space. The needle is inserted through the lower eyelid, just superior to the lateral third of the inferior orbital rim and advanced in parallel to the orbital floor. Once the needle is inserted about half an inch, the angle of insertion is shifted medially and superiorly allowing the needle to enter the intraconal space. Clinically, several confirmatory "pops" can be felt as the needle penetrates first

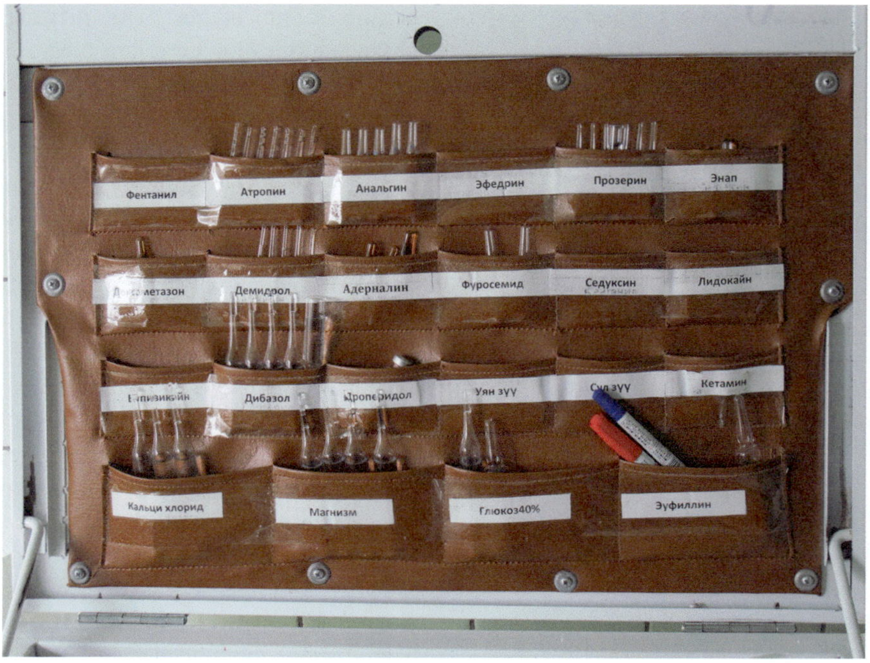

Fig. 15.1 When relying on a local supply of medications, it is imperative to foresee a mechanism to identify each drug appropriately

the skin, then the orbital septum, and finally the orbital cone. It is paramount to pull on the plunger prior to injection to avoid inadvertent intravascular injection of anesthetic.

The peribulbar block is administered by directing the needle parallel to the floor of the orbit. It may be given in a single inferior injection at the lower orbital rim; or a superior injection may also be used, given nasally above the medial canthus. For the inferior injection, the needle is inserted through the fornix below the lateral limbus or percutaneously through the inferior eyelid and directed back, laterally and slightly downwards. If a second injection is used, the needle is advanced between the caruncle and medial canthus in a medial direction, away from the globe. Studies suggest there is no particular benefit to one approach versus the other in terms of anesthesia, akinesia, or the development of severe complications [16].

Basic supplies required include sharp small gauge needles (typically 24–26G) and 5- or 10-mL syringes. Various needle lengths are available. The use of shorter needle lengths decreases the risk of needle passage beyond the ciliary ganglion. For the retrobulbar block, a 1.25 in. (31-mm) needle is sufficient; for the peribulbar block, a ¾ inch (19-mm) needle is adequate. For the retrobulbar block, a typical injection is 3–5 mL of anesthetic solution. For the peribulbar block, 5-mL to 12-mL of anesthetic solution is used, depending on whether the block is performed with one or two sticks.

Sub-Tenon's Block

The sub-Tenon's block involves injection of local anesthetic into the episcleral (sub-Tenon's) space, which then spreads circularly, providing anesthesia to the entire globe. It is sometimes performed as an adjunct to a retrobulbar or peribulbar block, or it may be used by itself for cataract or short vitreoretinal surgeries. Relative to topical anesthesia, sub-Tenon's block provides superior pain relief to patients undergoing cataract surgery [17]. However, for many patients, placement of the block is the most painful part of the procedure, with nearly half of patients reporting pain on injection [18]. In contrast to the retrobulbar or peribulbar

Table 15.5 Complications of regional orbital blocks

Symptom	Causes
Bradycardia	Oculocardiac reflex
Superficial hemorrhage	Circumorbital hematoma
Chemosis (conjunctival swelling)	Anterior spread of local anesthetic (more common after peribulbar and sub-Tenon's block)
Loss of vision	Retrobulbar hemorrhage
	Intraocular injection
	Central retinal artery occlusion
	Trauma to the optic nerve
Diplopia, strabismus	Extraocular muscle injury
Convulsions	Intra-arterial injection
Unconsciousness, muscle paresis, cardiopulmonary collapse	Injection of local anesthetic into the cerebrospinal fluid due to perforation of the meningeal sheath surrounding the optic nerve
Hypertension, tachycardia, angina	Epinephrine toxicity
Wheezing, hypotension, hives	Allergic reaction, e.g., ester-type local anesthetic

block, the sub-Tenon's block is usually performed using a specially designed blunt cannula rather than a needle. After placing topical anesthesia, a buttonhole incision is made into the conjunctiva and Tenon's capsule usually in the inferonasal quadrant using spring (Westcott) scissors. Anywhere from 2 to 5 mL of local anesthetic may be injected via this incision, with the degree of sensory and motor block produced proportional to the amount of volume of anesthetic utilized. Chemosis (conjunctival swelling) and subconjunctival hemorrhage are relative common complications with this block; the application of gentle pressure is helpful and neither generally causes intraoperative problems. The sub-Tenon's block may also be performed using a needle, but this approach is associated with more complications.

When performed by experienced providers, regional ophthalmic blocks are safe procedures. A summary of potential complications is provided in Table 15.5.

Orbicularis Oculi Block

The muscles of the eyelids are controlled by the orbicularis oculi, a division of the facial nerve. To prevent a rise in IOP due to squeezing of the eyelids, temporary paralysis of the orbicularis oculi is sometimes required for cataract or other ophthalmologic procedures. Because of the large volume of local anesthetic applied extraconally, paralysis of the orbicularis oculi is often a secondary consequence of peribulbar block. However, a retrobulbar block leaves the facial nerve untouched.

The facial nerve arises from the stylomastoid foramen and passes into the substances of the parotid gland. Various methods for blocking the orbicularis oculi have been described, including the methods of O-Brien, Van Lint, Atkinson, and Nadbath-Ellis. The O'Brien method is fairly popular owing to its easy landmarks and high efficacy. It aims to block the nerve at its proximal trunk through injection of local anesthetic at the condyloid process of the mandible, which may be located by asking the patient to open and close his or her mouth. After infiltration of the skin with local anesthesia at the site of injection, a 25G 1-in. needle should be passed directly to the periosteum. Injection of 2–3 mL of local anesthesia is usually sufficient to provide paralysis of the orbicularis oculi within 5–10 min. The use of this block warrants close attention to the status of the eyelids following surgery, as the normal blink response is suppressed. A compressive eye patch generally can prevent corneal exposure until eyelid function returns.

Topical Anesthesia

Topical anesthesia involves installation of local anesthetic eye drops onto the eye surface. This approach has several advantages including avoiding the risks associated with regional blocks, as well as reducing case turnover time. However, cases that require globe immobility or interventions beyond limited corneal incisions generally require denser anesthesia. Furthermore, the patient must have sufficient linguistic and cognitive skills to follow directions and maintain steady gaze during the procedure. Topical anesthesia is ideal for standard phacoemulsification procedures performed by experienced surgeons.

Options for eye drops include the shorter-acting agents such as proxymetacaine 0.5 %, and oxybuprocaine (benoxinate) 0.4 %; and longer-acting drugs such as lidocaine 1–4 %, bupivacaine 0.5–0.75 %, and tetracaine 0.5–1.0 %. All topical local anesthetics sting on application owing to their acidic pH; the longer-acting anesthetics are relatively more painful on instillation, so some providers use a combination of short-acting drops first followed by longer-acting agents to reduce patient discomfort [19]. The intracameral injection of a small volume (0.1–0.3 mL) of 1 % preservative-free lidocaine is an option for enhancing the analgesia provided by topical drops [20]. An alternative to drops is the use of anesthetic gels, including lidocaine 2.0 %. The gel may be mixed with dilating medications, antibiotics, and nonsteroidal anti-inflammatory drugs and applied before surgery [21].

Local Anesthetics

The choice of local anesthetic depends on the requirement for onset of action, desired duration of anesthesia, and degree of akinesia required by the procedure. Lidocaine 2 % and bupivacaine 0.5 % are the two most commonly used local anesthetics; sometimes used in a 50:50 mix to combine the benefits of quicker onset and longer duration. Other local anesthetic agents used include 2-chloroprocaine 2–3 %, mepivacaine 1–2 %, bupivacaine 0.25–0.75 %, levobupivacaine 0.25–0.75 %, prilocaine 3 %, ropivacaine 0.75 %, and articaine 2–4 %. Table 15.6 provides a comparison of the properties of the local anesthetics commonly used for anesthetic surgery [22]. Table 15.7 provides typical anesthetic solutions used for the most common regional and topical ophthalmic blocks.

Table 15.7 Typical anesthetic solutions for regional and topical ophthalmic blocks

Technique	Solution
Retrobulbar/peribulbar/sub-Tenon's	Lidocaine 2 %
	Lidocaine 2 % + Bupivacaine 0.5 or 0.75 % in a 50:50 mixture
	Lidocaine 2 % + Ropivacaine 0.5 or 1 % in a 50:50 mixture
Topical	Oxybuprocaine alone OR with Tetracaine or Lidocaine for longer procedures
	Viscous lidocaine 2 % or tetracaine 4 % gel ± 4 gtts tropicamide, 4 gtts 1 % cyclopentolate, 10 % phenylephrine, 10 gtts moxifloxacin, 4 gtts ketorolac
Intracameral	Lidocaine 1 % (preservative-free) + Bupivacaine 0.5 % eye drops (preservative free)

Adapted from Malik et al. Local anesthesia for cataract surgery. *J Cataract Refract Surg* 2010;36:133–152. (Table 2, page 135)

Table 15.6 Local anesthetics commonly used for ophthalmic surgery

Agent	Onset	Duration	Toxicity
Procaine	Slow	Short	Low
2-chloroprocaine	Rapid	Short	Low
Tetracaine	Slow	Intermediate	Intermediate
Cocaine	Slow	Long	Very high
Oxybuprocaine	Slow	Short	Intermediate
Bupivacaine	Slow	Long	High
Levobupivacaine	Slow	Long	Intermediate
Lidocaine	Rapid	Intermediate	Low/intermediate
Ropivacaine	Intermediate	Long	Intermediate
Etidocaine	Rapid	Long	High
Articaine	Rapid	Long	Low
Proxymethacaine	Rapid	Intermediate	Low
Prilocaine	Rapid	Intermediate	Low
Mepivacaine	Rapid	Intermediate	Low

Modified from Malik et al. Local anesthesia for cataract surgery. *J Cataract Refract Surg* 2010;36:133–152 and Jackson et al. 2006

Several additives may be used to modify the effect of local anesthetics. Epinephrine 1:200,000 (5 μg/mL) may be added to increase the duration and quality of the block by causing local vasoconstriction; this effect is most prominent with bupivacaine. However, it should be avoided in patients with coronary artery disease and has been implicated in retinal artery thrombosis secondary to vasoconstriction. Sodium bicarbonate is thought to speed the onset of action of bupivacaine and may help reduce pain on injection. Hyaluronidase (15 IU/mL of local anesthetic) is an enzyme that helps facilitate the spread of local anesthetic thereby decreasing the amount needed to achieve a desired effect and improve the quality of the block. Its use remains controversial since rare, but serious allergic reactions have been reported [23, 24].

Allergic Reactions to Local Anesthetics

Although uncommon, allergic reactions to local anesthetics occur and may be caused by (1) the local anesthetic or its metabolite; (2) the methylparaben preservative used in multidose vials; or (3) antioxidants added to some formulations of local anesthetics. There are two classes of local anesthetic based on chemical structure: esters and amides (Table 15.8). Esters are associated with a relatively higher incidence of allergic reactions due to one of their metabolic by-products—para-amino-benzoic acid (PABA), which is structurally similar to methylparaben. Amide local anesthetics do not metabolize to PABA; therefore, patients allergic to the ester local anesthetics are generally able to tolerate the amide local anesthetics. However, even with amides, methylparaben is used to preserve the multidose vial and patients who are allergic to PABA will have reactions. Sulfites are another potential allergen used in some formulations of local anesthetic solutions, notably those containing vasoconstrictors such as epinephrine. Therefore, in patients with a known sulfite allergy, it is best to avoid solutions containing additives such as sodium bisulfite and metabisulfite.

Table 15.8 Classification of local anesthetics

Ester	Amide
Procaine	Lidocaine
Tetracaine	Mepivacaine
Chloroprocaine	Bupivacaine
Cocaine	Ropivacaine
Benzocaine	Levobupivacaine
Oxybuprocaine	Etidocaine
	Prilocaine
	Articaine

The first step in treatment of an allergic reaction is recognition of its occurrence. The inciting agent should be removed or discontinued if possible and additional assistance should be summoned. Initial attention should focus on the airway, breathing, and circulation. The patient should be placed in a recumbent position with the legs elevated to offset vasodilation and maximize perfusion to vital organs. Intravenous access should be obtained as soon as possible. Supplemental oxygen should be administered by face mask. Ideally, the patient should be monitored with continuous electrocardiogram (ECG) and pulse oximetry as well as routine blood pressure and heart rate assessment. Pharmacologic treatment usually includes administration of histamine-1 and histamine-2 antagonists such as diphenhydramine 25–50 mg IV (1 mg/kg for patients <40 kg) and ranitidine 50 mg (1 mg/kg for patients <40 kg), respectively. Albuterol nebulizers or inhalers are useful in the treatment of bronchospasm. Refractory bronchospasm or hypotension is best treated with epinephrine. Epinephrine may be administered intramuscularly in the outer thigh. When administered intramuscularly, a concentration of 1 mg/mL (1:1,000) is used, and the dose is 0.3–0.5 mg per dose (0.01 mg/kg per dose in patients <50 kg). Epinephrine may also be given intravenously in a concentration of 0.1 mg/mL (1:10,000), usually as a continuous infusion 2–10 μg/min, titrated to blood pressure. Owing to their long onset of action, glucocorticoids are not useful in treating the initial symptoms of an allergic reaction; however, they may be given to prevent late-stage responses. Typical treatment is methylprednisolone 1–2 mg/kg daily for a maximum of 72 h.

Monitored Anesthesia Care

Monitored anesthesia care (MAC) as an adjunct to local or regional anesthesia is a widely used approach for ophthalmologic procedures. Supplemental oxygen is required, and the patient should be monitoring for satisfactory respiratory effort—ideally with end-tidal carbon dioxide monitoring. For patients requiring retrobulbar or peribulbar block, a brief period of general anesthesia using a bolus dose of propofol (30–75 mg) or methohexital (30–75 mg) is frequently employed just prior to performing the block. The patient is then allowed to awaken spontaneously. Propofol as a continuous infusion (25–75 μg/kg/min) is sometimes used to provide deeper sedation in younger or more anxious patients. This technique offers the benefit of reduced awareness and anti-emetic properties.

The main role of the anesthesiologist during MAC for eye surgery is to monitor the patient's vital signs and attend to the patient's comfort. Deep sedation is unnecessary and best avoided owing to the risk of airway obstruction with the airway in the operative field far from the anesthesiologist, prolonged recovery time and possible disinhibition or confusion, especially in the elderly population. Verbal reassurance is often all that is required; however, for some patients, a small dose of anxiolytic (midazolam 0.5–2 mg) is advantageous. An oral or nasal dose of midazolam (0.5 mg/kg) may also be given to children (2–10 years) prior to minor ophthalmologic procedures. Diphenhydramine, a histamine-1 antagonist that has sedative, antiemetic, and anticholinergic properties is an alternative to midazolam. However, owing to its long half-life (3–6 h), Diphenhydramine tends to prolong recovery times and may cause confusion in the elderly.

Occasionally, intravenous narcotics are used as a supplement for pain control; short-acting agents such as fentanyl (0.5–1.0 μg/kg), remifentanil (0.5 μg/kg), and alfentanil (3–7 μg/kg) are commonly employed. Owing to its lower potency and greater safety margin, fentanyl is the most commonly use agent.

Other less commonly used drugs include clonidine and dexmedetomidine. Both are alpha-2-agonists with anxiolytic and sedative properties.

Table 15.9 Example of procedure-specific ophthalmic surgery preoperative orders

Extraocular procedures
– Check vital signs – Midazolam or Diazepam po or IV according to size of patient – Chloroprocaine gtt every 3 h until surgery – If patient to have general anesthesia: IV insertion with 500–1,000 mL preload, if adult; weight-based for pediatric patients
Intraocular procedures (cataract, lens placement)
– *Check vital signs* – Midazolam or Diazepam po or IV pre-op according to size of patient – Chloroprocaine gtt every 3 h until surgery – Diamox 250–500 mg pre-op – Dilating drops: mydriacyl or phenylephrine gtt pre-op – Cyclopentolate gtt per MD orders – If patient to have general anesthesia: IV insertion with 500–1,000 mL preload, if adult; weight-based for pediatric patients

Adapted from Moos DD. Perianesthesia nursing at an ophthalmic hospital in the Middle East. *Journal of perianesthesia nursing: official journal of the American Society of PeriAnesthesia Nurses/American Society of PeriAnesthesia Nurses*. 2005;20(2):83–91. Table 3 [27]

A benefit of these drugs is that they do not impair respiratory effort. However, they may cause cardiovascular depression. Dexmedetomidine is also expensive and unlikely to be available in hospitals with limited resources.

Ketamine is a low-cost anesthetic with analgesic properties that has the benefit of causing little respiratory depression or hemodynamic instability. Therefore, it is theoretically ideal for MAC where resources are scarce. However, patients who receive ketamine often suffer unpleasant psychomimetic emergence reactions; in addition, they may develop intraoperative hypertension. In small doses (10–20 mg), these side effects can usually be avoided. When higher doses are used, it is best to pretreat with an anxiolytic such as midazolam.

Table 15.9 provides an example of procedure-specific preoperative orders for extraocular and intraocular procedures.

General Anesthesia

General anesthesia is usually reserved for pediatric patients, adults who are unable to lie flat or still, as well as for strabismus surgery and more complicated oculoplastic procedures. General anesthesia is indicated for emergency procedures, such as penetrating eye injuries ("open globe"). The experience and skill of the anesthesiologist is often the limiting factor in smooth inductions and emergence. An endotracheal tube (ETT) is preferable in patients at risk for aspiration. Specifically, a Right Angle Endotracheal (RAE) Tube may be best as it protects the airway, facilitates mechanical ventilation, if necessary, and angles down towards the chest away from the surgical field. The installation of intratracheal lidocaine (2–4 % solution; 1 mg/kg) or intravenous lidocaine (1.5–2.0 mg/kg) may be considered in an attempt to reduce coughing on insertion or removal of the ETT. A supraglottic airway (e.g., laryngeal mask airway) may be suitable for some ocular procedures. Compared to an endotracheal tube, insertion of a supraglottic airway may be associated with less of an increase in intraocular pressure (IOP). In addition, its use may reduce bucking on emergence. Spontaneous respiration can be maintained during general anesthesia, avoiding the need for a mechanical ventilator, which may be in scarce supply in limited resources areas. Ultimately, the choice of ETT versus LMA should be left to the anesthesiologist.

Inhalational anesthesia (e.g., halothane, sevoflurane, isoflurane ± nitrous oxide) is most commonly used for maintenance of general anesthesia, although total intravenous anesthesia (e.g., propofol and narcotic infusion) may be used as well. Nitrous oxide should not be used in procedures requiring instillation of intravitreal gas.

Strabismus Surgery

Strabismus surgery is most commonly performed on pediatric patients although it may be indicated in the adult population as well. Strabismus surgery typically requires general anesthesia. Muscle relaxation may be requested by the surgeon to reduce tone in the extraocular muscles. Non-depolarizing agents are preferred to succinylcholine because the latter interferes with the forced duction test (FDT), an intraoperative maneuver that helps distinguish the cause of impaired eye muscle function.

Special considerations during strabismus surgery include the propensity for surgical manipulation of the eye to induce bradycardia (oculocardiac reflex) and the relatively high incidence of postoperative nausea and vomiting (oculogastric reflex). If bradycardia occurs intraoperatively, the best approach is to ask the surgeon to temporarily discontinue ocular manipulation; however, glycopyrrolate and atropine should be available as well. The avoidance of narcotics helps to minimize the risk of postoperative vomiting, as does the use of total intravenous anesthesia with propofol; however, this approach may be impractical in developing countries, owing to cost considerations. The nonsteroidal anti-inflammatory agent ketorolac is a suitable alternative to narcotics for postoperative analgesia.

The prophylactic administration of antiemetic agents at induction has been shown to reduce the incidence of postoperative vomiting. Droperidol had been well-studied for this indication, though its use in the USA has decreased dramatically since the Food and Drug Administration's "black box" warning concerning the risk of QT interval prolongation. Alternative antiemetics include serotonin antagonists (e.g., ondansetron) and glucocorticoids (e.g., dexamethasone, 0.25 mg/kg). There is an increased incidence of malignant hyperthermia in patients with strabismus. Therefore, it is important to be vigilant about monitoring of temperature and end-tidal CO_2.

Open Eye Surgery

Special considerations in the management of anesthesia for open eye injuries include the need to minimize aspiration risk and the desire to avoid increases in IOP that could cause extrusion of vitreous contents from the damaged eye. While succinylcholine offers the safest option for rapid intubating conditions, concern exists over its potential to temporarily increase IOP. High-dose rocuronium (1.0 mg/kg) is an alternative to succinylcholine, but due to its intermediate duration of action, the use of rocuronium may be dangerous in patients with known or unrecognized difficult airways. It is also often not available in developing countries. In a patient with a known difficult airway, options are limited to awake fiber-optic laryngoscopy, topical or regional anesthesia. Fiber-optic laryngoscopy requires skill as well as expertise in anesthetic airway blocks to obviate increases in IOP. The fiberoptic scope is expensive, fragile and requires sophisticated processing for sterilization; therefore, it is not likely to be available on a mission. The management decisions for this type of emergency should be made in consultation with the ophthalmologist and decisions made based on the probability of saving the injured eye.

It is prudent to administer an H2-receptor antagonist such as ranitidine prophylactically prior to general anesthesia in the non-fasted patient. Given intravenously, ranitidine is effective within 60 min and lasts for up to 9 h. Non-particulate antacids, such as 0.3 M sodium citrate raise gastric pH within 15–30 min, and are therefore also useful for patients presenting for emergency surgeries. Metoclopramide, a dopamine antagonist that increases gastric motility and gastroesophageal sphincter tone may be considered. It is optimally administered via infusion within 15–30 min of induction. Contraindications include patients with a bowel obstruction and should be used with caution in the elderly, because of possible side effects such as confusion and drowsiness.

Postanesthesia Recovery

In many developing countries, there is no designated postanesthesia recovery area and no direct nursing or medical oversight for recovering patients. Instead, on emergence, the patient is transferred from the operating table to a stretcher and moved to an area outside the operating theatre; and the anesthesia provider remains responsible for recovering the patient, even as he or she prepares for or begins another case.

Recovery from an uneventful cataract surgery should take less than 20 min. The degree of postoperative recovery is directly related to the sedation given during the procedure. When postoperative care resources are limited, it is beneficial to minimize sedation required to provide a satisfactory patient experience. Compared with a regional block, topical anesthesia also allows for more rapid vision recovery, which is important in patients with poor vision in both eyes [24].

Most pediatric patients undergoing ophthalmic procedures will have uneventful recoveries. Postoperative breath-holding and episodic bradycardia may be a problem in procedures performed on preterm infants (e.g., surgery for retinopathy of prematurity). Close monitoring is warranted in these patients.

Documentation and Communication

Documentation

In order to achieve the humanitarian objective of medical missions, it is fundamental to maintain administration and documentation standards. Each patient should be registered with a unique identifier, and on the day of surgery, the patient should wear that identifier at all times. Digital photography can be especially useful to maintain a centralized visual identifier of patients and their chart. Furthermore, photographs can easily be printed and used as a means to verify patients' identities and treatment plans. The WHO recommends the use of a surgical safety checklist to ensure availability of necessary equipment, confirmation of patient, procedure and surgical site, and review of anticipated critical events, etc. [25] Basic components of a surgical medical record should include: (1) preoperative assessment; (2) consent in the local language; (3) operative note; (4) anesthesia record; (5) postanesthesia recovery record; and (6) discharge plan. All patients should be assessed postoperatively and a treatment plan needs to be established by the surgical team that allows for a practical transition of care to local health personnel.

An anesthesia record should be completed for every procedure. This should include the surgical procedure and its length, interval recordings of oxygen saturation, heart rate, respiratory rate, blood pressure, as well as the length and type of anesthesia, and drugs and fluids administered [26]. This record should also note any unusual intraoperative events, such as intubation difficulties, hypotensive episodes, etc. An appropriate hand-off should be given to a care provider in the postanesthesia care unit (PACU), and this area should be supervised by an anesthesiologist. Postanesthesia orders should include provisions for pain medications as well as routine measurement of vital signs.

Communication, Ethical, and Cultural Considerations

While obtaining surgical consent, it is imperative that the risks, benefits and alternatives to surgery be adequately explained in a language that is accessible to patients. Arranging for translation prior to the mission is useful in order to avoid misunderstandings that can lead to catastrophic outcomes. Consent documents should be read to patients in consideration of high rates of illiteracy.

Ideally, medical missions are performed in conjunction with local specialists who may assume postoperative care of the patients when the visiting team departs. If such local support is lacking, patient selection should be limited to those who can be treated with limited aftercare. For example, cataract surgery can be performed with minimal follow up in most cases whereas glaucoma surgery requires frequent follow-ups and close monitoring. In cases where no after care support is available locally, it may be more appropriate to help transfer the patient to a different facility rather than risking visual complications due to inappropriate postoperative care.

Planning for a medical mission presents unique challenges to the medical team. Patient selection often depends on a number of factors including the availability of local support, the nature and difficulty of the operation and the utilitarian value of a particular intervention. In the authors' experiences, two types of operations are ideally suited for medical missions: (a) Surgery for common conditions that can be treated by the local physicians with minimal capacity building and knowledge transfer (e.g., cataract surgery) and (b) rare serious conditions for which local know-how or available equipment may be lacking (e.g., orbital decompression). The authors have found that a prescreening triage with priority assignment allows patients and the local providers to have clarity with regard to the nature and scope of cases that are to be performed.

Before incision, it is also useful to conduct a verbal "time out" to verify the patient's identity, confirm the procedure to be performed (including laterality) and any special equipment or prosthetics needed, determine antibiotics that need to be administered, and review any critical issues expected during the procedures.

Conclusion

Providing anesthesia support to ophthalmic surgeries presents both unique challenges and opportunities. With adequate preparation and foresight, life-transforming operations can be safely provided to millions of individuals in need. In places where healthcare infrastructure is scarce, the anesthesiologist must not only be able to improvise with limited means but also continue to remain intimately involved in the patient's recovery outside the operating room.

References

1. Nouvellon E, Cuvillon P, Ripart J. Regional anesthesia and eye surgery. Anesthesiology. 2010;113(5):1236–42.
2. McQueen KA, Magee W, Crabtree T, Romano C, Burkle Jr FM. Application of outcome measures in international humanitarian aid: comparing indices through retrospective analysis of corrective surgical care cases. Prehosp Disaster Med. 2009;24(1):39–46.
3. Li G, Warner M, Lang BH, Huang L, Sun LS. Epidemiology of anesthesia-related mortality in the United States, 1999–2005. Anesthesiology. 2009;110(4):759–65.
4. Ouro-Bang'na Maman AF, Tomta K, Ahouangbevi S, Chobli M. Deaths associated with anaesthesia in Togo, West Africa. Trop Doct. 2005;35(4):220–2.
5. Hodges SC, Mijumbi C, Okello M, McCormick BA, Walker IA, Wilson IH. Anaesthesia services in developing countries: defining the problems. Anaesthesia. 2007;62(1):4–11.

6. Hansen D, Gausi SC, Merikebu M. Anaesthesia in Malawi: complications and deaths. Trop Doct. 2000;30(3):146–9.
7. Thoms GM, McHugh GA, O'Sullivan E. The Global Oximetry initiative. Anaesthesia. 2007;62 Suppl 1:75–7.
8. Merry AF, Cooper JB, Soyannwo O, Wilson IH, Eichhorn JH. International Standards for a safe practice of anesthesia 2010. Can J Anaesth. 2010; 57(11):1027–34.
9. World Health Organization. 2013. WHO Model List of Essential Medicines. Available: http://www.who.int/medicines/publications/essentialmedicines/en/. Accessed 26 Jan 2014.
10. Sanmugasunderam S, Khalfan A. Is fasting required before cataract surgery? A retrospective review. Can J Ophthalmol. 2009;44(6):655–6.
11. American Society of Anesthesiologists. Practice guidelines for preoperative fasting and the use of pharmacologic agents to reduce the risk of pulmonary aspiration: application to healthy patients undergoing elective procedures: an updated report by the American Society of Anesthesiologists Committee on Standards and Practice Parameters. Anesthesiology. 2011;114(3):495–511.
12. Vann MA, Ogunnaike BO, Joshi GP. Sedation and anesthesia care for ophthalmologic surgery during local/regional anesthesia. Anesthesiology. 2007;107(3):502–8.
13. Kallio H, Rosenberg PH. Advances in ophthalmic regional anaesthesia. Best Pract Res Clin Anaesthesiol. 2005;19(2):215–27.
14. Alhassan MB, Kyari F, Ejere HO. Peribulbar versus retrobulbar anaesthesia for cataract surgery. Cochrane Database Syst Rev. 2008;3, CD004083.
15. Davison M, Padroni S, Bunce C, Ruschen H. Sub-Tenon's anaesthesia versus topical anaesthesia for cataract surgery. Cochrane Database Syst Rev. 2007;3, CD006291.
16. Jeganathan VS, Jeganathan VP. Sub-Tenon's anaesthesia: a well tolerated and effective procedure for ophthalmic surgery. Curr Opin Ophthalmol. 2009; 20(3):205–9.
17. Kumar C, Dowd T. Ophthalmic regional anaesthesia. Curr Opin Anaesthesiol. 2008;21(5):632–7.
18. Ezra DG, Allan BD. Topical anaesthesia alone versus topical anaesthesia with intracameral lidocaine for phacoemulsification. Cochrane Database Syst Rev. 2007;3, CD005276.
19. Cass GD. Choices of local anesthetics for ocular surgery. Ophthalmol Clin North Am. 2006;19(2): 203–7.
20. Jackson T, McLure HA. Pharmacology of local anesthetics. Ophthalmol Clin North Am. 2006;19(2): 155–61.
21. Kumar CM, Dowd TC. Complications of ophthalmic regional blocks: their treatment and prevention. Ophthalmologica. 2006;220(2):73–82.
22. Malik A, Fletcher EC, Chong V, Dasan J. Local anesthesia for cataract surgery. J Cataract Refract Surg. 2010;36(1):133–52.
23. World Alliance for Patient Safety. 2008. Surgical Safety Checklist. Available: http://www.who.int/patientsafety/safesurgery/ss_checklist/en/. Accessed 27 Jan 2014.
24. Chackungal S, Nickerson JW, Knowlton LM, Black L, Burkle FM, Casey K, et al. Best practice guidelines on surgical response in disasters and humanitarian emergencies: report of the 2011 Humanitarian Action Summit Working Group on Surgical Issues within the Humanitarian Space. Prehosp Disaster Med. 2011; 26(6):429–37.
25. Moos DD. Perianesthesia nursing at an ophthalmic hospital in the Middle East. J Perianesth Nurs. 2005;20(2):83–91.

Cardiothoracic Anesthesia and Intensive Care: What Is the Role of Missions?

16

Peter M.J. Rosseel and Carrie L.H. Atcheson

Introduction

Some might say practicing cardiovascular anesthesia and intensive care in a low-resource setting is overly ambitious and unrealistic and that having a chapter on cardiothoracic anesthesia in a book on anesthesia missions opens up many contradictions and ambiguities. Addressing these contradictions and ambiguities is necessary, however, as hospitals in low- and middle-income countries (LMICs) across a variety of geographic and socioeconomic contexts develop and expand surgical and anesthesiology services.

The field of cardiovascular anesthesiology in a global health setting touches on so many domains that it deserves a text of its own covering epidemiology, prevention, accessibility to cardiac surgery and anesthesia, postsurgical care, supply chains, and quality control, just to name a few. Furthermore, the domains of cardiovascular anesthesiology and intensive care have developed so broadly that they cannot be rightly practiced without specific knowledge, expertise, and skills developed through teaching and mentorship. Cardiothoracic anesthesiology is well covered in other texts,[1] and within the field there is a circumscribed chain of surgical care. Thus, the expertise and evidence presented elsewhere should serve the provider well when adapted and implemented in a global health context. Intensive care is also a broad field that is well described in other texts,[2]

P.M.J. Rosseel, M.D. (✉)
Department of Cardiothoracic Anaesthesia and Intensive Care, Amphia Hospital, Molengracht 21, Breda 4818 CK, The Netherlands
e-mail: peterrosseel@telenet.be

C.L.H. Atcheson, M.D., M.P.H.
Oregon Anesthesiology Group, Department of Anesthesiology, Adventist Medical Center, Portland, OR, USA

[1] Suggested resources for cardiac anesthesiology include, but are not limited to: *Kaplan's Cardiac Anesthesia*, A Practical Approach to Transesophageal Echocardiography by A. C. Perrino, S. T. Reeves (ISBN-13: 978–1451175608), the updated clinical practice guidelines maintained by The Society of Thoracic Surgeons found at http://www.sts.org/resources-publications/clinical-practice-credentialing-reporting-guidelines, the Transoesphageal echocardiography e-learning certification course from the European Association of Cardiovascular Anaesthesiologists http://www.eacta.org/education/eacademy and the lecture series maintained by the Society of Cardiovascular Anesthesiologists at http://www.scahq.org/FellowshipCareerOpportunities/Adult Cardiothoracic Anesthesiology Fellowships/FellowshipLectureSeries.aspx (must be a member to access, and membership costs $40 USD for fellows and residents).

[2] Suggested resources for critical care medicine include, but are not limited to: Paul Marino: The ICU Handbook, fourth edition, ISBN 13–1451121186; *Murry & Nadel's Textbook of Respiratory Medicine*, the American Thoracic Society Reading List found at http://www.thoracic.org/career-development /residents/ats-reading-list/, the treasury of review articles in The Clinics series found at http://www.chestmed.theclinics.com/, and—for procedures—the video library of the New England Journal of Medicine found at http://www.nejm.org/multimedia/medical-videos and that maintained by Cook® Medical at https://www.cookmedical.com/web/critical-care?id=Educational_Video.

R. Roth et al. (eds.), *The Role of Anesthesiology in Global Health: A Comprehensive Guide*, DOI 10.1007/978-3-319-09423-6_16, © Springer International Publishing Switzerland 2015

and therefore this chapter focuses on the special provisions and minimum standards of care needed to provide appropriate intensive care for safe cardiovascular anesthesiology services.

Additionally, for many of the lowest income countries (LICs), the resources required to develop safe cardiovascular surgical and anesthesia services are too great. Therefore, in this chapter, we further narrow the scope to focus on those countries where the conditions are somewhat more favorable, e.g., middle-income countries (MICs). Cardiovascular disease is one of the greatest public health concerns, even when limited to those forms that are amenable to surgery. Surgery has been called the neglected stepchild of global health because of its dependency on a well-functioning hospital structure including laboratory and blood banking services [1]. This applies especially to cardiac surgery. Short term, self-contained surgical trips are described elsewhere in the text, but his chapter focuses on the building of a sustainable service of cardiovascular anesthesiology and intensive care, staying away from voluntarism without a clear objective.

This chapter brings together expertise from cardiovascular anesthesiology and intensive care gained in High Income Countries (HICs) and the experience and knowledge of the humanitarian context of LMICs. Although practical clues for organizing a mission will be provided, this chapter aims more to convey a way of thinking and provide a framework that can be adapted to the local situation. Explicitly the authors want to thank the pediatric and adult cardiac anaesthesiologists who contributed their experiences and reviewed this manuscript and want to pay their deepest respect to those who are practicing cardiothoracic anesthesiology and intensive care in more difficult and less comfortable conditions.

Cardiac Surgery and the Global Burden of Cardiovascular Disease

Global Burden of Cardiovascular Disease

In a landmark article in 2001 Yusuf describes how during the twentieth century the epidemiology of cardiovascular disease has shifted from a predominantly nutritional and infectious origin to degenerative causes and how this shift paralleled socioeconomic development. In medical terms, cardiac surgical disease went from being predominantly rheumatic in origin among a young population to ischemic coronary disease and degenerative valve disease causing heart failure in middle aged or elderly patients (Table 16.1) [2]. According to Yusuf et al., this disease pattern differs throughout the world, depending on the socioeconomic status and evolution of a particular country or region, and a well-developed health care system can regress due to a changing socio economic event, e.g., war or natural disaster. The following section traces the impact of socioeconomic status on cardiovascular disease and surgery through three different scenarios.

Table 16.1 Adapted from (Yusuf et al. [2]). Mortality from Cardiovascular Disease and Infectious Causes in 1990, by region and gender (in thousands)

Region	Cardiovascular causes in men	Infectious causes in men	Cardiovascular causes in women	Infectious causes in women
India	611	429	481	240
China	576	158	439	89
Other Asian and Pacific Island	289	147	226	140
Commonwealth of Independent States	416	20	253	6
Sub-Saharan Africa	183	215	211	228
Latin America/Caribbean	186	62	147	48
Middle East Crescent	258	56	215	35
Established Market Economies	483	42	227	12
Total	3,028	1,128	2,201	798

In 2001, Yusuf and colleagues demonstrated in their landmark article series "The Global Burden of Cardiovascular Diseases" that, even in regions with the lowest per capita incomes, mortality from cardiovascular disease is high and growing. Only in sub-Saharan Africa did mortality from infectious causes exceed that from cardiovascular disease.

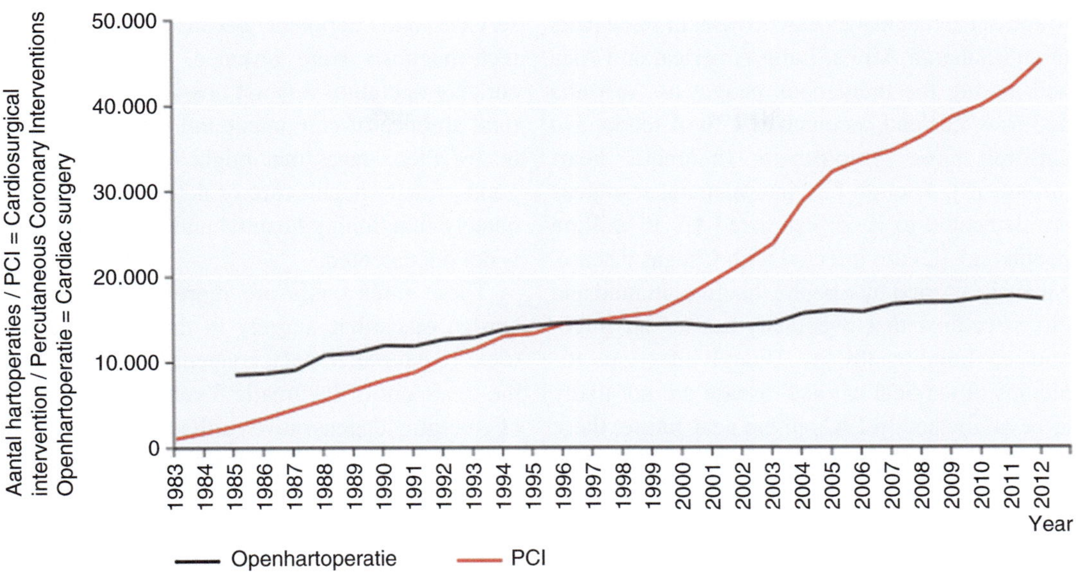

Fig. 16.1 The increase in the absolute number of percutaneous coronary interventions versus the number of open heart surgeries from 1983–1985 to present. *X* axis: year. *Y* axis: number of interventons. According to the 2013 report of the "Nederlandse Hartstichting" (Dutch Cardiac Foundation). *Black lines* depict absolute number of annual cardiosurgical intervention (open hart operaties) as compared to the number of percutaneous coronary interventions (PCI) represented by the *red line*

Situation in Developed Countries

The Netherlands is a country on the high end of development and income with an exemplary and highly accessible health care system that focus on disease prevention. The number of cardiac surgeries is only slowly increasing while the number of percutaneous procedures in octogenarians remains stable due to increased life expectancy (Fig. 16.1).

In 2012, 17,293 open heart operations were performed on a total population of 16.7 million, which represents 104 open heart operations per 100,000 inhabitants [3]. Fifty-five percent of these were isolated coronary artery bypass grafting (CABG) and 42 % were isolated valve surgery. The remainder of the cases were for combined valve with CABG surgery, or other less prevalent forms like repair of the thoracic aorta, heart transplants, and congenital cardiac surgery [3]. Most valve surgery is for degenerative valve disease, and the proportion of valve operations due to delayed consequences of rheumatic fever is scant and mainly among patients born in other countries with a higher incidence of rheumatic fever in childhood. In the Netherlands, only 761 of the 17,293 cases of cardiac surgery were performed for children younger than 14 years.

Lowest Income Countries

On the other end of the spectrum are the poorest countries that have few local, national, or private sector resources and are categorized by the World Bank as Low Income Countries (LICs). Sixty percent of the burden of cardiovascular disease is borne by LICs, and the epidemiology of cardiac surgical disease is different in these countries [4].

According to the World Heart Federation (WHF), the burden of rheumatic heart disease—which is a consequence of an untreated or undertreated streptococcal upper respiratory infection—falls disproportionately on the children and young adults in LICs. In LICs alone, 15.6 million people are affected by rheumatic heart disease, two million per year require hospitalization, and 233,000 deaths per year are attributable to end-stage rheumatic heart disease. In some parts of sub-Saharan Africa, Latin America, and Asia and among the indigenous people of Australia and New Zealand, as much as 1 % of school age children have symptomatic rheumatic heart disease [5]. Though few international resources are dedicated to it, an estimated 16–18 million people in LICs are infected with Chagas disease, a parasite carried by a beetle that lives in mud and dirt structures that eventually causes an infectious cardiomyopathy [6]. Though infectious etiologies of surgical cardiac disease are not likely to be eradicated in LICs in the near future, these countries are beginning to confront ischemic heart disease due to the obesity epidemic and ischemic heart disease is expected to grow more quickly in LMICs than in HICs [6, 7]. According to the World Health Organization (WHO), in 2011 "Coronary disease killed more than 7 million people and stroke killed nearly 6 million. Most of the deaths were in developing countries" [4]. Thus, the burden of surgical cardiac disease will continue to fall disproportionately on the people with the least access to medical care and surgical services.

This author (PR) can easily recall three cases from Médecins Sans Frontières (MSF) emergency response humanitarian projects:

- In Somalia, a pregnant woman presented at the emergency department in overt cardiac failure clinically diagnosed as aortic insufficiency.
- In Liberia, a middle aged male visitor in the hospital suffered sudden cardiac death, presumably from a myocardial infarction.
- In Somalia again, a newborn infant remained cyanotic after birth, a condition that did not improve with oxygen by face mask and a clinical diagnosis was made of cyanotic heart disease of unspecified cause.

In these cases, as in many cases of cardiac disease encountered in LICs, "clinically", "presumably" and "unspecified" are the key words. As this author did, visiting anesthesiologists and local practitioners alike find themselves feeling ignorant and impotent in such clinical situations—"ignorant" because the exact diagnosis cannot be known without ECG and echocardiography equipment and an appropriate laboratory services, and "impotent" because even if the correct diagnosis were revealed, resuscitation or curative operation was not possible because of a total absence of equipment and tools. The number of these cases that might be prevented by good primary health care or detected by an adequately functioning hospital and cardiology care is not documented.

These three cases are representative of the burden of cardiac surgery in the poorest countries. To have an impact, congenital heart disease, the treatment of rheumatic fever, and the causes of emerging degenerative cardiac disease such as aging, urbanization, and lifestyle changes (smoking, decreased physical activity, obesity, and nutrition must all be addressed from a public health perspective. Goal oriented resource management can only be achieved when adequate data regarding existing health conditions are provided for low- and middle-income countries [8].

Middle-Income Countries

BRICS Countries

In between these socioeconomic extremes, on the top of the bell curve, lie the middle-income countries. This group is too diverse to describe as a whole. On one hand there are the so-called BRICS—Brazil, the Russian Federation, India, China, and South Africa—the countries representing three billion habitants of our planet. This term was first coined in a white paper by a Goldman-Sachs executive in 2001 to describe the investment opportunities in these up-and-coming economies [9]. This group of countries holds a yearly international summit; Argentina, Indonesia, Turkey, Iran, Nigeria, Syria, and Egypt are sometimes practically grouped in the same category, but do not take part in the BRICS economic summit [10].

Though the level of health care is considerably better than in the developing countries, it is far below what would be expected in the G7 countries, the most important differences being a marked disparity in the quality of health care provided and even more important unequal access to health care [11]. The disparity in access occurs for a variety of reasons such as a lack of universal social security system as in India and China or a marked urban–rural quality of life disparity as in South Africa and Brazil. Lack of health insurance providers in countries like India and China is also a primary cause of unaffordability in treating cardiac surgical cases [12]. Still many hospitals and university centers in BRICS nations may provide advanced medical care including advanced cardiac surgery at a standard of care comparable to that offered in so-called developed nations. The case mix is different from what may be seen in the developed countries with a substantial proportion of valve surgery due the late consequences of rheumatic fever and a much younger population of CABG patients owing to unhealthy lifestyle and "iceberg phenomenon" of diabetic patients [11].

BRICS countries have the personnel and expertise to improve the quality of their cardiosurgical care and the political potential to improve accessibility, but cooperation between practitioners and institutions in BRICS countries and HICs can still be fruitful. For host countries, these partnerships sharpen new techniques and improve academic rigor, and the visiting practitioners profit from the rewarding teaching and learning experience of helping a growing anesthesiology department or cardiac surgical program. Indeed the creative and innovative solutions employed by practitioners and health care systems in BRICS in order to invest limited resources effectively will be of interest to all health care practitioners. Health care professionals universally face the changing landscape created by the global economic crisis and can subsequently implement these measures in their home country.

Other Middle-Income Countries: The Target Group?

At the lower end of the MIC group, are the countries that have less immediate economic potential or are lagging behind in development as compared to these BRICS countries. Very probably realpolitik will drive the majority of cardiac surgical missions to these countries where primary and secondary care is sufficiently developed to be able to consider doing cardiac surgery (Fig. 16.2).

Congenital Cardiac Surgery

Discussing cardiac surgical disease is incomplete without mentioning congenital cardiac heart disease. Structural heart disease affects infants and adults in high-, low-, and middle-income countries with relatively the same genetic prevalence—8–12 cases/1,000 live births, with the rate depending on the method of detection—but the burden of disease falls disproportionately on the lowest income countries [13–15]. This disparity exists not only because of lower per capita income to support expensive care but because

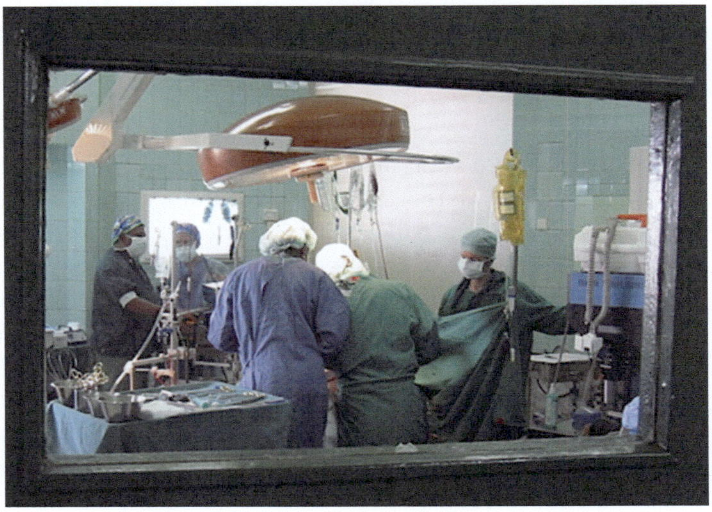

Fig. 16.2 Peeping through the window of the cardiac OR in Suriname. Suriname is considered an upper middle income country by the World Bank, which means the Academisch Ziekenhuis of Paramaribo, the academic hospital, has sufficient resources to support a cardiac surgical mission

higher fertility rates in LICs translate to more cases of congenital heart disease per wage earner [13]. Although only a small proportion of cardiac surgical care in any setting is provided to infants and children, the effect of treatment can provide 20–50 Disability adjusted life years (DALYs)[3] per case treated in the population in question [16]. Timely detection followed by curative surgical treatment may normalize life expectancies as well as improve neurodevelopmental outcomes for a considerable proportion of congenital cardiac malformations as well as cardiac disease due to infectious causes [15, 17]. The problem of congenital heart disease must be addressed from several angles with increased attention for mother and child survival campaigns, improved capacity of medical and diagnostic services, and finally improved access to cardiac surgical services [6]. As we discuss below, for successful treatment of any cardiac surgical disease—including congenital heart disease—several layers of care and capability must be in place to detect congenital cardiac malformations in an early stage, provide timely treatment, and to propose appropriate follow-up programs.

Summary

Cardiovascular disease has a huge impact on the global burden of disease, an impact that will continue to grow in particular among the populations of LMICs, who are not only affected by infectious cardiac disease, but have an increasing incidence of ischemic and degenerative disease. Although the largest impact in many countries will come from a focus on primary prevention, cardiac surgical care is an indisputable part of public health concern. The particular burden of disease and capacity to build surgical services will be different in every country and how that should be organized will very much depend on the specific context of the country. Typically a minimal level of primary and secondary health care will be necessary in order to be able to deploy a cardiac surgical development program. For more comprehensive review the reader is referred to an excellent article of Pezzella et al. [18] In the next section, we discuss the task of assessing capacity, forming partnerships, and making goals for a cardiac surgical program.

Cardiac Surgical Mission Goals and Preparation

Goals and Modalities of a Cardiac Surgical Mission

When one is choosing to participate in a humanitarian surgical mission, it is a good idea to think about how one's personal goals and the goals of the organization align. Especially for a cardiac surgical mission, the goals of the trip will dictate the daily activities and responsibilities, which may range from simply providing the anesthetic to helping plan the case schedule to providing postoperative ICU care. These can also include teaching a team of local practitioners how to expand their practice to implement the new procedures performed.

Defined goals of cardiac surgical missions may include:

- Bringing patients with advanced disease from LMICs to a cardiac surgical center in HIC and repatriating the patient after recovery.
- Performing cardiac surgery and anesthesia in a well-equipped but temporary structure, e.g., an empty wing of a hospital.
- Performing cardiac surgery and anesthesia in a local facility in conjunction with local practitioners.
- Assisting in setting up or planning a new cardiac surgical facility.
- Providing education for local practitioners, residents, fellows, nurses, or perfusionists.

Participants should look for programs where the host institution has a voice in the design and implementation of the program. Reputable programs will also be recognized by the host country Ministry of Health (MoH) and host national

[3] See the chapter in this text entitled "Comparative Economics of Anesthesia Care and the Global Anesthesia Workforce" for a thorough discussion of the Disability Adjusted Life Year (DALY) measure.

professional associations. Often local or international nongovernmental organizations (NGOs) will play a role in the organization and logistical support. The technical expertise can come from international specialty associations (in anesthesia and surgery). Regardless of who the players on the ground are, looking for an organization that emphasizes sustainability and self-sufficiency of the host team and training of specialists as opposed to substitution of roles will ensure the best experience for the visiting practitioner, host institution, and ultimately the population of the host country.

The Premise of a Mission

Making Voluntarism Meaningful and Impactful

Many authors in this text have spoken out against medical tourism in its many forms. That argument will not be repeated here; however, it is worth noting that more than any other subspecialty care, the treatment and care of cardiac surgical diseases requires long-term care from a team of health care providers including: cardiologists, cardiac surgeons, cardiothoracic anesthesiologists, perfusionists, intensivists, operating room technicians, and last but certainly not least nurses with experience in the OR, ICU, post-anesthesia care unit (PACU), and clinic.

Dr. Aldo Castañeda[4] noted in his address to the World Society for Pediatric and Congenital Heart Surgery (WSPCHS) in Antigua, Guatemala in 2010, "occasional visits of traveling teams performing a few diagnostic tests, interventions, and operations...will not solve the permanent needs of a cardiac unit in a developing country" [19].

Dr. Castañeda's work is one of the best examples of holistic surgical service capacity building. Since 1997, the Fundación Aldo Castañeda has facilitated growth of the Paediatric Cardiac Surgical Unit of Guatemala, expanding the capacity for outpatient consultation, echocardiography diagnostics, preoperative, intraoperative, and postoperative care of cardiac surgical patients, and graduate medical education [20, 21]. As of 2012, the Paediatric Cardiac Surgical Unit of Guatemala had tripled the number of surgeries performed annually, had become an international referral center for pediatric cardiology, and had begun to train subspecialist physicians in pediatric cardiac anesthesiology, pediatric cardiology, pediatric critical care, and cardiopulmonary perfusion [20]. Whether it is through "developing a functioning, independent local effort" [19] as Dr. Castañeda has done in Guatemala and as Surgeons of Hope® has done in Nicaragua, through ongoing collaboration between university departments in HICs and LICs, or by a establishing a meaningful, long term education program, enhancing the ability of local practitioners to safely care for the needs of their community should be the ultimate goal.

The most explicit example of this philosophy is described by the organization Children's HeartLink®, which was founded by Drs. Frank Johnson and Joseph Kaiser cardiovascular surgeons at Swedish Hospital in Minneapolis, Minnesota. In the early 1990's, Children's HeartLink® transitioned from providing care for children from LMICs in the USA to partnering with local hospitals and practitioners. Currently Children's HeartLink® practices a well-delineated process of local surgical capacity building with its sites; during this 6- to 10-year process they call the "Phased Support Approach," they work with sites on three continents to achieve a state where local practitioners are able not only to perform surgeries with acceptably low complication rates, but to train other practitioners [22, 23].

The transition from service substitution to independence often evolves organically without a well set plan, as in the example of the experience of one of the authors (PR) with the setup of a cardiac surgery program in Suriname. Until the late

[4] Aldo Casteñeda, MD is a humanitarian and a pediatric cardiac surgeon of unparalleled achievement who has contributed over 400 scholarly articles and advanced the field of pediatric cardiac surgery in the areas of heart-lung transplantation and neonatal correction of complex cardiac malformations. He is the William E. Ladd Professor Emeritus of Child Surgery at the Children's Hospital of Boston. Since his retirement from Harvard Medical School and the Children's Hospital of Boston, he has worked as founder and leader of the Fundación Aldo Casteñado centered in Antigua, Guatemala.

nineties Suriname cardiac patients were operated in The Netherlands, through a program which was financed by the Dutch Government. When this agreement was stopped for political reasons, one German and three Dutch cardiac surgical departments joined efforts with the Academic Hospital of Paramaribo to organize three to four 3-week missions per year. During these missions, an average of 35 patients were operated upon; these patients were pooled in advance by Suriname Cardiologists. The effort required to keep up this frequency of missions was challenging and required dedicated perseverance in particular from a single cardiac surgeon (GJ Kootstra) from Breda, The Netherlands, Gradually more coordinated efforts for collaboration and training of cardiac anesthesiologists and perfusionists were introduced involving three one-year fellowships in Amphia Hospital, supported by a grant from the European Association of Cardiothoracic Anaesthesiologists (EACTA). This additional training bolstered the ICU, pharmacy, and organization of the cardiac surgical mission (Fig. 16.3).

Through 10 years of collaboration with Surinam Hospital management and cardiologists, what started a volunteer-based and externally financed project ended in a fully independent cardiac surgical department in Suriname fortuitously staffed by a Dutch cardiac surgeon eager for the opportunity to direct a fully functional cardiac surgical unit in his native country.

Partnering for Sustainability

Unless the organization's mission is explicitly dedicated to cardiac surgery—as is the case with several organizations mentioned above—local nongovernmental organizations (NGOs) often have profound knowledge of the local context but lack specific expertise in cardiac surgery. The advantage of partnering with local NGOs is that the surgical team gains entrée into the community. In the experience of the author (PR), the disadvantage is that local NGOs will be driven by their funding streams, which are tied to achievement of short- and medium-term goals with high impact or great visibility. Partnering with local NGOs may mean an open time schedule if no interest exists in finalizing funded project.

Hospitals have access to all of the supply chains and structural implements for surgical missions, but administrators often lack knowledge of the larger national context as they are focused on maintaining private practices, serving the patients in need, and keeping the doors open. In working with any hospital, one also must deal with the microcosm of personalities and habits governing health care business as usual.

As successful university collaborations and NGOs such Children's HeartLink®, Surgeons of

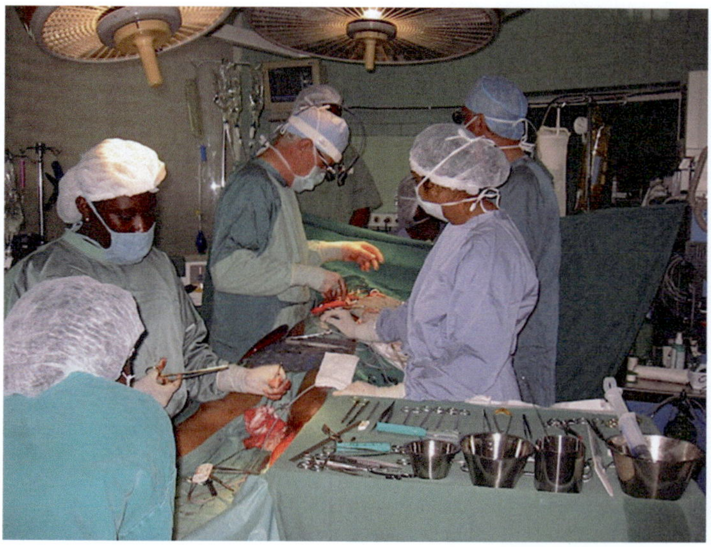

Fig. 16.3 A mixed surgical team at work on a coronary artery bypass graft (CABG). Local OR nurses are harvesting the venous graft while the visiting surgeons prepare the arterial target sites. This is an example of the middle stages of transition from a substitution team to a fully trained local team

Hope®, and Fundación Aldo Castañeda have demonstrated, the ideal situation may be the hybrid approach of connecting a host hospital where practitioners are ready to build a program with a functional team of practitioners with the support of an NGO or professional association. The Surinam example shows that this can be done without an NGO, but considerable effort will be need to overcome administrative and logistical hurdles.

With all of this in mind, physicians and nurses who are inspired to serve need not wait for the ideal situation to act or volunteer on a cardiac surgical mission—many anesthesiologists have had very fulfilling volunteer experiences in the absence of one or more of the conceptual elements described here [24–26]. No volunteer experience, even a surgical mission, comes with the guarantee of success and future productive academic relationships. Not all sites will become fully functioning independent adult or pediatric heart centers. But in order to help patients, one does need to know that minimum standards of quality and safety will be met. These standards are discussed in the next section.

Table 16.2 WHO Objectives of Safe Surgery

	Objective
1	Operate on correct patient and site
2	Use anesthetic methods known to prevent harm and treat pain
3	Be prepared for airway emergency or respiratory failure
4	Avoid or appropriately treat adverse drug reactions
5	Recognize and treat large volume blood loss
6	Minimize risk of surgical site infections
7	Prevent retention of surgical instruments or implements
8	Label all specimens correctly
9	Communicate effectively for the exchange of critical information
10	Establish and participate in routine surveillance at the hospital system level

The WHO Safe Surgery Saves Lives campaign encourages hospitals around the world to use the WHO Safe Surgery Saves Lives Checklist (SSLC) to help hospitals and practitioners meet these ten basic objectives.

Cardiac Anesthesia: Providing Optimal Care in Low Resource Settings

In 2008, the World Health Organization (WHO) published guidelines identifying multiple recommended worldwide safe surgical practices (see Table 16.2) [27]. In order to be able to practice any type of surgery in LMICs, these minimum conditions need to be fulfilled. In 2010, the World Federation of Societies of Anaesthesiologists (WFSA) updated the existing international standards for a safe practice in anesthesia and correlated these standards with the three levels of a hospital structure as defined by the WHO [28]. Although the WFSA guidelines were created for anesthesia for non-cardiac surgery, a cardiac anesthesia unit or visiting medical team should comply with all grades of suggestions and recommendations applicable for a level 3 hospital structure (see Table 16.3).

Donabedian described in 1988 how the quality of medical care could be assessed and assured in a three dimensional model [29]. He described three criteria that should be addressed to achieve an acceptable level of quality: structure, process and outcome criteria.[5] In order to discuss specifically the minimum standards for cardiac anesthesia, the Donabedian model will be used.

Structure

The Regional Context

The socioeconomic environment will have some bearing on the type of cardiac surgical care that can be provided. Given the nature and the extent of the investment needed in cardiac surgery, local cardiologists must have infrastructure in place to be able to identify patients in sufficient numbers, prepare them for surgery, and support them after visiting practitioners leave. Often this will imply that a cardiac surgical mission is best planned in an urban area. In particular staff, equipment

[5] See the chapter in this text "Quality Care: Maintaining Safety through Minimum Standards" for an in-depth discussion.

Table 16.3 Standards for infrastructure, supplies, and anesthesia at the Referral Hospital Level

Level 3 (Should meet at least *highly recommended*, *recommended* and *suggested* anesthesia standards) Referral hospital
A referral hospital of 300–1,000 or more beds with basic intensive care facilities. Treatment aims are the same as for Level 2, with the addition of: Ventilation in OR and ICU
Prolonged endotracheal intubation Thoracic trauma care Hemodynamic and inotropic treatment Complex neurological and cardiac surgery
Basic ICU patient management and monitoring for up to 1 week : all types of cases, but possibly with limited provision for: multi-organ system failure
Hemodialysis Prolonged respiratory failure Metabolic care or monitoring
Essential procedures Same as Level 2 with the following additions: Facial and intracranial surgery Bowel surgery Pediatric and neonatal surgery Thoracic surgery Major eye surgery Major gynecological surgery, e.g. vesico-vaginal repair
Personnel Clinical officers and specialists in anesthesia and surgery
Drugs Same as Level 2 with these additions: Propofol Nitrous oxide Various modern neuromuscular blocking agents Various modern inhalation anesthetics Various inotropic agents Various intravenous antiarrhythmic agents Nitroglycerine for infusion Calcium chloride 10 % 10 i.m. injection

Adapted from Merry et al. Can J Anesth/J Can Anesth (2010) 57:1027–1034 (Springer)

These are the minimum standards recommended by the WSFA for anesthesia for complex non-cardiac surgery, including thoracic surgery. The authors suggest these can also be considered as minimum standards for an institution hosting a cardiac surgical mission

requirement and on-site logistical support will necessitate good geographic accessibility (good roads, proximity to airport).

The Hospital

Cardiac surgery and anesthesia can only be performed in a qualified hospital structure, preferably a referral hospital. As a cardiac surgical project or mission will create a spin-off effect that might benefit or draw on the resources other departments, affiliation with a university or teaching hospital should be actively sought out. It is perhaps out of touch with reality to say that the hospital should be well organized and functional—as there are so many hospitals in HICs that are not—but a thorough check on a secure water supply, electricity, medical gasses and waste management should be performed and confirmed to comply with minimal standards.[6] An adequate number of qualified medical and support staff from the host site should be available around the clock. A reliable telecommunication system (within the hospital and outwards) needs to be in place (Fig. 16.4).

The hospital should offer most major categories of specialty care (at minimum cardiology, internal and pulmonary medicine, general surgery and paediatrics). Intensive care staffing and work patterns for monitoring postoperative patients may be considered adequate by the host team, but will not meet standards of care of the visiting team [26]. Specific inquiries should be made to determine if intensivists needs to be added to the visiting team. Specifically for cardiac surgery, the availability of transesophageal echocardiography (TEE) machines and probes and bronchoscopy equipment appropriately sized for the surgical population needs to be determined.

In an ideal situation, cardiology department should be fully functional with a qualified staff of interventional cardiologists, equipped with a cardiac catheterization laboratory and echocardiography equipment and expertise. A local cardiologist must be available for postoperative care and for emergency interventional procedures. Ideally, the hospital would have a dedicated ICU and cardiac surgical ward with 24/7 nursing staff. If this is not available, provisions must be made so all cardiac surgical patients can be hospitalized and monitored preoperatively and postoperatively. If a ward or a smaller hospital will be repurposed for PACU, ICU, and ward, this space should be equipped with ventilators, oxygen saturation and invasive blood pressure

[6] See the chapter in this text "Planning a Mission, Fundraising, and Building a Team: the Kybele experience" for further discussion of site evaluation.

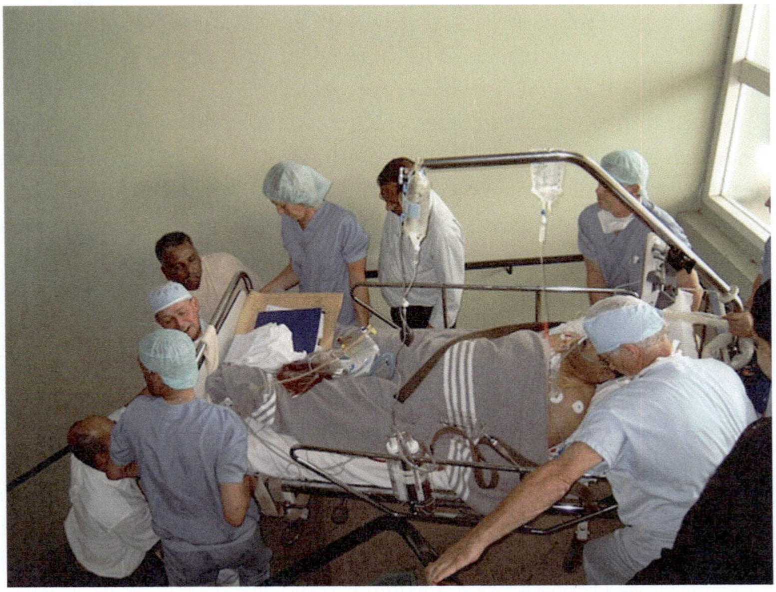

Fig. 16.4 Even with a thorough site evaluation, one must always be ready for the unexpected change in the infrastructure. Here, for example, the whole team transports a patient—stretcher and all—one floor downstairs from the OR to the ICU because the electricity and therefore the elevator had gone out

monitoring, a telemetry system, a central oxygen supply system, medical air and vacuum pipeline system for connecting suction drainage systems.

Laboratory and Imaging Services

A well-staffed laboratory that can perform chemistry, hematology, and hemostasis tests will be needed providing service around the clock. Substituting an accurate Point of Care (POC) laboratory unit for hemoglobin, glucose, blood gases with electrolytes, and/or dynamic hemostasis may prove to be effective and efficient. Radiology services need to be available on a daily basis for diagnostics [30–32].

Pharmacy Services

The local pharmacy should dispense a regular, secure supply of essential drugs contained in WHO Model List of Essential Medicines for adults or children, whichever is appropriate for the surgical population [33]. The surgical and anesthesia team can agree that a few drugs not on the WHO lists need to be brought from the home institution or purchased in-country, e.g., different synthetic opioids, subcutaneous heparin preparation for venous thromboembolism (VTE) prophylaxis, milrinone, phenylephrine, sevoflurane, and hemostatic agents (protamine, antifibrinolytics, desmopressin) [24–26]. This expanded pharmacy list should only contain drugs that have proven evidence-based efficacy. It is tempting to import an entire pharmacopeia to provide "optimal care," but in the setting of global health, optimal care is the care that will be available when the team leaves, so some consideration should be given to using and training local providers to use the drugs most readily available.

Transfusion and Blood banking

The Society of Thoracic Surgery (STS) identified three groups of patients who are at increased risk of perioperative bleeding and transfusion during cardiac surgery: patients of advanced age, patients with small blood volume due to small body size, and patients having emergent or complex operations [34]. Practitioners are unlikely to encounter patients of advanced age or to undertake emergent or redo procedures in a global health setting. Thus, aiming for a low transfusion exposure should be a primary objective of every cardiac surgical program.

The local blood bank should be able to guarantee a secure supply of properly tested blood products according to the 2010 recommendations by the WHO (Screening donated blood for transfusion transmissible infections (TTI) [35]. This document describes universal and country-specific requirement for screening. Blood products that should be available are packed cells (all blood groups), fresh frozen plasma (FFP), thrombocyte concentrate (TC) and maybe cryoprecipitate. Component therapy—with a growing body of evidence—may be an effective solution to decrease the dependency on FFP and TC but probably depend on import [36]. With a growing arsenal of equipment required to maintain blood component therapy, a maintenance department with qualified biomedical engineers will be needed by the hospital.

Intensive Care and Monitoring

The staffing and capacity of host facility to provide intensive care may be variable, and even if intensive care services are readily available, the host institution may not have capacity to expand to accommodate the increase in volume from a week of cardiac surgery. Consideration should be given to including one or two intensivists and up to four critical care nurses with experience caring for the surgical population on the visiting team [24, 25]. The extent of the requirement for postoperative ventilator support must not be overestimated. Mechanical ventilation has both indications and risks [37, 38]. Most cardiac anesthesiologists would prefer to ventilate their patients for a few hours postoperatively but cardiac anesthesia can be performed with extubation in the OR, and this can have considerable advantages in a setting when electricity is not a guarantee. Early extubation and "fast-track" programs have been implemented in LMICs where they were associated with decreased morbidity and mortality and should be implemented if possible (Fig. 16.5) [39, 40].

For postoperative intensive care, one must check the number and availability of up-to-date bedside monitoring equipment including: two selectable ECG channels (five lead system), invasive pressure monitoring (two channels), pulse oximetry, capnography (side stream or main stream). In addition, number and maintenance of artificial ventilators able to provide different modes of ventilation (Volume and pressure control and pressure support) should be determined. Defibrillators, enteral and parenteral nutrition should be routinely available. Dialysis either intermittent or continuous hemofiltration (CVVH) should be available either as an in hospital use service or in agreement with a nearby dialysis centre.

The Operating Room and Extracorporeal Circulation

An equipped and functional OR including a sterilization unit is a mainstay, and the functionality and reliability of electricity, OR table, lights, and climate control should be discussed. Specific equipment should consist of diathermy devices,

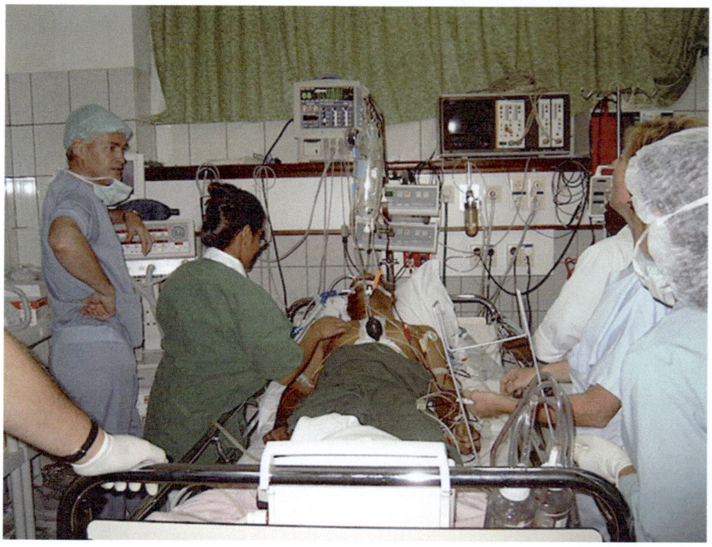

Fig. 16.5 The resources required for proper postoperative management and monitoring are substantial. Here the patient is mechanically ventilated, but "fast-track" anesthesia, which aims at extubation in the OR or in the immediate postoperative period is the goal in a global health setting

OR tables, and a method of charting. Particular care should be given to the presence of a few sets of cardio-surgical instruments and disposables. At minimum, two identical cardiopulmonary bypass (CPB) machines for extracorporeal circulation (ECC)—one for use and one to serve for spare parts are essential, along with a sufficient supply of ECC circuit sets and disposables. A CellSaver® for red cell salvage and autotransfusion, if available, will be of paramount importance.

Historically the CPB unit was known as the Heart-Lung Machine (HLM) and is colloquially known as a "pump." CPB has become safer and better controlled than ever, but with the incorporation of sophisticated electronics, it is particularly vulnerable in the context of LMICs. Biocompatible and prepacked sterilized low volume circuits including membrane oxygenators have rendered bubble oxygenators and blood priming obsolete, but machines with these features may still be in operation in LMICs (Fig. 16.6).

Monitoring for cardiothoracic surgery has evolved a great deal from the age of simple monitoring to the advent and use of very invasive monitors and now a return to simplicity courtesy of technology. In addition to the standard monitors enumerated above, transesophageal echocardiography (TOE) should be available. Mandatory pulmonary artery catheterization and measurement of cardiac output by thermodilution has been abandoned in routine practice as benefits have failed to be proven [41, 42]. TOE is a superior monitor, providing more information and more insight than pulmonary artery catheterization. TOE equipment and proficient use of it at an advanced level is essential in every cardiac surgical program, but the purchase and maintenance of TOE machines and probes may prove challenging for the host institution. Visiting providers may have access to probes in the host facility, but maintenance and sterilization should be discussed prior to arrival. If well-maintained equipment will not be available, vendors from the home institution may be a good source of probes or equipment for loan and use during the surgical mission [24].

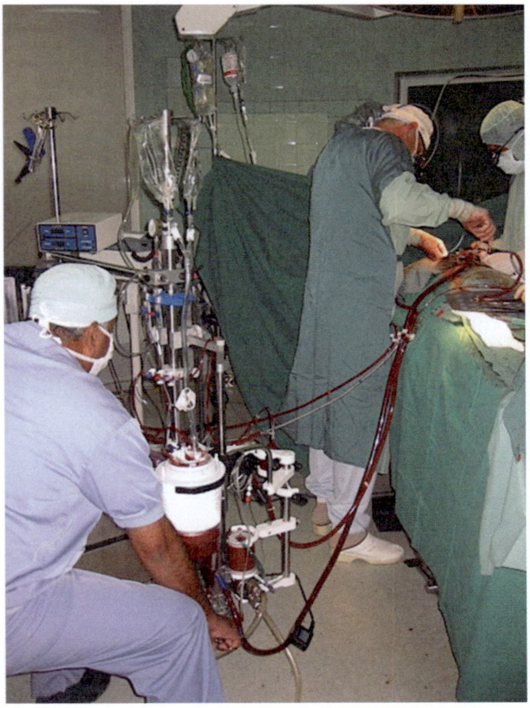

Fig. 16.6 A simple but functional extracorporeal circulation (ECC) cardiopulmonary bypass machine run by a local perfusionist in use during a coronary artery bypass grafting surgery

Newer and simpler noninvasive monitoring concepts are being proposed and although their benefits are not proven yet may appear as interesting concepts in particular in low resource settings. Near-infrared spectroscopy (NIRS) monitoring may prove to become a reliable trend monitor of cardiac output and mixed venous O_2 saturation and may provide additional (limited) information on brain saturation [43, 44]. At this stage, disposables are expensive, and without a strong industry partnership, are likely not yet practical in the global health setting. However, one author (PR) has experience safely reusing NIRS disposables; single use sensors provided though by the manufacturer can be adhered to the forehead of several patients until the transducer finally becomes defective.

It is always best to use local equipment when possible. The anesthesia machine should be a "modern" ventilator (different ventilations modes with PEEP and variable bypass vaporizers for, in order of increasing preference: halothane, isoflurane, or sevoflurane). The availability of syringe and infusion volumetric pumps should be in sufficient quantity and thoroughly checked. Two to five syringe pumps will be needed per OR. Again, vendors from the home institution may prove to be helpful in obtaining donation or loan of such durable medical equipment. Temporary pacemakers and a defibrillator with internal pads will complete the list of essential equipment. One may discuss with the team the necessity of having an intra-aortic balloon pump in the light of lack of evidence, but in the likely absence of ECMO outside the OR, most cardiac anaesthesiologist and surgeons would feel more comfortable with having IABP at hand.

Personnel: The Anesthesia Department and the Cardiac Surgical Team

Again the framework set forth by the 2010 WFSA international standards for a safe practice in anesthesia, though designed for anesthesia for non-cardiac surgery, is an excellent lens through which to evaluate the status of the host anesthesia department. In order to offer cardiac services, a cardiac surgical unit should at least comply with all recommendations for a level 3 hospital structure [28].

In the early stages of a mission, the cardiac surgical team will be flown in from abroad. The team should be carefully selected and consist of qualified and experienced staff: at least one cardiovascular surgeon, one cardiac anaesthesiologist with one cardiac anesthesia resident or nurse, one or two cardiac surgical scrub nurses or technicians, and between three and four nurses with critical care training experienced with the cardiac surgical population. This personnel is in addition to any needs for critical care physicians, critical care nurses, or cardiologists from the local hospital required for safe preoperative and postoperative care. The staffing will depend heavily on the experience and comfort level of the host practitioners, with staffing on the higher side for the initial visit of a paediatric cardiac surgical mission [24–26].

Supplies: Assuring a Secure Logistical System

The difficult logistics of securing a reliable supply chain for disposables and drugs is a *conditio sine qua non* of a cardiac surgical mission. In developed countries there is a whole system in place assuring used to well-functioning supply systems in the hospitals and even if a shortage or stock rupture occurs we can easily fall back on a reliable commercial and industrial network. In the LMIC countries such a backup network system is often lacking or not reliable. Furthermore, for cardiac surgery, anesthesia, and intensive care, specific drugs and equipment are needed (valve implants, catheters, extracorporeal circuits) for which there is no other local market.

Because of spatial and financial impacts of maintaining high stocks and the potential for diversion of supplies the common HIC practice of "having it available" is not practical. Creativity and flexibility will need to be employed with respect to materials and supplies. Budgeting for and using the disposables from within the local hospital will strengthen the supply chain within the host country. In the event that specific and essential items are not available, they will need to be secured from outside sources or imported prior to arrival. Supply and back up should be secured. Expiration dates and shipping will need to be taken into account [24].

Bringing in equipment and leaving it in the local structure is a delicate proposition. Equipment from the home hospital must work under the conditions in the local hospital, it must be reliable and well maintained equipment; and it must be delivered with essential spare parts. In donation, uniformity is the golden rule, and different types or brands of equipment should be avoided. The equipment and monitors used in HICs is increasingly digital which makes it more sophisticated, fragile and expensive to maintain. Older equipment, such as that often found in BRICS countries, may have a more robust and suitable construction.

The process for obtaining the vast array of drugs and disposables for surgery, anesthesia and perfusion begins with maintaining a detailed

Table 16.4 Adopting the KISS principle

	Home institution	Local project
Ventilators	Sophisticated, digital	Local brand, search outside Europe or USA
Opioids	Remifentanil, sufentanil	Morphine sulphate
Anesthetics	Sevoflurane	Halothane, isoflurane
Pulmonary dilution catheters	Different brands	Skip, use NIRS, TOE
Intravascular pressure monitoring	3–4 channels	1–2 channels
Mixed venous saturation	Lab	NIRS
Classical coagulation tests	APTT, PTT, INR, fibrinogen	Dynamic POC coagulation testing

Practitioners working in a global health setting will benefit from applying the KISS (Keep It Simple Stupid) organizational principle to their pre-trip planning and in-country activities

inventory and finding a reliable source for each item. Then the whole logistic chain from purchase (often abroad) through use and disposal must be monitored and assured. The KISS principle ("Keep It Simple, Stupid") should prevail at all time. Some examples are given in Table 16.4. Securing a supply line offers some control of or preparedness for financial and administrative hurdles that will inevitably come with planning a cardiac surgical mission.

The FDA accepts the reuse of medical devices and disposables under strict conditions [45]. In August 2000, FDA released a guidance document on single-use devices reprocessed by third parties or hospitals. In this guidance document, FDA states that hospitals or third-party re-processors will be considered "manufacturers" and regulated in the same manner [45, 46]. Thus, reprocessing of medical equipment is possible but is a significant undertaking that is probably outside the abilities of a single mission team. For a thorough discussion, see the chapter on "Materials Management" within this book.

Sorting and salvage of waste material is an easily overlooked aspect of logistics. Though it can be reliable in state-of-the-art hospitals, in LMIC countries appropriate waste disposal can be a source of infection in regular hospitals. There exists no international standard for disposal and there is a dire need of infectious waste disposal management. There is a trend for disposal of medical wastes in landfilled sites which requires strict quality control from the local health authorities and local health department [12].

Processes

The processes include all medical and administrative tasks performed during the cardiac surgical mission. It involves the medical and surgical care from the preoperative period to the patient's discharge and recovery. Guidelines are readily available, and evidence based care should prevail above personal convictions. The processes of care are often presented or enumerated in written documents, usually called policies. Each policy should aim at providing effective surgical care, where, as the adage goes "better" can be the enemy of good." The challenge in global health is not only to respect the host practitioners' opinions but to actually adapt to the local conditions. Visiting practitioners may feel secure in their own habits, and it is tempting for the visiting team to impose their own ways, techniques, equipment and drugs. However, it is a sign of true professionalism to respect the local perspective, help the host team to adapt evidence based recommendations to local conditions (such as local medication availability), and be prepared to learn new techniques in the process.

A major problem may arise when different host teams are involved who all might try to impose their particular habits (and drugs and equipment). It is in the interest of the program to search for a modus vivendi to which all teams commit.

Surgical Planning

The determination of surgical indications differs little in a low resource setting from the high resource setting of the home institution. The difference is in the risk-benefit analysis because the team must determine if the risks within the local conditions outweighed the benefits of the surgical intervention.

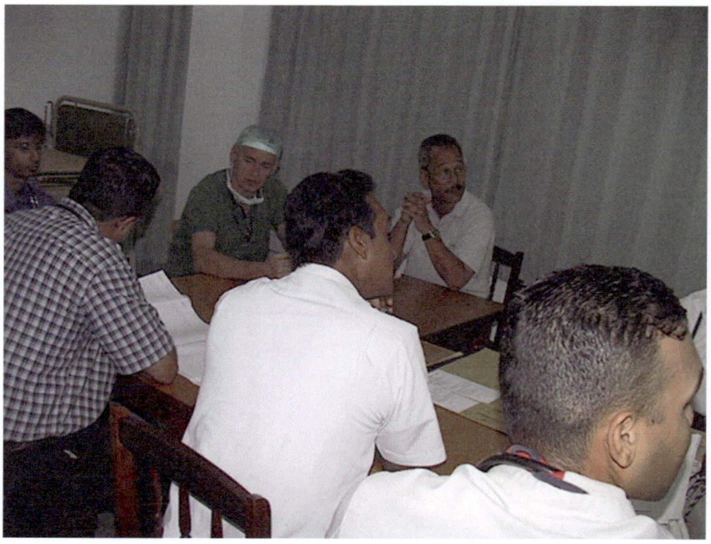

Fig. 16.7 A multidisciplinary case conference with representatives from all specialties and professions held prior to and after arrival in-country will help provide the most rational plan for the operating room

These are difficult decisions that are best made as a group.

Many practitioners have described the value of a multidisciplinary conference in operative planning for humanitarian surgery, especially for pediatric cardiac surgery [23, 24, 26, 40]. This multidisciplinary approach includes input from practitioners from cardiothoracic anesthesiology, cardiac surgery, cardiology, critical care, nursing, and perfusionists who have access to the patient's history, imaging, testing, and context from the primary care physician (see Fig. 16.7) [23–25, 40]. In global health, the proposed surgery will succeed or fail based not on technical skill or perioperative care but on issues like family situation, housing, and working environment, and economic constraints. For example, a patient may be an excellent candidate for valve replacement, but lifelong anticoagulant therapy might not be tenable for the patient who lives in a remote area. Safety should prevail and alternatives offered.

Surgical technique will be meticulous and should aim at the safest global outcome. This might mean that at times a simpler intervention may prove "better" than the "best" or most complete treatment. Complications like the requirement for a permanent pacemaker or coagulopathy from a long bypass time may jeopardize the global success for a given patient.

In adult cardiac surgery, the SYNTAX trial has clearly shown that fewer major adverse cardiac events (MACE) occur after coronary artery bypass grafting (CABG) than after percutaneous coronary intervention (PCI) among American and European patients with three vessel coronary artery disease [47]. However, this study has yet to be repeated in BRICS or MICs, where surgical morbidity and mortality may be higher than with percutaneous interventions. In addition, CABG performed without ECC (a so called "off pump" procedure) may be preferable over a CABG with ECC (an "on pump" procedure) and may be particularly suited to the context in BRICS and MICs [48]. As another example, though recent data suggests there is no difference in outcome between mitral valvuloplasty and mitral valve replacement [49], in the global health context valvuloplasty may be the preferable option in particular if there is no atrial fibrillation as lifelong anticoagulation may be avoided. In the pediatric surgical population, though a patient might benefit hemodynamically from a Fontan procedure, if there are no cardiologists in the country capable of medically managing such a patient postoperatively, it is not the best operation [24].

In order to provide evidence based surgical care in a low resource setting, each individual practitioner on the surgical team must exercise not only good, experienced and individualized clinical judgment but a holistic approach to applying the evidence and making the surgical plan.

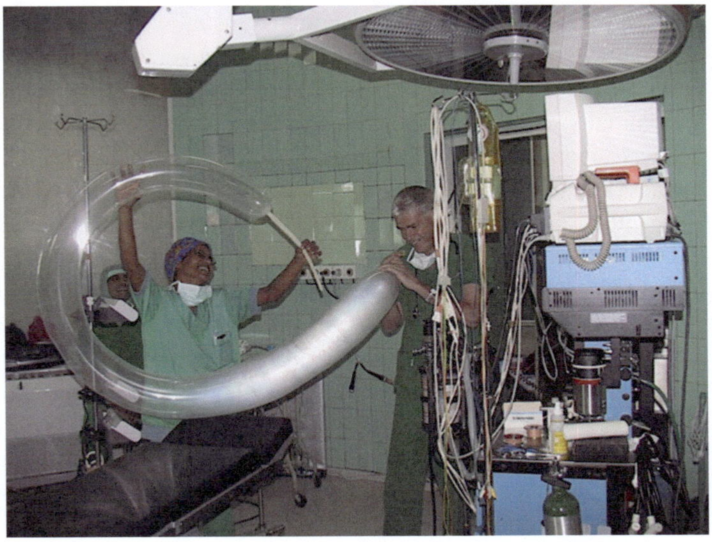

Fig. 16.8 A novel use for a transoesophageal echo (TOE) probe cover keeps the mood light in the OR. TOE is an essential function of the cardiac anesthesiologist in all settings

Embracing Advances in Cardiac Anesthesia

Currently, progress in cardiac anesthesia by the refinement of anaesthetic techniques from deep anesthesia to high dose opioids and progressing to a balanced anaesthetic technique is not too different from anesthesia for non-cardiac surgery. Fast-track anesthesia techniques can—depending on the study—include utilization of a balanced anesthesia technique with short-acting opioid, early extubation in the OR or ICU, and rapid normalization of the patient with early mobilization and removal of lines and tubes [40, 50–52].

Meta-analysis has shown decreased complication rates and larger retrospective studies have shown efficacious resources (reduced duration of postoperative ventilation or decreased length of stays in ICU and hospital) [53]. It is tempting to attribute the merits of fast track anesthesia to the use of ultrashort acting opioids, anaesthetics with speedy pharmacokinetics, and increasing availability of intermediate-acting muscle relaxants, though fast-track anesthesia can be provided with older pharmacologic agents [40, 50]. Longer acting and much cheaper drugs have been used successfully (e.g. morphine or fentanyl, halothane or isoflurane and pancuronium) [54].

An essential diagnostic skill for the cardiac anesthesiologists is transesophageal echocardiography (TOE) monitoring (see Fig. 16.8). The indications and uses for (TOE) is constantly evolving and expanding, and these guidelines are well described elsewhere [55]. Many professional anaesthesiology associations like the Society for Cardiovascular Anesthesiology (SCA), European Association of Cardiothoracic Anaesthesiologists (EACTA) and the Asian Society of Cardiothoracic Anesthesia (ASCA) offer certified training programs at beginner, advanced and expert levels.

One study of implementation of TOE in a low-resource setting concluded that the major challenges were "(1) limited availability of equipment and trained personnel in either the public or private facilities in the region (2) restricted movement of skilled manpower in the region to support enhanced service delivery and (3), low level of awareness of providers and patients of the clinical utility of this procedure" [56]. Beginning or enhancing a program for TOE in the host country is an excellent opportunity for the visiting anaesthesiologist to work with local practitioners on this essential skill.

Patient Blood Management Programs

Patient Blood Management Programs (PBMP) contributed substantially to the progress in cardiac anesthesia and surgery. Cardiac surgery used to consume an important fraction of blood usage in developed countries. Nevertheless, the benefits of transfusion have not borne out in the evidence, while the data surrounding transfusion-related morbidity and mortality is accumulating [57, 58]. PBMP have proven to substantially decrease transfusion requirements, and have contributed to the safety and cost effectiveness of both adult or congenital cardiac surgery [59]. This result was achieved without an increase in morbidity and mortality and with a decreased cost on top, both being important reasons to make PBMP a high priority of any cardiac surgical unit. Modern patient blood management is focuses upon three axes: (1) optimizing the patient's preoperative condition in particular hemoglobin and coagulation, (2) minimizing hemodilution, blood loss, and transfusion, and (3) maximizing blood salvage. The evidence based guidelines for blood conservation are well summarized elsewhere [34].

Having an appropriate algorithm for preoperative patient optimization, appropriate transfusion indications, minimizing blood loss, blood recuperation (red cell salvage), and point of care (POC) dynamic coagulation are essential for a successful PBPM. If possible, POC testing should be implemented as it provides considerable advantages above the classical coagulation tests [34].

For a surgical mission, a blood conservation policy can be agreed upon by the anesthesia and surgical team prior to travel. Efforts for blood conservation are an excellent opportunity to work with local practitioners to achieve a common goal, especially in the area of patient preparation. The prevalence of anaemia in LMICs is very high—perhaps 30 % in some areas, and patients with anaemia have a higher rate of requiring transfusion during cardiac surgery [34, 60]. Furthermore preoperative anemia significantly contributes to postoperative morbidity [61]. Collaborative effort will be required to identify patients that are at risk, to provide goal-directed treatment with vitamin K for an abnormal coagulation profile and/or iron supplementation for anemia in the weeks prior to surgery, to monitor for and treat any infectious aetiologies, and to assure that patients are monitored while discontinuing antiplatelet drugs preoperatively. Erythropoietin may only rarely be necessary to optimize preoperative hemoglobin.

Intraoperatively, tranexamic acid and desmopressin, which are on the WHO Essential Medications list, may be more available in LMIC cardiac surgical units; this is less the case for fibrinogen and factor concentrates (prothrombin complex) [62]. Still many cardiac anesthesiologist will be glad to have this at hand, especially with an insecure supply of platelets and fresh frozen plasma. If available, the use of a CellSaver® as standard technique of a cardiosurgical program, its absence resulting in a substantial increase in consumption of transfusion products [34, 63]. The surgical and anaesthetic technique should be judiciously used as unrestricted use of cell salvage will result in a depletion of coagulation factors and platelets with a likely increase in blood loss. A Cell Saver® will need disposable components but the reservoir of the ECC circuit may be used for a dual purpose if appropriately adapted.

Perfusion Medicine

Some would say cardiac surgery cannot be performed without a cardiopulmonary bypass (CPB) machine for extracorporeal circulation (ECC), but in reality, these surgeries cannot be performed without the services of a perfusionist. The safety and quality of ECC has improved dramatically over the last two decades because of rapid technologic developments, academic research into the science of ECC, and the professionalization of perfusion medicine.

Perfusionists have a variety of professional backgrounds from paramedical training (nursing, lab technicians), to a dedicated three-year postgraduate degree in perfusion medicine, to medical school and anaesthesiology residency (as in France and in Poland). In most European countries training of perfusionist is nationally regulated. National training institutes can apply for certification on a European level by the European Board of Clinical Perfusionists (EBCP). At this moment the EBCP applies with the European Commission for recognition as a

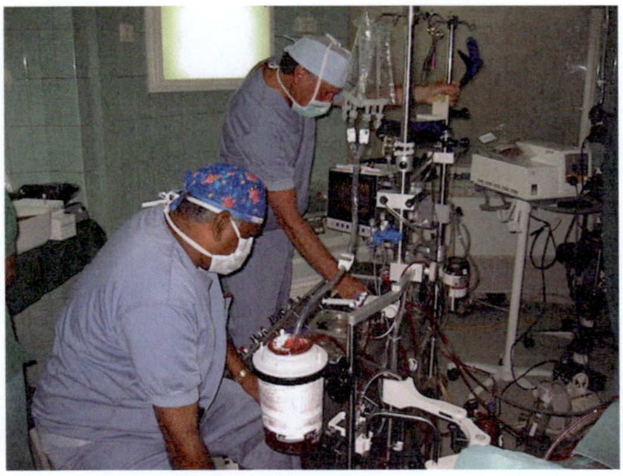

Fig. 16.9 Local and visiting perfusionists work together to prime the ECC circuit for the next case. Perfusionists from different backgrounds will have different education and training

separate specialty with its own requirements and responsibilities (Fig. 16.9).

Whatever her/his background, the perfusionist will need to combine knowledge and understanding of the physics and physiology of ECC and a wide array of technical skills to assure the ECC machine is functioning and interfacing well with human circulation and respiration. At times, the perfusionist must recommend the appropriate cannulas to the surgeon, manage the CellSaver® for blood conservation, perform point of care dynamic hemostatic testing, and assist with transfusion management. S/he will monitor the ECC including going on and coming off bypass and intervene if necessary in close collaboration with cardiac anaesthesiologist and surgeon. Likewise, the cardiac anaesthesiologist should have a thorough understanding of ECC because s/he is the physician ultimately responsible for maintaining oxygen delivery and homeostasis. Particular attention should be given to assure that the patient's temperature is normal at the end of surgery, as hypothermia causes and exacerbates coagulation abnormalities and increases postoperative morbidity.

Intensive Care and Recovery

Cardiac surgical patients will almost invariably need intensive care postoperatively, irrespective of the location or nomenclature of the facility where this care will be provided. The main objectives of this phase of care are to monitor, assure optimal hemodynamic stability, prevent complications (especially bleeding and coagulation disturbances), and facilitate an advantageous and quick return to the surgical ward and eventually home.

Dynamic coagulation testing may be useful but coagulation test disturbances without bleeding should not be treated. Lactate measurements, NIRS and TOE may be useful techniques to respectively monitor hemodynamics. The importance of early recovery and weaning of controlled ventilation cannot be over stated as awake and alert patients provide excellent clinical clues to evaluate their hemodynamic and respiration. More over the needs for fluid loading and vasoactive drugs will be greatly reduced in the awake and pain free patient as compared to the sedated and artificially ventilated patient (Fig. 16.10).

Complications of cardiac surgery will put additional stress on the capability and capacity of an ICU. Peri-operative myocardial infarction, dysrhythmias, kidney disturbances or renal failure, and respiratory complications may require additional diagnostic and therapeutic interventions like heart catheterization, bronchoscopy, hemodialysis or CVVH, and pleural drainage. Any cardiac surgical program needs to be capable of handling these challenges. One of the greatest opportunities of a cardiac surgical program occurs in the relationship between the hosting team and the local critical care teams, which can have a positive effect on the local ICU.

Outcome and Quality Control

Every cardiac surgical program should monitor its results and clinical statistics should be proactively registered, monitored and analyzed and lead to further improvement according the "plan–do–check–act or adjust" cycle proposed by Deming [64].

This should follow the Donabedian's principles. Appropriate indicators for structure, process,

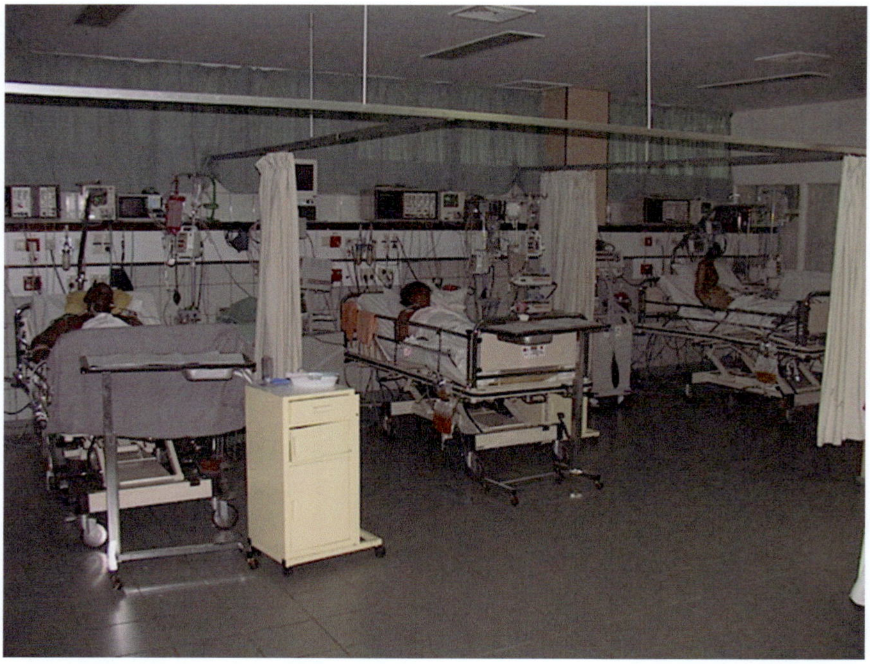

Fig. 16.10 A view on the cardiac surgical side of the ICU of the University Hospital in Paramaribo (AZP) shows that all patients are awake. Also of note here is the heterogeneity of equipment, which was a mix of host institution and donated equipment

and outcome should be identified and registered for preoperative, intraoperative, and postoperative phases. Preoperatively besides the normal patient identifiers gender, age, weight, length, preoperative blood count and creatinine, diagnostic descriptive elements should be recorded, and a recognized risk assessment should be used. The EuroSCORE is one of the most universally used and best known risk assessment systems and can be found at www.euroSCORE.org). Intraoperatively, data describing surgical technique and relevant processes like duration of clamp time, ECC time, use of special techniques, and transfusions given should be registered.

Postoperatively process indicators as length of stay in intensive care and hospital, use of adjuvants (IABP, renal replacement therapy) should be assembled together with outcome indicators including crude and risk adjusted mortality, morbidity (including renal failure, myocardial infarction, re-intervention, surgical site infection, mediastinitis), transfusion and a description of the patient's condition at discharge. Finally, special attention may be needed to assemble data to evaluate the financial burden and impact of the project or mission.

Conclusion

In conclusion, setting up a cardiac surgical project positively impacts a local health care system and population. Very likely a successful cardiac surgical and cardiac anesthesiology project will result in unanticipated benefits to the whole local hospital. However, it is highly demanding on the expertise, flexibility, and organizational power of the visiting practitioners in collaboration with the local hospital and team. This chapter has outlined the specific clinical and logistic considerations for this type of high yield global health project, which are summarized in Table 16.5.

Table 16.5 Checklist for considerations for a pediatric or adult cardiac surgery humanitarian mission

Preparation

- ✓ Site evaluation
- ✓ Definition of host team and visiting team composition and goals. Roles/needs (with minimum number of personnel) include:
  - Cardiac surgeon (1)
  - Cardiothoracic anesthesiologist (1)
  - Anesthesia nurse, tech, or resident (1)
  - Perfusionist (1)
  - Cardiologist (1, optional if competent and available local interventional cardiologist.)
  - OR nurse (2 – may substitute 1 scrub tech)
  - Intensive care physician (1) or cardiac anesthesiologist with IC expertise
  - Recovery/ICU nurse (4 – 2 day shift, 2 night shift)
  - Site coordinator (1)
- ✓ Logistics: inventory and sourcing of supplies and equipment; defining need for additional equipment and disposables
- ✓ Pre-trip case conference to create preliminary OR schedule
- ✓ Education: determination of mentorship, training, and/or lecturing requested by host team

Structure

- ✓ Safe physical structure with consistent electricity, water, sanitation, compressed oxygen, and climate control
- ✓ Safe supply of banked blood/blood components
- ✓ Laboratory (24 hours/day) and radiology services (daily)
- ✓ Durable medical equipment including, but not limited to:
  - Anesthesia machine + backup* (suitable for neonates/children)
  - IC ventilators
  - 2 sets of surgical instruments
  - OR and ICU monitors including: pulse oximetry, telemetry, 2 channels of invasive pressure monitoring, noninvasive blood pressure monitoring, capnography if not incorporated in ventilator, temperature, +/- near infrared spectroscopy (NIRS)*
  - Syringe pumps 2-5 per OR*
  - Transoesophageal echocardiography (machine and 2 probes)*
  - Extracorporeal circulation (ECC) machine (including evaluation of type, maintenance, and back-up)*
  - Patient warming
  - Point of care testing (blood gas, glucose, Hb, electrolytes, dynamic haemostasis)
- ✓ Single-use† supplies (number sufficient for planned surgeries + several extras)
  - Circuits and cannulas for ECC
  - Invasive pressure monitoring (catheters, transducers, ...)
  - Central venous catheters

* Photos helpful in determining compatability

† See chapter entitled "Materials Management" for a discussion of re-use of disposable medical equipment.

(continued)

Table 16.5 (continued)

- IV, pressure, and syringe pump tubing
- Cell saver + equipment
- Echocardiography and TOE probe (optional: probes for transthoracic and epicardial echo and vascular access) .
- Supplies for neuraxial anesthesia technique (+/- according to team preference)

✓ Pharmacy
- Anesthetics, analgesics, inotropes, chronotropes, vasodilators
- IV fluids
- Priming solution for ECC
- Cardioplegia solution

✓ Dedicated space to store equipment and disposables and pharmaceuticals

Process

✓ Policies for:
- Blood conservation and transfusion management

✓ Standing order set
- Preoperative testing
- Postoperative/ICU management

✓ Surgical safety checklist

Outcome

✓ Who will keep/maintain outcome database?, prepare forms (paper or excel)

✓ To whom will data be reported?
- Home institution
- Local cardiac surgical unit
- Hospital/hospital system
- Ministry of Health
- Sponsoring organizations

References

1. Farmer PE, Kim JY. Surgery and global health: a view from beyond the OR. World J Surg. 2008;32:533–6. http://www.pubmedcentral.nih.gov/articlerender.fcgi?artid=2267857&tool=pmcentrez&rendertype=abstract. Accessed 25 May 2014.
2. Yusuf S, Reddy S, Ounpuu S, Anand S. Global burden of cardiovascular diseases: part i: general considerations, the epidemiologic transition, risk factors, and impact of urbanization. Circulation. 2001;104:2746–53.
3. Vaartjes I, Koopman C, Visseren F, Bots M. Hart- en vaatziekten in Nederland 2013. Hart- en vaatzieketen in Nedrerland, cijfers over levensstijl, risicofactoren, zikete en sterfte. Hart Bull. 2013;43:24–8.
4. World Health Organization. The atlas of heart disease and stroke. 2013. http://www.who.int/cardiovascular_diseases/resources/atlas/en/. Accessed 20 May 2014.
5. World Heart Federation. Cardiovascular disease in youth and children, vol. 3. Geneva: World Heart Federation; 2012.
6. Yacoub MH. Establishing pediatric cardiovascular services in the developing world: a wake-up call. Circulation. 2007;116:1876–8. http://www.ncbi.nlm.nih.gov/pubmed/17965402. Accessed 14 May 2014.
7. Gaziano T, Bitton A, Anand S, Abrahams-Gessel S, Murphy A. Growing epidemic of coronary heart disease in low- and middle-income countries. Curr Probl Cardiol. 2010;35:72–115. http://www.pubmedcentral.nih.gov/articlerender.fcgi?artid=2864143&tool=pmcentrez&rendertype=abstract. Accessed 28 April 2014.
8. Watters D, Hollands MJ, Gruen RL, Maoate K, Perndt H, McDougall RJ, Morriss WW, Tangi V, Casey KM, McQueen K. Perioperative mortality rate (POMR): a global indicator of access to safe surgery and anaesthesia. World J Surg. 2014. http://www.ncbi.nlm.nih.gov/pubmed/24841805. Accessed 25 May 2014.

9. O'Neill J. Paper No. 66: building better global economic BRICs. London, 2002:1–16.
10. Wikipedia. BRICS – wikipedia, the free encyclopedia. 2013. http://en.wikipedia.org/wiki/BRICS. Accessed 13 May 2014.
11. Gomes WJ. EACTS in the future: second strategic conference. The view from the BRICS countries. Eur J Cardiothorac Surg. 2013;43:238–40. http://www.ncbi.nlm.nih.gov/pubmed/23148073. Accessed 28 May 2014.
12. Mukherjee C. Personal communication. 27 May 2014.
13. Hoffman JI. The global burden of congenital heart disease. Cardiovasc J Afr. 2013;24:141–5. http://www.pubmedcentral.nih.gov/articlerender.fcgi?artid=3721933&tool=pmcentrez&rendertype=abstract. Accessed 1 May 2014.
14. Lloyd-Jones D, Adams R, Carnethon M, De Simone G, Ferguson TB, Flegal K, Ford E, Furie K, Go A, Greenlund K, Haase N, Hailpern S, Ho M, Howard V, Kissela B, Kittner S, Lackland D, Lisabeth L, Marelli A, McDermott M, Meigs J, Mozaffarian D, Nichol G, O'Donnell C, Roger V, Rosamond W, Sacco R, Sorlie P, Stafford R, Steinberger J, et al. Heart disease and stroke statistics – 2009 update: a report from the American Heart Association Statistics Committee and Stroke Statistics Subcommittee. Circulation. 2009;119:480–6. http://www.ncbi.nlm.nih.gov/pubmed/19171871. Accessed 8 May 2014.
15. van der Linde D, Konings EEM, Slager MA, Witsenburg M, Helbing WA, Takkenberg JJM, Roos-Hesselink JW. Birth prevalence of congenital heart disease worldwide: a systematic review and meta-analysis. J Am Coll Cardiol. 2011;58:2241–7. http://www.sciencedirect.com/science/article/pii/S0735109711030798. Accessed 29 April 2014.
16. Harris RE. The Epidemic of Chronic Heart Failure in the United States. In: Epidemiology of Chronic Disease; 2013. p. 25–33.
17. Marino BS, Lipkin PH, Newburger JW, Peacock G, Gerdes M, Gaynor JW, Mussatto K, Uzark K, Goldberg CS, Johnson WH, Li J, Smith SE, Bellinger DC, Mahle WT. Neurodevelopmental outcomes in children with congenital heart disease: evaluation and management: a scientific statement from the American Heart Association. Circulation. 2012;126:1143–72. http://www.ncbi.nlm.nih.gov/pubmed/22851541. Accessed 1 May 2014.
18. Pezzella AT. Global aspects of cardiothoracic surgery with focus on developing countries. Asian Cardiovasc Thorac Ann. 2010;18:299–310. http://www.ncbi.nlm.nih.gov/pubmed/20519304. Accessed 28 May 2014.
19. Castañeda A. Final thoughts. World J Pediatr Congenit Heart Surg. 2011;2:115–8. http://www.ncbi.nlm.nih.gov/pubmed/23804942. Accessed 28 May 2014.
20. Fundación Aldo Castañeda. http://www.fundacionaldocastaneda.org/index.php?page=logros. Accessed 2 May 2014.
21. Vida VL, Sade RM, Stellin G, Castañeda AR. Cardiol Young, 2006;16:221–8. http://www.ncbi.nlm.nih.gov/pubmed/16725061. Accessed 28 May 2014.
22. Children's HeartLink. Phased support approach. 2013. http://www.childrensheartlink.org/phased-support-approach. Accessed 23 May 2014.
23. Dearani J, Neirotti R, Kohnke EJ, Sinha KK, Cabalka AK, Barnes RD, Jacobs JP, Stellin G, Tchervenkov CI, Cushing JC. Improving pediatric cardiac surgical care in developing countries: matching resources to needs. Semin Thorac Cardiovasc Surg Pediatr Card Surg Annu. 2010;13:35–43. http://www.ncbi.nlm.nih.gov/pubmed/20307859. Accessed 28 May 2014.
24. Hollinger I. Personal interview. 8 May 2014.
25. Schwartzenberger J. Personal interview. 14 May 2014.
26. Rosen D. Personal interview. 25 May 2014.
27. Surgery S, Lives S. WHO Guidelines for Safe Surgery 2009. 2009.
28. Merry AF, Cooper JB, Soyannwo O, Wilson IH, Eichhorn JH. International standards for a safe practice of anesthesia 2010. Can J Anaesth. 2010;57:1027–34. http://www.pubmedcentral.nih.gov/articlerender.fcgi?artid=2957572&tool=pmcentrez&rendertype=abstract. Accessed 28 May 2014.
29. Donabedian A. The quality of care: how can it be assessed? JAMA. 1988;206:1743–8.
30. Hollinger I. Email communication. 26 May 2014.
31. Schwartzenberger J. Email communication. 27 May 2014.
32. Rosen D. Email communication. 26 May 2014.
33. World Health Organization. WHO model lists of essential medicines. 2013. http://www.who.int/medicines/publications/essentialmedicines/en. Accessed 21 May 2014.
34. Ferraris V, Brown JR, Despotis GJ, Hammon JW, Reece TB, Saha SP, Song HK, Clough ER, Shore-Lesserson LJ, Goodnough LT, Mazer CD, Shander A, Stafford-Smith M, Waters J, Baker R, Dickinson T, FitzGerald DJ, Likosky DS, Shann KG. 2011 update to the Society of Thoracic Surgeons and the Society of Cardiovascular Anesthesiologists blood conservation clinical practice guidelines. Ann Thorac Surg. 2011;91:944–82. http://www.ncbi.nlm.nih.gov/pubmed/21353044. Accessed 23 May 2014.
35. World Health Organization. Screening donated blood for transmissible infections. Geneva, Switzerland, 2010. http://www.who.int/bloodsafety/ScreeningDonatedBloodforTransfusion.pdf. Accessed 26 May 2014.
36. Kozek-Langenecker S, Afshari A, Albaladejo P, Santullano CAA, Robertis E, Filipescu DC, Fries D, Görlinger K, Haas T, Imberger G, Jacob M, Lancé M, Llau J, Mallett S, Meier J, Rahe-Meyer N, Samama CM, Smith A, Solomon C, Van der Linden P, Wikkelsø AJ, Wouters P, Wyffels P. Management of severe perioperative bleeding: guidelines from the European Society of Anaesthesiology. Eur J Anaesthesiol. 2013;30:270–382. http://www.ncbi.nlm.nih.gov/pubmed/23656742. Accessed 28 May 2014.
37. Singh KE, Baum VC. Pro: early extubation in the operating room following cardiac surgery in adults. Semin Cardiothorac Vasc Anesth. 2012;16:182–6. http://www.ncbi.nlm.nih.gov/pubmed/22798230. Accessed 31 May 2014.

38. Sullivan BL. Con: early extubation in the operating room following cardiac surgery. Semin Cardiothorac Vasc Anesth. 2012;16:187–9. http://www.ncbi.nlm.nih.gov/pubmed/22825916. Accessed 31 May 2014.
39. Leon-Wyss JR, Veshti A, Veras O, Gaitán G, O'Connell M, Mack R, Calvimontes G, Garcia F, Hidalgo A, Reyes A, Castañeda AR. Pediatric cardiac surgery: a challenge and outcome analysis of the Guatemala effort. Semin Thorac Cardiovasc Surg Pediatr Card Surg Annu. 2009;12:8–11. http://www.ncbi.nlm.nih.gov/pubmed/19349009. Accessed 28 May 2014.
40. Novick WM, Aniæ D, Ivanèan V, Di Sessa TG. International pediatric cardiac assistance in Croatia: results of the 10 year program. Croat Med J. 2004;45:389–95.
41. Tuman K, Roizen M. Outcome assessment and pulmonary artery catheterization: why does the debate continue? Anesth Analg. 1997;84:1–4.
42. Marik PE. Obituary: pulmonary artery catheter 1970 to 2013. Ann Intensive Care. 2013;3:38. http://www.ncbi.nlm.nih.gov/pubmed/24286266.
43. Murkin JM, Arango M. Near-infrared spectroscopy as an index of brain and tissue oxygenation. Br J Anaesth. 2009;103(Suppl):3–13. http://www.ncbi.nlm.nih.gov/pubmed/20007987. Accessed 28 May 2014.
44. Fischer GW, Silvay G. Cerebral oximetry in cardiac and major vascular surgery. HSR Proc Intensive Care Cardiovasc Anesth. 2010;2(4):249–56.
45. U.S. Food and Drug Administration. Reuse of medical disposable devices policy. http://www.fda.gov/MedicalDevices/DeviceRegulationandGuidance/GuidanceDocuments/ucm106350.htm. Accessed 8 May 2014.
46. U.S. Food and Drug Administration. Reprocessing of single-use devices. http://www.fda.gov/medicaldevices/deviceregulationandguidance/reprocessing ofsingle-usedevices/ucm121465.htm. Accessed 8 May 2014.
47. Head SJ, Davierwala PM, Serruys PW, Redwood SR, Colombo A, Mack MJ, Morice M-C, Holmes DR, Feldman TE, Ståhle E, Underwood P, Dawkins KD, Kappetein P, Mohr FW. Coronary artery bypass grafting vs. percutaneous coronary intervention for patients with three-vessel disease: final five-year follow-up of the SYNTAX trial. Eur Heart J. 2014. http://www.ncbi.nlm.nih.gov/pubmed/24849105. Accessed 28 May 2014.
48. Yadava OP, Kundu A. "On" or "Off" pump coronary artery bypass grafting – is the last word out? Indian Heart J. 2013;65:187–90. http://www.pubmedcentral.nih.gov/articlerender.fcgi?artid=3861129&tool=pmcentrez&rendertype=abstract. Accessed 28 May 2014.
49. Acker M, Parides MK, Perrault LP, Moskowitz AJ, Gelijns AC, Voisine P, Smith PK, Hung JW, Blackstone EH, Puskas JD, Argenziano M, Gammie JS, Mack M, Ascheim DD, Bagiella E, Moquete EG, Ferguson TB, Horvath K, Geller NL, Miller M, Woo YJ, D'Alessandro D, Ailawadi G, Dagenais F, Gardner TJ, O'Gara PT, Michler RE, Kron IL. Mitral-valve repair versus replacement for severe ischemic mitral regurgitation. N Engl J Med. 2014;370:23–32. http://www.ncbi.nlm.nih.gov/pubmed/24245543. Accessed 24 May 2014.
50. Svircevic V, Nierich AP, Moons KGM, Brandon Bravo Bruinsma GJ, Kalkman CJ, Dijk D. Fast-track anesthesia and cardiac surgery: a retrospective cohort study of 7989 patients. Anesth Analg. 2009;108:727–33. http://www.ncbi.nlm.nih.gov/pubmed/19224776. Accessed 28 May 2014.
51. Howard F, Brown KL, Garside V, Walker I, Elliott MJ. Fast-track paediatric cardiac surgery: the feasibility and benefits of a protocol for uncomplicated cases. Eur J Cardiothorac Surg. 2010;37:193–6. http://www.ncbi.nlm.nih.gov/pubmed/19646888. Accessed 28 May 2014.
52. Ender J, Borger MA, Scholz M, Funkat A-K, Anwar N, Sommer M, Mohr FW, Fassl J. Cardiac Surgery Fast-track Treatment in a Postanesthetic Care Unit. Anesthesiology. 2008;109:61–6.
53. Myles PS, Daly DJ, Djaiani G, Lee A, Cheng DCH. A systematic review of the safety and effectiveness of fast-track cardiac anesthesia. Anesthesiology. 2003;99:982–7. http://www.ncbi.nlm.nih.gov/pubmed/14508335.
54. Deshpande CM, Mohite SN, Kamdi P. Sufentanil vs fentanyl for fast-track cardiac anaesthesia. Indian J Anaesth. 2009;53:455–62.
55. Hahn RT, Abraham T, Adams MS, Bruce CJ, Glas KE, Lang RM, Reeves ST, Shanewise JS, Siu SC, Stewart W, Picard MH. Guidelines for performing a comprehensive transesophageal echocardiographic examination: recommendations from the American Society of Echocardiography and the Society of Cardiovascular Anesthesiologists. 2014:21–68. http://www.ncbi.nlm.nih.gov/pubmed/24356157. Accessed 28 May 2014.
56. Madu EC, Tulloch-reid MK, Baugh DS, Potu C. Clinical utility of transoesophageal echocardiography in low resource environments: the Jamaican experience utilidad clínica de la ecocardiografía transesofágica en medios de bajos recursos. West Indian Med J. 2011;60.
57. England TN. A multicenter, randomized, controlled clinical trial of transfusion requirements in critical care. N Engl J Med. 1999;340:1056. http://www.nejm.org/doi/abs/10.1056/NEJM199904013401322.
58. Vincent JL, Baron J-F, Reinhart K, Gattinoni L, Thijs L, Webb A, Meier-Hellmann A, Nollet G, Peres-Bota D. Anemia and blood transfusion in critically ill patients. JAMA. 2002;288:1499–507. http://www.ncbi.nlm.nih.gov/pubmed/23184038.
59. Pattakos G, Koch CG, Brizzio ME, Batizy LH, Sabik JF, Blackstone EH, Lauer MS. Outcome of patients who refuse transfusion after cardiac surgery: a natural experiment with severe blood conservation. Arch Intern Med. 2012;172:1154–60. http://www.ncbi.nlm.nih.gov/pubmed/22751620. Accessed 31 May 2014.
60. World Health Organization. Micronutrient deficiencies. http://www.who.int/nutrition/topics/ida/en/. Accessed 23 May 2014.

61. Kulier A, Levin J, Moser R, Rumpold-Seitlinger G, Tudor IC, Snyder-Ramos S, Moehnle P, Mangano DT. Impact of preoperative anemia on outcome in patients undergoing coronary artery bypass graft surgery. Circulation. 2007;116:471–9. http://www.ncbi.nlm.nih.gov/pubmed/17620512. Accessed 27 May 2014.
62. Dietrich W, Faraoni D, von Heymann C, Daniel B, Ranucci M, Sander M, Rosseel P. ESA guidelines on the management of severe perioperative bleeding. Eur J Anaesthesiol. 2014;31:236–7. http://www.ncbi.nlm.nih.gov/pubmed/23812623. Accessed 28 May 2014.
63. Wang G, Bainbridge D, Martin J, Cheng D. The efficacy of an intraoperative cell saver during cardiac surgery: a meta-analysis of randomized trials. Anesth Analg. 2009;109:320–30. http://www.ncbi.nlm.nih.gov/pubmed/19608798. Accessed 28 May 2014.
64. Wikipedia. PDCA – wikipedia, the free encyclopedia. http://en.wikipedia.org/wiki/PDCA. Accessed 27 May 2014.

Anesthesia Considerations for Facial Deformity Repair in Lesser Developed Countries

17

Clifford Gevirtz

Introduction

The birth of a child with a facial deformity has a devastating effect on both the child and its family. In ancient history, such births were regarded as warnings from the deities of ill portent. In modern times, the ability to repair these defects can be life changing for both the child and family. Where before the child might have faced social ostracism and very limited prospects, now the child can be a fully active and productive member of society.

Fabricius and his student, William Harvey, spent countless hours dissecting fetuses and stillbirths, in which they observed the various stages of cleft lip and palate development. Using these observations, they developed the concept of arrested development. From these early observations, a more sophisticated understanding of the migration of fetal tissue and of the role of apoptosis has emerged. Using the knowledge of embryology, it was recognized that all of the essential tissue for repair is present, but it is out of place. Advances in plastic surgical technique allow for simple and dramatic correction of these abnormalities by moving the pieces back into correct position. Similarly, cystic hygromas are easily correctable with appropriate surgical management and small hemangiomas can also be remedied in the LDC setting.

The anesthesiologist is an essential member of the surgical team that can transform these children. By deciding who is an appropriate anesthetic risk, how the airway is to be secured during the procedure, maintaining perioperative homeostasis, and providing adequate postoperative analgesia, the anesthesiologist facilities the surgical repair and screens out problems before they arise.

In working in LDCs, a key principle is to avoid any complication that might require an increase in the level of care required, e.g., where in developed countries, a patient might be admitted to the ICU out of an abundance of caution; in the LDCs, such care might not exist or may slow the production rate of the entire team by occupying a recovery room bed for an extended period of time. The anesthesiologist must be on guard for patients who are not optimized. For example, in the developed world, a patient with profound anemia would be submitted to surgery knowing that there was a complete blood bank available to support the care of the child. In the LDCs, the only option may be direct person to person transfusion, an option not to be undertaken lightly.

C. Gevirtz, M.D., M.P.H. (✉)
Department of Anesthesiology, LSU Health Sciences Center, New Orleans, LA, USA
e-mail: cliffgevirtzmd@yahoo.com

Somnia, Inc., New Rochelle, NY, USA

R. Roth et al. (eds.), *The Role of Anesthesiology in Global Health: A Comprehensive Guide*,
DOI 10.1007/978-3-319-09423-6_17, © Springer International Publishing Switzerland 2015

Nomenclature

The nomenclature of congenital abnormalities has relevance in that specified diagnosis may signal other associated abnormalities of anesthetic significance. Useful terminology:

Malformation—a primary structural defect which results from a localized error of morphogenesis, e.g., isolated cleft palate or cleft lip.

Anomalad—a malformation that results in subsequent morphologic changes, e.g., The Pierre Robin anomalad of micrognathia, a U-shaped cleft palate, and glossoptosis. The proximate cause is the hypoplastic mandible which causes the tongue to occupy a higher position in the oropharynx which in turn leads to a failure of the palate to fuse in the midline.

Syndrome—a pattern of malformation arising from a common etiology, but resulting in more than one region being affected, e.g., trisomy 19.

Association—the occurrence of two or more morphologic patterns together with a frequency greater than would be predicted by chance, e.g., The VATER association: vertebral defect, anal atresia, tracheoesophageal fistula, renal dysplasia.

A child with any lesion more complex than a malformation should probably not be operated on-site in an LDC. Evaluation and consideration of transporting the child back to the more developed world where complex care is available are indicated. While it is disheartening to have to pass on difficult cases, such challenges can lead to catastrophes if undertaken without necessary sophisticated backup.

Examples of syndrome which are best operated in developed countries include:

1. Pierre Robin anomalad—micrognathia, cleft palate, and glossoptosis
2. Merkel-Gruber syndrome—microcephaly, cleft palate, cleft tongue and epiglottis, micrognathia, congenital heart disease, and renal abnormalities
3. Oral-facial-digital syndrome—micrognathia, hypoplasia of the nasal alae, cleft lip, cleft palate, and lobate tongue
4. Trisomy 18 syndrome—malformed ear pinna, micrognathia, cleft palate, congenital heart disease, diaphragmatic defect, inguinal hernia, and Meckel's diverticulum
5. Cri du chat syndrome—microcephaly, micrognathia, cleft palate, antimongoloid palpebral fissures, and strabismus.
6. Fraser's syndrome—middle ear malformation, defects in the ear pinna, cleft palate, laryngeal deformities, and renal abnormalities.

A cleft lip is defined as any defect in fusion that occurs anterior to the incisive foramen. This point can be easily located in the adult as a small depression in the anterior portion of the midline of the roof the mouth. A cleft palate refers to any defect from this point posteriorly. Thus a cleft lip may be anything from a minor incomplete skin cleft to a complete interruption of the skin, gingiva, alveolar ridge, and part of the primary palate.

Epidemiology of Clefts

Cleft lip and palate is the most common congenital craniofacial anomaly and the fourth most common birth defect after congenital heart deformities, spina bifida, and limb deformities. In the United States, cleft palate alone has a prevalence of 6.35 per 10,000. Cleft lip with or without cleft palate occurs in 10.63 per 10,000 [1]. There are distinct differences in the occurrence of cleft lip and/or palate between various ethnicities, with an incidence of 1 in 1,000 live births in Caucasians, 3.6 in 1,000 in Native Americans, 2.1 in 1,000 in Japanese, and only 0.3 in 1,000 in African Americans. The overall incidence of isolated cleft palate is 1 in 1,500 live births and shows no ethnic variation.

Two thirds of orofacial clefting involve the lip and/or palate, and nearly one third involve the palate alone. The majority of cleft lip and/or palate cases are unilateral (80 %), and are more common on the left side. Midline clefts of the nose and/or lip are rare deformities. Isolated cleft palate occurs twice as often in females, while cleft lip with or without a cleft palate occurs more frequently in males.

Tanaka et al. [2] studied the number of live births with cleft lip or other congenital anomalies by soliciting data from national and international organizations covering for American states and 30 countries for the years 2002 to 2006. All data were normalized and reported per 10,000 live births. Descriptive statistics, in addition to correlation and regression, were used for analysis. Over the 5-year period studied the overall congenital anomaly rate increased in the United States and decreased internationally. The states with the highest and lowest rates were Maryland (21.46 per 10,000) and West Virginia (2.59 per 10,000), respectively. The United States cleft lip national rate averaged 7.75 per 10,000. Countries with the highest and lowest rates were Japan (19.05 per 10,000) and South Africa (3.13 per 10,000), respectively. Internationally, the rate of cleft lip declined, with an average overall prevalence of 7.94 per 10,000. The trends diverged over the 5-year period, as the rate was stable in the United States and the international rate declined.

Preoperative Evaluation

When a mission arrives on-site, there are several priorities:

1. Unpack and set up the anesthesia equipment. As much as possible, the setup needs to be identical in each anesthetizing location as personnel may shift or breaks given during the course of the mission.
2. Medication stocks may need to be secured each night but it is best to forward-deploy stocks as much as possible so that the complete disposal inventory is used during the mission and any emergency drugs are readily available, i.e., it makes no sense to transport medications back to the home base. ACLS kits for pediatric patients should also be kept within the OR along with any defibrillators.
3. Waste flow is a difficult issue. In developed countries, single-use syringes, IVs, and endotracheal tubes are the standard of care. In LDCs, these disposable items are washed and reused even through there is clearly a risk of disease transmission. While missions to LDCs should adhere to the standards of the developed world, it is important to be aware that the waste bags will probably be thoroughly examined and scavenged by the local medical community.

Settings Up the Preanesthetic Clinic

First, the surgeon must evaluate the child to see if he/she is a suitable candidate for repair and, along with a logistics person, assess to see where the case can be scheduled. If running a 4 table setup (2 OR tables per room), a spreadsheet is created which lists the expected duration of surgery. The anesthesiologist with the most pediatric experience should manage the youngest cases. The duration of the operative schedule should not exceed the endurance of the team. While the urge is to book as many cases as possible, the reality is that after 10–12 h, vigilance decreases and risks increase. There are other concerns in making the schedule, i.e., the success of the mission may be judged on the total numbers of cases done, and it is immaterial if there were 16 difficult cleft palates rather than 40 cleft lips. Only the total number of cases performed counts. Since the duration of a palate may be two to three times the length of a cleft lip, if the case volume is of concern, then it is definitely easier to do cleft lips and/or revisions than more palates. The adage that younger and sicker patients go earlier in the day certainly holds true here. Another consideration is timing the OR carefully so that the children are not fasted for prolonged periods, although that should be less of a concern if current recommendations to drink clear fluids up to 2 h before anesthesia are met.

If a pediatrician is available, he/she should be the first to screen for obvious signs of infection while conducting a history and physical examination. Birth history is a key factor. Those born before 37 weeks gestation, i.e., preterm have an increased incidence of perioperative respiratory complications. Many of these babies experience episodes of idiopathic apnea (defined as cessation of breathing for 20 s or more) until approximately 60 weeks post-conceptual age and therefore require additional monitoring postoperatively. These apneic episodes can occur up to 12 h after the completion of surgery. Since the resources for post-op monitoring may be very limited in the LDCs, surgery in premature babies may be problematic and therefore best avoided.

The degree of maternal–child bonding should also be assessed as this may be utilized during the induction period, i.e., the mother can hold and calm the child while a mask induction is performed. The mother also needs to be questioned about feeding problems. In cleft palate cases, the normal separation between food and air is absent, resulting in the mixing and deposition of food in the turbinates. This abnormality may impair nutrition, which in turn affects growth and development.

Dehydration may also be of concern and manifest subtly on physical examination. These children often do not suck well and may be relatively dehydrated. In all but the mildest cases, the child should be fluid repleted before starting the case.

Chronic rhinorrhea, which is caused by the cleft palate, needs to be differentiated by history and physical examination from the new onset of an infectious process. If the patient has a new fever, is irritable, and has an elevated white blood cell count, rescheduling the case until the process is winding down is judicious.

Carefully weighing the patient is important to assure that accurate dosage calculations can be made. The overall length and head circumference should be measured with the result plotted on standard childhood development curves. Children who are below the 10th percentile in weight demonstrate significantly delayed development and the cause needs to be determined prior to surgery. While it is very rare for the anesthesiologist to be the first to recognize a previously unrecognized syndrome in a child, it should be remembered that the anesthesiologist in the LDC setting may be one of the few physicians to actually examine the child and issues may have been missed by other examiners.

With respect to laboratory studies, a spun hematocrit is the barest minimum required since these patients are often anemic. If the patient has a hematocrit below 30 %, due consideration has to be given to the potential blood loss of the proposed procedure. A cleioplasty rarely loses a significant amount of blood while a cleft palate repair can involve significant blood loss even with the use of vasoconstrictors. The decision to proceed requires careful discussion as the blood bank facility may be limited or nonexistent.

The physical examination of the heart must be carefully done. The presence of a murmur needs to be discerned and a diagnosis made on-site as there is often no other consultation or investigations available, i.e., no echocardiography or cardiology consultation. The most common cleft lip/and or palate-associated cardiac problem is a ventricular septal defect and less commonly, atrial septal defects. Other physical signs such as clubbing or cyanosis may not be present in an infant.

The rest of the physical exam should be devoted to looking for other congenital abnormalities as up to 10 % of these patients also have a second significant defect.

Fasting Guidelines for Children

The ASA standards for preoperative fasting were recently updated [3]. The European Society of Anesthesiologists (ESA) published guidelines [4] that closely mirror the ASA guidelines albeit with measures of common sense added, e.g., chewing gum or a cough lozenge is not a reason to cancel a case. These guidelines are summarized in Table 17.1.

It is appropriate to fast from intake of breast milk at least 4 h before elective procedures requiring general anesthesia, regional anesthesia, or sedation/analgesia.

Preoperative Fasting Status: Infant Formula

An evidence-based review [3] of preoperative fasting was published by the ASA. While many observational studies have been done, the evidence

Table 17.1 A summary of fasting guidelines

Clear liquids	2 h
Breast milk	4 h
Infant formula	6 h
Nonhuman milk	6 h
Light meal	6 h

is equivocal regarding the impact of ingesting infant formula 4 h before a procedure on the risk of higher volumes or lower pH levels of gastric contents during a procedure. The literature is insufficient to evaluate the effect of the timing of ingestion of infant formula and the perioperative incidence of emesis/reflux or pulmonary aspiration. However, the literature suggests that 4 h is a commonly accepted time limit.

A poll of consultants and a large number of ASA members found agreement that for neonates and infants, fasting from the intake of infant formula at least 6 h before elective procedures requiring general anesthesia, regional anesthesia, or sedation/analgesia should be maintained. Similarly, the expert consultants agree and the ASA members strongly agree that for children, fasting from the intake of infant formula at least 6 h before elective procedures requiring general anesthesia, regional anesthesia, or sedation/analgesia (i.e., monitored anesthesia care) should be maintained.

Preoperative Fasting Status: Solids and Nonhuman Milk

The evidence-based review also reviewed studies with nonrandomized comparative findings for children given nonhuman milk 4 h or less before a procedure compared with children who fasted for more than 4 h and found higher gastric volumes and equivocal gastric pH. Another important study [5], which was observational only, suggested that fasting for more than 8 h may be associated with hypoglycemia in children. So it is important to closely monitor the OR schedule, to avoid prolonged fasts in children. The literature was found to be insufficient to evaluate the effect of the timing of ingestion of solids and nonhuman milk and the perioperative incidence of emesis or reflux or pulmonary aspiration.

Polling showed that the expert consultants agree and the ASA members strongly agree that fasting from the intake of a light meal (e.g., toast and a clear liquid) 6 h or more before elective procedures requiring general anesthesia, regional anesthesia, or sedation/analgesia should be maintained. Both the consultants and ASA members strongly agree that fasting from the intake of a meal that includes fried or fatty foods 8 h or more before elective procedures requiring general anesthesia, regional anesthesia, or sedation/analgesia should be maintained.

Both the consultants and the vast majority of ASA members agree that for infants, fasting from the intake of nonhuman milk 6 h or more before elective procedures requiring general anesthesia, regional anesthesia, or sedation/analgesia should be maintained. The consultants agree and the ASA members strongly agree that for children and adults, fasting from the intake of nonhuman milk 6 h or more before elective procedures requiring general anesthesia, regional anesthesia, or sedation/analgesia (i.e., monitored anesthesia care) should be maintained.

Premedication

The need for premedication varies widely. A 6-month-old who is held in the mother's lap will not need any premedication for cleioplasty. A 3-year-old who requires a 4th procedure may benefit from heavy sedation. If prior anesthetic records are available, (something which larger organizations returning to the same site year after year may have), these should be reviewed. Older children who can communicate effectively may express a preference for "blowing up the balloon" or accept "just one shot." If ketamine is being used as the anesthetic, a benzodiazepine and a belladonna alkaloid will minimize intraoperative secretions and decrease the risk of postoperative delirium.

Oral premedication with midazolam (0.5 mg/kg p.o.) to a maximum volume of 20 cc is a convenient way of sedating an anxious child but it must be emphasized that the child must be carefully observed and monitored for signs of overdosage during the preoperative period.

Friesen et al. [6] have demonstrated that, at least for infants between 1 and 6 months of age, intramuscular atropine administered within 45 min of the procedure is associated with a lower incidence of hypotension as compared with those unmedicated. Above this age, there was no demonstrable effect.

A surprisingly large number of children fulfill the criteria of being at risk for pulmonary aspiration of gastric acid (i.e., gastric contents with a pH of less than 2.5 and a volume of greater than 0.4 ml/kg). However, pulmonary aspiration is an exceedingly rare event in routine pediatric cases and regular administration of histamine-2 blockers, proton pump inhibitors, or metoclopramide is not recommended.

Timing of Surgery

Closure of the cleft lip (cleioplasty) is usually performed at the age of 3 months or when the child meets Musgrave's rule of 10s. Musgrave [7] reviewed his institution's considerable experience in cleft lip and palate repair. He published a simple rule which seemed to avoid many complications when considering the timing of cleioplasty. Indeed, not following any one element of the rule increased the risk of serious complications fivefold. The rule states the child is ready for cleioplasty when the weight is greater than 10 lb (4.5 kg), the hemoglobin is greater than 10 g percent, and the white blood cell count is less than 10,000 per cubic mm. The combination of all of these elements seems to insure that the child has enough physiologic reserve to survive the surgery. While the method of repair and the choice of anesthesia do not predict morbidity or mortality, the absence of infection, adequate oxygen carrying capacity, and sufficient nutrition to achieve 10 lb of weight seem to predict an excellent candidate for repair.

Cleioplasty during the neonatal period has also been described but is ill advised in the LDC setting.

Soft palate repairs are often conducted between 12 and 18 months of age while hard palate repairs are performed as a series of flaps starting after 2 years of age. How many procedures are required depends on the size of the defect and the growth of the child. The goal is to have a functioning soft palate before the onset of speech. It should be noted, however, that there is a wide range of opinion about repairs in the neonatal period and many advocate as early a repair as possible. In the LDC the risks of neonatal repair appear to rule out its advisability.

Transfusion in Children

While cleioplasty rarely requires transfusion, cleft palate repairs can involve significant blood loss. Guidance on transfusion in children can be inferred from three clinical trials evaluating transfusion triggers. The first trial [8] evaluated 100 preterm infants weighing between 500 and 1,300 g. The patients were randomly assigned to a restrictive or liberal transfusion algorithm that considered respiratory status and hematocrit level. Infants in the liberal group received more RBC transfusions (5.2 ± 4.5 vs. 3.3 ± 2.9) in the restrictive group. Infants in the restrictive group were more likely to have intraparenchymal brain hemorrhage and frequent apneic episodes.

The second trial [9] enrolled 451 infants with gestational ages less than 31 weeks, ages less than 2 days, and weight less than 1,000 g. There were no significant differences in outcome. The third trial [10] recruited 637 children in a pediatric ICU, randomly allocated to 7 g/dL or 9.5 g/dL thresholds. Again, there were no significant differences in outcome. Overall, the results of these three trials in children suggest that a restrictive trigger of 7–8 g/dL is safe.

Antibiotic Prophylaxis in Children with Coincidental Congenital Heart Disease

If the decision is made that a child with congenital heart disease is to undergo cleft palate repair in the LDC setting, then antibiotic prophylaxis should be administered. The risk of bacterial endocarditis is a very real possibility, since the oral cavity is heavily populated with pathogens such as Streptococcus viridans and Enterococcus species. While the antibiotics are best administered 60 min prior to the start of surgery, the guidelines [11] suggest that if this is not possible, they may be given up to 2 h after surgery.

The current recommendations for prophylaxis are shown in Table 17.2.

Table 17.2 Antibiotic prophylaxis in children with coincident congenital heart disease (adapted from AHA guidelines)

Situation		
Able to take oral medication	Amoxicillin	50 mg/kg
Unable to take oral medication	Ampicillin *OR*	50 mg/kg IM or IV
	Cefazolin or ceftriaxone	50 mg/kg IM or IV
Allergic to penicillins or ampicillin—oral	Cephalexin[a,b] *OR*	50 mg/kg
	Clindamycin *OR*	20 mg/kg
	Azithromycin or clarithromycin	15 mg/kg
Allergic to penicillins or ampicillin and unable to take oral medication	Cefazolin or ceftriaxone[a] *OR*	50 mg/kg IM or IV
	Clindamycin	20 mg/kg IM or IV

IM indicates intramuscular, *IV* intravenous

[a]Or other first- or second-generation oral cephalosporin in equivalent adult or pediatric dosage

[b]Cephalosporins should not be used in an individual with a history of anaphylaxis, angioedema, or urticaria with penicillins or ampicillin

Induction and Maintenance

If the parent can be enlisted, the child can sit in his/her lap or on the OR table with the parent at the side. Upon entering the operating room, a pulse oximeter probe should be applied first. (Although pulse oximeters are not available in many ORs in LDCs, missions that perform these surgeries are all so equipped.) This unobtrusive device is usually readily accepted and is often a point of fascination for children as they look at their transilluminated finger. Induction is usually accomplished via mask induction with sevoflurane or halothane (still commonly available in LDCs). The mask may be flavored with vanilla, cherry, orange, or bubble gum extracts which are readily available in Western supermarkets. A few drops applied to the inner surface of the mask will greatly increase acceptance by the child. Using a Mapleson D, E or Bain circuit for infants or a circle system for the older child, the mask is gently brought into proximity with the child's face with the agent drifting over. As the child loses consciousness, the mask is secured over the nose and mouth. It is at this point where the most danger lies. The potent inhalation agent is building up, while there is no venous access in the child. If an agent analyzer is present, watching the end tidal concentration build will signal when it is safe to cannulate a vein. Spontaneous ventilation ensures deepening anesthetic levels. Some experts suggest self-ventilation to a depth of 2 MAC and then laryngoscopy without muscle relaxation, thus avoiding the use of succinylcholine or the use of a non-depolarizing agent that would need to be reversed. Others suggest using only a non-depolarizing agent to perform the intubation, holding succinylcholine in reserve for emergencies. During induction there is an increased frequency of laryngospasm due to secretions and frequent upper respiratory tract infections experienced by these children. A plan needs to be in place should the laryngospasm not respond to positive pressure.

If an intracardiac shunt has been missed, it will often manifest itself at this point. Cyanosis in the presence of good breath sounds is the key to diagnosis. A sudden increase in right-to-left shunt may occur when the systemic vascular resistance decreases. Trying to treat the cyanosis by increasing frequency and depth of ventilation is a natural reaction of most anesthesiologists. But hyperventilation and increased intrathoracic pressure may worsen the shunt. The treatment of choice is to increase the afterload as well as decrease the inhaled agent. If a shunt has been missed, the case should be cancelled and further work-up performed.

In Fig. 17.1, three blades are illustrated: the Robertshaw, the Oxford, and the Seward. These are designed to minimize the likelihood of having the upright flange of the laryngoscope engaging the cleft palate causing injury to the membranes.

Equipment Used for Drawover Anesthesia

In some locations, the anesthesia equipment may be rather rudimentary based on drawover principles. These vaporizers work by drawing a carrier gas over a volatile liquid for the purpose of adding the vapor from that liquid to the carrier gas.

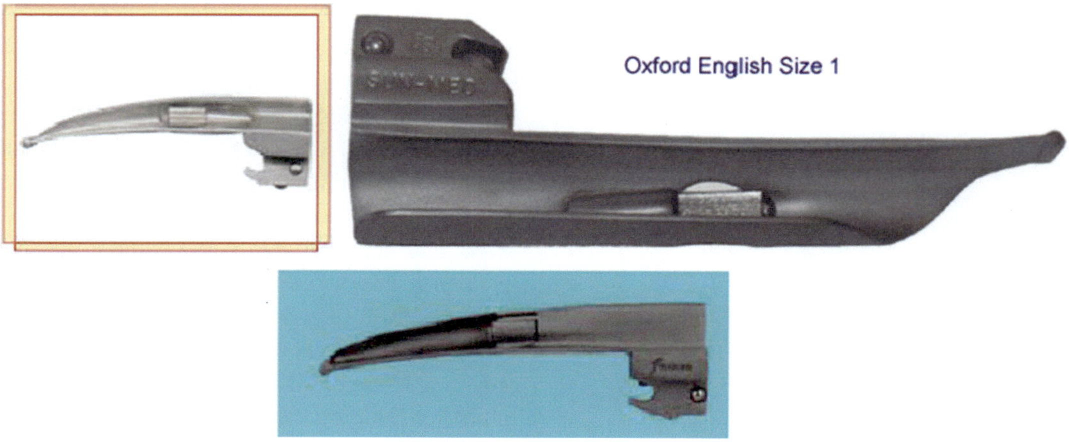

Fig. 17.1 The Robertshaw blade (*top*) has a 45° flange which curves back upon itself, The Oxford blade (*middle*) is tubular and the Seward blade has a low profile flange. The goal of each of these designs is to minimize the likelihood of engaging the cleft with the flange

This carrier gas/vapor mixture is then directed to the patient by a circuit. In drawover systems the carrier gas is drawn through the vaporizer either by the patient's own respiratory efforts or by a self-inflating bag or manual bellows with a one-way valve placed downstream from the vaporizer. Drawover systems operate at less than or at ambient pressure, and flow through the system is intermittent, varying with different phases of inspiration, and ceasing in expiration. A one-way valve prevents reverse flow in the circuit. This system differs from conventional plenum (continuous flow) anesthesia in which the carrier gas is sent through the vaporizer at a constant rate. In plenum circuits the anesthetic is then collected in a circuit with a reservoir bag or bellows. Pressure fluctuations in the circuit caused by patient respiration do not affect the vaporizer. Plenum systems operate at higher than ambient atmospheric pressure.

Drawover systems are simple to assemble and use, and can operate without fresh gas supplies. They are lightweight and portable. Plenum systems are much more technically complex, and need a well-regulated, constant, positive pressure gas supply which may not be available in LDCs. They require a sophisticated anesthesia machine to support them, which in turn needs regular preventive maintenance. The transport of gas cylinders for these systems is both expensive and potentially hazardous. Also, the cylinders in LDCs may be mislabeled or not carry medical grade gas. Therefore, drawover systems have obvious advantages in LDCs.

An important consideration is the respiratory physiological effects of general anesthesia which tends to reduce minute ventilation and increase shunting of blood within the lung (V/Q mismatch). These changes result in hypoxia when using halothane or isoflurane with spontaneous ventilation (SV) in air, and supplemental oxygen is necessary. The problem is reduced, but not totally abolished, by applying intermittent positive pressure ventilation (IPPV). Ether can be delivered in air (without supplemental oxygen), in IPPV mode, presumably because it causes less V/Q mismatch, and tends to stimulate ventilation, rather than depress it. When ether is used with just room air and spontaneous respiration, desaturation may occur.

In drawover systems supplemental oxygen is administered via a T-piece connection mounted to the intake port of the vaporizer. To maximize the inspired oxygen concentration a "reservoir tube" is attached to the T-piece. A 1 m length of corrugated tubing with an internal volume of 415 ml allows an FiO_2 of at least 0.3 % at an oxygen flow rate of 1.0 L/min, and 60 % at 4 L/min, at normal adult minute ventilation. Oxygen can be given from cylinders, or an oxygen concentrator.

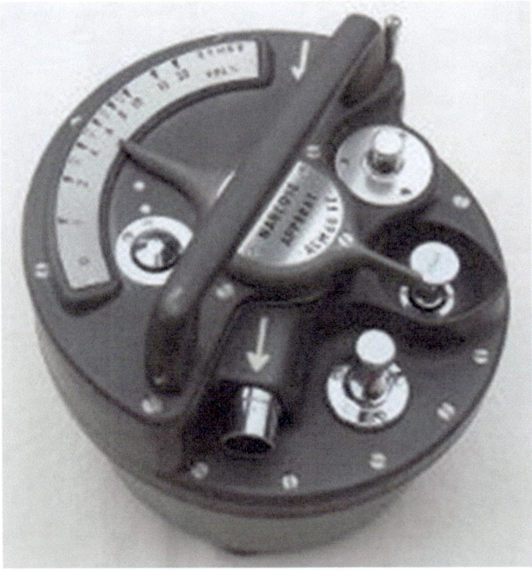

Fig. 17.2 The Epstein-Macintosh-Oxford (EMO) vaporizer is designed to deliver ether in known concentrations irrespective of the temperature of the ether. Used with a bellows, it can deliver the ether in a safe predictable manner

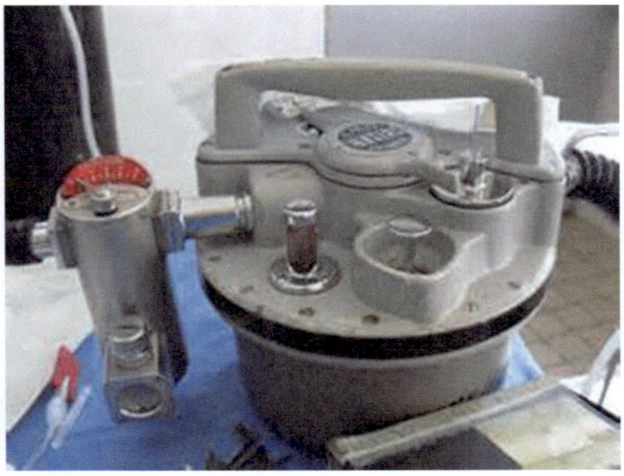

Fig. 17.3 The Oxford Miniature Vaporizer (OMV) in line with an EMO is used in a drawover system to provide anesthesia without requiring a supply of compressed gases. Atmospheric air is used as the main carrier gas and is drawn in by the patient's inspiratory effort. The OMV may also be used as a stand-alone vaporizer

If ether is used, absolutely NO cautery can be used nor can there be any open flames in the vicinity. This precludes doing cleft palate repairs as cautery is a frequent requirement. Cleft lips however can usually be done without the need of cautery.

The EMO (Fig. 17.2) and Oxford (Fig. 17.3) drawover vaporizers have low internal resistance to gas flow and allow easy spontaneous ventilation, while vapor output is fairly constant for a given dial setting over a wide range of minute volumes and ambient temperatures.

Complete operating instructions EMO and Oxford systems are available online through the World Anaesthesia Textbook.

Common Anesthetic Complications

Difficult intubations are fairly common in cleft palate patients due to the high arch, but can be managed successfully by the experienced providers, careful monitoring of oxygenation and capnography, positioning the patients by use of a shoulder roll to produce hyperextension, applying external laryngeal pressure to bring the chords into view, and routinely using a stylet. Intubation with a straight blade with a low or curve flange (see Fig. 17.1) should be used. Most cleft lip and palate repairs are performed using an oral RAE (Ring-Adair-Elwyn) endotracheal tube. The RAE tube is a preformed polyvinyl chloride endotracheal tube with a curve that fits easily into the natural curve of the pharynx. The RAE tube, however, is susceptible to kinking and mucous plugging at the curve. It is very important to reassess ventilation after tube fixation, oral packing and positioning, and after placement of a Dingman mouth gag (Figs. 17.4). Frequent checking of tube position will quickly alert the practitioner to misplacement, disconnection, or kinking. The final position of the child's head is hyperextended with 15° of Trendelenburg and often the surgeon may have the head suspended from a Mayo stand by the Dingman mouth gag with the occiput almost resting in the surgeon's lap. At the start of the procedure, the throat is packed by a roll of sponges tied with a long tailed suture that will remain outside the mouth (to help remember to remove the throat pack at the end). As the throat pack is advanced, the tube may be pulled along and a mainstem bronchial intubation may occur. Again, frequent checking of the breath sounds is necessary.

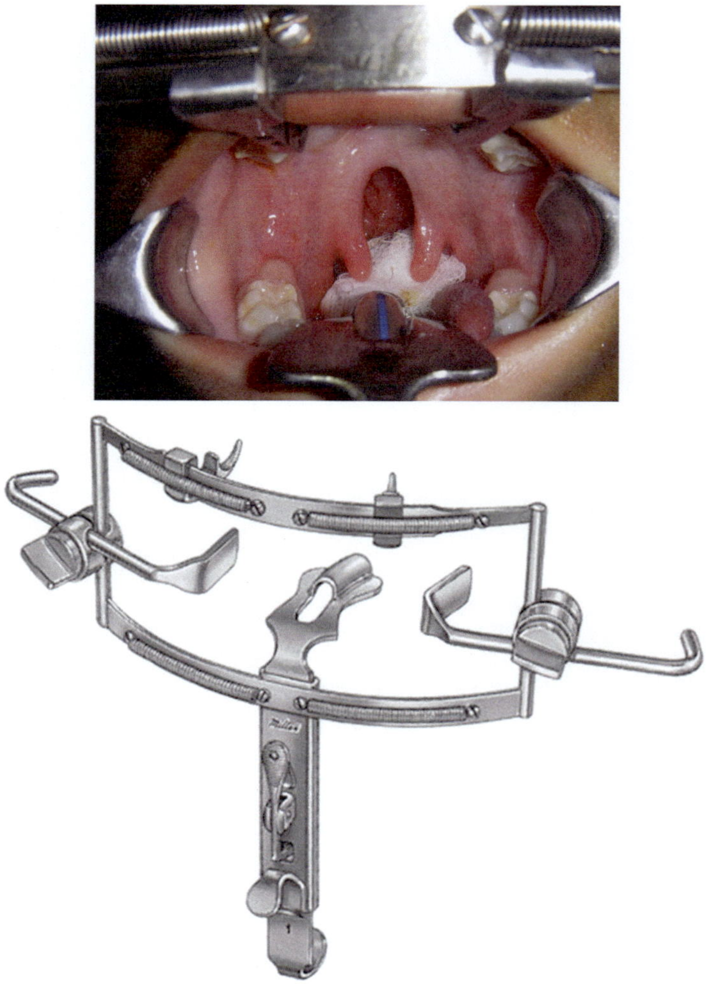

Fig. 17.4 The Dingman mouth gag in position for cleft palate repair. *Note Well*: The Endotracheal tube in located within the groove of the lower blade of the mouth gag. If the gag is rotated to gain better purchase on the incisors, the tube may become kinked. Similarly, if the gag is tilted from its normal blade, the endotracheal tube may advance or become kinked. (Reproduced with permission [17], Fig. 2)

The surgeon will place a traction suture (tongue tie) in the infant's tongue just before extubation. The ends of the suture are left long and tied in a loop that is easily grasped, providing an effective method of clearing the airway and at the same time providing a strong stimulus to breathe. Using the tongue tie at the end of the case allows the anesthesiologist to verify the removal of the throat pack and to assess whether the oropharynx needs further suctioning which should be carefully performed, midline, under direct laryngoscopy to avoid disrupting the repair.

Extubation is performed when the patient is relatively lightly anesthetized and can generate a negative inspiratory force of −30 cm H_2O or better. The infant's ability to raise his/her legs against gravity correlates well with adequate inspiratory strength. After completion of surgery, the patient is transported to the recovery room with the head turned to the side to allow the drainage of any blood or secretions.

Postoperatively, the most common cause of airway obstruction after extubation is due to failure to remove the throat packing. This cause should always be considered and ruled out by laryngoscopy if needed. The nursing staff in the recovery room should be instructed on the use of the tongue to aid in airway management.

The physiological changes that occur during anesthesia and surgery do not end immediately after completion of the procedure. Airway-associated complications are frequent during the first postoperative hour. Desaturation is most likely to occur. Few prospective studies exist and a 5 % rate of immediate upper airway obstruction has been reported [12] and occurs in children with associated syndromes because of critical decrease in size of a previous tenuous airway, excessive sedation, and laryngeal edema.

Airway edema may arise since the head is placed in extreme extension during palate repairs along with Trendelenburg positioning. These factors combine to increase venous pooling. With surgical manipulation of the airway, marked edema of the oropharynx may occur. The loose alveolar tissue of the glottis is also prone to edema after minor trauma or overhydration. If, after extubation, the child demonstrates signs of obstruction, namely retractions (suprasternal, subcostal, intercostal), nasal flaring, inspiratory stridor, and decreased or absent breath sounds, direct laryngoscopy should be performed. If the cause is not a retained throat pack (vide supra), the airway should be examined for signs of edema and the trachea reintubated. Keeping the child in reverse Trendelenburg position and the administration of dexamethasone (0.5 mg/kg) will be of assistance in reducing the edema.

According to Wood [13], children at ages between 44 weeks and 74 weeks after birth have demonstrated greater vulnerability to oxygen desaturation in the postoperative period. As compared to cleft lip surgery, palate is considered to be a high risk for postoperative hypoxemia.

Quershi et al. [14] have reported hypothermia as an important complication found most commonly in children with a bilateral cleft lip repair citing prolonged surgery as the cause. However, others [12] report that hypothermia was not observed as adequate preventative measures can be undertaken. Another important study [15] compared local anesthesia (LA) plus clonidine and LA alone in infraorbital nerve block (IONB). The study concluded that addition of clonidine as an adjunct to local anesthetic significantly decreased the requirements for other anesthetic drugs and significantly prolonged the duration of postoperative analgesia without any adverse effects.

Postoperatively the practice is to maintain the children in lateral or swimmers position to optimize air movement and to minimize the chances of aspiration. The arm restraints, which prevent elbow flexion, keep the child's hands away from the face to prevent rubbing at stitches, surgical site, and intravenous access site.

Coagulopathy

In a survey of 223 cleft lip and cleft palate cases (16 in India), anemia was seen in 83 % of cases with a majority being microcytic hypochromic and eosinophilia in 25 % of cases. The INR ratio was found to be elevated in 52 % of cases. While a normal bleeding time was seen in 70 %, 15.8 % had a prolonged prothrombin time. These abnormalities suggest the need for backup supplies of vitamin K as well as tubing and stopcocks for whole blood person to person transfusion if a bleeding diathesis is encountered.

Postoperative Analgesia

Because opiates are often in short supply, generous amounts of local anesthetic are injected as this may be the only postoperative analgesia available. Opiates should be locally sourced as transporting narcotics across international borders may be considered a severe criminal offense regardless of whether the transporter is a physician or that the drugs are destined for children submitted to surgery.

Morphine sulfate, given in 0.025 mg/kg increments intravenously, should provide excellent analgesia. Since airway obstruction is a concern, each administration needs to be carefully assessed and monitored. Standing orders for analgesia are not an acceptable approach as the monitoring can be very sparse on postoperative wards. Ketorolac tromethamine (1 mg/kg) i.m. also has been used, but there is always concern about the risk of bleeding from the cyclooxygenase inhibition effect.

Cystic Hygroma

Cystic hygroma, which originates from embryonic lymphoid tissue, is a benign tumor without potential for malignancy. It is commonly located in the neck area. Anesthetic management of a large neck mass may be challenging due to difficulty in intubation and the severe hemodynamic effects of surgical removal of a giant tumor. Serious consequences such as sudden airway occlusion resulting in hypoventilation and hypoxemia may arise.

Preoperative evaluation is similar to that of cleft lip and palate in that any co-existent abnormality needs to be detected prior to surgery. The hygroma may extend into the mouth and atropine can be used to dry secretions. If the hygroma obstructs the airway after induction, a "cannot ventilate, cannot intubate situation" can result, requiring an emergency surgical airway if simple maneuvers like placement of an LMA or other supraglottic device fail. While video laryngoscopy or fiberoptic scopes may be available on some missions, they may not always be accessible and awakening the patient needs to remain an option throughout induction. Partial aspiration of the cyst prior to induction may also help.

If there is thoracic extension of the hygroma, then positive airway pressure (PEEP) may be necessary to keep the airway open. However, positive pressure may alter the flow through the thoracic duct pushing more of the fluid into the neck.

If there was significant pre-tracheal involvement, there may be chondromalacia of the tracheal rings causing postoperative respiratory obstruction. Extubation in the upright position when the patient is fully awake may be beneficial.

Hemangiomas of the Face

A hemangioma is a benign and usually self-involuting tumor of the endothelial cells of the blood vessels and is characterized by increased number of normal or abnormal vessels. It usually is present at birth or appears in the first weeks of life and grows most rapidly over the first 6 months. Usually, growth is complete and involution has commenced by 12 months. Half of all infantile hemangiomas have completely involuted by age 5, 70 % by age 7, and most of the remainder by age 12. In more severe cases hemangiomas may leave residual tissue damage. If medical therapy of propranolol, steroid injection, laser therapy, and direct pressure application have failed, then surgical intervention may be attempted.

Patients with peri-orbital hemangiomas and lower lip hemangiomas should be transferred to facilities where there is an MRI available to assess the full scope of the lesion. These small abnormalities may be just the tip of the iceberg, i.e., a large vascular mass may extend back into the depths of the head and require extensive intervention that is not appropriate in the LDC setting.

Forehead hemangiomas, especially when located close to the hairline, tend to bleed profusely, spontaneously. The lesions can be excised through a direct incision. A bicoronal approach provides excellent exposure and allows for wide excision of the lesion with the scar hidden within the hairline. The anesthetic considerations include large bore venous access, the ability to turn the table 180° and the use of post-procedure restraints to keep the patient's hands away from the face post-procedure.

Nasal bridge and nasal tip lesions can be excised directly and supplemented with an open rhinoplasty.

Complications

Bleeding during the proliferative phase is of concern because there is high flow and erosions can occur with large amounts of sudden blood loss. Direct pressure can be a temporizing measure until surgical intervention can be implemented. Thrombocytopenia can also occur in large hemangiomas with a high flow (Kasabach–Merritt phenomenon). Significant thrombocytopenia (less than 100 K/cc) precludes surgical intervention in the LDC setting.

Conclusion

The anesthesiologist plays a central role in the repair of deformities of the face, allowing for plastic surgery interventions that could not otherwise occur. However, a significant portion of the preanesthetic assessment is determining which patient is an acceptable risk and determining if the patient be managed without the backup of a complete intensive care unit or blood bank. While this work is immensely satisfying, a key measure of success is the lack of serious complications. It is that goal upon which we must focus our efforts.

References

1. Parker SE, Mai CT, Canfield MA, Rickard R, Wang Y, Meyer RE, et al. Updated national birth prevalence estimates for selected birth defects in the United States, 2004–2006. Birth Defects Res A Clin Mol Teratol. 2010;88(12):1008–16.
2. Tanaka SA, Mahabir RC, Jupiter DC, Menezes JM. Updating the epidemiology of cleft lip with or without cleft palate. Plast Reconstr Surg. 2012;129(3):511e–8. doi:10.1097/PRS.0b013e3182402dd1.
3. American Society of Anesthesiologists (ASA) Committee on Standards and Practice Parameters, Jeffrey L. Apfelbaum, M.D. (Chair). Practice guidelines for preoperative fasting and the use of pharmacologic agents to reduce the risk of pulmonary aspiration: application to healthy patients undergoing elective procedures: an updated report by the American Society of Anesthesiologists Committee on Standards and Practice Parameters. Anesthesiology. 2011;114(3):495–511. doi: 10.1097/ALN.0b013e3181fcbfd9.
4. Smith I, Kranke P, Murat I, Smith A, O'Sullivan G, Søreide E, Spies C. Perioperative fasting in adults and children: guidelines from the European Society of Anaesthesiology. Eur J Anaesthesiol. 2011;28(8):556–69.
5. van Veen MR, van Hasselt PM, de Sain-van der Velden MG, Verhoeven N, Hofstede FC, de Koning TJ, Visser G. Metabolic profiles in children during fasting. Pediatrics. 2011;127(4):e1021–7.
6. Friesen RH, Honda AT, Thieme RE. Changes in anterior fontanel pressure in preterm neonates during tracheal intubation. Anesth Analg. 1987;66:874–8.
7. Musgrave RH. Surgery of nasal deformities associated with cleft lip. Plast Reconstr Surg. 1961;28(3):261–75.
8. Bell EF, Strauss RG, Widness JA, et al. Randomized trial of liberal versus restrictive guidelines for red blood cell transfusion in preterm infants. Pediatrics. 2005;115:1685–91.
9. Kirpalani H, Whyte RK, Andersen C, et al. The premature infants in need of transfusion (PIUNT) study: a randomized, controlled trial of a restrictive (low) versus liberal (high) transfusion threshold for extremely low birth weight infants. J Pediatr. 2006;149:301–7.
10. Lacriox J, Hebert PC, Hutchison JS, et al. Transfusion strategies for patients in pediatric intensive care units. N Engl J Med. 2007;356:1609–19.
11. Wilson W, Taubert KA, Gewitz M, et al. AHA guideline prevention of infective endocarditis guidelines from the American Heart Association: a guideline from the American Heart Association Rheumatic Fever, Endocarditis, and Kawasaki Disease Committee, Council on Cardiovascular Disease in the Young, and the Council on Clinical Cardiology, Council on Cardiovascular Surgery and Anesthesia, and the Quality of Care and Outcomes Research Interdisciplinary Working Group. Circulation. 2007;116:1736–54.
12. Jindal P, Khurana G, Gupta D, Sharma JP. A retrospective analysis of anesthetic experience in 2917 patients posted for cleft lip and palate repair. Anesth Essays Res. 2013;7(3).
13. Wood FM. Hypoxia: another issue to consider when timing cleft repair. Ann Plast Surg. 1994;32:15–8.
14. Qureshi FA, Kamran M, Ilyas M, Laiq N. Anesthetist experience for cleft lip and cleft palate repair: a review of 172 smile train sponsored patients at Hayat Abad medical complex, Peshawar. JPMI. 2011;23(1).
15. Jindal P, Khurana G, Dvivedi S, Sharma JP. Intra and postoperative outcome of adding clonidine to bupivacaine in infraorbital nerve block for young children undergoing cleft lip surgery. Saudi J Anaesth. 2011;5:289–94.
16. Singhal S, Negi G, Chandra H, et al. Hematological parameters in patients of cleft lip and cleft palate with special reference to eosinophil counts. J Craniofac Surg. 2014;25(1):103–5. doi:10.1098/SCS.0b013e3182a2eb3c.
17. Asegaonkar B, Kulkarni J, Totla R, et al. Perioperative Management of Cleft Palate Repair in a Patient with Williams Syndrome: A Case Report. Open J of Anaesth. 2013;3:57–60.

A Regional Anesthesia Service in a Resource-Limited International Setting: Rwanda

18

Alberto E. Ardon and Theogene Twagirumugabe

Introduction

As a CA-3 resident I was able to participate in a 1-month organized educational and clinical mission to Rwanda. Anticipating a fair amount of regional anesthesia, including peripheral nerve blockade, my supervising faculty and I had secured the loan of an ultrasound directly from a manufacturer. After 2 weeks of working in Rwandan surgical suites, however, we had not performed any peripheral nerve blocks and had used the ultrasound only once for central line placement.

One day a 23-year-old man presented for open reduction and internal fixation of a distal radius fracture. The patient had been admitted to the hospital 2 days prior and had been awaiting availability of the operating suite. He described eight out of ten pain in the right upper extremity, which improved with intravenous morphine. With the help of the Rwandan anesthesia resident, we confirmed an unremarkable medical and surgical history. The two-bay area where we conducted our preoperative interview was also the emergency room, with only one automated blood pressure cuff and pulse oximeter. Our anesthetic plan consisted of using a brachial plexus block for surgical anesthesia along with mild sedation. After learning that neither the Rwandan anesthesia resident nor faculty was facile with a nerve-stimulator infraclavicular technique, we decided to forego the ultrasound and use this opportunity to teach the nerve-stimulator approach. One vial of 0.25 % bupivacaine was available.

We brought the patient into the operating room to perform the nerve block, as no exclusive monitoring was available in the holding area. Additionally, even though the operating suite had been cleaned, the nursing staff still required an estimated 30 min to prepare appropriate instruments. After placement of ASA monitors, we successfully performed the brachial plexus block and complete surgical anesthesia was achieved. The patient received minimal additional sedation for the surgery and was thereafter taken to the eight-bed post-anesthesia care unit (PACU). He was comfortable and did not require analgesics or antiemetics. The single PACU nurse was appreciative of his unremarkable and abbreviated stay, as two of the beds were occupied by overflow patients from the intensive care unit.

From this experience we learned much of what is needed and what can work for anesthesia in orthopedic surgery in a limited resource center.

A.E. Ardon, M.D., M.P.H. (✉)
Department of Anesthesiology, University of Florida, 655 West Eighth Street, Jacksonville, FL 32209, USA
e-mail: alberto.ardon@jax.ufl.edu

T. Twagirumugabe, M.D.
National University of Rwanda, 3 Butare, Rwanda, Africa

R. Roth et al. (eds.), *The Role of Anesthesiology in Global Health: A Comprehensive Guide*, DOI 10.1007/978-3-319-09423-6_18, © Springer International Publishing Switzerland 2015

The Path to Safe Orthopedic Surgery in Rwanda

In 2006, an American Society of Anesthesiologists/ Canadian Anesthesiologists Society International Educational Foundation (ASA-CASIEF) mission to Rwanda was established to create a sustainable educational relationship between training programs in the USA and Canada and the cities of Kigali and Butare in Rwanda. A continuum of US and Canadian anesthesia teaching faculty from various institutions, including Dalhousie University and the University of Virginia was provided [1]. Another program, Human Resources for Health (HRH), is a multidisciplinary education initiative that provides faculty from nine US teaching hospitals to train Rwandan residents and mentor Rwandan faculty in anesthesia, surgery, obstetrics and gynecology, pediatrics, internal medicine, and family medicine. ASA-CASIEF and HRH faculty work in synchrony to support the development of Rwandan anesthesia training and clinical practice.

The World Health Organization estimates that, as of 2012, Rwanda has a total population of almost 11.5 million people, with a median age of 18 years and an annual population growth rate of 3 % [2]. It is the most densely populated nation in Africa. Unfortunately, the number of hospital beds is disproportionate, with an average of 0.0017 beds per 100,000 people [3]. Likewise, the number of physicians is less than 0.5 per 10,000 population. In contrast, the USA and Canada have 24.2 and 20.69 physicians per 10,000 population, respectively [3]. The Rwandan hospital system consists of 2 public referral hospitals and 1 private referral hospital, 34 district hospitals, and 402 health centers for the total population.

Despite limited physical and human resources, Rwandan medical capacity has steadily increased since the genocide of Tutsi and moderate Hutu in Rwanda by members of the Hutu majority and the civil war of 1994. Over the past 10 years, per capita health care expenditure has risen from \$9.49 per Rwandan citizen to \$55 per capita. Health expenditure as percentage of GDP has increased from 4 % in 2000 to 11 % in 2006 [4]. Many health indicators are better than those in the neighboring countries of Democratic Republic of Congo, and Burundi, as well as the African region overall (Table 18.1), yet they still fall behind global indices [2].

The capacity to perform safe surgery in Rwanda, while improving, is somewhat limited secondary to and inadequate infrastructure, surgical resources, and personnel. Up to 80 % of hospitals in the southern province reported absent or insufficient pulse oximetry, and 35 % reported no or inadequate oxygen supply [5]. Approximately 80 % of surgical procedures are performed at district level hospitals, which are typically less likely to have adequate capability for blood banking, amputations, closed or open fracture repairs, inhalational anesthetic administration, and chest tube insertion [5]. Many of the major surgical procedures are therefore performed at the referral hospitals. There are two public referral hospitals in Rwanda, the larger of which is Centre Hospitalier Universitaire, Kigali (CHUK). The other is Centre Hospitalier Universitaire, Butare (CHUB). These referral

Table 18.1 Mortality indicators in Rwanda [2]

	Rwanda	Burundi	Democratic Republic of Congo	Tanzania	Uganda	Africa	Global
Under 5 mortality rate (per 1,000 population)	55	104	146	54	69	95	48
Adult mortality (per 1,000 population)	317	345	384	342	385	383	176
Maternal mortality ratio (per 100,000 live births)	340	800	540	460	310	480	210

Adapted from www.WHO.int 2010 and 2012 data

Table 18.2 Surgical caseload by public referral hospital in Rwanda [5]

Hospital	Operating rooms	Major surgeries performed	Major and minor surgeries performed
University hospital—Kigali (CHUK) 2010 data	14	4,164	7,682
University hospital—Butare (CHUB) 2009 data	4	2,488	4,526

hospitals are equipped with eight and four general operating rooms, respectively. As shown in Table 18.2, in 2009 approximately 4,164 and 2,488 major surgeries were performed at CHUK and CHUB, respectively [5]. Although referral hospitals have better surgical capacity than their district-level counterparts, they still have some pragmatic limitations. On occasion, either of these large referral centers may have limited or absent surgical or anesthetic supplies, such as consistent capnography, local anesthetic agents, or banked blood products.

Limited personnel are also an issue. As of 2013, Rwanda has only 10 licensed anesthesiologists; the national anesthesia residency program currently has 16 trainees. In a continuing effort to build up Rwanda's anesthesiology capability, organizations such as ASA/CASIEF and HRH provide a significant contribution to the anesthesia workforce. These visiting anesthesiologists not only participate in daily clinical care but also teach and mentor residents and Rwandan staff. A recent surgical capacity national collaboration meeting emphasized the important role of international efforts in enhancing the education of Rwandan health care providers and therefore increasing Rwandan health care in a sustainable manner [5].

Lack of medical supplies, electricity, or appropriately trained staff is of course a problem not exclusive to Rwanda. Infrastructure analyses across sub-Saharan Africa show common themes of inadequate supplies and equipment, limited monitoring, lack of appropriate training for anesthesia providers, and few qualified anesthetists [6, 7]. In one 2006 survey among 97 non-private hospital anesthesia providers in Uganda, only 23 % stated they had the minimum monitoring requirements to conduct a safe anesthetic in an adult patient. The most frequently unavailable items included pulse oximetry and oxygen source; running water and electricity were also described as not always available [7].

This shortage of physical and personnel resources directly impacts the type of anesthesia and analgesia available for orthopedic surgery. As orthopedic procedures account for approximately 40 % of the surgical caseload at CHUB, and orthopedic surgery is amenable to regional anesthetic techniques, this chapter focuses on regional anesthesia for orthopedic surgery. Despite the decrease in postoperative opioid consumption and improvement in patient satisfaction that is associated with peripheral nerve block techniques [8], few orthopedic surgery patients in Rwanda receive such blocks. Whereas 99 % of lower extremity surgery at both CHUB and CHUK is performed under spinal anesthesia, only 10–15 % of these patients receive supplemental peripheral nerve blockade for postoperative pain control. Although approximately 55 % of orthopedic cases at CHUB involve upper extremity fractures, very few patients are offered brachial plexus blockade either for surgical anesthesia or postoperative analgesia [9]. Frequently cited reasons by Rwandan anesthesiologists are lack of needles or local anesthetic solution and lack of skills regarding peripheral nerve block techniques [1]. The low prevalence of brachial plexus blockade is particularly unfortunate given its benefits when compared to general anesthesia, including decreased postoperative pain, improved readiness for discharge, and decreased nausea and vomiting [10]. In a setting such as Rwanda, where both material and personnel resources are significantly limited, the impact of a consistent regional anesthesia service may be substantial. Economical, clinical, and training spheres may all be positively affected.

Economic Impact

Regional anesthesia has the potential to be cost-effective. For example, spinal anesthesia, which is already used in Rwanda for virtually all lower extremity and many intra-abdominal and pelvic procedures, can provide significant cost savings when compared to general anesthesia. Spinal anesthesia has been shown to improve cost-effectiveness in orthopedic as well as gynecologic surgery [11, 12]. A study conducted in Sweden from 2007 to 2009 compared the potential perioperative and recovery costs involved with each type of anesthetic. As shown in Table 18.3, a significant cost-savings per patient can occur with an estimated savings of approximately US$800 per patient when combined with a multimodal pain control regimen and minimization of opioids.

The use of peripheral nerve blockade, though, has been associated with considerable start-up costs. Some of these costs can be prohibitive in a limited-resource setting. While one study has shown that an ultrasound-guided brachial plexus block can be a cost effective anesthetic for arthroscopic shoulder surgery, resulting in a savings of approximately $220 USD per case [11], the use of ultrasound-guided blocks in a developing country hospital has its own challenges. Ultrasound machines are very expensive, usually costing more than $10,000 USD. While the initial cost of the machine may be recuperated over several years in a high volume practice, such an economic plan might not be feasible in a Rwandan hospital that, on average, provides 70 anesthetics a week, of which less than half would be considered potential candidates for peripheral nerve blockade. In addition, ultrasound machines require specialized maintenance and repair, which often is not readily available in a developing country.

Table 18.3 Economic impact of spinal versus general anesthesia in hysterectomy patients in Sweden (in US$) [12]

Costs	General anesthesia	Spinal-morphine anesthesia	Difference in costs
Time in operating theater	1,362	1,305	57
Anesthetic drugs	42	22	20
Time in post-anesthesia care unit	263	218	45
Sick leave	3,856	3,172	684
Total cost	5,523	4,717	806

Adapted from Woodlin et al.

Most studies regarding the cost-effectiveness of peripheral nerve blockade seem to indicate, however, that time involved with the block, as well as overall anesthesia-care time is the largest determinant of cost-effectiveness [13–15]. One retrospective study examining orthopedic and trauma patients found that brachial plexus blockade was less cost-effective than either general anesthesia or spinal anesthesia, particularly during short surgery [13]. A small prospective study suggested that use of brachial plexus block for outpatient hand surgery is associated with greater cost when compared to general anesthesia [14]. In these studies, increased cost is secondary to: (a) the more extensive time required to perform the block, and (b) the nursing time needed for patient monitoring after the block is completed and prior to entry into the operating room. Another prospective analysis from workers at Duke University, however, indicates that a regional anesthesia nursing team (block nurses) in fact increases operating room efficiency [15].

Translating this data to the situation in Rwanda requires special consideration of the work flow and day-to-day resources available. In both referral hospitals in Rwanda, there is no designated preoperative regional anesthesia "block" area, nor is there sufficient nursing staff to monitor a patient in such an area. However, average operating room turnover time at the Rwandan referral hospitals is 1–1.5 h, which is significantly greater than turnover times at the Canadian, German, and US hospitals where these studies were conducted. The patient could, therefore, be brought into the operating room while the surgical team is preparing instruments for the case. The regional anesthesia resident or faculty would be responsible for performing the nerve block and thereafter the patient could be monitored by the anesthesia provider assigned to the case. This method could minimize any potential delay in surgical start

Table 18.4 Criteria for safe peripheral nerve blockade administration [31]

Battery-operated EKG, pulse oximetry, noninvasive blood pressure monitoring prior to, during, and after nerve block
Supplemental oxygen available
Resuscitation supplies—including 20 % fat emulsion (Intralipid)—available to treat local anesthetic toxicity
Patient history, laboratory values (when available), and surgical procedure compatible with peripheral nerve block
Informed consent present
Proper patient identification prior to nerve block, with confirmation of anesthesia and surgical laterality
Hand washing by staff prior to performing block
Mask and hat worn by all staff involved
Sterile technique using sterile antiseptic prep and gloves; drape when applicable
Ability by staff to identify potential nerve injury or other complications
Ability to confirm block efficacy

Adapted from Smith et al.

time. Additionally, the more frequent use of peripheral nerve blockade could have an effect on post-anesthesia care. Recovery room space is restricted to eight PACU beds in Butare. Unfortunately, these beds are also used for emergency room and ICU overflow, thus actual recovery space can be even more limited. Staffing for PACU consists only of one nurse and an anesthesia technician (who also provides sedation for minor procedures and responds to cardiopulmonary arrest events throughout the hospital), and supervised by the ICU anesthesiology attending physician. A patient who received a peripheral nerve block as the surgical anesthetic would have an abbreviated PACU stay and lessen the burden on recovery room staff.

Another potential mechanism of cost-savings and operating room efficiency relates to oxygen, electricity, and capnography unavailability. In the Rwandan referral hospitals, loss of electricity or central oxygen supply occurs occasionally. Much like in developed country surgical suites, induction of general or spinal anesthesia is not carried out under these circumstances. However, peripheral nerve blockade could be performed and surgery could proceed as long as certain safety criteria could be satisfied, as shown in Table 18.4. Even with loss of a central source oxygen or electricity, simple upper extremity surgery, which does not require the use of a tourniquet, for example, could be performed safely under a peripheral nerve block with the support of E-cylinder oxygen tanks and battery-operated monitors. Regarding capnography, half of the operating rooms in Butare did not have capnography during our visit. The use of a brachial plexus block and maintenance of a natural airway during surgery, however, would obviate the need for capnography. Safe peripheral nerve block anesthesia under appropriate monitoring maximizes the available resources to meet the greater surgical need.

Clinical Impact

Regional anesthesia is associated with decreased blood loss, lower risk of nausea and vomiting, less likely unanticipated hospital admission, better postoperative pain control, and less postoperative opioid consumption as compared to general anesthesia [16, 17]. The 20 % decrease in likelihood of transfusion associated with neuraxial anesthetics is especially advantageous in a hospital such as CHUK, where only a dozen units of blood are available for the entire patient population [16]. Regarding both neuraxial and peripheral nerve anesthetics, a decrease in postoperative nausea and vomiting and immediate postoperative opioid consumption can decrease length of stay in the PACU and thus decrease cost for the anesthesia department while improving patient satisfaction [10]. In a small study conducted in Butare hospital in 2009, patients who underwent femur fracture repair and received a fascia iliaca block had less postoperative pain and opioid requirements in the first 12 h when compared to patients who received a sham block [18]. While the use of perineural catheters would be ideal for postoperative pain control and minimization of opioid consumption, the cost and necessity for close follow-up would be prohibitive in this setting.

Besides postoperative analgesia, peripheral nerve blockade can also provide improved *preoperative* analgesia to certain Rwandan surgical patients. In both Rwandan referral hospitals, orthopedic trauma patients may have to wait more than 48 h until their fractures can be surgically addressed. Femoral nerve or fascia iliaca blockade can be used to decrease pain and suffering associated with hip fractures prior to surgical intervention [19, 20] without the need for a large amount of opioids. Additionally, blockade of the femoral nerve can facilitate proper positioning for spinal anesthesia in the operating room. The relative ease of femoral nerve block and fascia iliaca block placement using a nerve stimulator or loss-of-resistance technique also makes these blocks useful.

While some orthopedic surgeons are quite concerned about the potential impact of continuous nerve blockade on the diagnosis of compartment syndrome, current data and numerous case reports suggest that peripheral nerve blockade, even if given continuously, does not affect the timeliness or adequate diagnosis of this complication [21–23].

Training Impact

In addition to its economic and clinical benefits, regional anesthesia can have a significant impact on a continually evolving anesthesia training program limited by low resources. Adequate training in regional anesthesia hinges on an adequate case load to master technical skills as well as clinical application of anatomy, physiology, and pharmacology [24]. Evidence suggests that learning nerve-stimulator-guided techniques may require more repetition that ultrasound-guided techniques [25]. As nerve-stimulator peripheral nerve block techniques are more practical in a limited resource setting, adequate patient volume becomes a key issue to developing proficiency. In Rwandan referral hospitals, where anesthesia residents train, approximately 30 patients a week are anesthetized for orthopedic or extremity trauma procedures. While certainly the evaluation of candidates for peripheral nerve blockade needs to be done on a case-by-case basis, quite often many of these patients have the potential to benefit from peripheral block techniques. The ultimate impact of learning these techniques during residency training would be evident as the Rwandan residents graduate and practice regional anesthesiology throughout the country.

Since visiting anesthesiologists and anesthesiology residents contribute a great deal to the development and implementation of the anesthesia training curriculum, they are poised to not only empower local anesthesiologists with techniques that can enhance anesthesia delivery but also improve their own training. By applying clinical knowledge to situations that are not likely to be encountered at their home institutions, visiting anesthesiologists and trainees can work with local staff to gain insights into clinical circumstances that may be unique to that specific country or region. For the resident in particular, this experience may prove invaluable. International encounters broaden differential diagnoses, improve physical exam skills, enhance cultural competence, decrease the use of routine lab tests, and enrich an appreciation for health systems [26, 27]. Specifically, the act of teaching may stimulate self improvement, improve clinical skills and perceived professional competency, as well as expand the teacher's knowledge base [28]. In the Rwandan ASA/CASIEF and HRH missions, there is a strong sense of cooperation among visiting and local anesthesiology staff, enhanced by the realization that both parties stand to benefit from the relationship.

Limitations/Barriers

One of the most frequently encountered limitations to consistent performance of neuraxial and peripheral nerve block techniques in a developing country is lack of materials. While hyperbaric bupivacaine for use in spinal anesthesia is available in Rwandan referral hospitals, ropivacaine, mepivacaine, and bupivacaine for peripheral nerve blockade are quite often in extremely short supply. Likewise, nerve stimulator needles and appropriately functioning nerve stimulators are also not consistently available. Regarding safety, the ability to treat local anesthetic toxicity also needs to be addressed, as currently there is no Intralipid in either referral hospital. The shortage of supplies for peripheral nerve blockade is multifactorial but mostly related to cost and thus largely depends on international donations. However, as health care expenditure grows and advocacy for regional anesthesia expands, anesthesia in Rwanda will hopefully be less reliant on external influence.

Another significant limitation is a low level of proficiency in peripheral nerve block techniques among Rwandan anesthesiologists. Currently there is a strong dependence on expatriate anesthesiologists to perform nerve stimulated or (when available) ultrasound-guided blocks. Herein lies the importance of teaching within the framework of a nascent regional anesthesia service. International academic partnerships benefit from mutual learning, in which visiting faculty commit to teaching local faculty and residents, thus perpetuating local capacity [29]. Thus, a continual stream of visiting faculty who are interested both in teaching needle-handling techniques and functioning as clinical consultants is required over an extended period of time. While this demand is graciously being met at the present time in Rwanda, the process is ongoing and reliant on long-term commitment.

As described by Schnittger with regards to the example of Zambian hospitals, low availability of local anesthetics can create a low level of training in regional techniques, which can thereafter lead to low prevalence of peripheral nerve block use. This low usage can in turn lead to less demand for regional anesthesia and thus eventually inspire less demand for regional anesthetic supplies [30]. Based upon our Rwandan experience, we would emphasize that both material supplies and training are both initially essential for the establishment of a regional anesthesia service and also for its sustainability. Concomitant adequate supplies and continual training are indispensible.

Conclusion

The establishment of a regional anesthesia service in a limited resource setting such as Rwanda may positively impact local anesthesia capacity as well as clinical, economical, and training aspects. We have learned valuable lessons from our experiences:

- Procuring regional anesthesia supplies including local anesthetic, nerve stimulators, and needles is a priority.
- To initially increase local resource supply, visiting anesthesiology faculty and residents may need to provide local anesthetics, needles, etc. until a more reliable local supply chain is secured.
- Improved preoperative and postoperative analgesia, decreased inflammatory and stress response, minimization of opioids, and decreased nausea/vomiting are some of the benefits of regional anesthesia that would be of value to this patient population.
- The use of ultrasound-guided nerve blockade is potentially not ideal given current resources and infrastructure.
- Working within the local framework is important for implementation of any new clinical endeavor. Utilizing available resources, while introducing new modalities and means within that framework, positions a visiting clinical mission for a better chance of success.
- The lasting impact of an international anesthesia effort relies on the sustainability of the effort, i.e. the impact must be present after the visiting anesthesia faculty have returned home. As equipment and supplies are procured and local staff become proficient in regional anesthetic techniques, the clinical environment depends less on international educational aid.
- Continued international collaboration and research are needed to properly improve anesthesia capacity in nations with limited resources.

References

1. Twagirumugabe T, Carli F. Rwandan anesthesia residency: a model of north-south educational partnership. Int Anesthesiol Clin. 2010;48:71–8.
2. World Health Organization Statistics Summary 2010–2012. www.who.int
3. Notrica M, Evans F, Knowlton L, McQueen K. Rwandan surgical and anesthesia infrastructure: a survey of district hospitals. World J Surg. 2011;35:1770–80.

4. ABT Associates. Health Systems 20/20 Report: National Health Accounts: Rwanda 2006, 2008.
5. Petroze R, Nzayisenga A, Rusanganwa V, Ntakiyiruta G, Calland J. Comprehensive national analysis of emergency and essential surgical capacity in Rwanda. Br J Surg. 2012;99:436–43.
6. Grady K. Building capacity for anaesthesia in low resource settings. Br J Obstet Gynaecol. 2009;166: 15–7.
7. Hodges S, Mijumbi C, McCormick B, Wlaker I, Wilson I. Anaesthesia services in developing countries: defining the problems. Anaesthesia. 2007;62: 4–11.
8. Kettner SC, Willschke H, Marhofer P. Does regional anesthesia really improve outcome? Br J Anaesth. 2011;107(S1):i90–5.
9. Personal communication with Twagirumugabe T, program director University of Rwanda Anesthesiology Residency; Kigale and Butare referral hospital data.
10. Hadzic A, Arliss J, Beklen K, Karaca PE, Yufa M, Claudio RE, Vloka JD, Rosenquist R, Santos AC, Thys DM. A comparison of infraclavicular nerve block versus general anesthesia for hand and wrist day-case surgeries. Anesthesiology. 2004;101:127–32.
11. Gonano C, Kettner S, Ernstbrunner M, Schebesta K, Chiari A, Marhofer P. Comparison of economical aspects of interscalene brachial plexus blockade and general anesthesia for arthroscopic shoulder surgery. Br J Anaesth. 2009;103:428–33.
12. Wodlin N, Nilsson L, Carlsson P, Kjolhede P. Cost-effectiveness of general anesthesia vs. spinal anesthesia in fast-track abdominal benign hysterectomy. Am J Obstet Gynecol. 2011;205:326. e1–7.
13. Schuster M, Gottschalk A, Berger J, Standl T. A retrospective comparison of costs for regional and general anesthesia techniques. Anesth Analg. 2005;100: 786–94.
14. Chan V, Peng P, Kaszas Z, Middleton W, Muni R, Anastakis D, Graham B. A comparative study of general anesthesia, intravenous regional anesthesia, and axillary block for outpatient hand surgery: clinical outcome and cost analysis. Anesth Analg. 2001;93: 1181–4.
15. Russell R, Burke K, Gattis K. Implementing a regional anesthesia block nurse team in the perianesthesia care unit increases patient safety and perioperative efficiency. J Perianesth Nurs. 2013;28:3–10.
16. Mauermann W, Shilling A, Zuo Z. A comparison of neuraxial block versus general anesthesia for elective total hip replacement: a meta-analysis. Anesth Analg. 2006;103:1018–25.
17. Greenberg C. Practical, cost-effective regional anesthesia for ambulatory surgery. J Clin Anesth. 1995; 7:614–21.
18. Twagirumugabe T, Midonze D, Uwambazimana M. Efficacy of a single fascia iliaca block in postoperative pain management of femoral shaft or neck fracture repair. Poster Presented at All Africa Anesthesia Congress; 2009; Nairobi, Kenya.
19. Fletcher A, Rigby A, Heyes F. Three-in-one femoral nerve block as analgesia for fractured neck of femur in the emergency department: a randomized, controlled trial. Ann Emerg Med. 2003;41:227–33.
20. Rashiq S, Vandermeer B, Abou-Setta A, Beaupre L, Jones A, Dryden D. Efficacy of supplemental peripheral nerve blockade for hip fracture surgery: multiple treatment comparison. Can J Anaesth. 2013;60: 230–43.
21. Mar G, Barrington M, McGuirk B. Acute compartment syndrome of the lower limb and the effect of postoperative analgesia on diagnosis. Br J Anaesth. 2009;102:3–11.
22. Cometa M, Esch A, Boezaart A. Did continuous femoral and sciatic nerve block obscure the diagnosis or delay the treatment of acute lower leg compartment syndrome? A case report. Pain Med. 2011;12:823–8.
23. Mannion S, Capdevila X. Acute compartment syndrome and the role of regional anesthesia. Int Anesthesiol Clin. 2010;48:85–105.
24. Neal J. Education in regional anesthesia: caseloads, simulation, journals, and politics: 2011 Carl Koller lecture. Reg Anesth Pain Med. 2012;37:647–51.
25. Luyet C, Schupfer G, Wipfli M, Greif R, Luginbuhl M, Eichenberger U. Different learning curves for axillary brachial plexus block: ultrasound guidance versus nerve stimulation. Anesthesiol Res Pract. 2010;2010:1–7.
26. Grudzen C, Legome E. Loss of international medical experiences: knowledge, attitudes and skills at risk. BMC Med Educ. 2007;7.
27. Hau D, DiPace J, Peck Jr R, Johnson W. Global health training during residency: the Weill Cornell Tanzania experience. J Grad Med Educ. 2011;3:421–4.
28. Busari J, Scherpbier AJ. Why residents should teach: a literature review. J Postgrad Med. 2004;50:205–10.
29. Riviello R, Lipnick M, Ozgediz D. Medical missions, surgical education, and capacity building. J Am Coll Surg. 2011;213:572.
30. Schnittger T. Regional anaesthesia in developing countries. Anaesthesia. 2007;62:44–7.
31. Smith H, Kopp S, Jacob A, Torsher L, Hebl J. Designing and implementing a comprehensive learner-centered regional anesthesia curriculum. Reg Anesth Pain Med. 2009;34:88–94.

Management of Pain in Less Developed Countries

19

Clifford Gevirtz

Introduction

Progress in acute pain management over the last 30 years has demonstrated that effective pain relief can be achieved by the use of inexpensive drugs and therapies, yet the vast majority of patients in less developed areas of the world have little or no access to even the most limited of therapies that could alleviate the suffering from acute and chronic pain.

The World Health Organization (WHO) [1] estimates there are 5 billion people living in countries with little or no access to pain medicines, including 5.5 million terminal cancer patients and millions of others suffering from acute illness and end-of-life suffering. Among patients with terminal cancer, 80 % are estimated to experience moderate to severe pain due to inadequate access to medicine.

Obstetric services in the developing world are lacking [2] with an estimated 99 % of all maternal deaths occur in the developing world and prolonged obstructed labor producing obstetric fistulae is a commonplace complication. The lack of obstetric services results in untold suffering of mothers, most of whom have no access to basic gynecological and medical care, let alone analgesia. A study [3] from the teaching hospital in Benin City, Nigeria, found that 85 % of women would request analgesia in labor if it were available. However, only 40 % of women received any analgesic intervention. In a large number of rural hospitals absolutely no analgesia is available to women with either normal or complicated labors.

The provision of analgesia is seen as a low priority by many aid organizations in comparison to the treatment of diseases such as malaria, tuberculosis, and HIV/AIDS. Since basic resources such as drinking water and electricity may not be available, it is not surprising that the provision of analgesic drugs is problematic and relegated to a lower priority. Although lack of finance is a significant barrier to improving this situation, better management of health care resources and infrastructure are also required.

Cancer Related Pain

A similar situation exists for the management of cancer related pain. An international survey [4] on the availability of opioids for cancer pain management was conducted by the European Society for Medical Oncology (ESMO), the World Health Organization (WHO), in collaboration with 17 leading cancer and palliative care organizations worldwide. The survey focused on the legal, regulatory, and social barriers that impact the availability and access to seven essential opioids for cancer pain management in Africa, Asia, Latin America and the Caribbean, and the Middle East. The opioids selected

C. Gevirtz, M.D., M.P.H. (✉)
LSU Health Science Center, New Orleans, LA, USA

Somnia, Inc., New Rochelle, NY, USA
e-mail: cliffgevirtzmd@yahoo.com

R. Roth et al. (eds.), *The Role of Anesthesiology in Global Health: A Comprehensive Guide*,
DOI 10.1007/978-3-319-09423-6_19, © Springer International Publishing Switzerland 2015

were all on the WHO Model Essential Medicines List and the International Association for Hospice and Palliative Care list of essential medicines for palliative care. The seven essential opiates are: morphine immediate release, morphine controlled release, morphine injectable, oxycodone oral tablets, methadone oral liquid, and fentanyl transdermal patch. The survey was conducted between December 2010 and July 2012. Clinicians in 81 countries and 25 Indian states completed an in-depth questionnaires on formulary availability, cost and barriers to accessing essential opioids, to measure current national standards against the reality in the communities. In LDCs, a majority of the seven essential opioids were on the national essential medicines lists. Oxycodone, methadone, and fentanyl were less consistently included on the national formularies. However, analysis of the availability data revealed that in many of the surveyed countries and all of the Indian states surveyed, fewer than three of the seven medicines were routinely available for use in hospital and pharmacies. In the Indian states, despite codeine, three morphine formulations and transdermal fentanyl being on state level essential medicine lists, only codeine was always or usually available. The six other opiates considered essential for pain management were either only occasionally or never available. All regions of the world show inconsistencies between the adoption of the essential medicine list at the national policy level and the actual range and availability of essential opioids to patients.

There is also a major gap in clinician attitudes and education. Although not a focus of the ESMO survey, there is a broad consensus among the international medical community and the WHO that inadequate education of health care providers is one of the most pervasive and urgent obstacles to address. A recent Human Rights Watch survey [5] on palliative care barriers in 40 countries found that most countries had inadequate medical education in palliative care and pain management and four of the countries surveyed had no relevant curriculum in these areas at all.

On the Ground Reality

It appears that analgesia has a lower priority than many other aspects of health care in developing countries so that effective pain relief is unavailable to a large numbers of patients. While comprehensive data about the incidence and management of pain are lacking, it is clear that, even when patients do access health care facilities, the degree of pain relief still seems to be inadequate.

Administration of available drugs may also not be managed appropriately. Doctors and nurses often receive little training in analgesic management. In rural hospitals in South America and Africa, it is not uncommon to have two nurses looking after a ward of 50 patients; the overstretched nursing staff may be unavailable to administer analgesic drugs and, indeed, the safety of administering potent analgesics in this setting has to be questioned as there may be little monitoring and no reversal agents are available should a problem arise. Lack of training manifests itself as an unreasonable fear on the part of the medical and nursing staff of side-effects or addiction, which may in turn propagate a culture of non-intervention. Doctors and nurses can become so used to doing nothing for patients in pain that non-treatment becomes the standard approach. Further, patients begin to believe that nothing can be done, or adopt a fatalistic attitude and suffer in silence, with little more than family members to offer comfort.

Therapeutic Agents

Opioids

Opioid analgesics are the gold standard for treating moderate to severe pain, drugs such as morphine being low cost and highly effective. However, the availability and use of opioids is not uniform across the globe.

Cleary et al. [6] studied the mal distribution of opiates and found in 2013, that 90 % of the world's morphine was consumed by ten major industrial countries: Australia, Canada, Denmark, France, Germany, Japan, Spain, Sweden, the UK, and the USA; 85 % of the world's population shared the remaining 10 % of the world's morphine.

In 1996, in a seminal publication [7], entitled "Cancer Pain Relief: A Guide to Opioid Availability," the WHO contributed a framework for developing or improving palliative care and pain relief within a country that comprised three key components:

1. Government policies that ensure the integration of palliative care services into the structure and financing of the national health care system.
2. Educational programs that provide support for the training of health care professionals, volunteers, and the public.
3. Drug availability supported by appropriate drug control policies and their administration to ensure the availability of essential medicines for the management of pain and other symptoms, in particular, opioid analgesics for pain relief.

Now almost 20 years later, many barriers remain to correct opioid use in the developing world. There may be concerns at government level over risks of addiction and abuse. Import restrictions may be overly stringent and the laws regarding prescribing and dispensing opioids can make it virtually impossible to get opioids to patients. Of the governments that responded to the International Narcotics Control Board survey, 43 % said that they require physicians to report to the government those patients who are prescribed opioid analgesics; this acts as a powerful disincentive to prescribe opioids.

Currently, the cost of importing morphine to developing countries is disproportionately high. A survey of opioid costs [8] in 2003 showed that opioid drugs were up to ten times more expensive in the developing world than in the developed world, after adjustment for differences in gross domestic product.

National legislation in individual countries [9] can have a massive effect on opioid consumption. In India, the introduction of a piece of legislation that resulted in a significant increase in the bureaucracy associated with purchasing opioids led to a 97 % fall in consumption of morphine from 716 kg in 1985 to 18 kg in 1997. The WHO estimates that if barriers to accessing morphine in the developing world could be removed, then a reasonable estimate of the cost of morphine would be just one US cent per milligram.

In an ideal world, assessment of pain should become as basic an observation as measuring pulse and blood pressure. The US Veterans Health Administration was the first to popularize the concept of pain scales as the fifth vital sign. Simple pain assessment tools such as the visual analog scale as well as the memorial pain card have been translated into nearly every language on the planet demonstrating that pain measurements can be adapted to local circumstances in LDCs.

Therapeutic Interventions

Psychological Interventions

Training programs in LDCs should encourage the discussion of pain management as part of the routine medical and surgical care of the patient. A simple explanation of the cause and likely duration of pain can noticeably improve a patient's ability to cope, even when other material interventions may be difficult to provide. Patients may have a limited understanding of their condition and assume that pain may be inevitable or not treatable in any measure. At this point, the palliative care training programs in the LDCs do not address chronic non-malignant pain.

Drug Treatment

The benefits of techniques such as patient-controlled analgesia have been clearly demonstrated in the developed world, but the lack of equipment and the lack of careful monitoring of these devices mean that in developing countries their use is impracticable and unsafe. However, administration of effective analgesia does not need to depend on sophisticated technology.

The original WHO analgesic ladder outlines simple techniques using minimal resources to combat cancer pain. This model has been applied to acute pain by the World Federation of Societies of Anesthesiologists (WFSA), which has produced a modified ladder for acute pain [10] (see Fig. 19.1).

Starting with strong parenteral opioids, ketamine, and/or local anesthetic, there is then a step down to oral opioids and finally to nonsteroidal anti-inflammatory drugs and acetaminophen on its own. All of these drugs appear on the WHO

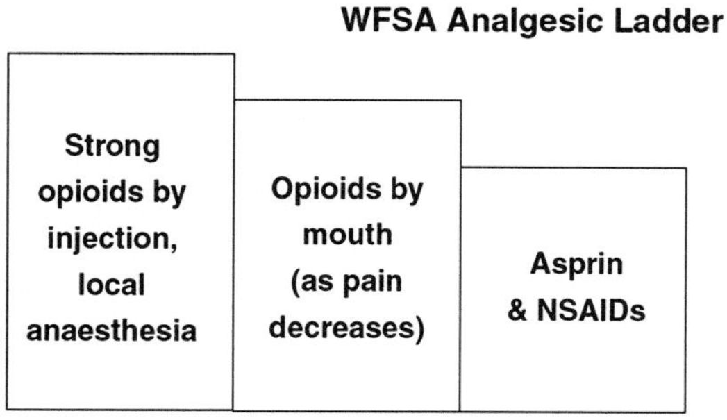

Fig. 19.1 WFSA Analgesic Ladder

list of essential drugs. This ladder should be coupled with multimodal analgesia techniques including local anesthesia blocks with longer duration agents, and prescribing regular analgesics with provisions for breakthrough pain. Ideally, the oral route should be used for postoperative analgesia, including the use of oral morphine when available and feasible.

Simple analgesics such as acetaminophen, ibuprofen, and diclofenac are cheap and readily available in most countries of the world. However, access to drug supplies may be limited within the hospital; a common solution is to pre-prescribe analgesics to be purchased by patients or relatives from local pharmacies prior to elective surgery. Unfortunately, patient may be unable to afford even the cheapest of analgesics.

Ketamine is the mainstay of anesthesia in many parts of the developing world, particularly for children. It is also an effective analgesic when administered in sub-anesthetic dosages (e.g., 10 mg i.m.) and can be used to provide immediate postoperative analgesia. It is particularly potent in combination with parenteral opioids, where it has a significant opioid-sparing effect.

Opioid use should be encouraged where possible, but this must include introduction of effective systems for opioid administration—reliable systems for purchase, safe storage, recording of use and training regarding effects and side effects. An example of success [11] in this area is in Nigeria where through several years of advocacy for availability of opioid analgesics at central government supply level, public enlightenment, and education (including undergraduate, postgraduate, and other health professionals) there has been a dramatic improvement in pain management achieved by the safe use of opioid analgesics.

Local Anesthetics

Local anesthetic techniques can provide excellent postoperative pain relief and their use should be encouraged whenever possible, by whichever route possible, even if only by local infiltration. Limited postoperative facilities and equipment shortages limit some of the more advanced options (epidurals and continuous plexus blockade), but simple techniques remain underutilized and have a low incidence of adverse effects.

Single shot techniques including spinal anesthesia, plexus blockade, caudal anesthesia in children, and infiltration of local anesthetic into wounds can be accomplished with minimal resources but great effectiveness. These techniques work most effectively using bupivacaine if it is available, but the use of shorter acting drugs such as lidocaine with epinephrine is also effective. The use of additives such as ketamine and clonidine should be encouraged, if available, but it is important to avoid additives with preservatives. Both surgeons and anesthesiologists need training to develop the use of these straightforward techniques. Liposomal bupivacaine offers the opportunity to provide more than 24 h of analgesia.

Many anesthesiologists in LDCs do not own an anesthesia textbook. Publications such as *Update in Anaesthesia* and the *Tutorial of the Week* published by the World Anaesthesia Society show how simple, cost-effective, practical information can be made available to isolated anesthesiologists in LDCs, both in hard copy and via the Internet. Open access journals are a newer approach to presenting information in the LDCs. Encouraging links between developed and developing countries (e.g., by linking academic anesthetic departments) can lead to the sharing of ideas and problems, and exchange visits of personnel, and may even help with the supply of essential equipment and drugs.

Refresher courses provide invaluable opportunities to share ideas about analgesia (Please also see details of the NYSSA Visiting Scholar program in the vignettes section) and can reach a large number of staff. Materials can be modified for the level of resources found in the country, local protocols developed, and expertise can be brought to bear on particular local problems.

On a cautionary note, care should be taken to ensure that training programs are relevant to the problems that are encountered in everyday practice. For instance, it is important to include consideration of the side-effects of different drugs, especially in hypotensive patients. Intramuscular opioids should be used carefully in such patients (i.e., it is preferable to titrate intravenous opioids) and trainers should be aware of the limitations or lack of monitoring in ward areas.

Although classroom teaching can improve knowledge, the best way of improving practice is to be taught in the operating room or recovery area by an anesthesiologist. As well as providing personal attention and mentorship, it allows anesthesiologists to act as role models and to stress the effectiveness of basic techniques and the importance of patient safety. In addition, it may help to recruit young doctors in training into a career in anesthesia. Training the local trainers and adding to the anesthesia workforce are important steps on the route to sustainability in developing countries.

Chronic pain management requires pharmacological and non-pharmacological therapies with attention to other needs of the patient (psychosocial and spiritual). In Nigeria, a pain clinic [11] was first established at the University College hospital, Ibadan, by the Department of Anesthesia in 1979 but the clinic failed to survive the period of specialist medical manpower exodus from the country in the late 1980s. The clinic was reestablished by a multidisciplinary group as a Pain and Palliative Care Clinic in 2005 to treat cancer and non-cancer pain. The analgesics available were mainly non-opioids until recently, when opioids including oral morphine solution have become available and used for cancer patients. Both physical and psychological therapies are offered by the multidisciplinary team.

A major challenge of that clinic is that patients expect to be cured and dropped out from the clinic after a few visits because of a lack of understanding that chronic pain may persist for years. The lack of pain specialists and specialized pain clinics along with the lack of training among health professionals constitute the major impediment to chronic pain services in the LDCs.

Unaddressed Pain Challenges

Dengue Fever (Break Bone Fever)

Dengue is an infectious disease caused by dengue viruses, which are transmitted to humans by mosquitoes. The rising number of dengue infections and the expanding range has become a serious international concern. Each year, the WHO reports that approximately 50 million people are infected with dengue. Typically, dengue causes a severe flu-like illness with high fever, headache, and severe body and joint pains (hence the name break bone fever).

A more dangerous form of dengue infection, however, called severe dengue, hospitalizes an estimated 500,000 people—most of them children—every year. In some regions of the world, severe dengue is fatal in more than 5 % of patients. An estimated 2.5 billion to 3 billion people around the world are currently at risk of dengue infections, and most of these people live in tropical, urban regions of Southeast Asia, the Americas, Africa, and the Pacific. The risk of dengue is higher in urban regions than in rural areas.

Babies and young children infected with the dengue virus typically have mild symptoms such as a fever and a rash over their entire bodies, but no other symptoms of dengue. Older children and adults may also have these mild symptoms, or they may have classic symptoms of dengue, including a high fever that lasts for 2–7 days, severe pain in the muscles, bones, and joints, pain behind the eyes, severe headaches, nausea and vomiting, and a rash [12]. Dengue fever is characterized by a fever response with two peaks. Near the beginning of the infection, the patient experiences a very high body temperature, which then starts to drop and then suddenly climbs again for a second time. Other symptoms of dengue fever include a decrease in the number of white blood cells and thrombocytopenia. Patients with dengue fever may have frank purpura. Dengue fever can also cause bleeding from the skin, nose, and gums. Recovery from dengue fever is often lengthy, lasting several weeks, and patients can experience lingering pain, fatigue and depression. The pain symptoms associated with dengue can be managed with pain relievers that do not increase the risk of bleeding (acetaminophen, opiates). There is currently no vaccine and treatment is mainly supportive.

Pain in Leprosy (Hansen Disease)

Stump et al. [13] reviewed the prevalence of neuropathic pain in leprosy patients. While the introduction of multidrug therapy by the WHO has dramatically reduced the world prevalence of leprosy the disease is still a public health problem in many countries, with a world prevalence of almost 600,000 cases in 2001. Damage to peripheral nerves is a key component of leprosy and the sensory and motor loss that follows is the basis for many of the classical features of this disease, such as skin wounds, cracks, plantar ulcers, clawed hands, drop foot, and incomplete closure of the eyelids. One of the most remarkable aspects of leprosy to lay persons and health care workers alike is that patients are reputed to feel no pain. However, neuropathic pain is arising as a major problem among leprosy patients. It can be nociceptive due to tissue inflammation, which mostly occurs during episodes of immune activation or neuropathic due to damage or dysfunction of the nervous system. In Stump's study [13] of 358 leprosy patients, there was a considerable prevalence of neuropathic pain, which suggests that this common problem should be a high priority of those in charge of leprosy control programs. Therapy with gabapentin or tricyclic antidepressants would be first line therapy.

Pain in Victims of Torture

According to Amnesty International, government-sanctioned torture is verified in one-third of the countries in the world. The physical and psychological sequelae are numerous. Thomsen et al. [14] studied the pain diagnosis, characterizing pain types as nociceptive, visceral, or neuropathic. Torture victims from the Middle East, treated at the Rehabilitation and Research Centre for Torture Victims (RCT) in Copenhagen, participated in the study. The patients were referred to a pain specialist for evaluation of unsolved pain problems. Eighteen male torture victims were examined. Twelve patients experienced pain at more than three locations. Nociceptive and neuropathic pain were demonstrated in all patients. Specific neuropathic pain conditions were related to the following four types of physical torture: Palestinian hanging, falanga, beating and kicking of the head, and positional torture. When treating torture victims, it is important to know about torture methods, to think differently than normal on etiological and pathogenetic factors and always consider the presence of neuropathic pain.

Ongoing Efforts

The IASP offers visiting lectureships and consultations to assist nascent pain programs in the LDCs. It also has a "adopt a member" program, to pair members in the developed world with those in the LDCs to encourage ongoing educational and experiential exchange. The IASP also offers translation and publication of monographs into various languages as well as travel grants to attend its world congress.

The World Institute of Pain (WIP) (founded 1993) has helped train and provide a global forum for pain physicians from around the world. In 2010, the WIP Foundation was established and provides fellowships for physicians from LDCs to attend programs conducted by the WIP.

Conclusion

It is indeed frustrating that 20 years on from the first recognition of the paucity of pain management in the LDCs, only modest improvements have been made. Anesthesiologists must take the opportunity to teach pain medicine in LDCs along with supporting efforts to establish pain clinics.

References

1. World Health Organization Briefing Note. Access to controlled medications programme. Developing WHO clinical guidelines on pain treatment. Feb 2009. Medicines Access and Rational Use, Department of Essential Medicines and Pharmaceutical Policies Health Systems and Services, World Health Organization.
2. Graham WJ, Cairns J, Bhattacharya S, et al. Maternal and perinatal conditions. In: Jamison DT, Breman JG, Measham AR, et al., editors. Disease control priorities in developing countries. 2nd ed. New York: The World Bank and Oxford University Press; 2006. p. 499–529.
3. Imarengiaye CO, Ande AB. Demand and utilisation of labour analgesia service by Nigerian women. J Obstet Gynaecol. 2006;26:130–2.
4. The First International Survey on Availability of Opioids for Cancer Pain Management: Data Results for Africa, Asia, Latin America & the Caribbean and the Middle East. Data available by region from: http://www.esmo.org/Policy/International-Access-to-Opioids-Survey
5. Human Rights Watch. Global State of Pain Treatment: Access Palliative Care as a Human Right. May 2011. Available from: http://www.hrw.org/sites/default/files/reports/hhr0511W.pdf
6. Cleary J, for the Pain and Policy Study Group. Improving opioid availability for pain and palliative care: a guide to a pilot evaluation of national policy. Madison, WI: University of Wisconsin Carbone Cancer Center; 2013.
7. World Health Organization. Cancer pain relief with a guide to opioid availability. Geneva: World Health Organization; 1996. p. 43.
8. De Lima L, Sweeney C, Palmer JL, Bruera E. Potent analgesics are more expensive for patients in developing countries: a comparative study. J Pain Palliat Care Pharmacother. 2004;18:59–70.
9. Rajagopal MR, Joranson DE, Gilson AM. Medical use, misuse, and diversion of opioids in India. Lancet. 2001;358:139–43.
10. Charlton E. The management of post operative pain. Update Anaesth. 1997;7:1–7.
11. Akinyemi OO, Famewo CE. Pioneering a Pain clinic in a developing country. The first two years. J Pain Suppl. 1981;1:299.
12. Dengue Fever. Centers for Disease Control and Prevention. National Center for Emerging and Zoonotic Infectious Diseases. Atlanta, GA. http://www.cdc.gov/dengue/. Accessed 28 May 2014.
13. Stump PR, Baccarelli R, Marciano LH, Lauris JR, Teixeira MJ, Ura S, Virmond MC. Neuropathic pain in leprosy patients. Int J Lepr Other Mycobact Dis. 2004;72(2):134–8.
14. Thomsen AB, Eriksen J, Smidt-Nielsen K. Chronic pain in torture survivors. Forensic Sci Int. 2000;108(3):155–63.

Living the Mission in Serbia and Other Less Affluent Worlds

20

Miodrag Milenovic

Introduction

Teaching, learning, and anesthesia practice has changed globally, together with medical science during the last few decades. An important development has happened, especially in economically prosperous regions. Recent years have been more dynamic and have produced more professionally challenges for anesthesia societies in less affluent countries, than occurred in the previous half century. Globalization of knowledge, dynamic communication, and transfer of technology saved some time, efforts, planning, and resources but still takes significant effort to ensure that anesthesia in low-income countries can reach internationally accepted standards. It is difficult to standardize access to medical service, quality, and safety in highly populated areas without an organized modern health system [1].

Evolution and undoubted improvement in everyday clinical practice was scientifically, but also strategically guided by international professional organizations. National anesthesia societies, universities, and anesthesia departments mostly were helpful, but crucial was the personal initiative of proactive individuals with a strong vision. International professional societies, charitable associations, nongovernmental and governmental organizations, philanthropic efforts, together with industrial and pharmaceutical development facilitated changes the basic needs of the vast majority of the global population, as well as in less-affluent parts of the world [2]. A lot of educational possibilities, ethical dilemmas and safety issues came along with undoubted good intentions. Outreach medical missions are a significant part of these efforts. A number of various models of medical outreach have shown the ability to create sustainable change through education, which is much more needed than episodic impact [3].

History

Some fields of Anesthesia, Intensive Therapy and Pain in Serbia and the region were organized in the early 1950s of the last century. Good structured and sufficiently founded anesthesia, synchronised with the latest modern standards at that time was achieved in the late 1970s and 1980s [4]. Theoretical background was obtained by the pioneers and teachers of Anesthesia trained abroad, at the best modern medical systems at that time. Later on, during the 1990s together with political instabilities, isolation, wars, and economic crisis in the region, all the deterioration and devastation happened [5]. Nearly a million refugees and internally displaced persons became a hard burden for the public health system.

M. Milenovic, M.D. (✉)
Department Anesthesiology and Intensive Care Medicine, Emergency Center, Clinical Center of Serbia, Pasterova 2, Belgrade 11000, Serbia
e-mail: milenx@eunet.rs

R. Roth et al. (eds.), *The Role of Anesthesiology in Global Health: A Comprehensive Guide*,
DOI 10.1007/978-3-319-09423-6_20, © Springer International Publishing Switzerland 2015

Education

Investments in education are strongly related to the economic system of one country and Gross Domestic Product (GDP), so less affluent parts of the world suffer a lot and sustain serious human resource problems in education. Life expectancy, mother and infant mortality rate, recognition and treatment of curable illnesses on time, pain treatment, and other variables are measurable in the process of quality evaluation of the education and medical care. There is no doubt that strong influence in education is possible during short-term medical missions. In an increasingly globalized world, it is not likely that medical missions will be less needed in the near future. What should be changed in strategy if possible is that health care professionals instead of tending to treat patients with illnesses do more in education, prevention and earlier detection [6] (Fig. 20.1).

Outreach Anesthesia Team Benefit

Surgical and anesthesiology education as a part of the international mission's curriculum with the basic aim to provide help to those who work in resource-poor areas of the world and care for underserved populations may be significant for the anesthesia professionals practicing in well-equipped and well-provided, resourceful environment. The visiting mission teams have an opportunity to learn as much as the people they are helping and teaching, because this is a two-way process [3] (Fig. 20.2). The importance is in the opportunity to practice anesthesia with a less developed technology and older generation of anesthesia drugs, which are mostly abandoned because of safety issues, new and improved products, or simply because they are much cheaper than recently developed [7]. The level of infrastructure development on the European ground, especially in the non-European Union nations are so divergent, that some of the anesthesia techniques considered as a part of anesthesia history are still in use (e.g., "blind" landmark-based regional anesthetic techniques; eliciting paresthesia regional anesthesia techniques; or "blind" central venous catheter insertion techniques etc.) [8, 9].

Some other areas of the less affluent world are still struggling with the lack of basic needs like running water, electric supply, oxygen, and anesthetic gas supply, as well as no physician anesthesiologists, so training and teaching experience for the anesthesia professionals in that circumstances are priceless because of the constant safety challenges of the modern world (major climate changes, tectonic disorders, terrorism, etc.) [10].

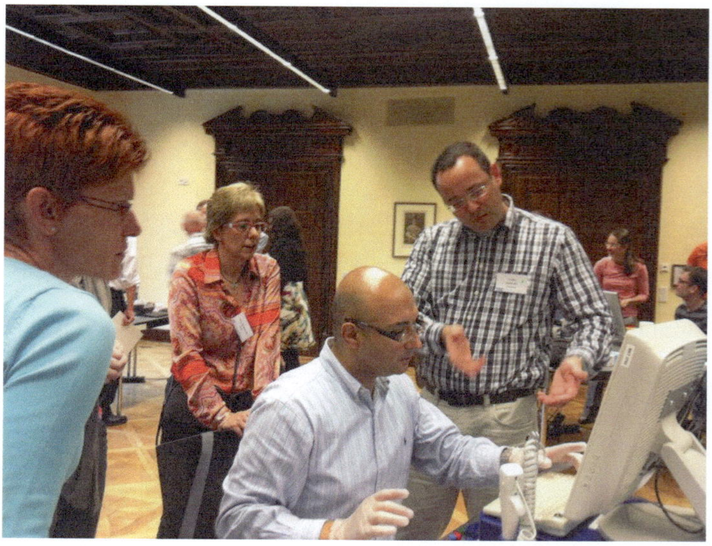

Fig. 20.1 AAF Salzburg medical seminar "Severe Bleeding Management" and point-of-care testing workshop, Salzburg, Austria, July 2012

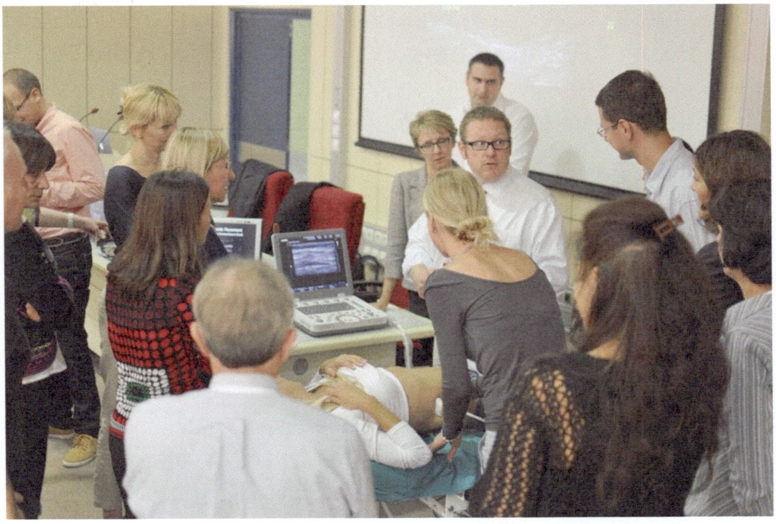

Fig. 20.2 International School of Obstetric Anesthesia, supported by WFSA, ultrasound guided regional anesthesia techniques workshop, Novi Sad, Serbia, September 2013

In the moderately developed, but still less-resourceful societies, there is significant experience with donation of necessary equipment and simultaneously organized training with the priority of teaching skills (operative or anesthesia technique), as opposed to just performing operations by the mission team, it is possible to achieve sustainable surgical care after missions are officially concluded [11].

The problems are ubiquitous. State-owned and public universities in less-affluent and post-"Iron-Curtain" societies, dominantly affiliated with public hospitals, have the tradition and exclusive rights in teaching and education of healthcare providers and future professional leaders. Archaic inherited rigid rules in education in former East European and Ex-Yugoslavia countries, as well as negative selection in teachers and leaders in anesthesia through generations, influenced the basic structure and moral views. Open-minded, intellectually independent individuals, exhausted by a long post-conflict period and economic transition, migrated and became part of the post-"Iron-Curtain" intellectual exodus named "Brain Drain." A small minority made a difficult and insecure choice, to stay and try to influence the system. All the others simply "floated with the mainstream" to become a silent part of the structure.

Local Priority Change

Health authorities detected the local need for priority change and some efforts and necessary changes have been made recently, but not enough. Private initiative in the teaching and education of healthcare providers is insufficient and not nationally standardized yet. This will be hard to achieve under the present human recourse policy. Negative and intransparent human resource selection dominates in anesthesia university departments, so now they have manpower problems relating to useful applied knowledge. Real change would be electing hard working professionals and devoted teachers with the knowledge and vision to emphasize quality, safety and professionalism, together with introducing region-specific teaching methods and problem-based learning techniques [12]. Hospitals have a dramatic problem keeping a sufficient number of trained anesthesiologists. Public sector without stable funding suffers significant governmental and international creditors influence on reduction of personal incomes and on numbers employed. Added are all previous challenges that opened the space for unethical and unmoral corrupting elements. The most vulnerable part of society and the ultimate victims are the youngest, the oldest, and the critically ill part of the population [13].

Migration of Professionals

The most important and hardest part was to detect the local needs and the people willing to facilitate the transition of knowledge and practice. The demands differed in various parts of the world and depended on the stage of development and the number of educated individuals [14]. Language barriers, not enough IT trained people and prolong periods of segregation are constant problems. Even so, a number of anesthesiologists from less affluent countries participated in international trainee exchange programs, and visited a number of university hospitals with highly developed and structured educational system [10]. They acquired personal knowledge and skills and then decided to stay permanently, instead of returning to the home country. They utilized the opportunity to change a personal lifestyle and offered to their families a better and certainly more predictable future. The personal free choice cannot be questioned, but investment in that "one-way" migration has to be considered as substantial loss of human resources [15]. The legal background of those actions came along with the opening of the European borders and the establishment of a European job market for the health care professionals [16].

Teach the Teachers in Anesthesiology

The area with obvious difficulties and a huge quality and safety gap that was detected between West and the former East European nations was anesthesiology. Some original ideas of visionary people with huge experience in education and strategically guided system development, supported and funded by WFSA Education Committee and ESA later on, offered original solutions. Systematically chosen young people from former East European nations and less-affluent parts of Europe, with teaching and leading capabilities were delegated from their national anesthesia societies (Fig. 20.3). They were exposed to practice of the modern theory of teaching and adult learning in the form of originally created "Teach the Teachers" (TTT) courses and techniques, to upgrade already acquired knowledge and to adopt new and modern ways of planning, preparation, presentation, research planning, dealing with the difficulties they can meet on the way and much more [17].

After the pilot project with participants from five national societies were concluded, more than 20 national societies delegated participants and they successfully completed the program.

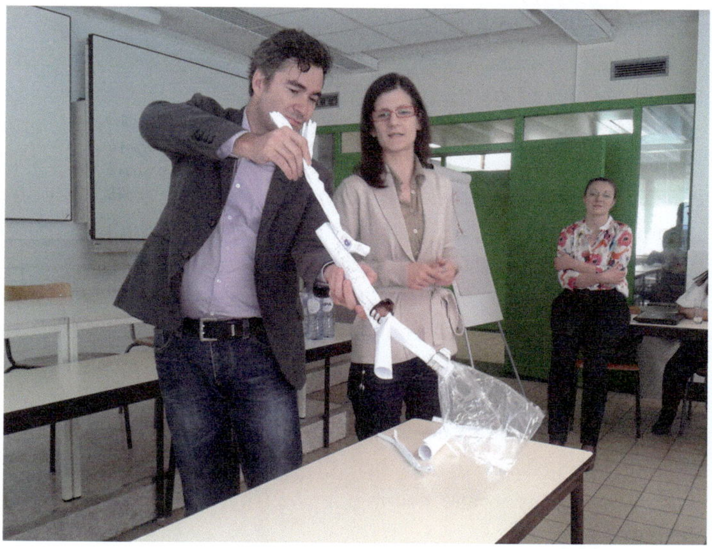

Fig. 20.3 Visual aids in teaching and simulation with low resources. "Double lumen tube and one lung ventilation simulation", by participants from Romania and Macedonia, ESA TTT course, Brussels, Belgium, April 2014

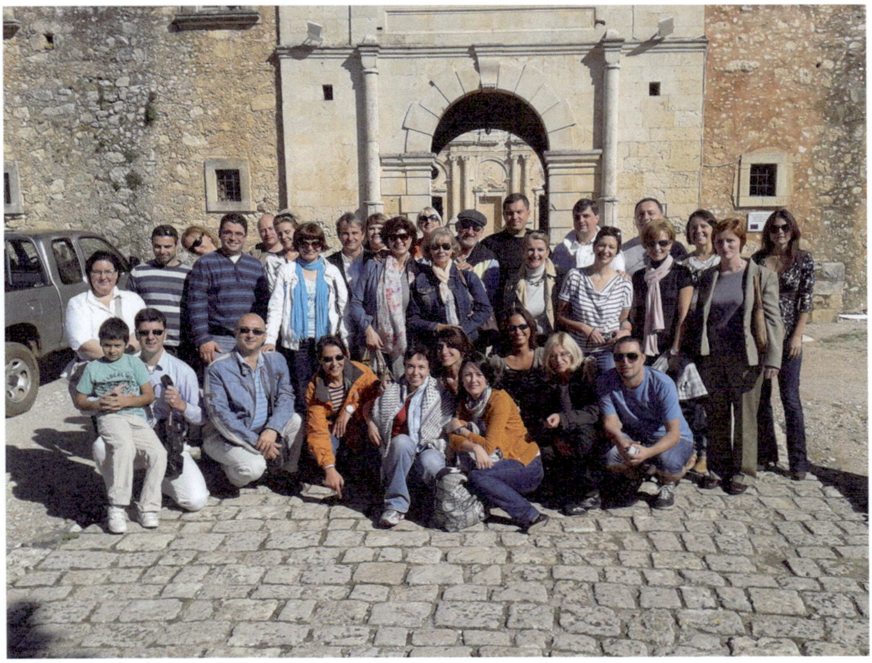

Fig. 20.4 European ISIA 3 (TTT) Course, cofounded by WFSA and ESA, Crete, Greece 2012. Participants from Latvia, Lithuania, Georgia, Croatia, Greece, Turkey, and Malta

The graduates took the obligation to detect local anesthesia needs and to start similar TTT or the original educational programs at the national level (Fig. 20.4). This strategy gave unexpectedly quick excellent results and exceeded previous format. Because of the high accomplished standards and excellent feedback from previous participants, a great number of other European nations asked to participate. Not all of the national teams gave the same results, but all have produced a substantial quality change in teaching and started the mission in their home countries. The graduates remain connected in between and have created a network of people with the same goal, to raise the level of education and anesthesia practice. They organized international events with the participants from the region, and hosted a number of quality CME programs: seminars, workshops, national congresses which created a "snowball effect."

Alumni of the TTT course named International School for Instructors in Anesthesiology (ISIA) have become devoted teachers and took leading roles in their environment: hospitals, universities, professional societies and contributed to raising the level of quality care and patient safety. The next step is to start calling for reform of postgraduate medical training structures, to define excellence in anesthesia and to redefine the role of personal merits and responsibilities [18].

International Cooperation

Several international professional organizations, some friendly foreign humanitarian organizations as well as a number of nonprofit and nongovernmental organizations, offered their help. The Serbian Association of Anesthesiologists and Intensivists (SAAI) regained its position in international professional organizations. World Federation Of Societies of Anaesthesiologists (WFSA), European Society of Anaesthesiology (ESA), the New York State Society of Anesthesiologists (NYSSA), as well as university exchange programs of the European Commission as a promotion of harmonization of education in Europe and a great number of international

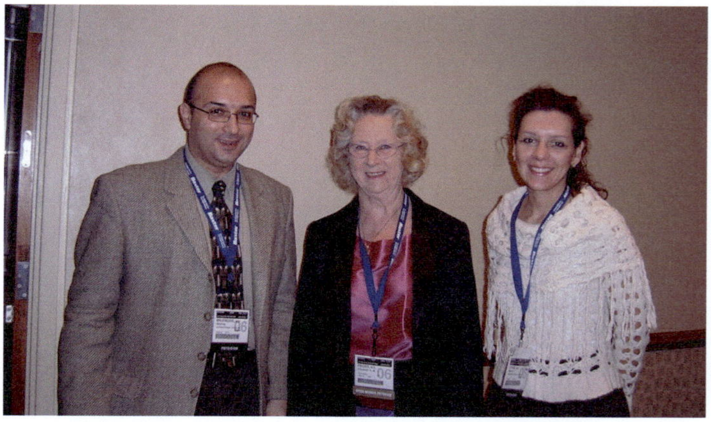

Fig. 20.5 Prof. Elizabeth Frost, chairperson of the PGA International scholar committee, with the scholars from Serbia, New York, December 2006. From the *left*: Miodrag Milenovic, Elizabeth Frost, Marina Lukic

organizations and foundations offered independent international scholarships and awards (Fig. 20.5) [19].

With intention to help in bridging the gap in medical knowledge and practice between the affluent and less-affluent worlds, significant help came from the American Austrian Foundation. Thousands of medical doctors from all over the world and hundreds from Serbia used that opportunity and spent some time for education in the highly ranked Austrian university hospitals. That gave an opportunity to gain priceless knowledge and experience and establish good interpersonal relations with the experts from abroad [20]. Our national organizations and universities hosted, co-organized, and endorsed a number of international scientific meetings and hands-on training workshops in Anesthesia subspecialty fields (pediatric, obstetric, pain, etc.), with the significant regional influence and international professional recognition.

Safety Issues

Epidemiology and safety issues of anesthesia related complications, for long were not in the focus of health authorities in less affluent societies. A number of perioperative and post-procedural crisis in anesthesia, intensive care medicine and pain therapy that might have been expected were not avoided, majorly because of inconsistency of a education and medical system and insufficiency of health authority. Numerous of unsynchronized attempts have been made globally to improve patient safety, with partial success. It is time for the health authorities of nations with developing or transitional economies to treat the patient safety issue with the greatest concern [21].

A number of former East and South European nations made great efforts to achieve a sufficient level of trained anesthesia professionals, equipment, and safety regulations, but long period of political instability and economic crisis slowing down the process. Pioneer efforts have been made to unite the political and professional influence, knowledge, and experience and to launch the first international declaration on patient safety—The Helsinki Declaration on Patient Safety in Anaesthesiology. The main initiative came from the two prominent European Anesthesia bodies: European Board of Anaesthesiology (EBA) and the European Society of Anaesthesiology (ESA). The endorsement of this important initiative came from the World Health Organization (WHO), the World Federation of Societies of Anaesthesiologists (WFSA), and the European Patients' Federation (EPF). The Declaration gave strategic foundation and short term plan for improvement to all parties in the safety process: anesthesiology professionals, industry, and patients [22, 23].

Cultural and Ethical issues

Cultural and religious background of the targeted population and ethical challenges should be considered when planning outreach missions in less affluent parts of the world. Careful planning may help in avoiding conflict with local traditions and religious beliefs. Sometime local regulations or habits are not compliant with modern western medical approach and often neglected during planning. It does not mean that certain changes for the better are not wanted or possible. Some level of reserve can be expected in the very conservative or religiously influenced societies (e.g., reproductive health and sexual behavior).

References

1. Enright A. Review article: safety aspects of anesthesia in under-resourced locations. Can J Anaesth. 2013; 60(2):152–8.
2. Eichhorn JH. Review article: practical current issues in perioperative patient safety. Can J Anaesth. 2013; 60(2):111–8.
3. Hughes SA, Jandial R. Ethical considerations in targeted paediatric neurosurgery missions. J Med Ethics. 2013;39(1):51–4.
4. Simić D, Dragović S, Budić I. History of pediatric anesthesiology. Srp Arh Celok Lek. 2007;135(1–2): 111–7.
5. Vucovic D. The development of anaesthesia in Serbia. The newsletter of the association of anaesthetists of Great Britain and Ireland. ISSN 0959-2962. The history page – Anaesthesia News June 2008 Issue 251, 17–18. http://www.aagbi.org/sites/default/files/june08.pdf. Accessed 18 Apr 2014.
6. Martiniuk AL, Manouchehrian M, Negin JA, Zwi AB. Brain gains: a literature review of medical missions to low and middle-income countries. BMC Health Serv Res. 2012;12:134.
7. Adudu OP, Isa I, Longway FO. Trends in intraoperative pain relief in anesthesized Nigerian pediatric patients: implications for a developing economy. Ann Afr Med. 2011;10(3):233–7.
8. Howe KL, Malomo AO, Bernstein MA. Ethical challenges in international surgical education, for visitors and hosts. World Neurosurg. 2013;80(6):751–8.
9. McDermott G, Korba E, Mata U, Jaigirdar M, Narayanan N, Boylan J, Conlon N. Should we stop doing blind transversus abdominis plane blocks? Br J Anaesth. 2012;108(3):499–502.
10. LeBrun DG, Chackungal S, Chao TE, Knowlton LM, Linden AF, Notrica MR, Solis CV, McQueen KA. Prioritizing essential surgery and safe anesthesia for the post-2015 development agenda: operative capacities of 78 district hospitals in 7 low- and middle-income countries. Surgery. 2014;155(3):365–73.
11. Duenas VJ, Hahn EJ, Aryan HE, Levy MV, Jandial R. Targeted neurosurgical outreach: 5-year follow-up of operative skill transfer and sustainable care in Lima, Peru. Childs Nerv Syst. 2012;28(8):1227–31.
12. Dubowitz G, Evans FM. Developing a curriculum for anaesthesia training in low- and middle-income countries. Best Pract Res Clin Anaesthesiol. 2012; 26(1):17–21.
13. Paredes-Solís S, Andersson N, Ledogar RJ, Cockcroft A. Use of social audits to examine unofficial payments in government health services: experience in South Asia, Africa, and Europe. BMC Health Serv Res. 2011;11 Suppl 2:S12.
14. Lipnick M, Mijumbi C, Dubowitz G, Kaggwa S, Goetz L, Mabweijano J, Jayaraman S, Kwizera A, Tindimwebwa J, Ozgediz D. Surgery and anesthesia capacity-building in resource-poor settings: description of an ongoing academic partnership in Uganda. World J Surg. 2013;37(3):488–97.
15. Blacklock C, Ward AM, Heneghan C, Thompson M. Exploring the migration decisions of health workers and trainees from Africa: a meta-ethnographic synthesis. Soc Sci Med. 2014;100:99–106.
16. Costigliola V. Mobility of medical doctors in cross-border healthcare. EPMA J. 2011;2(4):333–9.
17. Bould MD, Naik VN, Hamstra SJ. Review article: new directions in medical education related to anesthesiology and perioperative medicine. Can J Anaesth. 2012;59(2):136–50.
18. Smith AF, Glavin R, Greaves JD. Defining excellence in anaesthesia: the role of personal qualities and practice environment. Br J Anaesth. 2011;106(1):38–43.
19. Pallikarakis N, Bliznakov Z, Miklavcic D, Jarm T, Magjarevic R, Lackovic I, Pecchia L, Stagni R, Jobaggy A, Barbenel J. Promoting harmonization of BME education in Europe: the CRH-BME Tempus project. Conf Proc IEEE Eng Med Biol Soc. 2011; 2011:6522–5.
20. AAF, Newsletter of the American Austrian Foundation. Healing, Harmony, Honesty…and Hope. http://www.aaf-online.org/tl_files/externals/downloads/publications/docs/AAF_image_folder_2007.pdf. Accessed 18 Apr 2014.
21. Wilson RM, Michel P, Olsen S, Gibberd RW, Vincent C, El-Assady R, Rasslan O, Qsous S, Macharia WM, Sahel A, Whittaker S, Abdo-Ali M, Letaief M, Ahmed NA, Abdellatif A, Larizgoitia I, WHO Patient Safety EMRO/AFRO Working Group. Patient safety in developing countries: retrospective estimation of scale and nature of harm to patients in hospital. BMJ. 2012;344:e832.
22. Mellin-Olsen J, Staender S, Whitaker DK, Smith AF. The Helsinki Declaration on patient safety in anaesthesiology. Eur J Anaesthesiol. 2010;27(7): 592–7.
23. Staender S, Smith A, Brattebø G, Whitaker D. Three years after the launch of the Helsinki Declaration on patient safety in anaesthesiology: the history, the progress and quite a few challenges for the future. Eur J Anaesthesiol. 2013;30(11):651–4.

Anesthetic Management During the Lebanese Civil War

21

Anis Baraka

Introduction

The American University of Beirut (AUB) and the Faculty of Medicine and its Medical Center have been the major lifeline for the local population and foreign communities during two world wars and several local and regional crises [1]. The 15-year civil war in Lebanon caught us unprepared and stretched our resources beyond belief [2, 3]. Conflict had started after the balance of power in Lebanon became uneven. Before 1975, the Sunni dominated the coastal regions; the Shias were more in the South and the Druze in the Central Chouf. The government was in the hands of Maronite Christians and had been pro-Western since the end of the French occupation. With a large influx of Palestinians, Muslim numbers increased and opposition to the government grew. The war may have started after the fishermen in Sidon went on strike and the government moved to take over the port. Matters quickly escalated and foreign countries like Israel, Syria, Jordan, and Germany became involved. Several communist groups formed along with other more militant organizations. Alliances were made and almost as quickly broken. Chaos soon reigned. During the war that followed there were an estimated 120,000 killed and an unknown number injured with enormous property damage (Fig. 21.1a–c).

A. Baraka, M.D., F.R.C.A. (Hon.) (✉)
Department of Anesthesiology, American University of Beirut-Lebanon, Bless Street, Beirut, Lebanon
e-mail: anisbaraka@live.com

Statistics

Between April 1975 and November 1976, 8,324 casualties came though the Emergency Room of AUB (Table 21.1). The age range was newborn to 76 years but most were adult males 14–30 years; only 20 % were >30 years and 10 % <14 years. Gender differences were males 87 %, and females 13 %. Shrapnel was the cause of injury in 66 %, bullet wounds in 29 %, and blast injuries and extensive burns in 5 % [2]. Abdominal injuries were most common at 35 %, followed by chest 21 %, extremities 20 %, head 13 %, spine 2 %, mandible 1 %, and multiple injuries 8 % (Table 21.2).

Dead on Arrival

Patients dead on arrival at the Emergency Room had usually succumbed immediately from overwhelming injury or from exsanguination (Fig. 21.2a–c) Death from trauma occurs in a trimodal fashion. Fifty percent of deaths in the theater of war are immediate and result from massive injury to a major vessel, the heart, the brain, or the spinal cord. After a hiatus period, sometimes called the "golden hour," 30 % of

R. Roth et al. (eds.), *The Role of Anesthesiology in Global Health: A Comprehensive Guide*,
DOI 10.1007/978-3-319-09423-6_21, © Springer International Publishing Switzerland 2015

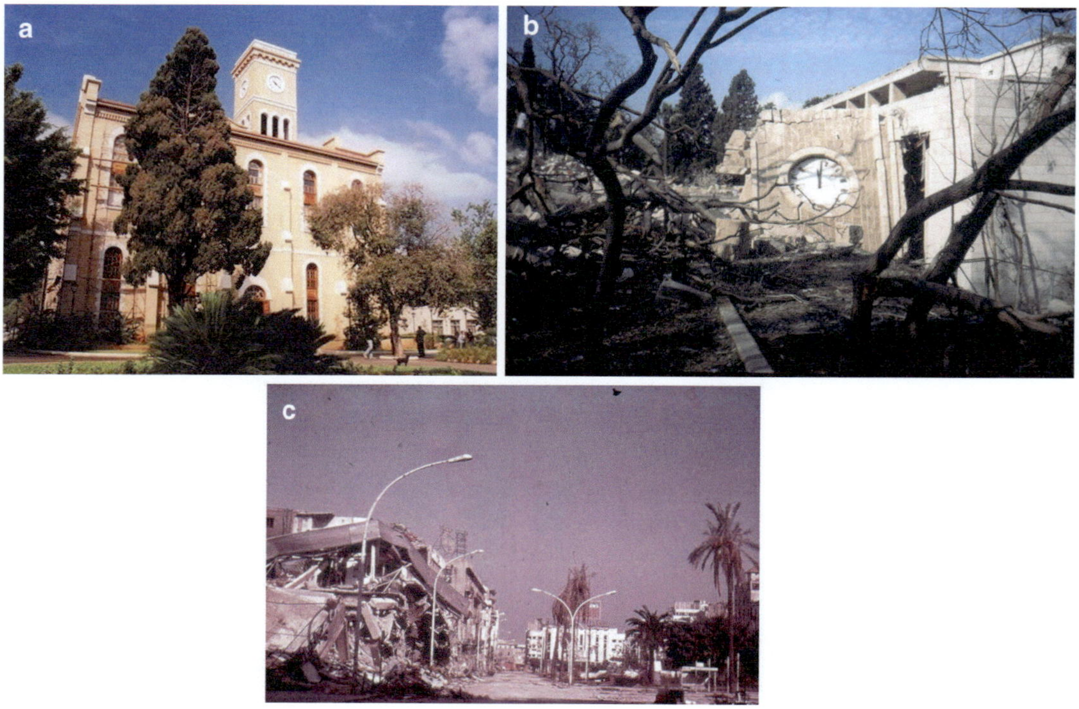

Fig. 21.1 (**a**, **b**) The AUB clock Tower before and after destruction. (**c**) Center of Beirut destroyed

deaths occur as a result of potentially treatable conditions such as hypoventilation, hemorrhage, hemopneumothorax, cardiac tamponade, or an expanding intracranial mass. Days to weeks later, 20 % of patients die from sepsis or multiple-organ failure, or both.

Triage

Triage in the emergency room (Fig. 21.3) consisted of assigning patients to one of the three categories:

1. Seriously injured patients were stabilized using measures such as fluid resuscitation, endotracheal intubation, and ventilation. They were then transferred for further investigation or surgery, or sent to the recovery room.
2. Patients with lesser injuries were taken to the outpatient department reception area, where interns and medical students managed minor problems. Patients were then discharged home.
3. Patients who were dead on arrival were transferred to the morgue.

Challenges of Anesthesia

Table 21.3 illustrates some of our challenges. Unprepared for such a massive onslaught personnel were afraid. Also, given the large exodus of many who were able to leave Lebanon, we were short not just of supplies but also of skilled people.

Oxygen and nitrous oxide were in shortest supply. We economized gas by using low flows via a carbon dioxide absorption circuit. All respirators driven by oxygen (Ohio, Bird, etc.) were retired. Finally we used compressors to feed room air into anesthesia machines. The noise of these machines compelled us to turn to simple draw over equipment such as the Epstein, Mackintosh, and Oxford (EMO) inhaler (Fig. 21.4a, b).

Table 21.1 Casualties received at the American University of Beirut Medical Center from April 1975 to November 1976

Month	Casualties treated in E.R.	Total deaths	Admitted to AUBMC from ER	Deaths in OR
1975				
April	60	1	24	0
May	38	7	9	1
June	28	0	12	0
July	41	1	24	0
Aug.	10	1	0	1
Sept	86	0	31	0
Oct.	110	1	58	1
Nov.	73	4	32	2
Dec.	235	5	58	1
1976				
Jan.	375	10	149	3
Feb.	92	4	25	2
Mar.	788	39	207	3
Apr.	609	22	135	9
May	1,114	76	243	12
June	1,131	49	245	7
July	793	52	132	1
Aug.	1,008	53	143	3
Sept.	631	33	92	2
Oct.	750	54	126	6
Nov.	352	17	57	0
	8,324	429	1,802	54
		5.15 %		2.99 %

Table 21.2 Statistical analysis of operated casualties according to their sex, age, cause, and site of injury

Sex	Male 87 %	Female 13 %
Age	70 % 14–30 years	
	20 % more than 30 years	
	10 % less than 14 years	
Cause of injury	Shrapnels 66 %	
	Bullets 66 %	
	Blast 5 %	
Site of injuries	Abdominal injuries	35 %
	Chest	21 %
	Extremities	20 %
	Head	13 %
	Spine	2 %
	Mandibular	1 %
	Multiple	8 %
Anesthesia	Ketamine induction	55 %
	Thiopentone induction	40 %
	Regional anesthesia	3 %
	No anesthesia	2 %
Blood transfusion	50 % received blood transfusion	
Intraoperative death		2.9

Reprinted from MEJA 7(1–2) 1983 by kind permission of Prof M.K.

Preoperative Assessment

As many as 150 casualties might come in simultaneously and we had to transfer more severely injured cases to the recovery room where they were assessed, resuscitated and triaged further (Fig. 21.5). Cardiac tamponade and major vessel injuries were given first priority. Life-threatening trauma cases were transferred directly to the operating room which was in close proximity to the recovery room. Table 21.4 lists our assessment.

Rapid infusion of lactated Ringer's solution via intravenous cannulae was initiated to correct hypovolemia and we proceeded with emergency surgery without waiting for blood. Blood transfusion was given in 50 % of cases usually with fresh blood donated by relatives and militia comrades. Simple clinical criteria such as adequate urine output, blood pressure, and pulse rate assessed replacement therapy.

Arterial blood gas analyses were available as were blood warmers. Metabolic acidemia was corrected by sodium bicarbonate according to the equation

$$\text{Base deficit}: \frac{\text{Body weight}\left(\text{kg}\right)}{5} \times \text{Base deficit}\left(\text{mEq / kg}\right).$$

Severely shocked patients were given 1 mEq/kg of sodium bicarbonate on arrival but routine bicarbonate administration according to the amount of transfused blood was not done because of the extreme variability in acid–base response to multiple blood transfusions. Rapid correction of acidemia was followed by cardiac arrest in two patients.

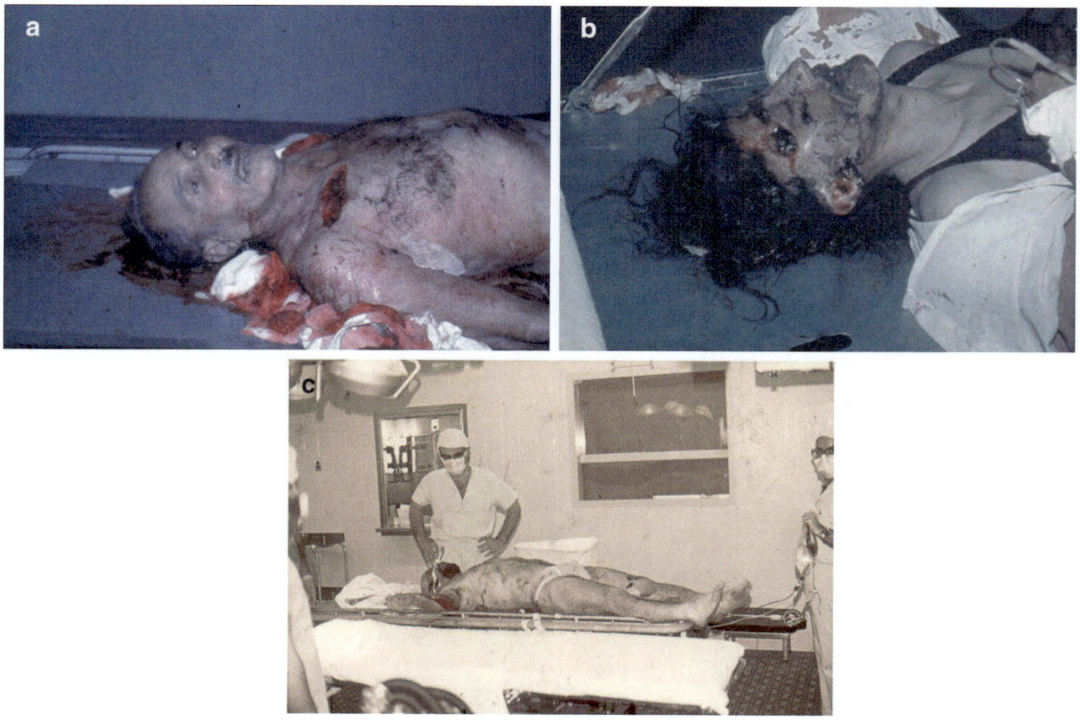

Fig. 21.2 (**a**, **b**) Death on arrival. (**c**) Death in the operating room

Fig. 21.3 Emergency room during an attack

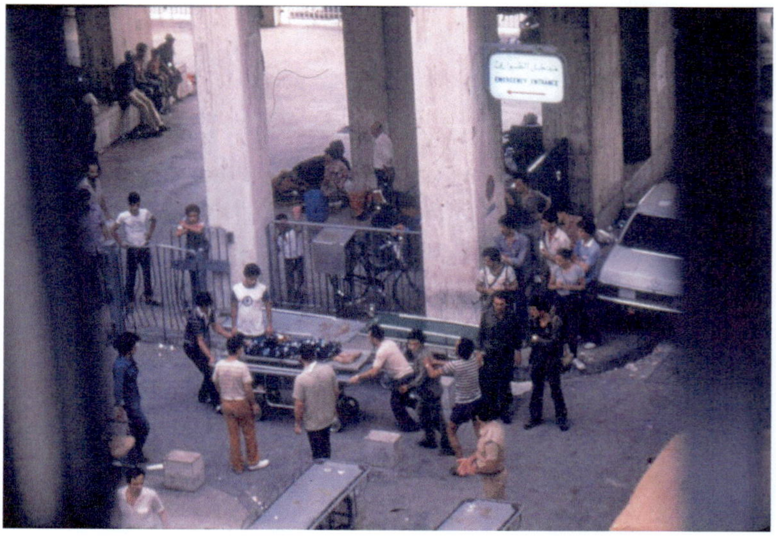

Many patients with head injuries required ventilator support and were intubated and hyperventilated before surgery in the hope of stabilizing intracranial pressure. Intubating patient with facial injuries was challenging, most surgeons preferred nasotracheal intubation, perhaps ill-advised in the presence of maxillary and basal skull fractures. Figure 21.6 shows the most severe facial injury we treated. Tracheotomy under local anesthesia was done before general anesthesia could be administered. Neck injuries often involved the spine, trachea, esophagus, and/or the great vessels.

Chest injuries included flail chest, hemothorax, and pneumothorax which necessitated tracheal intubation and underwater seal drainage. Cardiac injuries and cardiac tamponade were explored immediately [4]. Abdominal injury especially liver and splenic injuries required prompt attention to control internal bleeding.

Table 21.3 Statistical analysis of operated casualties according to their sex, age, cause, and site of injury

1. Problems related to the civil war itself
2. Personnel deficiency (death, exodus, isolation, and nervous exhaustion)
3. Deficiency of supplies particularly oxygen and nitrous oxide
4. Work load
5. Problems of anaesthesia of the seriously traumatized patients such as (a) respiratory failure (b) shock, cardiac tamponade, flail chest… (c) full stomach
6. Special problems (a) postoperative respiratory failure (b) tetanus (c) gas gangrene (d) decompression sickness

Reprinted from MEJA 7(1–2) 1983 by kind permission of Prof M. Khatib

Anesthetic Management of Head, Neck, and Faciomaxillary Injuries

Head and neck injuries secondary to bullets, shrapnel, and/or glass were frequent. These injuries involved the faciomaxillary structures, the upper airways and the carotid arteries, as well as the head and the cervical spine. Management of these patients followed a comprehensive approach that included safe transfer of the patient, airway management, and hemodynamic resuscitation.

Faciomaxillary Injury

At least one-third of the casualties suffered from faciomaxillary injury. The maxilla was the most commonly involved facial structure (24 %), followed by the mandible (18 %). Most maxillary fractures were of the compound comminuted type. Le Fort I (the transverse fracture), Le Fort II (the pyramidal fracture), and Le fort III (craniofacial disjunction) followed in order of decreasing frequency, but were rarely in the simple or classical forms. Also, most mandibular fractures were of the compound comminuted type. Mandibular fractures involved the body, the parasymphyseal area, the condyle, the alveolar margin, the angle, and ascending ramus and the

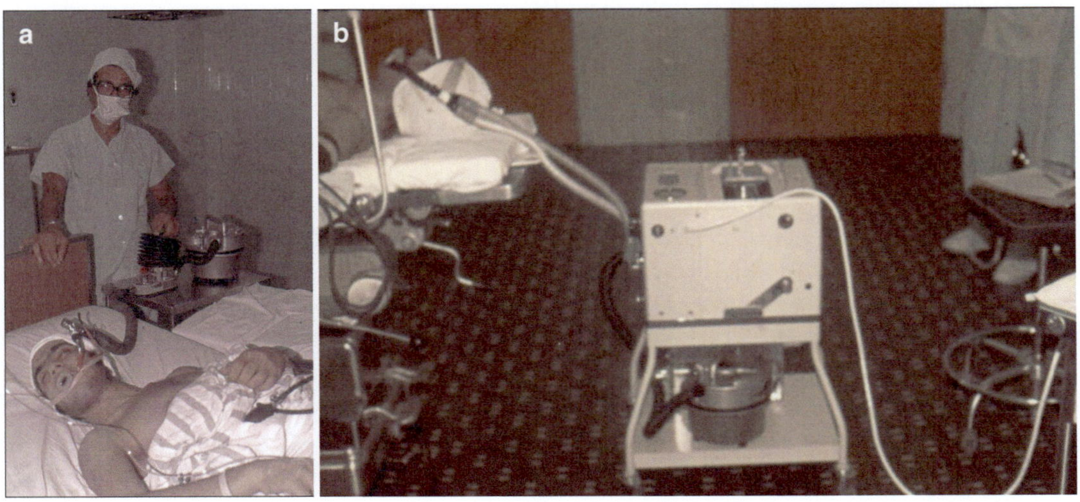

Fig. 21.4 (**a**, **b**) Patient anesthetized with ether using the EMO inhaler. The EMO inhaler connected to the Radcliffe respirator

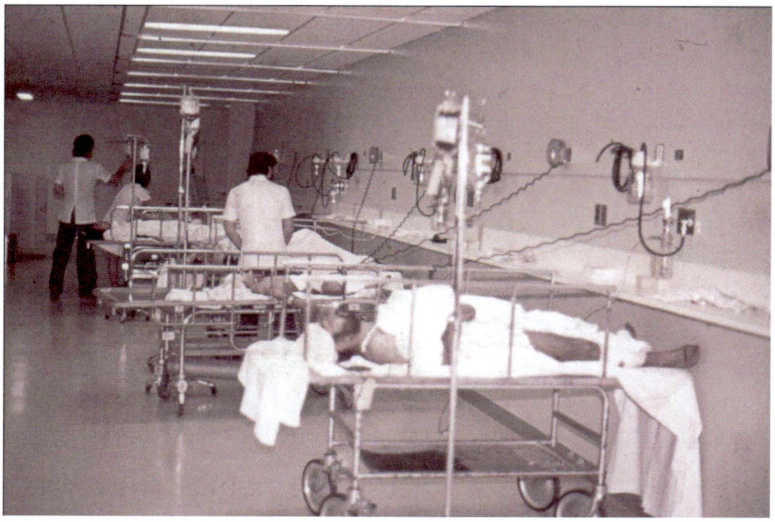

Fig. 21.5 The recovery room open 24 h, and accommodating up to 50 patients. Its function was often modified to serve as a preoperative and postoperative surgical intensive care

Table 21.4 Assessment of Injury

1.	Adequate respiration and patent airway
2.	Blood loss
3.	Tissue damage
4.	Possible fractures
5.	C.N.S. or spinal cord injuries
6.	Effect of injury on pulmonary, cardiovascular, renal, cerebral, and hepatic organs
7.	Evidence of recent use of alcohol as drug abuse

coronoid process in decreasing frequency. Since the mandible is a tubular bone, it is most vulnerable to fracture where the cortex is thin and, hence, most fractures occur in the ramus, while the second most common point of fracture is at the first or second molar.

Management of the Traumatized Airway

Adequate management starts with recognition of the traumatized airway and knowing the common patterns of disruption, as well as the different techniques of securing the airway. It must be emphasized that airway injuries are dynamic rather than static, and hence close observation is essential. Most catastrophes occur when possible difficulty with the airway is not recognized. It may be safer to consider all patients with upper airway injury as potentially hypoxic, with a compromised airway and as having recently eaten. Essential monitoring includes continuous ECG and pulse oximetry. Awake examination of the airway and preoxygenation must be carried out before any attempt is made to commence anesthesia or intubate the trachea.

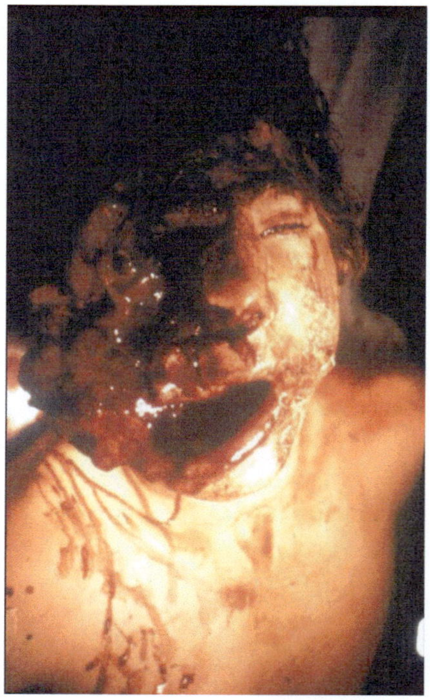

Fig. 21.6 Faciomaxillary trauma necessitating tracheostomy

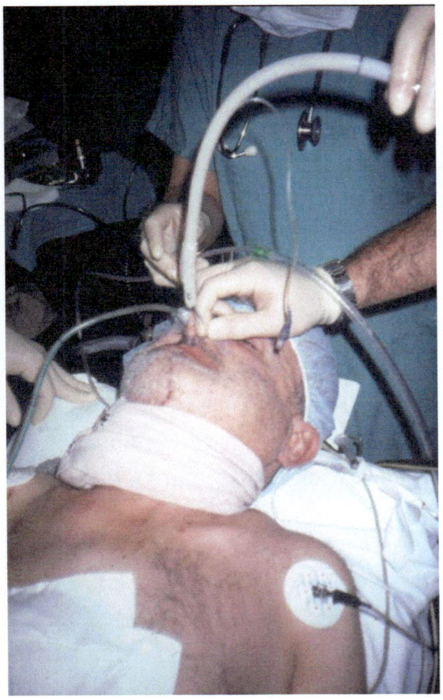

Fig. 21.7 A patient with faciomaxillary trauma. Following surgery, the TEC was reintroduced via the tracheal tube into the trachea . The trachea was extubated over the TEC which was left in situ

In patients with faciomaxillary injury, there may be airway obstruction from blood, teeth, soft tissue, vomitus, or edema. Incomplete closure of the airway will result in noisy, stertorous breathing; the patient is usually anxious, and may sit up and lean forward in order to allow gravity to assist in preventing a disrupted tongue and/or mandible from falling backward and impacting the upper airway. Placing the patient in the lateral or semi-prone position may also help to clear the airway. With severe disruption of the airway, emergency tracheostomy may be the safest method of securing the airway (Fig. 21.7).

In some patients with severe faciomaxillary trauma, the Cook tube exchange catheter (TEC) was inserted, following induction of anesthesia and direct laryngoscopy, into the trachea to facilitate tracheal intubation(Fig. 21.8). At the end of surgery, the TEC was reintroduced via the tracheal tube lumen before extubation, in order to facilitate tracheal reintubation if indicated, and to maintain postoperative oxygenation.

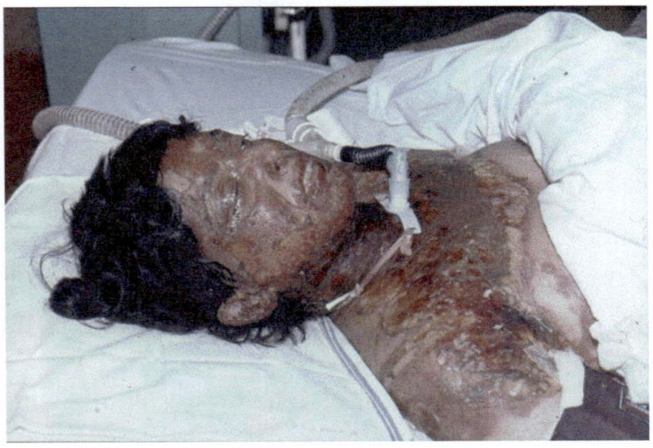

Fig 21.8 Extensive burn necessitating tracheostomy

Neck Injury

Injuries of the soft tissues were the commonest, followed by trauma to the laryngotracheal complex and the pharynx. The larynx is relatively superficial, and unprotected, and is thus vulnerable to injury, while the trachea is well protected by the thoracic cage and pulmonary tissue which will serve to cushion the effect of blunt trauma and even missile injury. Severe injury of the laryngotracheal complex mandated tracheostomy. Cervical spine fracture was always considered in patients with head and neck injury. As well, 10 % of neck injuries were complicated by carotid artery injuries. Most of the surviving patients had only carotid lacerations, but few patients reaching the hospital alive had total disruption. The patients presented either with severe hemorrhage from a neck vessel, or with a rapidly expanding neck hematoma compromising the airway. Neurologic deficits were present in about one-third of those cases. Most of the vascular injuries were repaired by end-to-end anastomosis, with or without a venous graft. A shunt was not used in the assumption that most victims were young healthy patients who had an adequate collateral circulation. Neurological deficit sequelae occurred in patients who were severely shocked, or who had a delayed transfer to the hospital.

Head Injuries

About 10 % of all casualties seen during the study period had an injury to the skull and a little more than half of them suffered a penetrating brain injury. There were three types of injury; high velocity, low velocity and tangential. Craniotomy whenever feasible was found to be superior to the accepted technique of craniectomy. It affords a wider field, better exploration, and greater decompression and does not have the disadvantage of requiring a second operation for cranioplasty. Mortality and morbidity rates were no higher than for craniectomy. Retained fragments of bone are not as dangerous as is widely believed. If a thorough debridement of the brain is carried out with perfect hemostasis, one or two deeply placed bone fragments have no deleterious effect, at least for the period of our follow-up ranging from 3 to 15 months. However, patients with retained bone fragments should be closely observed for at least 6 weeks. Traumatic aneurysms are not as rare as the literature indicated. Routine postoperative arteriography was carried out [5].

Spinal Cord Transection-Autonomic Hyperreflexia

Spinal cord injuries carried with them the risk of later development of autonomic hyperreflexia.

Traditionally, autonomic hyperreflexia has been attributed to massive unchecked reflex sympathetic discharge that occurs below the level of spinal cord transection in patients with chronic spinal cord injury. In neurologically intact individuals, spinal sympathetic outflow is modulated by inhibitory impulses from higher centers in the central nervous system. In patients with spinal cord transection, the spinal sympathetic outflow is isolated from restraining supraspinal influence, and hence stimulation below the level of cord transection initiates an exaggerated autonomic reflex, resulting in excessive vasoconstriction below the level of cord injury with marked elevation of the blood pressure. Elevation of the blood pressure will be sensed by the baroreceptors resulting in reflex bradycardia and vasodilation above the level of transection. About 85 % of patients with transection above T6 exhibit the reflex.

Moreover plasma catecholamines (epinephrine and norepinephrine) are subnormal in patients with cord transection. During autonomic hyperreflexia, the level of norepinephrine increases but still does not exceed the resting level of control normal patients. Thus, patients with chronic spinal cord transection have a subnormal sympathetic tone, even during an attack of autonomic hyperreflexia. The results suggest that the excessive reflex elevation of blood pressure in patients with spinal cord transection is not secondary to autonomic hyperreflexia, but is rather due to a denervation supersensitivity response to the released norepinephrine.

Although many patients with spinal cord injuries were not candidates for immediate surgery, they often developed later complications that required intervention, especially adequate anesthetic management [6].

Limb Injuries

No matter how efficient the eventual management of war injuries may be, good results depend on early proper treatment. Essential first-aid, energetic resuscitation, wound excision plus delayed primary closure and coverage of the wound with split thickness graft at the proper time, and immobilization are the essential principles that have been learnt from war surgery [7]. They must be applied to missile wounds in particular those resulting from high velocity bullets, and high velocity fragments from explosive blasts (Fig. 21.9). These principles must be understood by all who are concerned with the treatment of wounded patients. They have stood the test of time and sadly they have to be relearned the hard way in every war [7].

Techniques of Anesthesia

General anesthesia was used in 95 % of the cases, while regional analgesia was only used in 3 % and no anesthesia in 2 %. Regional analgesia was limited in the emergency situation because of the severity and multiplicity of trauma and because of the associated shock and/or respiratory failure.

All patients were considered as full stomachs and rapid sequence induction anesthesia was used in most with application of the Sellick maneuver [8].

Preoxygenation

Preoxygenation is widely accepted to increase oxygen reserves and delay the onset of arterial oxygen desaturation during subsequent periods of apnea. For many years, tidal volume breathing for 3–5 min has been commonly practiced as the standard technique for preoxygenation. However, eight deep breaths within 60 s can produce maximal preoxygenation, and is followed with slower desaturation than that following the traditional tidal volume preoxygenation [9, 10].

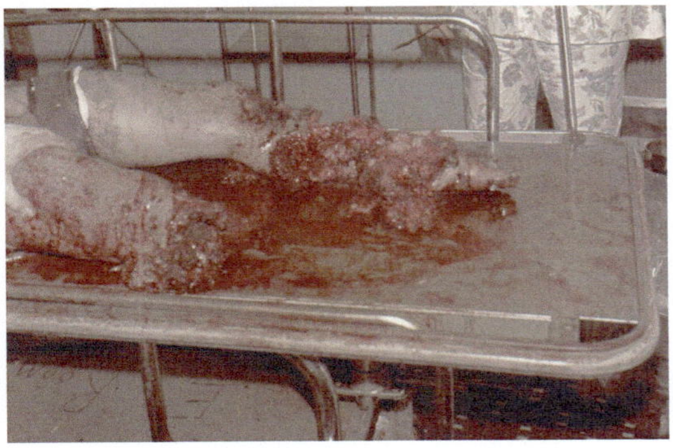

Fig. 21.9 Limb injury

Confirmation of Tracheal Intubation

Auscultation of breath sounds is the traditional technique for confirming tracheal intubation and end-tidal capnography has been used since the mid-1980s. Capnography was not available to us, and we relied on the self-inflating bulb of the esophageal detector devices to confirm tracheal intubation (Fig. 21.10a–c). The underlying principle is that the esophagus collapses when a negative pressure is applied to its lumen, while the trachea does not. Nunn utilized a self-inflating bulb (SIB) of 75–90 ml capacity. After tracheal intubation, the device is connected to the tracheal tube, and the bulb is compressed. Compression is silent and refill is instantaneous if the tube is in the trachea. In contrast, if the tube is in the esophagus, compression of the SIB is accompanied by a characteristic flatus-like noise, and the SIB remains collapsed on release [11]. The technique

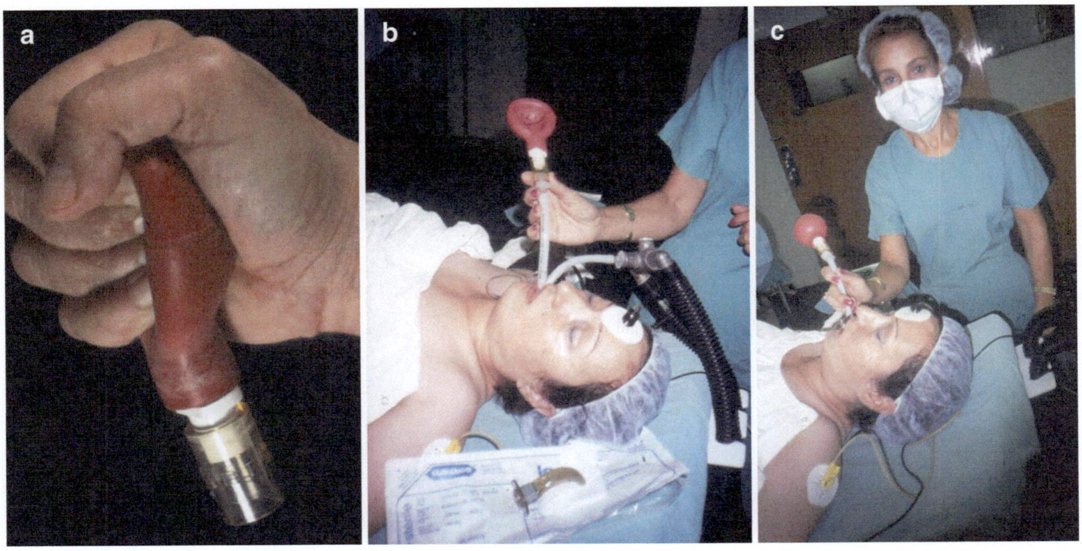

Fig. 21.10 The self-inflating bulb (SIB) for confirmation tracheal versus esophageal intubation. (**a**) SIB. (**b**) The bulb remained collapsed denoting esophageal intubation. (**c**) The bulb refilled denoting tracheal intubation

was modified by compressing the SIB before rather than after, connection to the tracheal tube connector [12].

Anesthesia

Anesthesia was induced in 55 % of patients with ketamine 2 mg/kg intravenously for induction and followed by 1 mg/kg every half an hour for maintenance. Tracheal intubation was facilitated by succinylcholine 100 mg. while pancuronium was used to maintain muscular relaxation. Controlled ventilation was achieved either manually by the Ambu bag, or by connecting the tracheal tube to an electrically driven respirator such as the Radcliffe or Emerson. No significant operative awareness or post-operative hallucinations were observed following pure ketamine anesthesia in shocked patients, despite the limitation of premedication to atropine. PaO_2 and $PaCO_2$ were adequately maintained, as spot checked by arterial blood gas analysis (Table 21.5).

The E.M.O. (Epstein, Macintosh, Oxford) draw-over ether inhaler proved itself during this crisis. Following intubation and connection to the E.M.O. inhaled anesthesia was maintained with 3 % ether and pancuronium, while controlling respiration manually. The E.M.O. could be also connected to the air inlet of a Radcliffe respirator (Fig. 21.11a, b). Both ether and ketamine anesthesia maintained stable circulation, provided the blood volume was maintained.

Such simple techniques of anesthesia proved their safety. In rush hours, one anesthesiologist might cover up to five operating rooms at the same time. The patient was anesthetized, monitored by EKG, attached to the respirator, and was left attended by a student, a nurse, or a technician and occasionally unattended except by the surgeon.

Table 21.5 Arterial blood gas analysis (PO2, PCO2, and pH) in traumatized and anesthetized patients ventilated

	PO2 (mm Hg)	PCO2 (mm Hg)	pH
	90	16	7.63
	65	37	7.45
	90	23	7.58
	92	21	7.6
	50	30	7.56
	100	19	7.7
	85	40	7.37
	90	41	7.4
	90	25	7.66
	110	30	7.49
	120	25	7.51
	118	17	7.6
	110	22	7.54
Mean	93.0	26.6	7.54

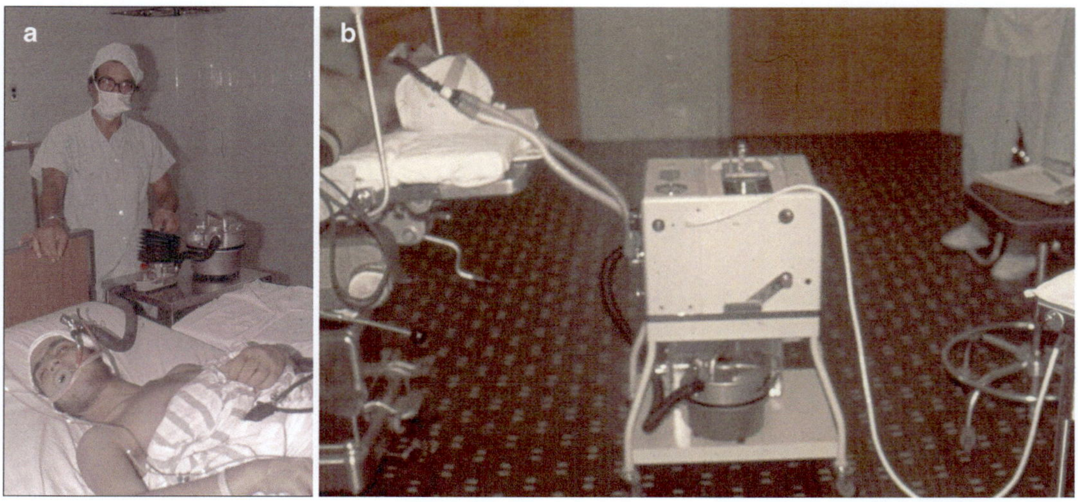

Fig. 21.11 (**a**) Ventilating with an EMO draw-over inhaler and (**b**) a Radcliffe respirator

Specific Problems Specific Problems

1. *Respiratory failure*

 Patients with multiple injuries and head injuries were artificially ventilated. Spinal cord injuries associated with quadriplegia, chest injuries, particularly those associated with flail chest and/or severe lung lacerations, and massive abdominal injuries also necessitated respiratory support. The "shock lung syndrome" resulting from multiple factors such as: aspiration, fat emboli, pulmonary edema, massive blood transfusion and/or shock all necessitated prolonged I.P.P.V. using PEEP and high FIO2. Weaning was sometimes delayed and problematic (Fig. 21.12).

2. *Tetanus*

 We treated 11 patients with tetanus following trauma. The cases were classified into mild, moderate, or severe according to the clinical picture, incubation period (injury-trismus), and onset period (trismus-convulsions) (Tables 21.6 and 21.7, Fig. 21.13). The severity of tetanus correlated better with the onset period rather than the incubation period. All cases of severe tetanus required intubation to be followed by tracheostomy, curarization, and intermittent positive pressure ventilation. The period on respiratory control varied between 5 and 55 days (average 4 weeks).

 None of the mild cases of tetanus died, while three of the moderate and severe cases died from secondary to sepsis, pulmonary embolism, and respiratory failure. Another case of severe tetanus developed a compression fracture of the dorsal spine during convulsions.

3. *Gas gangrene* (Fig. 21.14)

 Several patients developed gas gangrene. Anaerobic infections, particularly those due to clostridial organisms, respond dramatically to hyperbaric oxygenation. We did not have enough oxygen and could only manage ten patients using 7–9 sessions each limited to 2 h reaching

Table 21.6 Cases of tetanus classified according to incubation period

		Incubation period (injury-trismus)		
Severity	No.	14 days	10–14 days	10 days
Mild	3	2	1	0
Moderate	2	2	0	0
Sever	6	2	2	3

Table 21.7 Cases of tetanus classified according to onset period

Severity	No.	Incubation period (injury-trismus)		
		7 days	3–7 days	3 days
Mild	3	3	–	–
Moderate	2	–	1	1
Sever	6	–	–	6

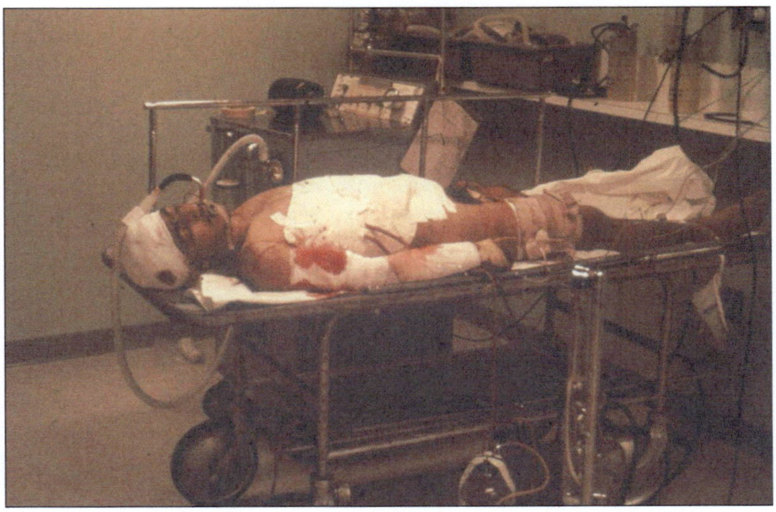

Fig. 21.12 Patient with multiple injuries necessitating respiratory support

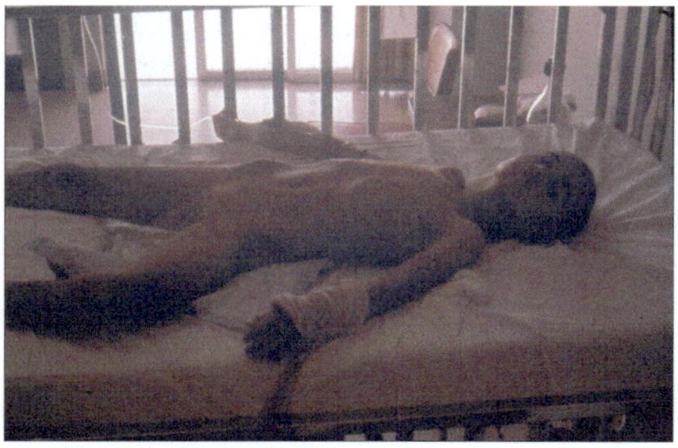

Fig. 21.13 Child suffering from tetanus

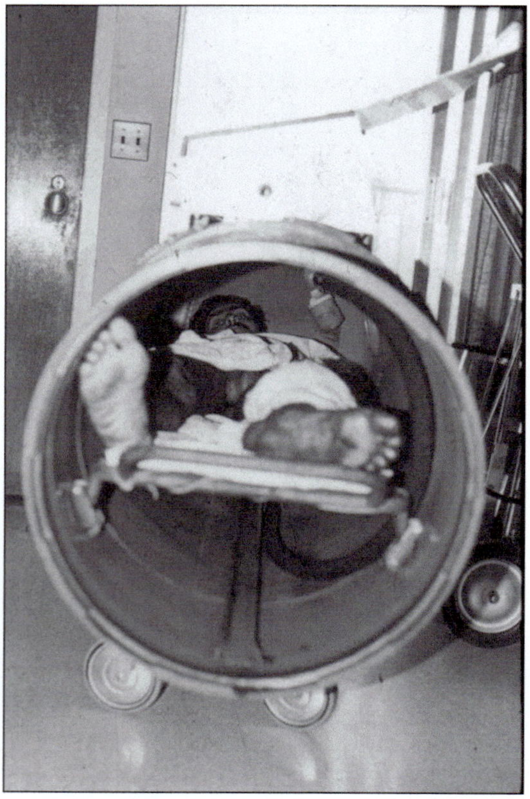

Fig. 21.14 A patient with gas gangrene inside the compression chamber to undergo hyperbaric oxygen therapy

three absolute atmospheres (3 AT.A.). Some surgeons amputated the affected areas first and then put the patient in the compression chamber, while others believed that the patient should be put first in the compression chamber.

Our compression chamber was small and portable and could only accommodate the patient (Fig. 21.14).

Brain Death

Because of the increasing number of casualties in face of the shortage of personnel, supplies, and space, some guidelines depending on brain function were established to be applied according to the injuries and circumstances:

1. Total support: normal brain function or brain failure with potential reversibility.
2. All but CPR (cardiopulmonary resuscitation): normal brain function or brain failure with potential reversibility + irreversible vital organ failure.
3. No extraordinary measures: severe irreversible brain failure with only minimal neurological activity + irreversible other vital organ failure.
4. Brain death.

Unfortunately, we could not manage all patients even those in the first two categories. Death was surrounding us, and often we could not prevent it.

Acknowledgement I am extremely grateful to Dr. Mohamad Khatib, Managing Editor of the Middle East Journal of Anesthesiology and Director of the Respiratory Therapy Department, for reviewing my report and granting permission to reprint several figures that are published in the Middle East Journal of Anesthesiology 7(1–2), pp 41–53, 1983.

References

1. Khuri RN. The summer of 1982. M E J Anaesth. 1983;7(1–2):107.
2. Baraka A. Anaesthetic problems during the tragic civil war in Lebanon. M E J Anesth. 1983;7(1–2): 41–53.
3. Shehadi SI. Anatomy of a hospital in distress. M E J Anaesth. 1983;7(1–2):21–7.
4. Slim M, Yacoubian HD, Dagher I. Penetrating injuries of the heart and great vessels. M E J Anaesth. 1983;7(1–2):94–104.
5. Haddad FS. (Wilder Penfield Lecture) Nature and management of penetrating head injuries during the civil war in Lebanon. M E J Anesth. 1983; 7(1–2):73–5.
6. Baraka A. Is it autonomic hyperreflexia or denervation supersensitivity. M E J Anaesth. 1989;10(2):95–7.
7. Nsouli A. War injuries of limbs. Basic principles of management. M E J Anaesth. 1983;7(1–2):137–40.
8. Baraka A. "Crash induction" in patients with full stomach. M E J Anaesth. 1979;5(4):283.

9. Baraka AS, Taha SK, Aouad MT, et al. Preoxygenation: comparison of maximal breathing and tidal volume breathing techniques. Anesthesiology. 1999;91:612–5.
10. Benumof JL. Preoxygenation. Best method for both efficiency and efficacy (editorial). Anesthesiology. 1999;91:603–5.
11. Nunn JF. The oesophageal detector device. Anaesthesia. 1988;43:804.
12. Baraka A. The oesophageal detector device. Anaesthesia. 1971;45:697.

Trauma, War, and Managing Vascular and Orthopedic Injuries

22

John Benjamin and John Rotruck

Introduction

There are marked differences in trauma anesthesia between the dedicated trauma center in the developed world and the care that is rendered under less than ideal conditions in the wartime environment. These differences include the variety of injuries that can be anticipated. While the clinical guidelines of US and NATO military medicine units are referenced here, similar protocols may be encountered among other military units. Preoperative evaluation and resuscitation of war-injured patients, their intraoperative care, and the postoperative environment along with considerations for transfer to other facilities are presented. Finally, the use of regional anesthesia techniques for wartime casualties with possible benefits extending beyond the operating room is considered.

The views expressed in this chapter are those of the authors, and do not necessarily reflect the official policy or position of the Department of the Navy, Department of Defense, or the US Government.

J. Benjamin, M.D. (✉) • J. Rotruck, M.D.
Department of Anesthesia, Walter Reed National Military Medical Center, 8901 Wisconsin Avenue, Bethesda, MD 20889, USA
e-mail: john.r.benjamin2.mil@mail.mil; john.r.rotruck.mil@mail.mil

Injury Patterns

There is considerable data on injury cause and location for US military forces in conflicts from World War I all the way to the most recent decade of war in Iraq and Afghanistan [1]. It can be reasonably extrapolated that the armed forces of other first-world nations experienced similar injuries over the same time period, both in the cause and affected parts of the body. Far less data exists on the injury patterns experienced by the civilian populations in these same conflicts, or for the combatants representing guerilla armies or insurgent forces not tied to a specific nation. Nevertheless, some general observations can be made on the evolution of wartime injuries for these various groups. For all of these groups, it is important to consider the rise in use of the improvised explosive device (IED) as a cause of injury in the modern era to be of equal or greater or importance than traditional weapons of war.

Nowhere is the shift to IED-related injuries more apparent than for the armies of developed nations. During World War II, a third of injuries were due to gunfire, with the remaining majority coming from mortar rounds, artillery, and grenades. In more recent conflicts in Iraq and Afghanistan, gunfire still accounts for a quarter of injuries, but two-thirds of injuries are now due to IEDs. The injury location and severity have also evolved. Although extremity injuries have always been prevalent, they are now much more likely to be traumatic amputations due to IED

R. Roth et al. (eds.), *The Role of Anesthesiology in Global Health: A Comprehensive Guide*, DOI 10.1007/978-3-319-09423-6_22, © Springer International Publishing Switzerland 2015

blasts rather than simple gunshot or fragment wounds. Significant penetrating injuries to the thorax and abdomen are less common, which is easily explained by the widespread use of high-quality body armor in these areas. Many potentially catastrophic exposures to IED blasts result in no fatalities due to the use of heavily armored vehicles, although traumatic brain injury of varying degrees is quite common for the occupants of these vehicles, as the blast can still easily overturn the vehicle.

In contrast, the civilian population and guerilla or insurgent forces can be considered together, as they often uniformly lack any sort of body armor, helmets, or armored vehicles. For these groups, wartime injuries can and do cross the entire spectrum. In the absence of any protective equipment, exposure to an IED blast results in more battlefield fatalities before these individuals can be brought to any level of medical care.

Preoperative Assessment

Preoperative evaluation of wartime casualties begins with ensuring that they can be safely treated by the surgical team. For friendly forces, this includes having a security team remove any weapons, ammunition, and other potentially dangerous items, preferably at a point prior to entering the medical facility. This security search should also look for unexploded ordinance (i.e., an unexploded grenade), which the casualty may not even be aware of depending on the extent of their injury. This search and clearing phase is even more critically important in the case of civilians and insurgent fighters, who are essentially indistinguishable from each other. It would be a simple matter for an insurgent to present a real or simulated injury in order to gain access to the medical facility, and then detonate concealed explosives or attack the health care team with hidden weapons.

Patients may arrive via ground vehicle or on aircraft, although those being transported by air are often met by a ground vehicle at the runway or helipad for final transport to the medical facility. The extent of post-injury pre-hospital care varies greatly by the skill levels of the individuals in the field, combined with their available supplies, and the extent of ongoing hostilities. In the event of active fighting, the priority will be on protecting the fighting forces and enabling medical evacuation instead of rendering care. Likely pre-hospital interventions include obtaining intravenous access and administering crystalloids, or sometimes packed red blood cells. Occasionally, advanced airways will also be placed in the field, whether intubation with an endotracheal tube (ETT) or percutaneously with cricothyroidotomy. For any in-situ advanced airway encountered, it is important to confirm that it is in the trachea. As would be expected, airway devices placed in field conditions have a higher failure rate than those placed in a medical facility. Confirmation should include the presence of end-tidal CO_2 and bilateral breath sounds, with the understanding that a pneumothorax or hemothorax might obfuscate the latter finding. For patients with facial or head injuries, sometimes advanced airways are placed in the field preemptively, despite the patient having a normal level of consciousness and adequate minute ventilation without signs of respiratory distress. In these instances, if the advanced airway from the field is not found to not be in the trachea, consideration should be given as to whether it needs to be urgently replaced.

Unless the patient is in respiratory or cardiac arrest on presentation, securing the airway without patient resistance is usually contingent on first obtaining intravenous (IV) access and administering the appropriate anesthetic and muscle relaxant agents. As with other trauma scenarios, one or more short, large-bore peripheral IV catheters are the most desirable form of initial access. However, in the patient with extensive injuries including multiple traumatic amputations as may be seen with IED blast exposure, peripheral IV access may not be available. These patients are often the ones most in need of early aggressive resuscitation with blood products, so IV access is a high priority. If central venous access is required, an introducer of at least 8.5 French diameter with one or more side arms should be used instead of long, multi-lumen catheters of smaller diameters. For central venous cannulation, any site where access may be obtained quickly is suitable, although there are advantages and disadvantages to each. The internal jugular vein is the easiest for the anesthesia provider to access, but it may be unavailable due to the presence of a cervical collar. The subclavian vein is also an option, although the haste with which these lines are placed in a trauma setting may increase the risk of known complications such as non-compressible vessel injury and pneumothorax. The femoral vein does offer some advantages in the trauma setting:

- Generally offers easy access for the surgeon to place the catheter.
- Although the femoral vein is considered a "dirty" site, central venous catheters placed in an emergent trauma setting are rarely inserted with ideal sterile technique and full body draping. Using the femoral site initially preserves the internal jugular and subclavian veins for later access in a controlled environment with the use of true sterile technique if central venous access is still required.
- In the event the femoral artery is inadvertently accessed, consideration should be given to advancing a guidewire, and then continuing on with accessing the femoral vein. Once the femoral vein has been successfully cannulated, a catheter can be advanced over the wire in the femoral artery to use for arterial pressure monitoring, as more peripheral arteries such as the radial can be difficult to successfully access in the setting of trauma and significant hypotension.

Once IV access is established, or immediately in the case of cardiac or respiratory arrest, the anesthesia provider's attention can turn to securing the airway. Indications for endotracheal intubation remain the same as other non-wartime trauma patients. All of these patients should be considered to be at increased risk for aspiration regardless of the timing of their last oral intake, so some version of a rapid-sequence intubation is recommended. It should be expected that any casualty exposed to an IED blast is at risk for cervical spine injury, so those patients should have airway management conducted with manual in-line cervical spine immobilization, regardless of whether they arrive to the medical facility with a cervical collar and other spinal precautions in place. Well-functioning suction and tools for managing difficult airways should be readily available at this time, to include the Eschmann tracheal tube introducer (aka bougie) and other adjuncts such as a video laryngoscope and/or a lighted intubating stylet. Once the patient is intubated, or for patients who arrive with an advanced airway in place, it is recommended to place them on mechanical ventilation in the preoperative phase in order to maximize the ability of the team to focus on other aspects of the patient's care. Most patients arrive tachypneic as an adaptive response to the trauma and shock. Respiratory rates should be maintained (at least 20 breaths per minute) on the ventilator and then adjusted as blood gas or end-tidal CO_2 readings become available.

Drugs to facilitate intubation for wartime casualties are similar to other trauma situations. Although any induction agent can be utilized, those with minimal hemodynamic effects are better suited for the trauma patient. In the absence of significant myocardial injury, Etomidate is hemodynamically comparatively stable as opposed to Propofol and the barbiturates. Ketamine is also an option, although the expected small increase in sympathetic tone to help support the blood pressure is usually not seen in significant trauma, as these patients already have high sympathetic output. For the severely injured patient, the expectation would be a single endotracheal intubation at the first medical facility providing surgical care, with the ETT remaining in place through most of the critical care phase of the patient's recovery, to include early follow-up surgeries. Therefore, relative contraindications to succinylcholine such as use more than 24 h after a significant burn or spinal cord injury generally will not apply to this population. If succinylcholine is used to facilitate the intubation, it will likely be of benefit to administer a longer-acting nondepolarizing neuromuscular blocking agent once the airway is secured.

Concurrent with appropriate airway management and following establishment of IV access, volume resuscitation must begin for severely hypovolemic patients with significant blood loss.

The later section on transfusion medicine will address issues such as the ratios of blood component therapy and the use of fresh whole blood. However, the preoperative phase is where aggressive resuscitation with blood products must begin for these severely injured patients, with the goal of minimizing the total amount of crystalloid infused. For patients deemed to be appropriate candidates for antifibrinolytic therapy, this is also the time to begin the initial bolus of tranexamic acid (TXA). If rapid transfusion devices are available, they should initially be used in the preoperative environment, and then follow the patient into the operating room to continue the resuscitation. It is critically important to administer supplemental IV calcium as needed to offset the chelating effect of the additives to various blood products. If time allows, point-of-care testing can be utilized to monitor and maintain the ionized calcium level in the normal range. However, in the midst of a massive transfusion, it may be necessary to simply administer IV calcium empirically, particularly in the setting of new or worsening hypotension without other obvious causes.

For patients with traumatic amputations, the surgeons may desire to release the tourniquets in the preoperative period for a number of reasons. First, they may want to better assess the extent of vascular injury and whether there is ongoing blood loss. In addition, from an orthopedic standpoint, minimizing tourniquet time also decreases the risk of nerve injury. Since the anesthesia provider is usually ultimately responsible for maintaining the patient's hemodynamics, it is critically important for the surgeons to communicate their intent to release a tourniquet. Likewise, the anesthesia provider should not consent to the release of a tourniquet unless the patient has adequate IV access to permit a massive transfusion, and the immediate availability of blood products to support that transfusion if needed.

Particularly with exposure to IED blasts, it is common for wartime patients to present with closed head injury and the risk of increased intracranial pressure (ICP). Closed head injury can be difficult to assess in the setting of other concomitant significant injuries. Blast victims with a Glasgow Coma Scale (GCS) score of less than 9 with one for both pupils fixed and dilated and asymmetric motor posturing are at the highest risk. In addition to standard efforts to avoid hypoxemia and hypotension, normocarbia should be maintained with a goal $PaCO_2$ of 35–40, unless there is a need to transiently hyperventilate the patient to acutely decrease the ICP in response to rapid clinical deterioration. In the absence of readily available POCT for arterial blood gases, an end-tidal CO_2 goal of 30–35 can be used for most patients. In addition, a bolus and infusion of 3 % saline can be administered, even to patients who are hypotensive, whereas the second-line agent Mannitol should not be used in the setting of ongoing hypotension and hypovolemia. If serum chemistries are available, the target serum sodium level is 155–160 mEq/L. Despite a long history of controversy in the literature, steroids are not currently indicated in the management of head injury [2]. Although aggressive measures are generally employed to prevent heat loss in trauma patients to prevent hypothermic coagulopathy, head injury patients are one subgroup who should not be allowed to become hyperthermic as a result of warming efforts.

Early on in the preoperative phase, it is important to make an overall assessment of the survivability of the casualty's injuries. This assessment is not based solely on the ability of the initial surgical team to keep the patient alive through transport to the next facility. It must take into account what follow-on surgical and intensive care is available for the particular patient. This level of care available may be dictated by the patient's status as a member of the armed forces of the host nation or a foreign government, or if the patient is a civilian or insurgent fighter who will be classified as a prisoner of war. Severe injuries that might be survivable with multiple surgeries and an extended ICU stay in the developed world may not be so in other parts of the world. If the injury is deemed non-survivable based on the access to follow-on surgical and critical care, the surgical team may need to make a difficult decision about how best to utilize limited resources in caring for these patients. For example, the team may elect to evaluate the likelihood of long-term survival after administering 10 units of blood products before deciding to continue with resuscitative efforts. This is a difficult decision that is very much dependent on the circumstances of both the individual patient and the health care system.

Intraoperative

For the anesthesia provider, the intraoperative management of the wartime casualty is mainly a continuation of what has been done in the preoperative period. If the airway was not secured before coming to the OR, that is usually the first step after applying the appropriate monitors. Resuscitation with blood products and fluids must continue, with the agreed upon ratios of packed red cells to fresh frozen plasma and platelets, or alternatively with the use of fresh whole blood.

The intraoperative phase is also the time to introduce the concept of damage control surgery (DCS). DCS has been growing in acceptance amongst both military and civilian surgeons. The fundamental principle behind DCS is attempting to minimize the time initially spent in the OR after injury, limiting interventions to attaining hemostasis and stopping further contamination. The focus is on getting the patient to an intensive care setting in order to restore coagulation, reverse acidosis, and regain normothermia, prior to returning to the OR for more definitive surgeries [3]. The corollary to DCS is damage control resuscitation (DCR), which further attempts to limit or prevent coagulopathy by using a combination of blood components, antifibrinolytics, and recombinant factor VIIa, while simultaneously avoiding dilution of these factors by excessive use of crystalloid. Each of these elements of component therapy is considered in more depth in the later section on Transfusion Medicine. A further principle of DCR is the notion of permissive hypotension until surgical control of bleeding is attained, with the exception of head injury patients [4]. While DCS begins in the OR, the principles of DCR begin as soon as IV access is obtained preoperatively in severely injured patients.

For maintenance of anesthesia during the surgical procedure, there are several options available. If calibrated vaporizers for volatile anesthetics and a delivery system are available, anesthesia can be maintained as for any routine case in the developed world. One challenge with this in austere environments is the ability to provide waste anesthetic gas disposal. As an alternative to volatile anesthetics, a balanced total IV anesthetic (TIVA) can be employed. In regular hospitals it might be common to do TIVA using a separate pump and tubing for each IV agent. In a wartime scenario, it may be simpler to mix varying ratios of Propofol, Ketamine, a benzodiazepine such as Midazolam, and an opioid such as Fentanyl into a 100 or 250 mL IV bag and use a micro-dripper in order to titrate the TIVA to effect. This technique requires no IV pump or electrical power, and any combination of the aforementioned drugs can be used at the practitioner's discretion.

If the patient will require longer-term central venous access for their postoperative care, the intraoperative setting is a good time to perform that cannulation under sterile conditions. Likewise, if regional anesthesia is being considered for post-operative pain management, this may be a good opportunity to employ that technique under controlled circumstances while the patient is still under general anesthesia.

Postoperative

Modern deployed trauma facilities are not designed to hold patients and need to be part of an extensive evacuation system. In Afghanistan and Iraq, seriously wounded US and allied casualties were evacuated the night of injury to either a larger facility in theater or to Landstuhl Regional Medical Center in Germany. From Germany, US patients proceeded either to the Walter Reed National Military Medical Center in Maryland or, particularly if significant burn injuries were present, to the Brooke Army Medical Center in Texas. Most combat hospitals are not designed to hold patients for any length of time. In many facilities, the anesthesiologist functions as the intensivist and trauma and perioperative nurses staff the ICU. It is critical that continual communication be maintained between the combat hospital and the evacuation and air asset command. If just a few critically injured patients require an extended stay in a small combat hospital, the ability of that facility to receive new casualties may be significantly degraded.

Both patient and aircrew safety are major factors in determining when a patient can be evacuated. Weather and enemy activity often prevent flight operations. Dust storms are often encountered in the Middle East and often ground flight operations. The asymmetric nature of modern warfare has blurred the concept of "front lines" and combat hospitals frequently come under attack by snipers and indirect fire (rockets and mortars). It is usually safest to operate medevac aircraft at night to lessen the risk of hostile fire. Given all of these variables, there is usually a limited period of time for aircraft to operate safely and patient transport may be delayed. As discussed above, trauma patients often undergo damage control procedures and can require return trips to the operative theater within several hours. Frequently those patients are manifested for evacuation the following day. The ability to monitor and intervene on an unstable patient is limited in an aircraft, particularly a helicopter; therefore, questionable patients often remain in a facility until they are deemed stable enough to survive a several hour flight.

Coordination with local host nation medical assets and capabilities is essential and must be constantly assessed and updated. A critically injured local patient may be stable enough for transport but the receiving facility may have inadequate equipment, such as ventilators, staffing (physicians able to perform vascular procedures) or technical knowledge (can they place an intramedullary nail or just apply an external fixator?). It is recommended that, if feasible and safe, site visits to local receiving hospitals be made frequently and, if a facility will be used often, a permanent liaison team set up. What may seem to be a universal standard of care—such as sending more than just a driver in an ambulance to retrieve a ventilated patient—is often not the case. Ethical issues such as code status and end of life issues on critically injured local patients can quickly overwhelm a small combat hospital. Family members are often difficult to locate to guide decision making. Knowledge of local customs and practices is necessary to avoid offending citizens of the host country. In addition, employing translators who have medical knowledge is often impossible. Using a translator who cannot comprehend the information that he is then conveying to a patient's family is fraught with complications and potential immeasurable misunderstandings.

Transfusion Medicine

Transfusion and resuscitation strategies are a combination of factors based on trauma literature, logistics, facility capability, and patient volume. Current practices advocate a "whole blood" and low crystalloid approach. Studies, mostly observational, call for a unit of plasma to be transfused with every unit of packed red blood cells (PRBC) and an apheresis unit of platelets (or "six pack" depending on transfusion medicine services) administered after every six units of PRBCs. This research largely came from data from the most recent conflict in Iraq [5]. Civilian data investigating similar practices are more equivocal [6, 7]. Most retrospective studies contain survivor bias, meaning that a patient enrolled in the high PRBC to plasma ratio group must survive long enough to receive thawed plasma. A recent randomized prospective trial in civilian trauma centers demonstrated a survival benefit at 6 h in patients receiving increased plasma and platelet to PRBC ratios but no benefit after 24 h and no survivor benefit in patients who were alive after the first day [8].

In a well-supplied, busy trauma hospital, thawed plasma can be stored in close proximity to the trauma bay and transfused in conjunction with PRBCs. Due to the short shelf life of thawed plasma, another option in lyophilized plasma. This is a freeze-dried formulation of human plasma that can be stored up to 1 month at room temperature and reconstituted when required. There appears to be only a slight decrease in clotting activity in lyophilized plasma when compared to thawed plasma [9].

Cryoprecipitate contains ten times the concentration of five clotting factors compared to a unit of plasma, several which are rapidly consumed in an exsanguinating, critically injured trauma patient. If available, cryoprecipitate should be administered:

- With every 6–8 units of PRBCs.
- If labs are available and fibrinogen levels fall below 100 mg/dL.
- If guided by point of care testing (see below).

Caution should be exercised when using rapid transfusion technology such as the Belmont Rapid Infuser®. The extremely high flow rates (in excess of 400 mL/min) may provide life-saving blood products to a trauma patient with uncontrolled hemorrhage. However, at this flow rate, blood products are being infused almost as quickly as new bags are hung. Any delays in a continual supply of new bags will often cause the operator to run saline while additional products are made ready because interruptions in flow cause the machine to alarm and require repriming the tubing. If the operator doesn't decrease the flow rate, several liters of crystalloid can be infused, in direct conflict with the goal of low crystalloid/high blood product resuscitation.

Walking Blood Bank

Even in a well-established trauma network with a robust supply system, platelets are routinely not available or must be obtained from donors at individual treatment facilities. In response to the numerous supply, storage, and limited shelf-life issues of component therapy, the US military instituted a walking blood bank policy. Significant observational data supports the use of fresh whole blood in bleeding trauma patients; however, this practice is not FDA approved and is used primarily when component therapy is limited or patient needs surpass blood bank capabilities. The primary concerns with implementing a walking blood bank are infection, ABO compatibility, and administrative implementation. Rapid HIV, HBV, and HCV tests exist and should be performed on every unit of whole blood prior to administration. While the sensitivity of these tests is high, other infectious agents may be transferred to the recipient, including bacterial contamination. With the chaos that normally surrounds a high volume of trauma admissions and the inherent hygiene issues that are present in a deployed environment, maintaining both aseptic technique and using sterile equipment does not always take place. Unlike transfusing Type O PRBCs, there is no universal donor with whole blood. Not only does donor blood need ABO/Rh typing performed, but the recipient's blood type must be confirmed. Patient recall and identification systems (i.e., "dog tags") are notoriously unreliable. The administrative burden in implementing, maintaining, and utilizing a walking blood bank is significant. Ideally, donors are pre-screened every 90 days for infectious diseases and their blood type is maintained on a roster. The frequent rotation of donors in a forward deployed camp mandates continued screening and updates to the roster. A reliable and prompt notification and response system must be in place for when blood is needed. If the walking blood bank is the primary source of blood products for a combat hospital, the call for donors must take place before arrival of casualties if at all possible due to the delay from notification to units ready to transfuse. This delay can be deadly to a bleeding patient. The nature of a combat trauma hospital means patients often arrive unannounced. In the excitement surrounding initial casualty assessment and treatment, clerical tasks such as ensuring donor blood is properly labeled and then subsequently verified prior to transfusion may be hastily done and thus prone to error.

Point-of-Care Testing

Portable blood analyzers such as the iStat® analyzer may help guide transfusion therapy in combat trauma victims. Rapid assessment of blood gas, hemoglobin concentrations and INR are available for interpretation. The US military also utilizes rotational thromboelastography (ROTEM®) in some of the larger deployed combat hospitals. While a review and interpretation on ROTEM® is beyond the scope of this chapter, ROTEM® can provide valuable data for the management of a coagulopathic trauma victim and guide transfusion of component therapy.

Tranexamic acid

Tranexamic acid (TXA) is an antifibrinolytic shown to decrease mortality in civilian trauma patients and is used in deployed US military trauma hospitals [10]. TXA's effects are believed to blunt the hyperfibrinolysis associated with the coagulopathy seen in trauma patients. Survivor benefits are most significant if administered within an hour of injury and there appears to be no benefit beyond 3 h post-injury. In a combat environment where evacuation is often delayed due to ongoing enemy activity in the landing zone or evacuation point, the 3-h window for TXA administration is not always possible. Current US military guidelines advocate administering TXA in concordance with the CRASH-2 trial recommendations. One gram of TXA is given intravenously over 10 min and a second gram is infused over 8 h. TXA should not be administered through the same line in which blood products are infusing. In addition, plasma volume extenders derived from starch, such as Hextend® or Hespan®, should not be used as a carrier fluid or infused through the same line as TXA. Some experts believe that hetastarch products may attenuate the antifibrinolytic activity of TXA.

The use of TXA with either recombinant factor VIIa (rFVIIa) or activated prothrombin complex concentrate (APCC) must be carefully considered given the theoretical risk of forming thrombotic complexes. In the CRASH-2 trial, a small number of patients in the TXA treatment group also received rFVIIa with no recorded thrombotic complications. However, it is difficult to draw any significant conclusions given the small sample size in a subgroup analysis.

Recombinant Factor VIIa

The use of recombinant factor VIIa (rFVIIa) during a massive transfusion is both off label and controversial given recent literature elaborating on the relatively high incidence of thrombosis [11, 12]. Administration during the resuscitation of a trauma patient should be on a case-by-case basis and not used as a routine. If bleeding is from an isolated source (i.e., inferior vena cava, femoral artery), the use of rFVIIa has little utility and surgical control is essential. However, blast injury patients often have dozens of penetrating wounds not amenable to rapid surgical intervention. The authors recommend use of rFVIIa in an exsanguinating patient with multiple injuries where rapid surgical control of bleeding cannot be obtained.

Regional Anesthesia

Regional anesthesia was once considered an intervention best utilized after patients were evacuated out of the combat zone and stabilized in a tertiary care center. Thanks to the works of Buckenmaier et al. and other military acute pain specialists, regional techniques are utilized early in combat trauma patients [13]. Although no formal studies have investigated the infection rate associated with regional techniques performed in combat hospitals, there appears to be no increased infection rate. There is data to support early intervention in the pain process to prevent both chronic and phantom limb pain [14]. While preemptive analgesia cannot be obtained in trauma patients, an effective nerve block that persists until central sensitization subsides may help prevent chronic pain. Patients with traumatic amputations require multiple wound wash outs before final closure. These repeated reinitiating events are best prevented, if possible, by a continuous nerve catheter rather than multiple single shot injections. In addition, there may also be mental health benefits as well. In Afghanistan, we were able to extubate many patients after the OR that traditionally would have remained intubated for their evacuation flight. Instead of squad members visiting an intubated and sedated patient, we often witnessed joyous reunions and conversations. It is our belief that this early "telling your story" may have later benefits and help prevent or lessen posttraumatic stress disorder.

In deciding between single shot peripheral nerve blocks and continuous techniques, whether peripheral or neuraxial, a safe delivery system for local anesthetic must be considered. The US military used pumps cleared for flight operations. Given the logistics of air evacuation and variables such as cabin pressure, pumps must undergo certification before use to prevent such disasters as runaway infusion. If a single shot technique is utilized, the timing of the block must coincide with evacuation to avoid loss of analgesia while airborne.

Controversy exists regarding regional anesthesia and masking compartment syndrome in extremity injuries. The literature does not support this belief [15]. The use of local anesthetic techniques to achieve a surgical block should not be continued into the postoperative period. Low-concentration infusions (i.e., bupivacaine 0.125 or 0.25 %) should provide analgesia while maintaining an examinable extremity. What is even more important is an educated surgical staff and an involved acute pain team. Whether a patient at risk for compartment syndrome is using opioids or a peripheral nerve catheter for post surgical analgesia, missing a change in the exam will delay the diagnosis of compartment syndrome. Vigilance on patients requiring more frequent pushes on a PCA or nursing intervention cannot be overlooked and a mechanism for identifying these patients and contacting a surgeon are paramount.

The Need for Future Research

The future of chronic pain prevention may lie in the aggressive management of acute pain. Clark et al. [16] found that using regional anesthesia and opiates lowered pain scales over the entire hospital course of veterans suffering from polytrauma and suggested that the incidence of chronic pain maybe decreased. Similarly, further research by Gironda et al. [17] suggested that in order to decrease the total pain experienced along with effectively treating associated comorbid conditions such as post-traumatic stress disorder and postconcussive syndrome will require the development of integrated approaches to clinical care which bridge traditional subspecialty divisions. Several of these multi-specialty teams are in operation and their long term effectiveness will be evaluated.

Summary

The modern combat hospital spans a few tents with a makeshift operating room and basic supplies to stabilize a patient all the way to hardened structures with modern facilities and capabilities such as interventional radiology and MRI scanners. Ideally, each hospital should be part of an established evacuation system to both receive and discharge casualties. Capabilities are often limited by logistics and therefore goals, such as blood product administration, must be established so a single patient doesn't exhaust the resources available. Combat hospitals see primarily penetrating injury trauma as opposed to civilian centers where motor vehicle and other blunt force trauma victims make up a majority of patients. In recent years, blast injuries have become the primary injury mechanism. In a modern combat force wearing body armor, extremity injuries are most common and the use of tourniquets has dramatically improved survival. Prompt evaluation, recognition, and treatment of injury are no different than in civilian trauma centers. What is more unique to combat hospitals is the frequent delay in treating casualties due to hostilities and the chance that the hospital itself may come under fire. The energy from a blast and the ensuing deep seated soil contamination often leads to wound infections that delay definitive treatment of fractures. The deployed military environment is uniquely well suited for the implementation of a walking blood bank. Early use of regional anesthesia may reduce the incidence of chronic pain and PTSD.

References

1. Borden Institute. Weapons effects and war wounds. In: Cubano MA, Lenhart MK, et al., editors. Emergency war surgery. Fort Sam Houston, TX: Borden Institute; 2013. p. 1–16.
2. Management of patients with severe head trauma. In: US Army Institute of Surgical Research joint theater trauma system clinical practice guidelines. 2012. http://www.usaisr.amedd.army.mil/clinical_practice_guidelines.html. Accessed 15 May 2014.
3. Duchesne JC, Barbeau JM, Islam TM, Wahl G, Greiffenstein P, McSwain NE. Damage control resuscitation: from emergency department to the operating room. Am Surg. 2011;77:201–6.
4. Damage control resuscitation. In: US Army Institute of Surgical Research joint theater trauma system clinical practice guidelines. 2013. http://www.usaisr.amedd.army.mil/clinical_practice_guidelines.html. Accessed 16 May 2014.
5. Holcomb JB, Jenkins D, Rhee P, et al. Damage control resuscitation: directly addressing the early coagulopathy of trauma. J Trauma. 2007;62:307–10.
6. Holcomb JB, Wade CE, Michalek JE, et al. Increased plasma and platelet to red blood cell ratios improves outcome in 466 massively transfused civilian trauma patients. Ann Surg. 2008;248:447–58.
7. Scalea TM, Bochicchio KM, Lumpkins K, et al. Early aggressive use of fresh frozen plasma does not improve outcome in critically injured trauma patients. Ann Surg. 2008;248:578–84.
8. Holcomb JB, del Junco DJ, Fox EE, Wade CE, et al. The prospective, observational, multicenter, major trauma transfusion (PROMMTT) study: comparative effectiveness of a time-varying treatment with competing risks. JAMA Surg. 2013;148:127–36.
9. Shuja F, Shults C, Duggan M, Tabbara M, et al. Development and testing of freeze-dried plasma for the treatment of trauma-associated coagulopathy. J Trauma. 2008;65:975–85.
10. CRASH-2 Trial Collaborators. Effects of tranexamic acid on death, vascular occlusive events, and blood transfusion in trauma patients with significant haemorrhage (CRASH-2): a randomized, placebo-controlled trial. Lancet. 2010; published online June 15. doi:10.1016/S0140-6736(10)60835-5.
11. Levi M, Levy JH, Andersen HF, Truloff D. Safety of recombinant activated factor VII in randomized clinical trials. N Engl J Med. 2010;363:1791–800.
12. Simpson E, Lin Y, Stanworth S, et al. Recombinant factor VIIa for the prevention and treatment of bleeding patients without haemophilia. Cochrane Database Syst Rev. 2012;3, CD005011.
13. Buckenmaier III CC, McKnight GM, Winkley JV, et al. Continuous peripheral nerve block for battlefield anesthesia and evacuation. Reg Anesth Pain Med. 2005;30:202–5.
14. Kissin I. Preemptive analgesia. Anesthesiology. 2000;93:1138–43.
15. Mar GJ, Barrington MJ, Mcguirk BR. Acute compartment syndrome of the lower limb and the effect of postoperative analgesia on diagnosis. Br J Anaesth. 2009;102:3–11.
16. Clark ME, Bair MJ, Buckenmaier CC, Gironda RJ, Walker RL. Pain and combat injuries in soldiers returning from operations enduring freedom and Iraqi freedom: implications for research and practice. J Rehabil Res Dev. 2007;44:179–94.
17. Gironda RJ, Clark ME, Ruff RL, Chait S, Craine M, Walker R, Scholten J. Traumatic brain injury, polytrauma, and pain: challenges and treatment strategies for the polytrauma rehabilitation. Rehabil Psychol. 2009;54:247–57.

23 Anesthesiologists' Role in Disaster Management

Debbie Chandler, Yenabi Keflemariam, Charles James Fox, and Alan David Kaye

Introduction

The field of anesthesiology provides life-supporting care regardless of the etiology or circumstances. The anesthesia provider occupies a crucial and essential role in initiating effective and efficient health care, serving as a link between surgical services and the Intensive Care Units (ICUs) in the provision of medical care and the coordination and/or implementation of a disaster response strategy. Given the anesthesiologist's familiarity with the two specialties, it is of little doubt that the specialty of Anesthesiology should embrace a key primary role in the event of a disaster. The responsibilities of the anesthesiologist would include, but not be limited to, frequently coordinating the care of patients in nearly all fathomable settings/scenarios, analyzing and problem solving, performing a systematic triaging of patients, providing or supervising optimal anesthesia for best patient outcomes, and helping to improve upon previous areas of deficiency as a region begins the process of rebuilding. The sheer essence contained with the definition of a disaster are the circumstances which prove that these instances are usually unforeseen and similarly exert catastrophic damage as a result from inappropriate preventative or preparative measures. In the face of disaster, the implementation of the aforementioned responsibilities of the anesthesiologist ultimately will attempt to save lives by blunting the associated morbidity and mortality common during disaster circumstances.

As history has proven, there are many etiologies that fall under the umbrella term *disaster*. More formally, these are categorized as natural disasters to include hurricanes, earthquakes, tsunamis, forest fires, and epidemic diseases, and unnatural events including plane crashes, explosions, and train and car accidents. With increasing occurrence rates, a new category has grown in significance. These types of disasters of malicious and/or ill intent have included airline hi-jackings and serial killings, especially seen in educational institutions, to the use of weapons of mass destruction. Some notable natural disasters of the last two decades include Hurricane Katrina (2005), the Haiti earthquake (2010), the Tohoku earthquake and tsunami (2011), and the forest fires of Southern California (2003). Of the un-natural disasters, most vividly remember, the tragedy of September 11th, 2001, which killed nearly 3,000 people and sent 10,000 people for medical treatment of injuries related to the event(s) [1] and the bombing of the Alfred P. Murrah Federal Building in downtown Oklahoma City, Oklahoma, in 1995.

D. Chandler, M.D. • Y. Keflemariam, M.D.
C.J. Fox, M.D.
Department of Anesthesiology, LSU School of Medicine Shreveport, Shreveport, LA, USA

A.D. Kaye, M.D., Ph.D. (✉)
Department of Anesthesiology, LSU School of Medicine, Room 656, 1542 Tulane Avenue, New Orleans, LA 70112, USA
e-mail: alankaye44@hotmail.com

R. Roth et al. (eds.), *The Role of Anesthesiology in Global Health: A Comprehensive Guide*,
DOI 10.1007/978-3-319-09423-6_23, © Springer International Publishing Switzerland 2015

Regardless of the underlying cause or mechanism of disaster, the ultimate goals of the Anesthesiologists or anesthesia providers are to maximize the number of lives saved while limiting the injury and impact upon the population at risk. Such outcomes require a systematic and coordinated interplay of all medical professionals involved with anesthesiology and surgical specialties at the reins. Specific plans of action with emphasis on pre-, intra-, and post-disaster management are crucial to the effectiveness of the distribution of medical expertise, manpower, and resources. In this chapter, we review the types of disasters and identify the important underlying principles and/or strategies for each circumstance from an anesthesiology perspective.

Classification of Disasters

A *disaster* is defined as "a sudden calamitous event which results in great damage, loss, or destruction" [2]. When applied to modern societies, it is understood that this definition is often associated with widespread destruction of the environment and the loss of human life. The categorizations of disasters, for the purpose of this chapter, are determined by the inciting event and have been described as natural or unnatural to include those disasters of malicious intent.

Natural Disasters

Natural disasters are any events or forces of nature that have catastrophic consequences such as avalanches, earthquakes, floods, forest fires, hurricanes, tornados, tsunamis, and volcanic eruptions. Examples of such natural disasters that have significantly impacted densely populated regions of the world include: Hurricane Katrina (2005), the Haiti earthquake (2010), the Tohoku earthquake and tsunami (2011), the forest fires of Southern California (2003), and the devastating floods that occur in Bangladesh annually.

Floods remain the number one nonterrorist-related disaster in the USA in regard to mortality and property damages [3]. Prior to 2005, floods were the cause of roughly 140 deaths and property damages estimated at 6$ billion US dollars every year over a 25-year period [3]. In the USA, flash flooding is the leading cause of weather-related mortality [3]. The overall impact of flooding is multi-faceted including the loss of safe water, crop losses, disruption of food, distribution, adequate sanitation, loss of shelter, and disruption of health-care services [3]. Hurricane Katrina was the most devastating hurricane of the 2005 hurricane season and the most costly natural disaster in the US history [3]. Hurricane Katrina made initial landfall in Florida before entering the Gulf of Mexico and gaining enough strength to become a Category 5 storm. Just prior to making its second landfall on August 29th, 2005, at the Southeastern portion of the state of Louisiana, the storm weakened and came ashore as a Category 3 storm. The subsequent storm surge caused massive widespread flooding which resulted in property damages estimated at $81 billion US dollars and took the lives of roughly 1,836 people with 135 people reported missing [4]. The majority of the deaths attributed to Hurricane Katrina were a direct result of flash flooding caused by catastrophic failure of multiple levees which made 2005 the third deadliest flood year in the US history [3]. See Fig. 23.1.

Worldwide demographic analysis has proven that many heavily concentrated populations are located along major fault lines [3]. Such population trends predispose large numbers of people to the risks and complications associated with earthquakes. The most common causes of injury and/or death are crush injuries and the development of compartment syndrome. It has been shown that patient survival is inversely related to the amount of time necessary for extrication from collapsed buildings and structures damaged by the seismic activity [3]. The Haiti Earthquake occurred on January 12, 2010, and registered as a catastrophic magnitude 7.0 M_w. Occurring roughly 16 miles from the capital city of Port-au-Prince, the earthquake was, paradoxically, not proven to involve slipping of faults, the major cause of prior significant earthquakes. This earthquake's effects were felt by over 3.5 million people. The earthquake's intensity was severe enough to cause moderate-to-heavy damage to structures deemed earthquake

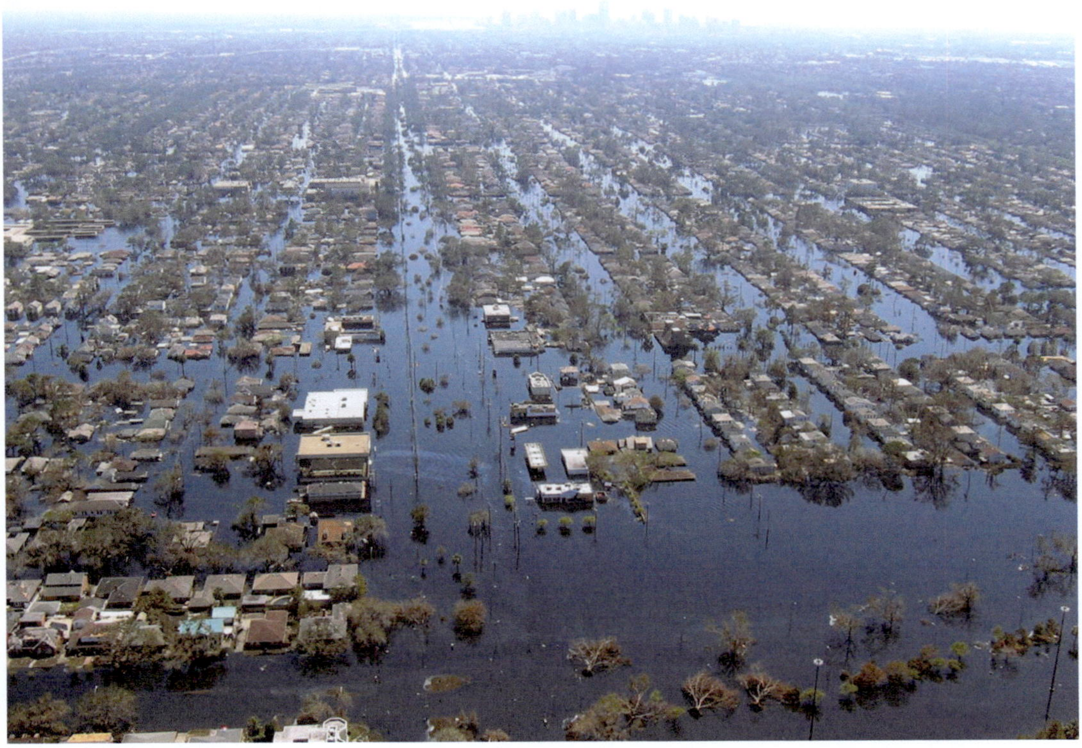

Fig. 23.1 Hurricane Katrina http://densitykatrina.wordpress.com

resistant. The shallow depth of the earthquake zone was postulated as the reason for its intensity [4]. It has been postulated that roughly 222,570 people lost their lives in this earthquake, while some 300,572 were injured. The estimated financial damage caused by this devastation tallied nearly $7.8 billion US dollars ($4.3 billion in physical damages and roughly $3.5 billion dollars in economic losses) [5]. Other notable causes of morbidity surrounding the initial devastation caused by an earthquake include secondary events such as fires, landslides, tsunamis, and exposure to toxic chemicals secondary to the destruction of chemical stores/plants [3]. See Fig. 23.2

March 11, 2011, was a day that changed the lives of many, if not most, on the eastern coast of Japan. The Tohoku earthquake, which registered at a magnitude of 9.0 Mw, compared to the Haiti earthquake which was recorded at a magnitude of 7.0 Mw, occurred nearly 43 miles off of the eastern coast of the Oshika Peninsula of Tohoku. The subsequent tsunami created waves as high as 133 feet which traveled nearly 6 miles inland. It is of little surprise that the devastation of such a massive earthquake and tsunami would top those created by the Haiti Earthquake of 2010. One year after the traumatic occurrence, reports had documented 16,273 fatalities, 3,061 missing, and 27,074 people injured with these numbers continually growing [6]. Unique to this particular disaster is the fact that there were two separate natural disasters which synergistically caused unimaginable destruction and changed the eastern coast of Japan forever. At the 1-year mark, damages were estimated roughly at $275 billion US dollars. It is now believed that the earthquake alone would have caused 40–45 % of the total damage surrounding this catastrophe [7]. See Fig. 23.3.

There have been many forest fires in the US, but the densest concentrations of these disasters

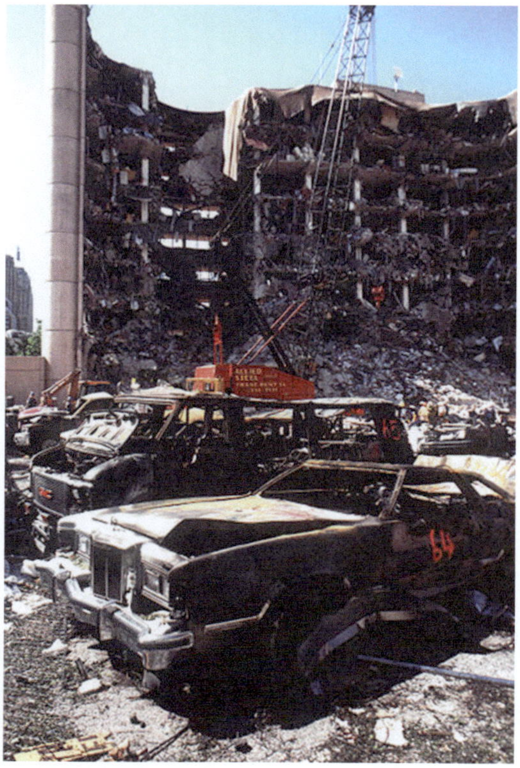

Fig. 23.2 Haiti earthquake destruction. http://www.scholastic.com/content/images/articles/sn_ts/sn_ts_011510_hdr.jpg

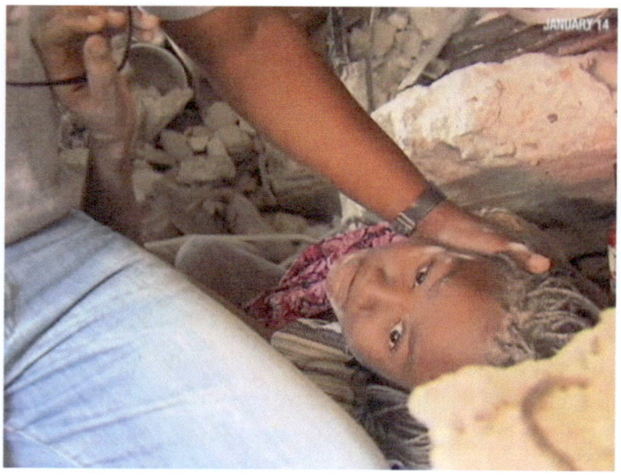

Fig. 23.3 Tohoku earthquake and Tsunami. http://www.elist10.com/wp-content/uploads/2013/03/T%C5%8Dhoku-Japan-earthquake-2011.jpg

have occurred on the Pacific coast. California has witnessed multiple incidents with the most devastating occurring between October 25th and October 29th of 2003. A series of 15 wildfires cumulatively coined the "2003 Firestorm" was noted to cause 24 deaths while destroying nearly 800,000 acres including 3,640 homes throughout the San Diego, Ventura, Riverside, and San Bernadino counties [8]. Although not as costly as the previously discussed natural disasters, there was widespread criticism by review committees as to the preparation and response to the disaster.

As a consequence of geographical location on the Ganges Delta, a tributary system which feeds into the Bay of Bengal, and the Himalayas, the country of Bangladesh is continually at risk for widespread destruction secondary to torrential floods during the monsoon season (June through September). 75 % of the landscape of Bangladesh is within 10 m of sea level with 80 % of this land being comprised of flood plains. With the rains provided by the monsoon season coupled with the rain and melting water runoff of the Himalayas, nearly two-thirds of the country are flooded annually despite ongoing attempts to improve the infrastructural stability designs specifically created to combat the well-known, recurring devastation. The most destructive flood witnessed by the country occurred in 1998 leaving 75 % of the country's land was left under water due to the rains occurring between August and September of that year. The heavier than normal rains led to the three-river system within Bangladesh reaching peak flow levels. The additional factors of global warming and above average melting of snowmelt on the Himalayas further exacerbated the annually anticipated flooding of the region causing over 1,000 deaths and forcing 30,000+ people to become homeless. Undercut by flooding and overcrowding, many victims perished as a consequence of everyday injuries and otherwise treatable medical conditions. Contamination led to both *cholera* and *typhoid* outbreaks. Crop and economic production and communication were crippled.

Unnatural Disasters and Malicious Disasters

Unnatural disasters and malicious/ill-intent disasters occur far more frequently than natural disasters but are generally not as catastrophic.

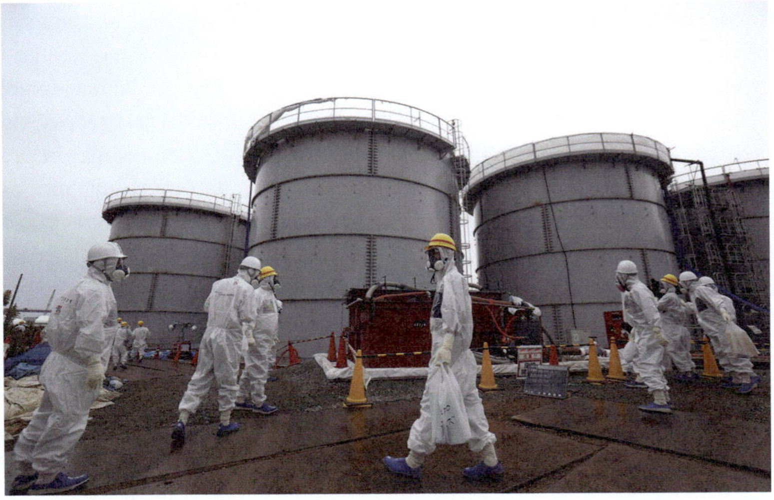

Fig. 23.4 Oklahoma City bombing. "Oklahoma City Bombing." *Wikipedia, The Free Encyclopedia, 2014*. Web. April 19 2014 http://en.wikipedia.org/wiki/2010_Haiti_earthquake

Examples of such include plane crashes, train and automobile accidents, explosions, and chemical spills. The most notable of these was the September 11th attacks of 2001 which occurred in New York, Virginia, and Pennsylvania which proved to be the most deadly terrorist-driven attack on United States soil. Four passenger airliners were hijacked and used as weapons to attack both the North and South towers of the World Trade Center, the Pentagon, and Washington D.C. The attacks on the World Trade Center involved two airliners making direct impact with the two towers eventually causing their collapse. The destruction of these two towers took the lives of 2,606 people, including 343 firefighters. The attack on the pentagon killed 125 people and there were a total of 246 people who lost their lives on the four passenger airliners. Estimates point to a total of roughly $2 trillion US dollars when including all economic losses from physical damages and the impact on the stock market [9].

On April 19th, 1995, the Alfred P. Murrah Federal Building in downtown Oklahoma City, Oklahoma fell victim to a domestic terrorist bombing which claimed the lives of 168 people, injured nearly 700 people, and caused roughly $650 million US dollars in damage [10]. Timothy McVeigh, and his co-conspirator Terry Nichols, were soon detained and charged with the crime. Upon interviewing McVeigh in search of a possible motive, he explained that the attack was greatly fueled by his hatred of the Federal Bureau of Investigation (FBI) as a result of what he believed to be mishandling of the Waco Siege which occurred 2 years prior in 1993 as well as the Ruby Ridge incident in 1992 [10]. The premeditated plan was to attack as many federal law-enforcement agencies as possible simultaneously making the Alfred P. Murrah Federal Building a leading target as it housed not only the FBI but also the Drug Enforcement Agency (DEA) and the Bureau of Alcohol, Tobacco, and Firearms (ATF). The man-made bomb harnessed the blast equivalent of 5,000 pounds of TNT and could be heard as well as felt more than 50 miles away upon detonation. See Fig. 23.4.

As the Iran-Iraq War came to a close in March of 1988, one of the world's worst genocidal massacres took place at the hands of the Iraqi regime under Saddam Hussein. The attack involved a series of more than 14 chemical bombings coordinated by helicopters of residential areas in the city of Halabja in Southern Kurdistan. The bombs were noted to contain combinations of sulfur mustard (also known as "mustard gas"), hydrogen cyanide, and other nerve agents. The effects of the nerve gas exposure led to the death of roughly 5,000 people and injured between 7,000 and 10,000 other civilians [11]. The devastation carried on for years after the initial attack as many more people perished from complications including diseases and birth defects. This attack, more commonly referred to as the Halabja Massacre or Bloody Friday, was the largest chemical weapon attack in history against a civilian populated region [11].

Pre-disaster Strategies

Some of the founding principles of the anesthesiology specialty include anticipation, thorough preparedness, hypervigilence, apt problem-solving skills, and sound decision making in critical situations. Anesthetic care providers must have a sense of discipline, dedication, empathy, and determination to respond to emergencies in an attempt to save the lives of victims and treat those injured in the face of catastrophic events. In order to maximize this initiative, there must be great emphasis and effort directed at being prepared. Such preparedness comes by way of identifying and organizing committees, resources, facilities, and personnel that can all be mobilized swiftly and efficiently.

Committees, Roles, and Communication

Organization is imperative to the success of disaster response. Because anesthesiology provides a key linkage between multiple specialties and also holds a central position in most medical care settings, providing the most efficient medical care to those in need should include the direction and coordination of an anesthesiologist. In ideal situations, there should exist a network of local and regional anesthesiology providers who are willing and able to provide their skill sets if called upon in the face of disaster. The creation of a core committee which includes these anesthesiologists as well as other subspecialties including, but not limited to, surgical subspecialties, critical care, nursing, emergency medicine, and internal medicine is essential. This committee will be the central unit in creating disaster management strategies to include pre-disaster awareness, disaster management planning, identifying resources and surplus availability, and creating mock-disaster trials. Given that the remainder of disaster strategy preparedness revolves around this central organization, there should also be elected/selected delegates of this group who hold ranking positions to ensure a tier-structure of command to facilitate instruction and direction in the event of impending catastrophe. The contact information of all ranking and registered providers should be available via various means in the case that activation of the group be needed and established lines of communication are jeopardized or destroyed entirely. Accordingly, all medical professional subspecialties should create similar registries with appointed ranking leaders and individual contact information should there be a breakdown in the ability for there to be a central organization coordinated disaster plan. Within each committee, rank should be appointed based on knowledge and experience within the particular specialty and subsequent positions should be appointed accordingly. It should be left to the discretion of committee leaders to determine the roles and responsibility given to each member. Creating individual committees, with their respective leaders, will ensure that once disaster is suspected or anticipated, all personnel, through a previously designed, or alternative, communication system will be informed and on high-alert that their individual skill sets may be called upon. The delegates of these groups should ensure that their registries are updated at least bi-annually and remain current to the best of their abilities. These appointed leaders would themselves join together to form a Disaster Management Board (DMB) which should similarly include senior ranking members/directors and administrators of all major hospital or health care facilities, local police and fire departments, and the local department of transportation. The DMB collectively formulates disaster plans and strategies built upon previous catastrophic experiences of all etiologies. Regularly scheduled meetings should be held in an attempt to review and update strategies and allocation of resources amongst many other facets of disaster management. These meetings may also be used to simulate potential disaster situations and test the abilities and limitations of the current policies and strategies. McIsaac et al. noted that the Joint Commission on Accreditation of Healthcare Organizations (JCAHO) requires all hospital to have biannual disaster exercises to help ensure proper coordination of operating room (OR) personnel and the department of anesthesiology [12].

It is also important to establish an organized group to be deemed "First Responders." Ideally this group would comprised a select group of anesthesiology providers as well as surgical specialists of each region. The primary goal of these health care providers is to make initial assessments based on:

1. The type of disaster and the most common types of injuries (crush, burn, chemical, etc.).
2. The need for particular types of medical specialists to be dispatched to the scene as well as sufficient numbers of such specialists.
3. Activation of all participating committees and hospital facilities needed based on the type of care required.

Once the initial assessments have been made and the disaster has been categorized, the DMB should activate predesigned protocols needed for the peri-disaster phase of management.

Communication amongst these committees is essential for initiation of proper disaster response. Particular attention should be given to the widespread distribution of a central set of contacts and contact numbers that others (professionals, administrators, media, etc.) may use for intergroup communication, reports, and updates. There should also be particular attention paid to the types of communications that may be lost given the type of disasters that are most likely to occur. In the event of widespread loss of electricity or cellular technologies, an alternative means for effective communication to facilitate and coordinate the disaster response is warranted. History has shown that the use of two-way radios provides a rather inexpensive means of communication in distances up to 12 miles. The Pan Am 103 flight bombing was an example of abilities of two-way radio communications as the pilots were able to make contact with the Shanwick Oceanic Area Control just seconds before the plane was subsequently destroyed by a terrorist bomb believed to be orchestrated by the regime under Libyan leader Muammar Gaddafi [13]. Ideally in disaster scenarios, the use of two-way radio communication would be able to provide key linkage between first responders and appropriate facilities or personnel in the event that other electricity-driven forms of media/communication were destroyed or rendered inoperable. The implementation of such alternative forms of communications would thus prove to be essential for execution of disaster strategies and providing up-to-date information regarding different aspects of disaster response(s).

Identifying Resources and Materials

Each DMB needs to identify potential resources and materials that can be mobilized in the event of a disaster which will require the input of hospitals and other medical facilities. Information that is usually needed includes, but is not be limited to, the numbers of hospital beds, including emergency room capacities, ICU and inpatient beds, functioning operating rooms (ORs), functioning mechanical ventilators, and emergency transportation vehicles (ambulances, fire trucks, other emergency vehicles).

It would be of great value to create a registry of approximate volumes of necessary resources particularly those that are more likely to be exhausted during a disaster situation. Of particular importance are the emergency medications that are specific to the treatment protocols of certain chemicals and nerve gases in the event of bio- or chemical disaster as well as those necessary to perform a wide array of anesthetics depending on the clinical scenario. The anesthesiologist must have the ability to treat patients both in and out of the hospital setting as it has been shown that the degree and types of injuries vary widely depending on the etiology of the disaster. The ability of the anesthesia provider to administer adequate clinical care for patients is

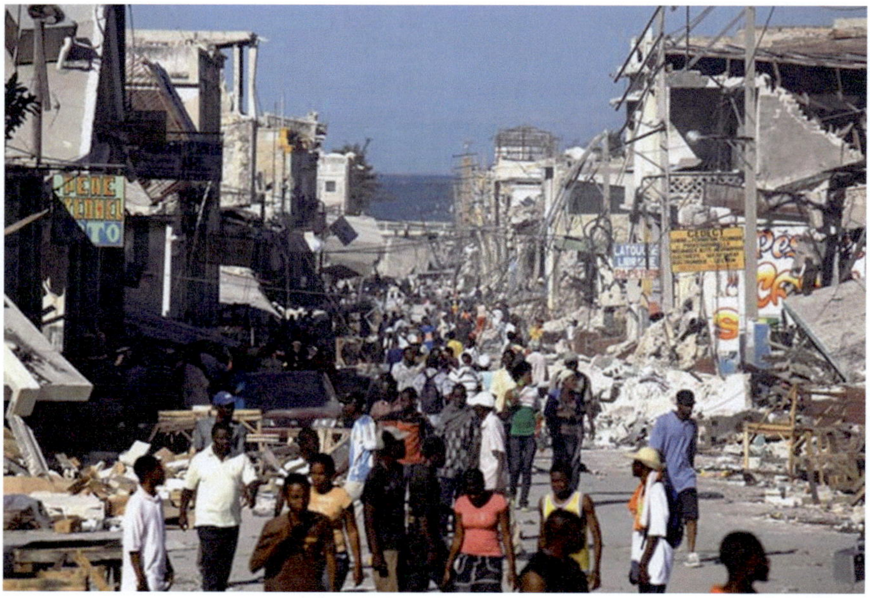

Fig. 23.5 Haiti earthquake http://www.cnn.com/video/world/2010/01/14/watson.haiti.trapped.girl.update.cnn.640x480.jpg

heavily dependent on his/her ability to construct anesthetic regimens based on individual clinical conditions. The anesthetic regiment may consist of particular drugs which provide better hemodynamic control in the face of severe traumatic injuries. Of particular note, patients who have succumbed to collapsing infrastructures and whose survival is dependent on emergency surgeries involving amputation of a limb pose a difficult, yet manageable, anesthetic scenario for the anesthesia provider as securing of a patient's airway may be impossible. In these dire circumstances, the anesthesia provider would be best served in utilizing medications whose side effect profile minimizes the possibility of respiratory depression (i.e. ketamine, non-steroidal anti-inflammatory drugs (NSAIDs)) but are capable of providing analgesia. See Fig. 23.5.

In the face of toxin or chemical exposure, the anesthesia provider will need to have sufficient quantities of disease-specific medications to appropriately treat exposed patients. There will also have to be sufficient protective apparel to be adorned by those providing medical care to prevent primary exposure and ultimately to maximize the efficiency of the disaster response [3]. The National Institute of Occupational Safety and Health (NIOSH) was designed to maximize workplace safety via a series of guidelines which define particular forms of protective equipment protocols based upon the type of chemical and/or biological disaster [3]. In the event that the initial supply of medications and/or personal protective equipment is exhausted with the first waves of treatment, secondary resources or supplies may need to be mobilized to supplement the deficits. For this reason, of the most plausible types of bio- or chemical exposure, it would be advantageous to identify depots or secondary outlets that would be able to provide any necessary medications or supplies based on the specific type of disaster. See Fig. 23.6.

Blood and blood products are often needed in the initial resuscitation of critically injured patients. For this reason, there should be a registry designed to monitor supply levels of such products. Most hospitals are associated with a coordinated blood bank system which monitors regional availability of blood and blood products. Given that patients will not be able to receive appropriate blood group matching strategies in such emergent/urgent scenarios, Type O-blood will be most commonly administered to decrease chances of ABO incompatibility. It is well-known that the transfusion of blood and

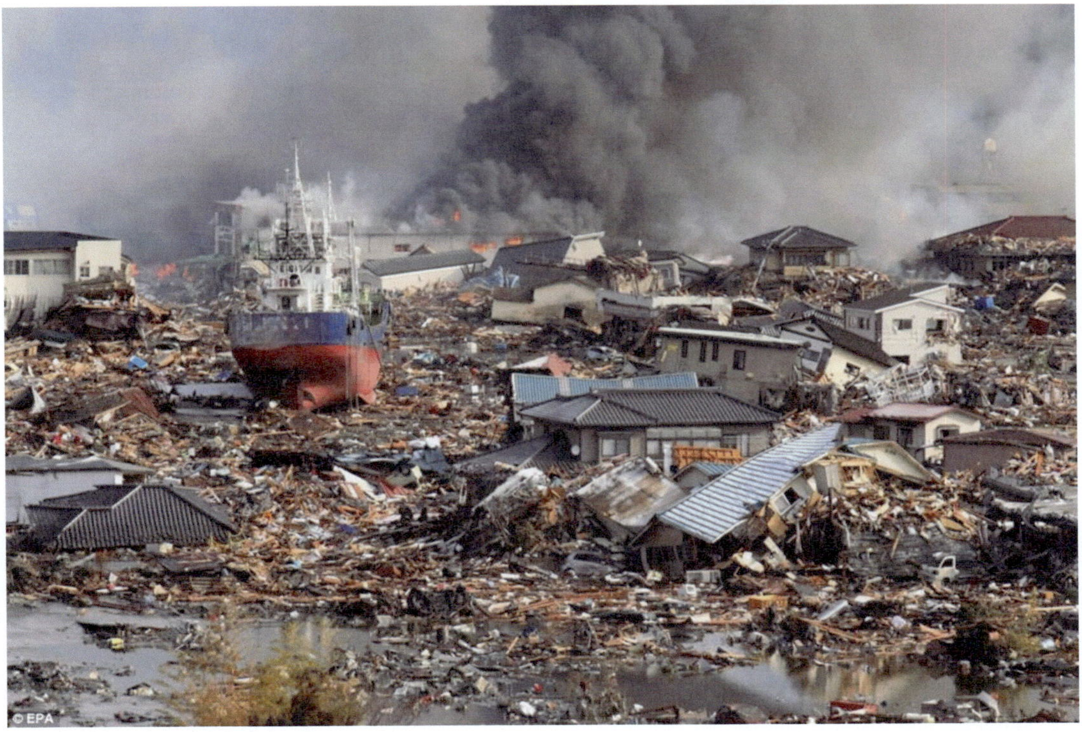

Fig. 23.6 Tohoku earthquake. http://jto.s3.amazonaws.com/wp-content/uploads/2014/03/p1-cleanup-a-20140309.jpg

blood products carries with it the risk of transmission of human immunodeficiency virus (HIV), hepatitis B virus (HBV), hepatitis C virus (HCV), Chagas disease, malaria, and other types of diseases [14]. In the event that an emergency transfusion is deemed necessary to provide oxygen-carrying capacity to patient's hemorrhaging or facing severe anemia, one must be mindful of the potential for complications associated with hypothermic transfusions including coagulopathy and hemolysis. For these aforementioned reasons, it is much safer to use non-blood substitutes (crystalloids, synthetic colloids, etc.) and, in some circumstances, more cost effective [14]. Anesthesiologists are aware of such risks involved but it is without question that the ability to provide oxygen to at-risk tissues is best served by increasing the availability of circulating hemoglobin via red blood cell transfusions. In knowing this simple fact, blood bank registries should make great efforts to maximize the acquisition and appropriate storage of these blood products to increase the availability in the event that there is an exhaustive demand through voluntary blood drives. The DMB should be in constant communication with available local blood banks to help create community outreach initiatives to maximize public awareness.

When Disaster Strikes

There is a direct relationship between the overall dampening of the devastation caused by a disaster and the appropriate pre-planning and execution of disaster management strategies. If a disaster is imminent, it is imperative that the DMB coordinate meetings to review all avenues to protect and provide relief for people in harm's way. Medical personnel should be on high alert as well as all operational medical facilities that are capable of assisting (hospitals, surgical centers, outpatient clinics, etc.) The anesthesiology DMB members will assume the leading role in ensuring that all essential personnel are ready to act if and/or when swift action is needed.

Implementing an Initial Response Plan

If a disaster occurs, the anesthesiology DMB members should activate the response team(s). The notifications should be delivered through all forms of media (television, telephone, e-mail, and radio) and the emergency contact numbers should be used to alert all essential personnel. These persons should be delegated their roles and eventual destinations by the Anesthesiologist DMB members in direct coordination with the First Responders. The primary goal of the first responders is to identify the type and severity of the event, the most common anticipated types of injuries, and to determine whether there is a greater need for on-site medical treatment and facility establishment versus evacuating and transporting patients to more appropriate and capable medical facilities. If transportation is deemed impossible, the appropriate course of action must be taken to bring medical professionals, supplies, and resources to the scene under the guidance of the local department of transportation and police authorities.

Triage Strategies

Upon establishing a plan, the anesthesiologist(s) within the first responder group should begin a survey of those most severely injured and immediately begin to triage these victims based on their individual injuries and clinical condition. From a broad approach, these individuals should be categorized as:

1. *Critical*—Prognosis is very poor and are beyond medical treatment.
2. *Severe*—Those in need of immediate medical attention and treatment on-site.
3. *Moderate*—Those who are clinically stable and not requiring emergency medical attention/treatment.

The Simple Triage and Rapid Treatment (START) system has been used in the USA since its creation in the 1980s. Its principles have been adopted by many other countries including Canada, Saudi Arabia, Israel, and parts of Australia [3]. The START system was designed to allow the healthcare provider to perform a patient assessment within 60 s and to identify those victims in need of immediate medical attention/intervention. Patients are assigned a colored ribbon dependent upon the severity of their injuries. The categorization of these patients is based upon respirations, perfusion/pulses, and mental status. Patients who remain apneic after initial airway repositioning are tagged as "deceased" and subsequently have a black label placed upon their body. Those patients who have a respiratory rate greater than 30 breaths per minute, have a capillary refill greater than 2 s, or are unable to follow simple commands are deemed "immediate" and are assigned a red label. The remaining patients are deemed "delayed" and are given a yellow label. Many other triage systems have been created and implemented based on the determination of each regional disaster management board. See Table 23.1.

Table 23.1 START triage [3]

Red	Any of the following
Immediate	Respirations >30 breaths/min
Priority 1	Capillary refill <2 s or no palpable radial pulse
	Not able to follow commands
Yellow	Non-ambulatory patients who do not meet black or red criteria
Delayed	
Priority II	
Green	Able to walk to a designated safe area for further assessment
Minor	
Priority III	
Black	Not breathing despite one attempt to open the airway
Deceased	
Priority IV	

Patients should be registered upon arrival in any type of medical care facility as they would be in the event of any naturally occurring hospitalization or clinic visit. In the event of a catastrophic event/emergency, some patients may not be competent clinically to provide such information. These patients should be assigned temporary medical record numbers (MRNs) that will be used to identify them as they receive different phases of medical care. The MRN numbers of current patients should be given to the hospital coordinator to help maintain an up-to-date census of those victims receiving care at their institution. These MRNs will also help ensure that the each patient receives his/her appropriate medication optimizing continuity of care. The effectiveness of this care is often derived from attentive and coordinated supervision provided by anesthesiologists whether on-site or in ICU and/or hospital settings. Anesthesiologists must be able to diligently and efficiently provide goal-directed medical care whether it is via direct patient care or through a guided supervisory position.

Initial Treatment Considerations

Once the triage assessments have begun, coordinated groups should begin prioritizing treating patients according to their categorization and/or severity. Ideally, these cohort groups should consist of an anesthesia provider, a surgical specialist, and at least three assistants if available: one dedicated to each specialist and one to serve as needed. If the clinical situation requires emergency surgery, these assistants will help the specialists however possible with particular emphasis on the provision of supplies/equipment. The anesthesiologist will briefly assess the patient's current clinical condition as it may be impossible to implement the standard American Society of Anesthesiologist standards for monitoring in these disaster situations and will develop an anesthetic plan. Of primary importance to the Anesthesiologist is to be able to control and/or assist the patient's airway, breathing, and circulation (ABCs). If unable to properly secure the airway, the anesthesia provider will be wary of using drugs that may potentially cause respiratory depression or apnea while still being able to provide analgesia to the patient. Securing intravenous access may also be very difficult in these situations hence the use of intramuscular (IM) drugs that will greatly facilitate the ability to provide anesthesia. *Ketamine*, an *N*-methyl-D-ASPARTATE (NMDA) receptor antagonist, has been the drug of choice in these dire circumstances given its clinical profile which includes its lack of cardiovascular depression, the ability to maintain spontaneous respiration, amnesia, and analgesic potential in sub-therapeutic dosages. It is also able to be administered via an IM route which greatly facilitates its use. An assistant will be needed specifically for the anesthesiologist especially in the event that significant amounts of intravenous fluids (blood and blood products, crystalloids, colloids) are needed for resuscitation of these patients granted there is intravenous (IV) or intraosseous (IO) access. Urgent plans should be made with ICU capable medical facilities for the transportation of these patients immediately after surgical intervention. The on-site anesthesiologist should communicate appropriate hand-off ideally directly to the anesthesiologist at the receiving hospital or facility. Of importance is the type of procedure, resuscitation requirements, and anesthetic management provided.

In the event of chemical or toxin exposure, the anesthesiologist must ensure protection to all medical personnel primarily to allow for medical care to be provided to victims, including availability and distribution of biohazard suits and masks. The first responder group should also include infectious disease specialists and/or specialists knowledgeable in the chemistry and chemical warfare. Treatment requirements should be assessed based on estimates of the number of victims involved. These resources should be mobilized to the scene as well as to designated facilities. Of the anesthetic medications, the Oximes (Pralidoxime chloride, Obidoxime) as well as Pyridostigmine should be readily available in mass quantities in the event of toxic nerve gas exposure.

Patients who are deemed "delayed" by initial triage should be evacuated and assisted to predesignated centers for secondary assessment and subsequent transfer to medical facilities. The continual reporting and updating of disaster coverage, the ongoing need for anesthesiologist(s) as well as other specialists, capacities of medical facilities, and inventories of supplies are essential functions to stay ahead of the curve in continually providing appropriate care and maximizing patient outcomes. There should be a designated official within each hospital facility whose primary objective is to continually review the availability of operating rooms, ICU rooms, and hospital beds. Transfer of critical patients to capable medical facilities without delay or the potential for the lack of essential resources to provide necessary care will greatly improve patient outcomes. The designated coordinators at each facility should continually update the status of their capacity to the central DMB so as to avoid overcrowding or deficiencies in provision of appropriate medical care to victims.

There is much to be learned from previous disasters to improve outcomes in the event that another disaster is to occur in particular regions. For example, there have been multiple reviews of the intricacies of Hurricane Katrina and its overall impact on New Orleans, Louisiana as well as the Gulf Coast. Great emphasis has been placed on certain essential points that correlate with those discussed in this chapter. In areas which are more likely to experience severe flooding secondary to geographical location, there should be meticulous review of previous data that serve to identify those areas most prone to being heavily impacted. Once these highly susceptible regions have been identified, the management of these lands should be monitored very closely. Prohibiting new development and flood-proofing existing structures will significantly decrease the amount of damage in the event of a flood as seen by the Gulf Coast during Hurricane Katrina [15]. If certain preventative and/or protective measures have previously been constructed (dams, levees, storm channels, etc.), it is of great importance to ensure these structures are of the highest standards of modern construction [15]. This point is emphasized by the catastrophic failures of the levees in New Orleans which were overpowered by the flood waters caused by Hurricane Katrina. A review of construction efforts centered around these levees revealed a chilling fact that these levees had not been assessed formally since 1985 when the Lake Pontchartrain and Vicinity Hurricane Protection Project (LP & VHPP) was re-evaluated and the decision was made to replace the existing surge barriers with a taller levee system [16]. Over 20 years after initial construction, new developments and changes in climate patterns were not enough to prompt review of the infrastructure of New Orleans' levee system and this lack of attention proved to be catastrophic when challenged by Hurricane Katrina flooding. Ideally, there should be a regulatory body of officials who are responsible for the maintenance of such structures which tests the integrity of such protective structures to ensure their quality and effectiveness. As in the case of the torrential annual flooding in Bangladesh which is necessary for the revitalization of fertile lands for crop productions, efforts should be placed on minimizing the damage of such floods while ensuring that the damages incurred by such are limited as much as feasibly possible.

Post-disaster Management

Without a doubt, victims of a wide range of disasters will often need medical and psychological care provided from initial triage to eventual return back to an approximation of life pre-disaster. There are many facets of recovery that should be addressed beyond the initial triage and medical attention. Long term issues that are equally important in addressing in order to allow a disaster-stricken region a more global recovery include infection rates/epidemics, psychological issues (i.e., post-traumatic stress disorder (PTSD)), as well as a retrospective review of the chronology of the actual disaster(s) and the subsequent disaster response.

Infectious Disease Transmission and Outbreaks

The majority of mortalities post-disaster are most often directly related to the initial disaster impact. As previously mentioned, crush injuries, blunt trauma, and burn injuries are those identified to place victims at higher mortality risk. Beyond the initial catastrophe, the prolonged detrimental impact on health has been proven to be multifactorial. The associated destruction or interruption in healthcare facilities and systems, the limitations to securing stable food sources secondary to disruptions in farming, livestock, or the usual importation of foods into the region, or the scarcity of medications or interruptions of ongoing treatments. Identified risk factors for infectious disease transmission or outbreaks include overcrowding and unplanned shelters, poor water conditions or sanitation, poor nutritional status, and inadequate provisions to maintain an appropriate level of hygiene (Fig. 23.7).

The infectious disease outbreaks witnessed in previous disaster situations have allowed researchers to categorize the associated events into phases. Given that disease transmission can occur hours, days, or even months after the initial disaster, three clinical phases have been described to chronologically categorize the health effects of survivors and those injured.

Phase 1 or Impact Phase: 4-day period when most victims are extricated and initial treatment strategies are implemented.

Phase 2 or Post-impact Phase: Period extending from day 4 up to 4 weeks when most infectious diseases (airborne, waterborne, and food-borne etiologies) would surface.

Phase 3 or Recovery Phase: Period starting at 4 weeks post-disaster when symptoms of latent-type of infections become clinically apparent. This period is noted to be when infectious diseases begin to grow into epidemics.

It is extremely important to realize that it is not the initial disaster that causes the infectious disease transmission and/or outbreaks but rather the exacerbation of the risk factors that exist in the disaster region(s). It has been postulated that there should be a rapid disease risk assessment performed within the first week post-disaster impact to identify risk factors and health needs. Utilizing case management and systems of surveillance can significantly limit infectious disease burdens associated with catastrophes.

The psychological impact of disaster is a topic of much interest as it can prove to be a significant burden to the mental health of disaster victims and witnesses alike. In reviewing the potential impact of such traumatic experiences, we look towards the experiences of victims of Hurricane Katrina and the Haiti Earthquake.

Post-Katrina-Health Issues

New Orleans and surrounding cities experienced massive flooding due to multiple levee breaks. Because of this, more than 100,000 homes were inundated with 4 or more feet of water. Many Mississippi or Louisiana coastal areas (within one mile of the Gulf of Mexico) lost all structures. Additionally, this natural disaster resulted in over 1,800 deaths. This combination of events created unimaginable stress for inhabitants left to deal with the aftermath [18].

Over 500,000 people were in possible need of mental health treatment after Hurricane Katrina according to The Substance Abuse and Mental Health Service Administration (SAMHSA). It was determined later that only 1.6 % of those in need received mental health treatment. First responders were surveyed 2–3months after the event; 19 % of police officers reported symptoms of posttraumatic stress disorder (PTSD) and 26 % reported symptoms of major depression, while amongst firefighters surveyed 22 % reported symptoms consistent with PTSD and 27 % reported major depressive symptoms [18–20].

Most associate PTSD when thinking of major mental health issues experienced by a community rebounding from a natural disaster; however, common anxiety and depressive disorders are more prevalent while long-term chronic stress may result in cognitive impairment. The term "*Katrina Brain*" was coined to describe the common impairments in concentration and memory experienced by many left to rebuild their lives under long-term chronic stress [22].

Ken Sakauye, MD, professor of Psychiatry at Louisiana State University Health Science Center in New Orleans, before and after Hurricane Katrina, described the effects created by long term stress. Diurnal regulation of cortisol is lost in these individuals and persistently high cortisol levels eventually lead to hippocampal atrophy, short term memory impairment and may contribute to the

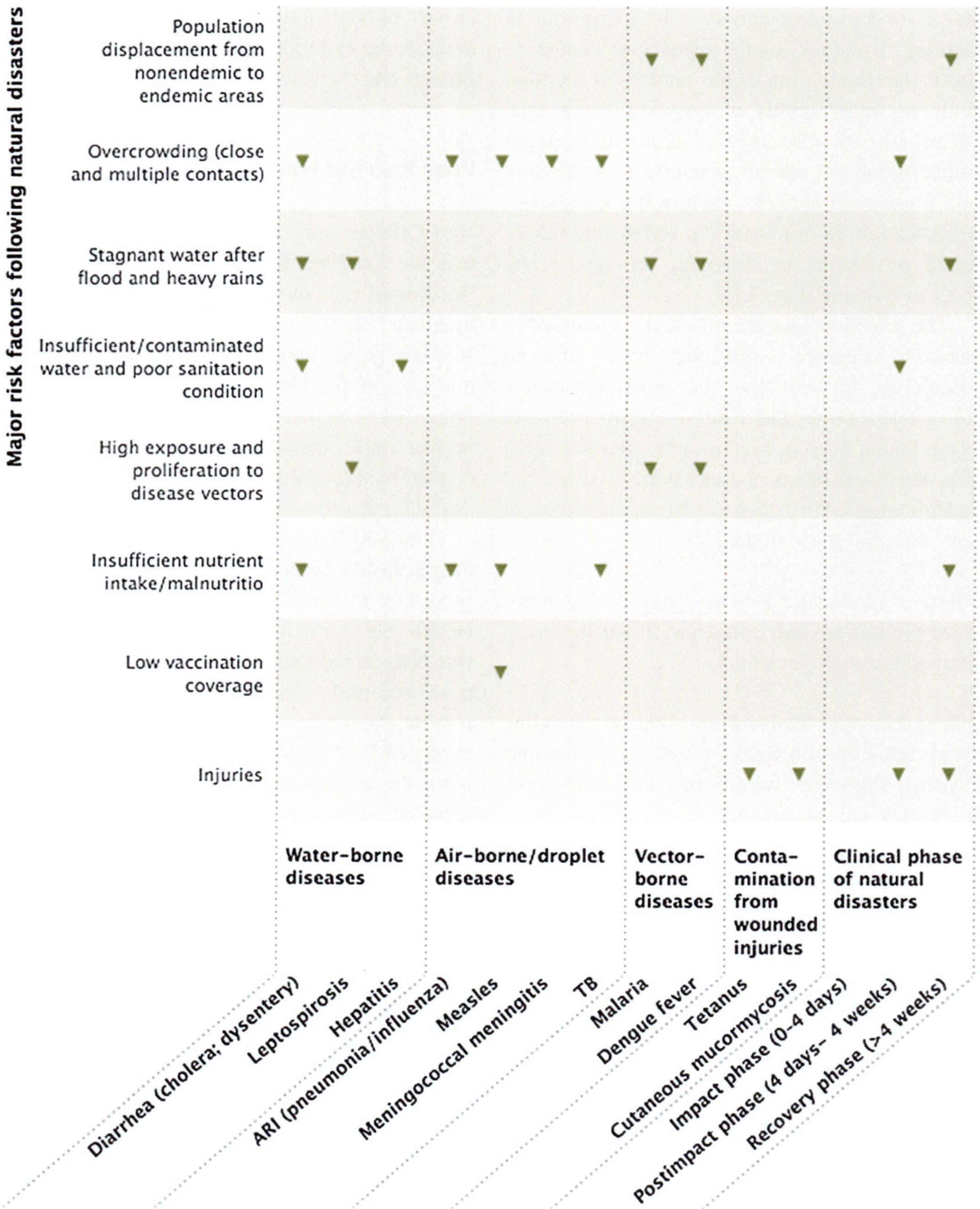

Fig. 23.7 Risk factors and onset of communicable diseases following natural disasters [17]

high health morbidity and death rates experienced by communities after a natural disaster occurs [22]. Additionally, Dr. Sakauye theorized that the loss of the support network (family and friends scattered), healthcare network and feeling of governmental abandonment compounded daily stress.

Months after Hurricane Katrina, with 50 % of the population gone, crisis helpline calls for psychiatric issues increased by 61 %. Dramatic changes in death, murder and suicide rates occurred in Orleans parish. From the previous year, death rates increased by 25 %, murder rates doubled for Orleans parish, while suicide rates tripled. Additionally, new mental health problems for children increased significantly [23].

The majority of initial reports and studies involved those individuals and families who returned to the New Orleans area to rebuild after Hurricane Katrina. It is now recognized that those displaced experienced even higher rates of mental health and substance abuse issues after Hurricane Katrina. The Center for Disease Control and Prevention surveyed individuals living in the New Orleans area in October 2005 and those living in trailers or hotels in 2006 and found that adults displaced from their dwelling for greater than two weeks post Katrina had higher drug use, cigarette use, serious psychological distress, major depressive episode and unmet need for mental health treatment or counseling than those not displaced. A recent study concluded that of the 20,000 children displaced by Hurricane Katrina, 60 % have serious emotional disorders, behavior issues or housing instability [23, 24].

Much is known about the psychological consequences of Hurricane Katrina; however, the effects on one's physical health are now emerging [25–27]. A retrospective study was conducted at Tulane Medical Center involving patients admitted with acute myocardial infarction (AMI) 2 years before Hurricane Katrina and in the 5 years afterward. The two groups were compared and the post-Katrina group had a higher prevalence of known coronary artery disease, prior coronary artery bypass grafts, hyperlipidemia, psychiatric comorbidities, smoking, and substance abuse. Also, the post-Katrina group was more likely unemployed and uninsured. Overall, they found a threefold increase in the incidence of AMI and believe the prevalence of these clinical and psychological factors have and will continue to have a profound impact on the community's cardiovascular health [28].

HIV disease progression has been measured post Katrina. A year after Hurricane Katrina, 145 HIV-infected patients returned for care at the HIV Outpatient Program clinic in New Orleans. They were interviewed and blood was drawn. Clinical factors pre and one and two year's post-Katrina were obtained. Of the 145 patients, 37.2 % had PTSD. Those HIV patients with PTSD were more likely to have CD 4 cell counts <200/mm [3] 2 years post disaster and have detectable viral loads at both follow-up sample times post-disaster [29].

Outside Aid

Medical capabilities of local or regional hospitals are sometimes overwhelmed when disasters occur. Because of this, medical aid from surrounding states or countries is needed to meet demands. Many hospitals have provided medical supplies or medical talent to aid those facing obstacles post-disaster. Some hospitals and universities medical centers have developed mission programs to help those in need. Those creating a pre-disaster plan should create a list of these programs, so that all contingencies are addressed.

Protocol Improvements

As the region affected by disaster begins the process of recovery and rebuilding, it is imperative that the details of the catastrophe be reviewed meticulously. It is of utmost importance for certain details to be addressed so as to improve upon current protocols and/or treatment strategies for future unforeseen disasters. The type of disaster(s) should be identified and individualized (in the event that multiple events occurred concurrently or sequentially) as well as the initial responses to each. Both tasks that were efficiently executed as well as those which lacked in strength should be identified and reconstructed if needed. Different strategies should be proposed and tested for their integrity when hypothetically applied to the previous events. The DMB, and more importantly the anesthesiologists, should identify the strengths and weaknesses of their primary role and identify areas that need improvement to ensure better outcomes in future scenarios.

It would be of great benefit for committees to review the statistics and data directly related to the disaster. Statisticians should calculate all important data in order to quantify the toll that was inflicted upon that particular region by the events. Data should be compiled to review many different facets of the disaster including the number injured, most common types of injuries, number/type of emergency surgeries needed, length of hospital stays, number of medical providers, types of medications used, overall cost burdens, and the types of resources required and used in the care of all victims regardless of clinical severity. These reviews will help to identify strengths and weaknesses in previous disaster strategies and plans. Once identified, these protocols can be strengthened or changed altogether so that in the unfortunate event of future catastrophes, a region will be optimally prepared and better equipped to address the immense burden of providing medical care in an unforeseen, uncontrolled environment. All of this information can be reused in formulating improvements upon the former disaster management strategies.

References

1. Casualties of the September 11 attacks. Wikipedia, the free encyclopedia, 2014. Web. 7 April 2014. http://en.wikipedia.org/wiki/ Casualties_of_the_September_11_attacks.
2. Disaster – definition and more from the free Merriam-Webster dictionary. Merriam-Webster, 2014. Web. 7 April 2014. http://www.merriam-webster.com/dictionary/disaster.
3. Koenig and Schultz. Disaster medicine.
4. Hurricane Katrina. Wikipedia, the free encyclopedia, 2014. Web. 7 April 2014. http://en.wikipedia.org/wiki/Hurricane_Katrina.
5. 2010 Haiti Earthquake. Wikipedia, the free encyclopedia, 2014. Web. 7 April 2014. http://en.wikipedia.org/wiki/2010_Haiti_earthquake.
6. Key statistics. U.N. Office of the Secretary-General's Special Adviser on Community-Based Medicine & Lessons From Haiti, 2012. Web. 7 April 2014. http://www.lessonsfromhaiti.org/relief-and-recovery/key-statistics/.
7. Armand V, James D. Japan – 366 days after the Quake… 19000 lives lost, 1.2 million buildings damaged, $574 billion. Earthquake-Report.com, 2012. Web. 7 April 2014. http://earthquake-report.com/2012/03/10/japan-366-days-after-the- quake-19000-lives-lost-1-2-million-buildings-damaged-574-billion/.
8. Worst U.S. Forest Fires. Infoplease, 2014. Web. 7 April 2014. http://www.infoplease.com/ipa/A0778688.html#ixzz2wo84ODyP.
9. The cost of September 11. Institute for the Analysis of Global Security, 2004. Web. 7 April 2014. http://www.iags.org/costof911.html.
10. Oklahoma City bombing. Wikipedia, the free encyclopedia, 2014. Web. 19 April 2014. http://en.wikipedia.org/wiki/2010_Haiti_earthquake.
11. Halabja chemical attack. Wikipedia, the free encyclopedia, 2014. Web. 19 April 2014. http://en.wikipedia.org/wiki/2010_Haiti_earthquake.
12. Joseph M. Chapter on emergency preparedness – manual for anesthesia department organization and management. ASA Committee on Trauma and Emergency Preparedness, American Society of Anesthesiologists, 2010. Web. 7 April 2014. http://www.asahq.org/For-Members/About-ASA/ASA-Committees/~/media/For%20Members/COTEP/MADOM-Edited-by-McIsaac-6.ashx.
13. Pan Am Flight 103. Wikipedia, the free encyclopedia, 2014. Web. 19 April 2014. http://en.wikipedia.org/wiki/2010_Haiti_earthquake.
14. Iserson, Kenneth V. Improvised medicine.
15. http://www.un.org/esa/sustdev/publications/flood_guidelines_sec02.pdf.
16. http://www.journalofamericanhistory.org/projects/katrina/resources/levee.html.
17. http://unu.edu/publications/articles/preventing-and-controlling-infectious-diseases-after-natural-disasters.html#info.
18. Weisler RH, Barbee IV JG, Townsend MH. Mental health and recovery in the Gulf Coast after Hurricanes Katrina and Rita. JAMA. 2006;296:585–8.
19. Agency for Toxic Substances and Disease Registry, 2005. Helping families deal with the stress of relocation after a disaster. http://www.atsdr.cdc.gov/publications/100233-RelocationStress.pdf. Accessed 22 Dec 2006.
20. Centers for Disease Control and Prevention. Assessment of Health Related Needs after Hurricanes Katrina and Rita: Orleans and Jefferson Parishes, New Orleans area, Louisiana, October 17–22. Morb Mortal Wkly Rep. 2006a;55:38–41. http://www.cdc.gov/mmwr/preview/mmwrhtml/mm5502a5.htm. Accessed 22 Dec 2006.
21. Centers for Disease Control and Prevention. Health hazard evaluation of police officers and firefighters after Hurricanes Katrina—New Orleans, Louisiana, October 17–28 and November 30–December 5, 2005. Morb Mortal Wkly Rep. 2006b;55:456–8.
22. Sakauye K. "Katrina Brain:" acute cognitive impairment. Program and abstracts of the 19th US Psychiatric & Mental Health Congress; 2006 Nov 15–19, New Orleans, Louisiana. Session 23–3.
23. Centers for Disease Control and Prevention. Assessment of health-related needs after Hurricanes Katrina and Rita—Orleans and Jefferson Parishes,

New Orleans area, Louisiana, October 17–22, 2005. Morb Mortal Wkly Rep. 2006c;55(2):38–41. http://www.cdc.gov/mmwr/preview/mmwr/mm5502a5.htm.

24. Abramson D, Redlener I, Stehling-Ariza T, Fuller E. The legacy of Katrina's children: estimating the numbers of hurricane-related at-risk children in the Gulf Coast States of Louisiana and Mississippi. NCDP Research Brief 2007_12. National Center for Disaster Preparedness, Columbia University Mailman School of Public Health, December 2007. http://www.ncdp.mailman.columbia.edu/files/legacy_katrina_children.pdf.
25. Madrid P, Grant R, Rosen R. Creating disability through inadequate disaster response: Hurricane Katrina and its aftermath. In: Disability: insights from across fields and around the world. Volume 2. Portsmouth NH: Praeger Press; 2009. p. 1–16.
26. Osofsky HJ, Osofsky JD, Kronenberg M, Brennan A, Hansel TC. Posttraumatic stress symptoms in children after Hurricane Katrina: predicting the need for mental health services. Am J Orthopsychiatry. 2009;79:212–20.
27. Children's Health Fund. Reforming disaster case management: national lessons learned from Louisiana. New York, NY: Children's Health Fund; December 2009.
28. Moscona J, Tiwari T, Munshi K, Srivastav S, Delafontaine P, Irimpen A. The effects of Hurricane Katrina on acute myocardial infarction five years after the storm. J Am Coll Cardiol. 2012;59(13s1):E354.
29. Reilly K, Clark R, Schmidt N, et al. The effect of post-traumatic stress disorder on HIV disease progression following hurricane Katrina. AIDS Care. 2009;21(10):1298–305.

Part III

Education at Home and Abroad

Surgical Mission Trips as a Component of Medical Education and Residency Training

24

Peter J. Taub and Lester Silver

Benefits

The benefits of global missions are numerous and students and residents can provide valuable assistance on such trips. Certainly, those who speak the language of the host country are at an obvious advantage and often serve as translators for those who do not. The education students and residents receive is immeasurable. They learn alternative models of health care delivery, how to manage health care with fewer resources, the effects of local culture on health care, and the management of disease entities they might not see back home, among other advantages. In the absence of sophisticated primary care and routine imaging studies, students and residents must rely more on their ability to perform thorough patient histories and complete physical examinations than they might at home where patients may have extensive medical charts documenting their entire medical history, including monthly clinic visits and numerous diagnostic studies.

Mission trips also foster problem solving (the "MacGyver effect"). Where resources might be abundant back home, they are often scarce abroad. When machines break, there might not be a technician on call to repair them or a backup machine ready to substitute. In such circumstances, ingenuity and decision making become valuable traits. Is the problem something that can be overcome with the available resources or do hard decisions have to be made about making alternate plans? These experiences have been shown to improve skills and confidence among students and residents, as well as increase their sensitivity to health care costs, awareness of reliability on technology, and need to improve communication across different cultures [1].

There are also benefits to the Departments that support and offer an international experience. Many students and residents have an interest in such programs and electively seek out and rank higher those programs that offer rotations or trips to foreign countries. The Department also creates a wider exposure for itself if their attendings, residents, and students carry with them the name of their institution as they travel abroad. Relationships with colleagues in foreign countries and at foreign medical schools are established and reinforced by future trips.

There are numerous examples where ongoing relationships outside of the single mission trip have developed between mentor programs in North America and a local university or hospital. As an example in Rwanda, a mutually beneficial relationship has been established between the Canadian Anesthesiologists International Education Foundation, the American Society of

P.J. Taub, MD, FACS, FAAP • L. Silver, MD (✉)
Division of Plastic and Reconstructive Surgery, Icahn School of Medicine at Mount Sinai, 5 East 98th Street, Box 1259, New York, NY 10029, USA
e-mail: peter.taub@mountsinai.org; lester.silver@mountsinai.org

R. Roth et al. (eds.), *The Role of Anesthesiology in Global Health: A Comprehensive Guide*, DOI 10.1007/978-3-319-09423-6_24, © Springer International Publishing Switzerland 2015

Anesthesiologists, and the National University of Rwanda. Volunteer faculty, often with residents from Canadian programs, travel to Rwanda to lecture and demonstrate in the local residency-training program. Similarly, Rwandan residents travel to Universities in Canada to enhance their training [2].

From these relationships, joint research projects and publications should be fostered. In many instances, academic endeavors by foreign clinicians are rare on account of limited resources but are certainly desired. Efforts should be made to include foreign colleagues on papers and presentations that relate to those conditions addressed on the trip.

Challenges

There are numerous challenges to developing a global health initiative and the amount borne by students and residents will relate to their level of involvement. Some students may not have ventured far from home for either college or medical school and may find it difficult to adjust to a different culture, as they will interact with people of different opinions, who speak different languages, and eat foods with different ingredients and flavors.

For some, the sheer numbers of patients that require care may be daunting. Students and residents who see a small handful of patients in clinics at home may be surprised to find large numbers of patients of all ages needing care. Such experiences may elicit feelings that the care provided on any one short trip is insignificant to the population on a global scale. Similarly, any one mission is limited by time and hard decisions often have to be made about which patients receive care and which do not. These decisions should probably not fall on students and residents who are the more junior members of a team, but are better left to attendings and local clinicians.

At home, team members have the luxury of any and all supplies they require and the opportunity to try out and use the latest equipment. Abroad, a lack of basic tools is usually the norm and team members have to bring what they feel they need to safely care for the patients or make do with what the host institutions provide. Thus scouting a location for a trip is critical and team members have to be flexible and resourceful in their decisions.

Some students may also be concerned with their own personal welfare, such as the safety of the housing and the cleanliness of the food and water supply. Again, housing arrangements should be scouted well in advance of the trip with a backup plan in hand. Smart food decisions should be made while abroad, including avoiding ice and freshly washed vegetables and drinking only bottled water in areas where gastrointestinal distress is common in those not used to the drinking water.

Students and residents may also have concerns about the costs involved in a mission trip. They should be aware of what is required of them up front so that there are no surprises during or after the trip. Some schools and organizations cover student and resident expenses, which alleviates this burden; others cover some or none of the costs. Funds may be available for travel alone while the students or residents cover housing and meals. However, meals and incidentals over the duration of a trip may prove costly.

Planning

The ultimate success of any medical mission lies in the completeness of the plan. Preparation should probably begin one or more years in advance of the actual mission. Medical students and/or residents with proper guidance and direction from more senior physicians should actually participate in the planning. Such actions serve as a valuable learning experience for international health care delivery. The plan should include the local problems to be addressed, the country and city, the medical facility, the length of the trip, team members, housing, transportation, and other critical information discussed herein.

The index population should have one or more medical conditions in which the team has an interest and familiarity regarding pathology and treatment. The condition(s) addressed abroad should be fairly straightforward, not requiring complicated preoperative studies, extensive equipment, or intensive postoperative care or rehabilitation. That being said, there are certainly successful mission trips that address the above, such as craniofacial malformations that require preoperative computed tomography, intraoperative drills and saws, and postoperative intensive unit care [3].

While medical students and residents may not have much familiarity with the medical conditions to be addressed, the attending physicians (surgeons, anesthesiologists, and others) should only treat those conditions that they manage at their home institution. International patients should be offered the same respect and high-level care that is offered at home. Medical missions should not serve as a venue to "practice" procedures that one does not do at home. The students and residents however may benefit from working with attendings from different subspecialties with whom they may not get to work at home until they are more senior.

The destination country should be decided upon based on several important factors. It should have a relatively stable governmental structure that does not place the team in significant danger from either the political climate or environmental concerns. The planners should be aware of any local customs/religions so as not to offend the host team members and patients upon arrival. The destination city should have a medical facility that has the resources needed for the safe treatment of patients, including a functioning blood bank and an intensive care unit. Also critical to international missions are "ground forces" (i.e., host team members) that can identify patients needing care and caring for these patients after the team returns home. The attendings from home should have an amicable, open relationship with the local host physicians since the latter are critical to the success of the mission. Contempt or derision between team members is an absolute recipe for disaster.

The destination institution/city should offer appropriate housing opportunities for team members. Accommodations should be in a safe neighborhood, clean, and situated not too far from the host institution to minimize the time needed for travel. If the housing is not within walking distance from the medical facility, transportation should be planned, either public transportation and/or a rental vehicle. Buses and taxis should be used with care and never alone. At least one team member should be comfortable driving in a foreign country, possibly in a vehicle with manual transmission. All local rules for driving should be known and followed as they are at home.

Currently, most institutions seek to approve mission trips in which their attendings, residents, or students are participating prior to embarking. The location, schedule, and overall plan will be reviewed by a global health committee and either approved or denied based on the merits of the proposed mission. Some institutions insist on a review of the travel advisories from the State Department to ensure that the region is safe. Most require proof of immunization for team members traveling abroad. Often, approval by the host institution is necessary for the institution to provide insurance for resident and student team members. Documentation should cover medical care for illnesses to team members while they are abroad, as well as emergency evacuation.

Financing an international mission often falls on the sponsoring organization or the team members. The budget generally includes costs for travel, housing, local transportation, food, and medical supplies. Students and residents can be asked to pay their own travel expenses and accommodations or the organization or school with which they are participating may cover them. Larger organizations often have the financial structure and clout to subsidize the travel and housing of all team members. Smaller organizations can benefit from fund raising efforts, which may be organized and run by students and residents.

Timing

In discussing the possible involvement of medical students and residents in international medical mission trips, an important question is "when." It could be argued that some minimal level of education/training should be completed at home prior to joining a medical mission. Is it better to take a first year resident as opposed to a fourth year student or are there students of any age that may be better able to participate? Perhaps, rather than the level of training, the decision to take a student should be based on prior global experience, the degree of maturity, and/or some demonstrated interest level. Since residents can potentially have more responsibility, higher PGY-level residents might be considered over interns and lower level residents. For surgical missions, residents in their chief year are preferred for their ability to add more technical expertise to the mission.

Any mission trip takes time to plan, time to prepare, and time to execute. The length of the trip must be considered in the planning. The trip itself is usually the least time intensive, usually spanning a week or 2. Attending physicians often dedicate a portion of their vacation time to such trips and cannot spend weeks or months away from their private practices or clinical departments. Students have curriculum concerns and residents have rotation schedules; thus a mission longer than 1 or 2 weeks may be too time consuming for some. Having a resident away from the program should not place undue stress on the work schedule or the call schedule of the remaining residents. Residents can often be scheduled for a month on a mission trip if it is part of a residency block. Vacation time may also be used for missions. It should be noted that longer missions also have potentially higher housing costs, meal costs, and equipment requirements.

Seasonality may also be important. Some countries have a rainy season, which participants may want to avoid. Local holidays are a double-edged sword: patients are off from work, which may be a good time for a trip, but they may also be away traveling. Similarly, key local personnel may not be available during the holidays.

Trips that involve operating on children may be better scheduled over the summer (winter back home if the destination is in the southern hemisphere) to minimize cancellations for ear infections and routine coughs and colds. Many schools are often on break over the summer so that children may not miss significant classwork if their surgery takes place at that time. Finally, summer missions allow team members to pack lighter than they would if the mission occurred over the winter when temperatures are colder.

Students may or may not possess the same freedom of time. The summer between the first and second years of medical school is often not filled with clinical requirements in the hospital and a couple of months can be dedicated to planning, preparation, or actual travel. Alternatively, a student or resident can take a year away from school or training to dedicate to a medical mission. This time commitment may be necessary in the early stages of development when approvals need to be obtained, contacts need to made, and planning is the most intense.

Travel

Travel can be a complicated endeavor if there are large numbers of personnel and a lot of equipment that needs to be taken. Medical students and residents can certainly participate in organizing travel plans. Airline flights and local transportation to and from the airport need to be arranged in advance. Team members often arrive from different cities, at different times, on different airlines, and often on different days. Key personnel should arrive in advance of days for equipment and patient screening.

If equipment needs to pass through customs, paperwork may be needed to prevent it from being confiscated or at least held up. Often, foreign countries fear that equipment is being brought it to be sold on the black market. Since time is valuable, delays can be quite detrimental to the mission. Students can coordinate the inventory of supplies that are being brought on the trip well in advance, including the serial numbers for all durable goods. This information should be sent to the Ministry of Health in the host country and copies of the receipts that it was received and approved should accompany any team members that will be traveling with the equipment so that they may have the information when they pass through the customs office.

Foreign countries are now more restrictive in what items are used during surgery. At one time, any suture material or medication could be used. Mission trips would gather expired suture at home throughout the year and bring it for use on the trip. Nowadays, foreign hospital administrators insist on using only products that have not expired and will inspect these products before allowing them into the operating suite. Similarly, durable goods may need to show proof that they have passed a mechanical inspection.

Preoperative Care

Once at the destination, the most important preoperative task is the screening and selection of patients to treat. Often the host clinicians have advertised and gathered possible surgical candidates before the team's arrival. Again, students and residents can play significant roles in the screening process with adequate supervision. Ultimately however, decisions regarding which patients will be scheduled for surgery will fall on the attending physicians. For surgical missions, the most junior members can participate in gathering medical histories, examining patients, speaking with families, and taking preoperative photographs. There can be a tremendous amount of organization that is needed in getting patients (and their families) to see the necessary team members in order to provide treatment or decide on the appropriateness of surgical intervention.

Prior to beginning a week or more of operative procedures, an inventory of the available equipment and supplies needs to be created. Some of the equipment may be brought from home, some may be left over from prior missions, and some may be provided by the host institution. Surgical instruments need to be left at the hospital in advance of the first day of surgery so that they may be properly sterilized. Again, students and residents can assist in creating the inventory and seeing that everything is returned at the conclusion of the trip. After the first operative day, the instruments again need to be sterilized for cases the following day. Often, some equipment can be left for the host institution's ongoing use.

Intraoperative Care

Intraoperatively, students and residents should be able to perform level-appropriate procedural tasks such as placing intravenous and intra-arterial lines, Foley catheters, intubation, emergence, and charting. Because of the critical nature of anesthetic and surgical care, vigilant supervision is paramount, especially during intubation, emergence, and key portions of any operation. This component of the mission trip has the greatest equipment requirements. Monitoring devices and ventilators may not resemble those at home and attendings and residents alike should be familiar with their use prior to starting a case that requires sedation or general anesthesia.

Similarly, the vast array of medications available at home and restocked by support personnel may not be available abroad. As part of the planning, a list of necessary medications and equipment should be drawn up and checked against availability at the institution. Anything that is deemed necessary at home should be brought with the team for use on the mission. In the case of medications and disposable devices (as well as sutures), supplies should be in their original, sterile containers and not expired. Durable equipment should be registered with customs both at home and abroad so that they may be brought into and out of the country without suspicion from the local government.

For surgical missions, junior members who plan to participate either in procedures, such as line placement, or the actual surgical procedure should have had some experience in an operative setting. They should understand the principles of sterile techniques and universal precautions. These practices will minimize the rate of infectious complications and the chance of inadvertent contamination by team members.

Postoperative Care

In the postoperative period, patient care remains paramount. The level of critical care monitoring may not be as thorough as it is at home and patients must be followed carefully. Here again, students and residents can play an important role. If a subsequent operative case is going, for which the attending must be present, a student and/or resident can periodically monitor the earlier patient in the recovery area and report back any changes that occur.

On the days following a surgical procedure, students and residents should employ the same practices abroad that they undertake at home. These functions include morning rounds before starting the days' cases to evaluate any postoperative patients. Of course, there should be adequate supervision so that complications may be recognized and promptly addressed.

Another excellent role for students and residents is to track outcomes. Patient demographics should be kept as a chart along with the anesthesia record, an operative note, and the record of the postoperative course, noting any complications. Since some complications do not manifest immediately, follow-up with the host medical team at some point after the trip is important to ascertain the health and outcome of the patients.

Didactics

For many reasons, a didactic program while in the host country is important (but not essential). Education and teaching reinforces the principle of reciprocal benefit to both those traveling abroad and those hosting foreign colleagues. Lectures can certainly be organized and planned, but also given, by students and residents. Host team members should be included in the program since they often have better knowledge and skill than their visitors. The student/resident is given an opportunity to delve into a particular topic and also build good will and bidirectional learning between host and visiting team members.

Concluding Statement

In today's medical training environment, global health missions should be considered an integral part of any medical student or residency-training program. The decision to begin a program however should not be taken lightly but requires significant foresight and planning. Today students and residents actively seek out programs with an international health component. Those with an interest in global health care should be encouraged to participate in such endeavors. Students or residents can be helpful in organizing the mission or participating as a team member. In either case, they are numerous, long-lasting benefits for both the trainee and the sponsoring institution.

References

1. Campbell A, Sullivan M, Sherman R, Magee WP. The medical mission and modern cultural competency training. J Am Coll Surg. 2011;212:121–9.
2. Twagirumugabe T, Carli F. Rwandan anesthesia residency program: a model for north-south educational partnership. Int Anesthesiol Clin. 2010;48(2):71–8.
3. www.komedyplast.org

25 Building a Global Health Education Program in an Urban School of Medicine

Natasha Anushri Anandaraja, Ram Roth, and Philip J. Landrigan

Introduction

Global health has become an increasingly important focus of education, research, and clinical service in medical schools and universities. Driven by rapidly growing student and faculty interest, by societal recognition of the importance of the field, and by increasing support from governments as well as from private donors and foundations, the number of academic global health programs in North American institutions has expanded from a handful 5 years ago to more than 80 today, and another 30 have formed in academic health centers in countries around the world [1]. Global health has become a focus of intense interest at the US National Institutes of Health (NIH), and NIH Director Francis Collins has named global health one of his top priorities.

Many of the new academic global health programs are interdepartmental and university-wide in scope. They have created curricula as well as field experiences in global health for trainees at multiple levels. The 2013 Consortium of Universities for Global Health (CUGH) Global Health Program Database lists 24 North American institutions as having global health tracks, pathways, certificates or other formalized global health opportunities within their medical school curricula [1]. Seventeen institutions were listed as having post-graduate, residency-based global health programs, most frequently involving Departments of Internal Medicine, Pediatrics, Family Medicine, and Emergency Medicine. There are currently no listings for global health residency offerings in either Surgery or Anesthesiology, although the authors are aware of the existence of several such programs. For example, the department of Anesthesiology at the Icahn School of Medicine at Mount Sinai has been providing international medical care for almost 20 years through several programs involving many specialties (Table 25.1). Impoverished and underprivileged children and adults receive world-class medical care and surgery in the fields of pediatrics, gynecology, orthopedics, otolaryngology, ophthalmology and general surgery.

N.A. Anandaraja, M.B.Ch.B., M.P.H.
Arnhold Global Health Institute, Mount Sinai Medical Center, One Gustave L. Levy Place, Box 1255, New York, NY 10029, USA

Departments of Preventive Medicine & Medical Education, Icahn School of Medicine at Mount Sinai, One Gustave L Levy Place, Box 1255, New York, NY 10029, USA
e-mail: natasha.anandaraia@mssm.edu

R. Roth, M.D.
Department of Anesthesiology, Icahn School of Medicine at Mount Sinai, New York, NY, USA

P.J. Landrigan, M.D., M.Sc., F.A.A.P. (✉)
Department of Preventive Medicine, Icahn School of Medicine at Mount Sinai, One Gustave L. Levy Place, Box 1057, New York, NY 10029, USA
e-mail: phil.landrigan@mssm.edu

R. Roth et al. (eds.), *The Role of Anesthesiology in Global Health: A Comprehensive Guide*, DOI 10.1007/978-3-319-09423-6_25, © Springer International Publishing Switzerland 2015

Table 25.1 Anesthesiologists from the Icahn School of Medicine have been participating in global outreach programs for almost 20 years

Year	Country	Organization	Year	Country	Organization
1997	Russia	Healing the Children North East	2007	Honduras	Gift of Life, Rotary Club
1997	China	Healing the Children	2007	Honduras	Medical Students Making Impact
1998	Russia	Healing the Children North East	2008	Liberia	Mount Sinai
1999	China	Healing the Children	2008	Dominican Republic	Healing the Children
2000	China	Healing the Children	2009	Vietnam	Gift of Life, Rotary Club
2000	Romania	Humana	2009	Liberia	Mount Sinai
2000	Dominican Republic	Healing the Children	2009	Thailand	Healing the Children
2000	China	Children of China Pediatric Foundation	2009	Ecuador	Healing the Children
2001	Romania	Humana	2009	Dominican Republic	Healing the Children
2001	Kenya	Healing the Children	2010	Guyana	Caribbean Heart Institute
2002	China	Healing the Children	2010	Liberia	Mount Sinai
2003	China	Children of China Pediatric Foundation	2010	Liberia	Mount Sinai
2004	Romania	Humana	2010	Haiti	Partners in Health
2004	Bolivia	Healing the Children	2010	Ecuador	Montefiore Medical Center
2004	Dominican Republic	Medical Students Making Impact	2010	Ecuador	International Surgical Health Initiative
2005	Honduras	Medical Students Making Impact	2011	Liberia	Mount Sinai
2005	Dominican Republic	Healing the Children	2011	Peru	Komedyplast
2005	Honduras	Medical Students Making Impact	2011	China	Healing the Children
2006	Vietnam	Rotary Club	2013	Peru	Komedyplast
2006	Honduras	Medical Students Making Impact	2014	China	Healing the Children
2006	Dominican Republic	Healing the Children	2014	Peru	Komedyplast
2006	Honduras	Medical Students Making Impact			

Recently, the hospital dispatched international medical teams of surgeons, anesthesiologists, and medical students to Central America, Africa, and the Caribbean. From Angola to Zimbabwe, these teams provide optimal health care to the population and teach local residents, nurses, and physicians, meantime forming enduring bonds of friendship. Our teams donate supplies to the local hospital operating theaters and clinics. Faculty team members pay their own expenses and time off from their regular duties is supported by their respective departments.

The department of anesthesiology at the Icahn School has also provided continuing support and mentorship for Medical Students Making Impact (MSMI), founded in 2001, orchestrating international medical/surgical teams that have completed service trips to Honduras, Belize, Zambia and Nigeria (Table 25.2). Anesthesiologists, surgeons, fellows, residents and a cadre of highly motivated medical students are currently raising funds and collecting donations of medical supplies for the next "Brigada" (a group of people organized for special activity) as they are called by the locals in San Pedro Sula, Honduras. Our teams demonstrate surgical techniques while providing care to as many people as possible by day. Evenings are spent with local government and health officials as well as medical school students and administration expanding our knowledge and understanding of global health issues and offering lectures and presentations to local colleagues. MSMI team members often gain first-hand knowledge of diseases, syndromes

Table 25.2 Anesthesiologist and medical students under their supervision have provided care in many countries over the past 14 years

Year	Country	Component of Mount Sinai
2000	China	MSSM & Children of China Pediatric Foundation
2003	China	MSSM & Children of China Pediatric Foundation
2004	Dominican Republic	Medical Students Making Impact
2005	Honduras	Medical Students Making Impact
2005	Honduras	Medical Students Making Impact
2006	Honduras	Medical Students Making Impact
2006	Honduras	Medical Students Making Impact
2007	Honduras	Medical Students Making Impact
2008	Liberia	Mount Sinai
2009	Liberia	Mount Sinai
2010	Haiti	MSSM & Partners in Health
2010	Liberia	Mount Sinai
2011	Liberia	Mount Sinai
2011	Honduras	Medical Students Making Impact
2011	Haiti	Mount Sinai
2012	Dominican Republic	Mount Sinai Global Women's Health
2012	Liberia	Mount Sinai
2012	Jamaica	Mount Sinai
2012	Bolivia	Mount Sinai Cardiac Anesthesiology
2013	Dominican Republic	Mount Sinai Global Women's Health
2013	Liberia	Mount Sinai
2013	Nicaragua	Mount Sinai Cardiac Anesthesiology
2014	Dominican Republic	Mount Sinai Global Women's Health
2014	Liberia	Mount Sinai
2014	China	Mount Sinai

and poverty that they would otherwise see only in textbooks.

Most dramatically, an e-mail was sent to all employees at Mount Sinai Medical Center asking for volunteers for an international surgical team to Haiti 2 days after the earthquake of January 2010. The rapidly assembled group included orthopedic and general surgeons, nursing staff to provide OR and PACU support and our anesthesiologists. Armed with narcotics and minimal equipment for performing regional anesthesia, we performed 75 procedures. We the providers of international surgical care gained much from the experience. The group returned to Mount Sinai with an understanding of the global burden of surgical need and a determination to affect sustainable change in Global Health.

We describe the development of a coherent, multi-level, interdisciplinary program in global health in the Icahn School of Medicine, a large, urban, hospital-based medical school in New York City. Our goal is to share lessons learned and offer guidance to programs in other institutions.

Evolution of Global Health at Mount Sinai

Phase 1: Initiating Factors and Design

The Global Health program at Mount Sinai School of Medicine was founded in 2005. Its creation was both catalyzed and supported by increasing trainee demand. This demand was evidenced by growing numbers of resident and student international electives and by expanding participation in student-led international health interest groups. Critical events were informal surveys of incoming, first-year medical students in which nearly two-thirds of these incoming students indicated an interest in spending at least a portion of their careers serving the underserved in low- and middle-income countries (LMICs). This response represented a dramatic increase from preceding years and was very important in demonstrating the need for global health programming to institutional leadership.

The global health initiative was developed and designed through a series of structured discussions among senior faculty from the Departments of Pediatrics, Preventive Medicine, and Medical Education as well as the Center for Community and Multicultural Affairs.

An important early decision was a plan to focus scarce program resources on education. A small grant was secured from a private foundation to support curriculum development. The intent was to develop a three-tiered educational program that may be visualized as an inverted pyramid:

Tier One: At the top of the inverted pyramid is the broadest of the three levels. It was designed to provide introductory courses for the entire medical school class. The goals were to introduce *all* of our students to key issues in global health and give them an introduction to the concept that these problems are soluble and that there exist rational approaches to problem solving.

Tier Two: In the middle of the inverted pyramid was seen a transitional tier. It consisted of elective offerings for those medical students and physicians who had become intrigued by the introductory material presented in Tier One. Through these electives, medical students, residents and physicians are given the opportunity to work for weeks or months in underserved areas either in the United States or abroad.

Tier Three: The tier with the fewest number of people at the bottom tip of the inverted pyramid consists of longer term training programs for physicians who have made a serious commitment to serving the world's poor. These could be special fellowships of 6, 12, or even 24 months in duration. They could be located geographically either in the United States or abroad, so long as the focus is on devising sustainable solutions to long-term health problems in poor communities.

To launch the program, four junior faculty members from four departments were recruited by the Dean of Medical Education based on their past experience in global health and their responsibilities for oversight of international activities within their home departments. These four junior faculty members each maintained a primary appointment within their own departments, that is, Pediatrics, Preventive Medicine, Emergency Medicine and Internal Medicine. In addition they were each given partial salary support from the global health planning grant to work on development of the multi-level global health training program. Leadership was provided by one of the senior founding faculty from the Department of Pediatrics and the Dean of Medical Education. The program was initially created as an Office of Global Health housed within the Department of Medical Education. The Dean of the Medical School provided a modest amount of funding through the Department of Medical Education to defray program costs as well as office space and administrative support.

To build a philanthropic base for the Global Health program, a Global Health Advisory Board was created. This board consisted predominantly of contacts of the senior founding faculty. The board had no fiduciary or programmatic responsibility for the program, but participated in fundraising and promotional events, including the hosting of an annual fundraising event. In 2006, a formal proposal was successfully presented to the family foundation which had granted the initial planning grant, and the program received a grant of $1,000,000 to be disbursed over 3 years. This grant gave the program the foundation for its growth. It supported part-time salaries for faculty, provided stipends to support global health field experiences for trainees, and supported travel expenses to allow faculty to build partnerships with organizations across the globe.

Phase II: Growth of Programs and Partners

Global Health in the Medical School

At the time of formation of the Global Health Office in 2005, student global health activities consisted of independently organized clinical electives in the third or fourth year of medical school and short clinical "mission" trips organized by volunteer faculty. With the exception of a brief preparatory curriculum for students participating in the clinical trips, there was no formal teaching in global health.

To address this gap in global health education, development of a formal curriculum was an early goal of the Global Health Office. Global Health faculty introduced many different curricular offerings over the succeeding 8 years, including a semester-long elective "Introduction to Global Health" course, a Global Health Career Speaker Series, and an annual Global Health Conference. All of these programs continue to the present, but have been continuously refined and improved in response to continuing program evaluation.

To introduce all of our medical students to core concepts in global health, the Global Health

Office developed a proposal to introduce an 18-h semester-long global health course to the first-year medical student core curriculum. This proposal was initially rejected by the Executive Curriculum Committee of the medical school in 2006. However, the Executive Curriculum Committee encouraged the creation of a global health "Course-without-Walls" with the aim of embedding global health topics into existing core courses. Through this "Global Health Course-Without-Walls," the content of the proposed stand-alone global health curriculum was delivered through a variety of core medical school courses including Epidemiology and Microbiology, as well as through clinical clerkships in pediatrics, OB-GYN and internal medicine.

Then in 2012, with the support of the Dean of Medical Education and following the placement of key Global Health faculty on the medical school Curriculum Redesign Committee, global health was accepted as a stand-alone course within the core medical school curriculum. This was a key development. Designed to be delivered over 3 weeks during the first and second year of medical school, the course titled "Global Health InFocus" is now a mandatory part of medical school education at Mount Sinai. Faculty for the GH InFocus collaborated with faculty from the Department of Health Policy and Evidence to create approximately 35 h of curriculum exploring themes of research, clinical care, public health intervention, human rights advocacy and policy change within the global health agenda. The first and second weeks of the new curriculum were delivered for the first time to the class of 2016. Evaluations from the launch of this program showed poor response to the largely lecture-based sessions on social determinants of health and health policy in the first week of the course. In response, the second week of the course was tailored to focus on more specific global health topics and included expert guest speakers, interactive small groups, and panel discussions. It was enthusiastically received.

Mentored fieldwork opportunities have been offered to medical students and Masters of Public Health (MPH) students through the Global Health program since 2009. These Summer Global Health Projects rely on relationships with partner organizations around the globe, and provide funded and closely mentored 8-week-long field experiences. An online system has been created through which students participate in a competitive application process. Applications are reviewed by faculty research mentors for each global partner site, and students are matched with a project site based on their interests, their level of prior global health experience, and their language skills. Successful applicants for the Summer GH Project are required to attend a semester-long "Preparation for Global Health Fieldwork" course. Over the years, this course has progressed through many revisions based on participant feedback and the evolving demands of the fieldwork. The course currently includes mandatory sessions on global health ethics, cultural competency and travel safety, plus elective sessions on survey design, needs assessment, database design, and qualitative methods, among others. In the months prior to their field placement, students and mentors work collaboratively with their partner organizations to develop research and educational projects. Research questions and educational interventions are designed to address the specific needs of the partner organization and community. Students and their mentors work together on the development of research methodology and tools, and obtain approvals from both Mount Sinai and local institutional review boards as needed. While in the field, students work under the supervision of a local mentor from the partner organization. Depending on the site and the nature of the project, the students may also be visited by their Mount Sinai mentor for a period of supervision.

On their return to Mount Sinai, students complete a number of post-trip requirements before receiving the last installment of their summer stipend. These include the submission of an abstract and poster for the Mount Sinai Medical Student Research Day, submission of a reflective journaling assignment, completion of a debrief interview, and submission of an online evaluation form. Following completion of their data analysis, students and mentors disseminate relevant information back to the partner organization.

Many students will go on to present their work at a national conference, and a smaller subset will produce an MPH thesis or a manuscript for submission to a peer-reviewed publication. Since 2009, 152 students have completed a Summer GH Project. This experience has proven to be the cornerstone of global health education for medical students at Mount Sinai. In contrast to field placements offered by many other institutions, the success of this program rests on individual mentorship, participation in a collaborative project rather than mere clinical observership, and the scholarly products required on completion of fieldwork.

To meet the increasing demand for practical experiences and to accommodate students whose academic schedule would not permit a full 2-month summer experience, a new opportunity for field placement was created in 2014. The "Global Health India Immersion Experience" provides an on-site learning experience focused on community-participatory healthcare in a rural underserved setting in India. The course was created in collaboration with the Comprehensive Rural Health Project (CRHP) in Jamkhed, India. It will be co-taught by Mount Sinai faculty and CRHP trainers. The first cohort of students has been selected and consists of 15 students from MD, PhD, MD-PhD, and MPH programs who will travel to India with three faculty members in July 2014.

In addition to summer field experiences, many students now independently undertake clinical global health electives during their third and fourth year of medical school. These experiences are organized independently by the students, but reviewed and approved by the Global Health program. Criteria for approval include the support of faculty mentors from Mount Sinai and the field site, adequate external funding, a robust plan for the student's on-site activities, and engagement with an underserved community.

Mount Sinai Global Health also supports students to undertake a year of Global Health Scholarly Leave between third and fourth year of medical school to pursue an in-depth global health research project. Some of these students will receive mentorship and funding for independent research at a global partner site. Others will be supported in the development and submission of an application to a structured fellowship or internship program. Historically, Mount Sinai students have had success applying for year-long internship and fellowship opportunities with the Doris Duke Foundation, the NIH/Fogarty International Clinical Research Scholars Program, and the Centers for Disease Control.

In keeping with the program's initial intention to provide advanced educational opportunities for a subset of committed medical students, the Global Health Dean's Scholar Program was launched in 2012. Each year the Scholars program recruits two candidates from the pool of accepted medical school applicants. The program provides successful applicants with a 5-year track which includes a combined MD-MPH degree, a Global Health Summer Project, the opportunity for global health clinical electives, a funded year of GH Scholarly Leave, and longitudinal mentorship. The GH Dean's Scholar Program is now in its third year of recruitment. The MPH component of the track is provided tuition-free for the Dean's Scholars, and fundraising continues towards the ultimate goal of full tuition coverage to allow scholars to graduate free of debt.

Global Health and the Graduate Program in Public Health

The directors of Mount Sinai's MPH program, like their colleagues in the medical school, quickly recognized the growing status of Global Health as a specialty within public health education. The MPH program is located within Mount Sinai's Graduate School of Biomedical Sciences. With their support a Global Health Concentration was launched within the MPH program in 2009. Guided by the standards of the Council for Education for Public Health, the GH Concentration consists of core course requirements in research, management and socio-behavioral topics in addition to specific global health coursework, a global health-related practicum and a thesis.

Many of the original courses within the Global Health Concentration were created and taught by the founding global health faculty, all of whom had completed their own MPH degrees.

Over time, each of the four founding Global Health faculty members also accepted faculty positions within the MPH program, and in 2011 the most senior of the group became the Director of the MPH program. These dual appointments created opportunities for sharing of resources and coordination of activities between the global health programs in the medical school, the MPH program and the global health residency programs.

To date, the Global Health Concentration of the MPH program offers ten courses plus a Master's thesis and practicum for a total of 30 credits. The designation of several institution-wide educational events as credit-earning MPH courses, including the annual Global Health Conference and the Global Health Career Speaker Series, creates further coursework opportunities. This strategy also allows faculty to earn recognition and compensation for their work on these events. Twenty-seven students have graduated from the Global Health Concentration in the 5 years since its creation.

Global Health for Residents

To support post-graduate training in global health, the multidisciplinary Global Health Residency Track (GHRT) at Mount Sinai was launched in 2006. The first four residency programs to participate were the home departments of the founding faculty: Pediatrics, Emergency Medicine, and Internal Medicine, with the addition of the Medicine-Pediatrics Combined Residency program.

The Combined Medicine-Pediatrics program later became a "Medicine-Pediatrics Global Health Residency" which specifically recruited candidates committed to global health as a focus of their residency and career. The program incorporated an MPH with a concentration in global health into the 4-year clinical residency, and provided support for extended field placements. This unique residency program graduated its last residents in 2014. Mount Sinai's Psychiatry and Obstetrics & Gynecology (OBGYN) residency programs also joined the GHRT soon after its creation. Due to scheduling difficulties, OBGYN eventually developed an independent global health track, but remained in close collaboration with the GHRT, sharing teaching resources and field sites. The support of Departmental Chairs and Residency Program Directors was essential to the creation of the GHRT. Internal pressure from residents for global health electives had already set the stage for this process, and the promise of a formalized administrative process, structured education, and provision of mentorship and funding was welcomed. A number of Departments were prepared to share the travel costs of their participating residents and to involve additional faculty in mentoring.

The GHRT recruitment process was designed with consideration of the pros and cons of pre- versus post-match recruitment, and with respect for the challenging schedule faced by interns from all specialties. Accordingly, GHRT participants are recruited through a competitive application process in the penultimate year of their residency program, allowing a focus on clinical medicine during the intern year and adequate time for global health coursework and field work during the less demanding latter years of residency.

Between one and four candidates are accepted annually from each residency program based on the ability of the program to meet educational and clinical coverage requirements. Selection of candidates is based on their commitment to a global health career as evidenced by past global health education and experiences and a personal statement of intent. Input from the candidate's residency director and chief resident are also sought as candidates must be in good standing clinically and professionally.

Once accepted to the GHRT, residents are matched with a research mentor and partner organization. They then work in collaboration with their Mount Sinai and on-site mentors over several months to identify and develop a research or educational project. This project is implemented in their final year of residency during a 6–10 week field placement. Although a small number of partner sites will provide an appropriate environment for clinical work, the focus of GHRT field placements is on developing skills for conducting research and implementing public health or educational initiatives in under-resourced settings. For many residents the global health field project will also fulfill a research requirement imposed by their clinical program. The residents' time in the field is protected by providing either call-free electives or supporting the resident to bank calls with their colleagues. For emergency medicine residents additional time may be available by manipulating clinical shifts, and many of these residents will go into the field twice during their residency. In preparation for their fieldwork GHRT residents are also mandated to participate in the "Preparation for Global Health Fieldwork" course.

The cooperation and guidance of the Mount Sinai Office of Graduate Medical Education has been essential in the creation of the GHRT. Co-creation of supervisory and educational standards for global health resident experiences has ensured that ACGME standards are adhered to while still providing for the unique circumstances of working in resource-poor communities.

To date, the Mount Sinai GHRT has graduated 71 residents from the GHRT.

The Arnhold Global Health Teaching Fellowship

The Arnhold Global Health Teaching Fellowship was established in 2011. The drivers for this initiative were both a deficit in post-residency global health training opportunities and the need for increasing teaching support at Mount Sinai and global partner sites.

Fellowship candidates are sought nationally with the only requirements being completion of an ACGME-accredited residency program, US licensure, and commitment to a career as a global health practitioner. In alignment with Mount Sinai's commitment to building the healthcare workforce in underserved areas of the world, the Fellowship program was designed to provide candidates with skills and experience as global health educators. To this end, Fellows are funded to complete short training courses relevant to their teaching role, to participate in the design and implementation of global health curricula at Mount Sinai, and to participate in educational initiatives for health workers at global partner sites.

The Teaching Fellowship is funded by a long-time donor whose contribution provides salary support and travel expenses for the year-long program. In comparison to other Global Health Fellowships which combine clinical responsibilities in the USA with international activities, the independent funding of this program gives Teaching Fellows complete freedom from revenue-generating clinical responsibilities, allowing for focus on global-health-related activities and fieldwork.

The first Arnhold Global Health Teaching Fellow was recruited in 2011. He worked with Global Health faculty on the design and delivery of new material for several global health courses within the medical school and MPH program, and played a significant role in the development of a new 300-h course in Tropical and Travel Medicine. The fieldwork component of his fellowship was carried out in Mozambique where he designed systems for evaluation of a Community Health Worker training initiative. While in the field he also supported GHRT residents in the design and implementation of their projects, which included training HIV Peer Educators and Mobile Clinic staff.

The second Arnhold Global Health Teaching Fellow was recruited in 2012 and came to the program with the intention to improve her teaching skills in underserved and cross-cultural settings. Her Fellowship was therefore designed to provide an extended experience in the field. Following language training in the capital of Mozambique, she became integrally involved at our rural partner site. Here she contributed to the training of several cohorts of health workers including traditional birth attendants, HIV peer educators, community health workers, local nurses, and a community-based Gender Based Violence taskforce. Importantly, she also developed connections at the academic level with the local schools of medicine and public health. Based on these relationships, Mount Sinai Global Health will now support Sinai faculty to teach at the local medical school and will match Mount Sinai MPH students with Mozambican MPH students for collaborative Summer Global Health Projects.

The program has just recruited its third Arnhold Global Health Teaching Fellow, who will be placed at a partner site in the Dominican Republic. In this role she will support the local Family Medicine Residency Program, design and deliver curricula for an urban Community Health Worker cohort, and coordinate field projects for Mount Sinai residents and students.

The Fellowship program, although in its early days, has already proven to be mutually beneficial for Mount Sinai and its global partner sites. The extended on-the-ground presence of our Fellows has been instrumental in the maintenance of partner site training initiatives, has provided opportunities for the development of academic partnerships, and creates a stable platform for Mount Sinai GHRT and student projects. Expansion of the Fellowship program is therefore a programmatic priority, with the ultimate goal of placing Fellows at each of our Flagship partner sites (see below).

The Annals of Global Health

In 2013, the Global Health program was invited to reconfigure and relaunch the *Mount Sinai Journal of Medicine* as a journal of global health. Under the leadership of the Dean and Associate Dean for Global Health, the 79-year-old *Mount Sinai Journal of Medicine* thus became the *Annals of Global Health*. The focus of the publication transitioned from translational research to the health issues of disadvantaged and low-income communities across the globe.

The *Annals of Global Health* is an open-access, peer-reviewed journal with a commitment to publishing authors from many institutions, countries, and disciplines. It will be accessible without cost to physicians, scientists, and concerned citizens in countries worldwide, including low- and middle-income countries and countries with distressed currencies. The journal represents an opportunity for Mount Sinai to support and promote global health scholarship and disseminate important new concepts in global health. The journal has a particular interest in publishing articles that critically examine the social determinants of health and disease and those that elucidate the connections between health and human rights. The inaugural issue focused on global cardiology and was published in January 2014.

Global Health Partner Sites

In 2006 an informal survey and interview process was conducted by Global Health faculty to poll "experts" in the field for their opinions on several education-related issues. These leaders of notable global health academic programs and non-governmental organizations (NGOs) were asked to identify organizations around the globe that could become partner sites for trainee field experiences. Based on these recommendations, several academic organizations and NGOs were contacted and site visits were conducted in the Dominican Republic, India, Uganda, Tanzania, and Kenya. Criteria for inclusion as "partner sites" were defined, memorandums of understanding (MOUs) were created, and trainees began to be placed at these partner sites to carry out collaborative research, public health, and educational projects.

Over the following years, maintenance of some sites and attrition of others occurred organically. Additionally, new partnerships arose through the preexisting connections of Mount Sinai faculty. As time passed the partner sites fell into one of two categories: (1) those where the partner organizations functioned independently of Mount Sinai's input but were able to provide high quality practical opportunities for Sinai trainees, and (2) those where Global Health Faculty were significantly involved in programmatic assistance and research with the partner organization, and where Mount Sinai engagement in health-worker training, research, and clinical care was needed and feasible. Programs falling into this second category were designated as "Flagship" sites. The strategic decision was made to focus programmatic resources at these sites to expand the scope of the partnerships and achieve greater impact on the healthcare capacity and health outcomes of the local communities. Flagship sites are currently under development in Mozambique, the Dominican Republic, Liberia, and North Dakota. Mount Sinai trainees will be preferentially channeled to these sites for fieldwork, with increasing commitment to the expansion of local health-worker training activities and the development of new collaborative funding and research efforts.

An important feature of Mount Sinai's global health partnerships has been the extent to which partner site projects are driven by the agenda of local organizations and communities. Due in large part to our predominantly private sources of funding and the broadness of our mission, the Mount Sinai Global Health program has had the freedom to prioritize local priorities over external agendas. This has created truly mutually beneficial and fulfilling relationships.

Global Human Rights

Over the past 3 years, Human Rights and advocacy have become a significant aspect of global health education at Mount Sinai. The addition of two faculty members with expertise in these fields has elevated these topics from a sidebar in overall global health education, as they are in many global health curricula, to a significant component at all levels of global health training.

Current human rights offerings for medical students include a semester-long elective course in Human Rights and Social Justice and a Human Rights and Social Justice Scholars Track, in addition to mandatory coursework in human rights and advocacy through the Global Health InFocus curriculum. Residents and students are also offered training in the assessment and management of survivors of torture. On completion of training they rotate through the Mount Sinai Survivors of Torture clinic to assist faculty in the examination of clients and preparation of affidavits for asylum application.

An initiative is now underway to integrate the human rights and advocacy approach across our Flagship partner sites. Multi-site research to investigate the health impacts of human rights abuses and support of local human rights education will further establish Human Rights as an integral activity of the Arnhold Global Health Institute.

Program Structure

In May 2010, to solidify the position of global health programs within the Mount Sinai School of Medicine, the Dean named two senior faculty members—one from Preventive Medicine and one from Cardiology—as Dean and Associate Dean for Global Health. Under their direction, the program was renamed Mount Sinai Global Health. This designation reflected the commitment of the medical school to global health. It resulted in a modest increase in internal funding, a substantial increase in program stature, and significantly enhanced the program's ability to raise funds from philanthropic sources.

The appointment of the Dean for Global Health, whose responsibilities include oversight of global health activities throughout the Mount Sinai Medical Center, Residency Programs, Graduate School and Medical School, also reinforced the centralized structure of global health at Mount Sinai. This centralization counters the formation of silos within the global health community, promoting efficient resource-sharing, collaboration, creation, and maintenance of standards for global work. The central governance and reporting system also enables a swift and coordinated institutional response to global health opportunities and educational needs within the Sinai community and its partner organizations.

In 2011, Global Health leadership, faculty and Advisory Board members participated in a strategic planning process to map out short-, mid-, and long-term programmatic and fundraising goals. Structural redesign at this stage resulted in the definition of four pillars of activity within the overall initiative: Research, Education, Patient Care, and Human Rights. Each pillar was appointed a Director who reported to the Dean of Global Health. Although providing a useful programmatic structure, the four pillars remained functionally connected with fluidity of faculty time and programmatic resources between them. Fundraising remained centrally coordinated with the assistance of the Mount Sinai office of Development.

Under the agenda of the Patient Care pillar, systems were developed to identify and oversee the activities of Mount Sinai faculty who were independently participating in clinical work in underserved communities around the globe. Codification of a set of requirements for Mount Sinai-affiliated global health projects was a necessary prerequisite to this process. These requirements included minimum standards regarding local supervisory and partnership capacity, completion by participants of online safety and health courses prior to travel, and creation of MOUs to be signed with local partnering organizations. Creation of databases to register faculty projects, and of systems to ensure adequate insurance and liability coverage for traveling faculty, was undertaken with the input of the Information Technology, Legal, Risk Management and Human Resources departments. A team of Global Health faculty members formed a Site Review Committee which meets monthly to review project applications submitted through the database. The Review Committee provides guidance to applicants as needed with the aim of bringing projects into alignment with the overarching mission of the Global Health program. This process has resulted in the transformation of existing short-term student-led clinical mission trips into public health-oriented learning experiences, and addition of local health-worker training strategies or research projects to faculty-led clinical mission trips.

In 2012 an External Advisory Board was recruited to provide expert guidance on the strategic development of the Global Health program. The board was composed of five leaders from a number of well-known academic, governmental and civil society organizations. The counsel of the Board and the program evaluations that they submitted to the Dean of the Medical School provided important insights and generated high-level support for the program. A critically important recommendation offered by this Advisory Board in 2013 was that Mount Sinai consider formation of a true Global Health Institute. The Dean of the School of Medicine accepted this recommendation and instructed the School's office of Development to make the formation of a Global Health institute a philanthropic priority.

In 2013, a founding donor to the Mount Sinai Global Health program made a generous endowment gift, allowing the program to be elevated to its current status as the Arnhold Institute of Global Health at Mount Sinai, the 16th cross-departmental institute to be created at Mount Sinai. The institute structure is critical to the continuing expansion of the global health mission at Mount Sinai. It will foster cross-departmental collaboration, increased internal and external visibility, and prioritization of Global Health as a focus for future philanthropy. Efforts are currently under way to define the levels, requirements, and privileges of membership in the new Institute, and to recruit a Founding Director.

Program Outcomes

Evaluation of the impact of the global health program at Mount Sinai has been a complex endeavor which is constantly being reassessed and modified. Several levels of evaluation are required, including the proximal outcome of trainee satisfaction with curricular offerings, the mid-term outcomes of impact on local partner site healthcare capacity, and long-term outcomes relating to the career choices of our graduates and changes in health outcomes in our partner communities.

Currently, evaluation of trainee satisfaction with global health curricular and extracurricular offerings occurs through existing medical school evaluation structures. These include individual course evaluations, a graduation survey, an intern survey, and a student council survey of satisfaction with medical school services. Participants in the GHRT participate in pre and post-track surveys to gauge the influence of the GHRT experience on their future training and career choices. The impact of training initiatives at Flagship partner sites is monitored with varying degrees of sophistication depending on the onsite capacity. These evaluations range from simple monitoring of numbers of health workers trained and services delivered, to systems which include data collection on both health-worker performance and the community-level impact of their work.

Although the evaluation of the most distal programmatic outcomes has proven challenging, there are ongoing efforts to investigate the impact of our global health training programs on participant career choices. Annual Alum Surveys are distributed to both graduated medical students who participated in a Summer Global Health Project and graduates of the Global Health Residency Track. Surveys of GHRT graduates to date showed that 55 % of respondents had participated in further global health-related training through Fellowship programs. 55 % of GHRT graduates continued to work with an underserved community abroad, and 90 % were working with an underserved population domestically. The response rates from graduated medical students was extremely poor, but it appears that a significant proportion (75 %) have remained engaged in global health work through their chosen residency programs.

Successes and Challenges

Institutional Structure, Funding, and Identity

The support of leadership within both the medical school and clinical residency programs has been a key factor for success since the inception of the Global Health program. This support was driven by an understanding of the rising demand for global health education from the Mount Sinai trainee population, and recognition of the power of a Global Health educational program as a recruitment tool. Internal support was also gained through the positioning of Global Health initiatives as central to Mount Sinai's longstanding commitment to social justice. Since its founding as the Jews' Hospital of New York in 1855, the institution's mission has reflected a commitment to the care of diverse and marginalized populations [2]. This alignment of values provides justification for ongoing engagement with underserved communities around the globe.

Unlike many global health ventures at larger academic institutions, the centralized leadership and governance structure at Mount Sinai supports cohesion, resource sharing, and synergy among the varied programs housed under the Global Health Institute. Weekly meetings involving the Directors of all four pillars, founding Global Health faculty and key administrators, ensure constant communication, group problem solving, and collaborative decision making. Bimonthly broader meetings involving faculty from throughout the institution promotes participation of the wider global health community. In addition, weekly meetings between the Dean of Global Health and the Dean of the Medical School ensure that the global health agenda is visible at the highest levels of leadership and allows for real-time feedback and support for emerging issues.

Although there are disadvantages in regards to branding and funding opportunities for a global health initiative that is not housed within a multi-school university setting, the relatively lean structure of Global Health at Mount Sinai creates efficiency. Short chains of communication and governance enable the program to be rapidly responsive to the changing demands of the academic environment and the needs of our trainees and partner organizations.

The recent acquisition of a sizeable endowment lends a strong foundation for the Institute. However, ongoing fundraising is essential to allow for growth of the program. Support for global health education and training has only recently appeared on the agenda of traditional Global Health funding agencies. Lack of university status has also limited the eligibility of our medical school-based program for funding options. However, significant support has been successfully obtained through private and family foundations, small government supported grants, and a dedicated group of private donors. As global health programs continue to emerge throughout US academic centers, competition for funding becomes more intense, and the importance of inter-institutional partnerships and public-private partnerships for funding increases.

An issue which influences the competitiveness of the Institute within the funding environment is that of "branding"—of establishing an identity for the program based on an area of expertise related to a specific global health topic, geographic location, population, or approach to global health work. As a significant function of the Mount Sinai Global Health program has been to convene a disparate group of global health activities under one institutional umbrella, the definition of a "brand" has been neither a simple task nor a priority. However, as the program has grown and a number of areas of expertise have arisen based on the strengths of key faculty and the priorities of our partner sites, the pros and cons of branding around one or a few of these areas has been debated. Other approaches to defining a brand could be identification of a niche area in global health as yet unclaimed by another major organization or academic institution, or a decision based on forecasting trends in funding for various global health topic areas. Benefits of branding include the ability to form a cohesive strategic plan for the Institute as a whole and to align funding priorities, programmatic decisions and evaluation metrics around a set of common goals. Increased clarity of messaging for fundraising and public relations purposes could also result from a successful branding campaign.

Disadvantages of branding the program may include loss of recruitment opportunities due to mismatch between trainee interests and the advertised brand of the Institute, limited ability to respond to evolving partner site needs, and reduction in broad donor appeal. Inability to engage with locally defined needs that are not in alignment with the brand of the Institute is a significant concern.

The balance between pros and cons of branding continues to be debated. However, in light of the recent formation of the Institute and the current search for an Institute Director, this issue is of increasing importance.

Faculty Development

A longstanding barrier to meeting demand for meaningful educational opportunities has been a shortage of mentorship for trainees. A significant input of time is required to prepare a student or resident for field work, to collaborate with partner organizations on the design of appropriate research methodology, to assist a trainee through local and US IRB processes, and, oftentimes, to visit that mentee in the field. Currently, a small and dedicated cohort of GH mentors work year-round to prepare trainees of all levels for practical field experiences and subsequent production of scholarly work. However, funds and official processes for compensation of mentor time and effort are limited. An institutional commitment to recognition and support of mentorship activities is required to incentivize and expand global health mentorship capacity at Mount Sinai.

As noted earlier in this chapter, global health training opportunities in medical school and schools of public health have emerged rapidly and recently into an environment where no formal global health career path existed. The challenge therefore becomes how to appropriately mentor Global Health trainees towards feasible and fulfilling careers, and how best to support junior faculty who wish to be involved in global health. The burden of debt incurred during a medical school education remains a significant hindrance to physicians seeking to dedicate their career to underserved populations. Many programs, including the one described here, seek scholarship funding to allow GH trainees to graduate debt-free. Some innovative new programs attempt to address this barrier by combining post-training Global Health service opportunities with loan forgiveness [3]. At Mount Sinai we also strive to create Global Health faculty appointments for our graduates. Provision of partial salary support can protect the time of these young faculty members, enabling them to maintain involvement in global health through roles as mentors and partner site project managers. Provision of scholarships for MPH tuition and additional Fellowship opportunities also broaden post-residency training opportunities and boost competitiveness in the global health employment arena.

Future Directions

Over the past 9 years a robust program in global health has been established at Mount Sinai. The Arnhold Global Health Institute now offers a multi-level interdisciplinary educational program, opportunities for research, human rights advocacy and patient care, and meaningful collaborations with international and domestic partner sites. Over the next 5 years we plan to strengthen engagement with our Flagship sites for increased impact on the growth of the local healthcare workforce. Reciprocal training activities will be expanded, including increased opportunities for health workers from partner sites to rotate through the Mount Sinai Medical System, as well as scholarship support for partnering health workers to obtain their MPH degrees from the Mount Sinai Graduate School. To support this commitment, increased funding and institutional support is sought for long-term placement of Global Health faculty at Flagship sites and expansion in the numbers of Global Health Teaching Fellows.

Many academic institutions with significant international presence have created offices to manage the multi-faceted issues around international engagement, including human resource and labor issues, liability and malpractice for physicians practicing abroad, and requirements around insurance, immigration and visa status, and international licensing. As Mount Sinai extends its international reach, not only in terms of global health activities but also for the purposes of academic and clinical exchange with institutions in high income countries, the establishment of a similar service within the Mount Sinai operations structure will likely be needed. An Office of International Affairs at Mount Sinai could provide this central body for the establishment of protocols and provision of support and regulation around all of these activities.

In addition, creation of a Global Entrepreneurship Team has been proposed to ensure that the expansion of activity also results in increased productivity in scholarship, fundraising and contribution to the global health knowledge base. Based on a model established by the Global Health Initiative of the Texas Children's Hospital and Baylor College of Medicine [4], the Global Entrepreneurship Team would consist of business, development and information technology support staff to provide assistance with planning, funding and execution of field projects, as well as creative approaches to dissemination of research findings and new educational resources. Specific areas of support would include assistance with creation of feasible business plans, identification of novel funding opportunities, and utilization of information technology for data collection, web-based educational platforms, and mobile health applications. It is proposed that the services of the Global Entrepreneurship Team be provided as a privilege of membership in the Arnhold Global Health Institute.

Conclusion

The success of the Arnhold Global Health Institute at Mount Sinai rests on the motivation provided by Mount Sinai's trainees, on the support of leadership, on the hard work of its faculty, and, most significantly, on the goodwill and collaboration of its global partners. The program's commitment to prioritizing partner's needs and local capacity building is the best example we can provide to our trainees for ethical global engagement. Over 9 years the program has grown immensely, yet continuous self-evaluation and modification are necessary to meet the changing demands of our trainees and partners. The global community is constantly growing in its awareness of the complexity of global health problems and its understanding of how best to create lasting solutions. Through our commitment to supporting the next generation of global health workers we hope to contribute to this slow but inspirational process.

References

1. Consortium of Universities for Global health. Available at: http://public.tableausoftware.com/profile/#!/vizhome/2013CUGHGlobalHealthProgramsDatabase/2013CUGHGlobalHealthProgramsDatabase. Accessed 20 May 2014.
2. Aufses AH, Niss BJ. This house of noble deeds: the Mount Sinai Hospital, 1852–2002. New York: New York University Press; 2002.
3. Seed Global Health. Available at: http://seedglobalhealth.org/seedglobalhealth.org. Accessed 27 May 2014.
4. Texas Children's Hospital, Global Health Initiative. Available at: http://globalhealth.texaschildrens.org/. Accessed 27 May 2014.

26 Closing the Gap in Europe Through Education: A Reverse Mission

Gabriel M. Gurman

The fall of the Soviet Union in late 1989, almost 20 years after immigration to Israel from Romania, found me as an Israeli citizen. At the time I emigrated, the overall situation in Romania was bearable and medicine was practiced at a level not too far behind what I found in Israel, a country in a stage of full development. In both countries medicine was somewhere on a level between the wealthy parts of the world and communist Eastern Europe.

The fall of the Soviet Union offered a glimpse into the over-all failure of health care. The system was unable to answer the huge needs of the population. There was a clear discrepancy between the degree of enthusiasm and dedication of the medical staff and the availability of modern modalities to treat patients. The situation in anesthesiology and critical care was no exception. There was a desperate need for modern equipment and drugs. Supplies produced in the Warsaw pact countries only partially covered the needs. The scarce aid coming from Western Europe was not enough to solve the problem. Contacts with medicine west of the Soviet bloc were difficult to achieve. The lack of funds, a very inconsistent command of foreign languages among young physicians, and the authorities' permanent fear of manpower defection to the free world, contributed to serious restrictions of free travel. Availability of textbooks and medical journals varied in different countries. Material could not reach remote, peripheral medical centers. In contrast, some physicians, scientists, and teachers from the western side of the continent regularly visited countries of the communist world, offering the local healthcare providers a chance to learn of new achievements in medicine and related fields of science.

At the same time, anesthesiology in the western part of Europe was leading the way to better patient care. In the second part of the twentieth century advances in anesthesia led to improvement in patient safety regulations, equipment and drug arsenals in the operating room (OR) and intensive care units (ICU), e.g., monitors, anesthesia machines, bedside lab, and X-ray availability. International organizations developed codes of ethical principles; significant basic and clinical research was taking place in large hospital centers, facilitated by easy and continuous access to information. The beneficial influence of developments on the North American continent was felt in the western part of Europe.

A palpable contrast, noticed during my short trips to some countries of the former Soviet empire, led me to search for a way to assist colleagues and friends to shorten the path towards modern medicine.

G.M. Gurman, M.D. (✉)
Professor Emeritus, Anesthesiology and Critical Care, Ben Gurion University of the Negev, Beer Sheva, Israel

Department of Anesthesia, Mayney Hayeshuah Medical Center, B'nai Brak, Israel

Soroka Medical Center, Beer Sheva, Israel
e-mail: gurman@bgu.ac.il

R. Roth et al. (eds.), *The Role of Anesthesiology in Global Health: A Comprehensive Guide*, DOI 10.1007/978-3-319-09423-6_26, © Springer International Publishing Switzerland 2015

The World Federation of Societies of Anesthesiologists (WFSA)–Beer Sheva Project

WFSA was aware of the problems arising from the continuous lack of contact between the two parts of the continent. In the years preceding and following the fall of the Iron Curtain, different world organizations including the WFSA tried to facilitate the process of harmonizing the level of the profession of anesthesia throughout the continent. After the fall of the communist bloc, many of Western Europe's leading anesthesiologists found their way to countries of the communist system. They took part in national congresses, organized teaching courses, taught new techniques, and invited young local specialists to spend periods of time in well-organized and equipped anesthesia departments [1]. Table 26.1 presents a short list of educational activities organized by various international organizations or individuals, with advantages and drawbacks delineated.

Based on this partially successful experience, we initiated two projects with different scopes. The aim of the first project was to expose a large number of young Eastern European anesthesiologists to the modern aspects of the profession by offering them a direct view of daily activities at a busy, up-to-date hospital. The project was situated in Beer Sheva, the largest city in the south of Israel. Beer Sheva is a university city, home to Ben Gurion University (BGU) of the Negev, which accommodates some 21,000 students in various faculties and research centers, including the Faculty of Health Sciences (FOHS). The FOHS includes a well-developed medical school that has clinical and teaching facilities for almost all fields of healthcare.

Table 26.1 Educational activities in anesthesiology promoted by individuals and professional international organizations in Europe in the first years after the fall of the Iron Curtain

Project	Advantages	Drawbacks
Training centers in some countries	• Economic • Teaching in accordance with the existing reality	• No use of up-to-date equipment • Paucity of teachers
Refresher courses	• Unlimited number of participants • Updating theoretical knowledge	• No immediate impact on the daily activity
Educational grants for various periods of time in various domains of the profession	• Wonderful contact with modern medicine	• Brain drain from the country of origin

The main teaching base was Soroka Medical Center (SMC), a 1,100-bed hospital, located in the immediate vicinity of FOHS. All its departments and clinics educate medical students and have established post-graduate and residency programs. At the time of initiation of this project, the SMC-FOHS Division of Anesthesiology and Critical Care employed 30 specialists and 35 residents, many of them holding academic degrees from BGU.

The project was proposed to the Committee for Education of the WFSA and was approved in 1992 [2]. The questions: Why Israel? And why Beer Sheva? Deserve special clarification. At that time Israeli medicine had an interesting place in the world of modern medicine. Its sophistication was well established. The quality of health care was high. Although characterized by easy access to up-to-date treatment for every citizen, cost was significantly less than that of many other developed countries. Even today health care accounts for a mere 8 % of the gross national product compared to 17.6 % in the USA (2012) [3].

The resolution of the BGU, FOHS, and SMC to host the program, together with the eagerness of the Division of Anesthesiology staff to teach and train, created the proper climate for implementing the project in Beer Sheva. One noteworthy detail is that the majority of the staff spoke numerous languages; in addition to Hebrew and English. Several were born in counties outside Israel and afforded native speakers of Russian, Romanian, Arabic, Hungarian, Bulgarian, Spanish, Italian, French, and Portuguese. In short, the young foreign anesthesia specialists visiting SMC were offered a chance to observe a reputable level of medicine, practiced at reasonable cost.

The Israeli system could be a source of inspiration for those who would try to improve the healthcare level in their own countries where the budget allocated to medicine was still low.

Another point is that according to Israeli regulations, a visiting physician is not allowed to remain in the country. They may only practice medicine with the necessary permits for a fixed and limited period of time and they require continuous supervision by an Israeli physician. This regulation was an assurance that the visitor would go back home after completing the training period. There would be no drain of qualified personnel from the countries involved in the project.

Implementation

As a result of the WFSA arrangement to sponsor the project, we approached the national anesthesiology societies of interested countries and planned interviews with candidates eager to take part in the program. Involvement of local society officers participating in the selection committee was vital. The local leaders were expected to know the candidates and assist in the process of selecting individuals with the highest potential to benefit from the observation period at SMC.

The interview, usually scheduled during an annual convention of the national anesthesia society, was in English and good command of this language was the first criterion in the selection of candidates. Equally important, the young anesthesia specialist was expected to explain what he/she anticipated from the observation period in Israel. In most cases the number of candidates exceeded the number of positions allocated to that specific country. The final decision was made after review by the committee members, which always included at least one SMC staff member.

WFSA decided to cover the cost of the foreign physicians' stay in Beer Sheva. BGU accepted the role of controlling the funds received from WFSA by opening a special account dedicated solely to this project. The BGU president at that time donated a substantial sum of money in order to ease the inauguration of the program. FOHS assisted the project by arranging accommodations for the foreign physicians in the immediate vicinity of SMC, in the premises of student dormitories. The walking distance between the apartments and the hospital eased the participants' approach to the special activities during the nights and weekends. The staff on duty would call and inform them about a special case or treatment deserving interest. Also, an agreement was reached with FOHS stipulating the right of the project participants to freely access the faculty library as well as the sport facilities of BGU.

We decided to ask each participant to cover his or her own travel expenses. This decision was based on the principle that the young physician involved in the program was supposed to be as invested as the sponsor in obtaining a place in the project. In discussions with the officers of the national societies we reached the conclusion that paying for the airplane ticket would not be too heavy a burden for any of the participants. The reality proved that this supposition was correct. During the 14 years of the project in Beer Sheva there have been no cancelations due to travel costs.

The decision to bring to Beer Sheva specialists in groups belonging to the same visiting country was taken after an intense discussion with WFSA officers. The alternative was to mix participants from different countries and offer everybody a chance to get information about other kinds of organizations in different parts of Eastern Europe. This would have also facilitated better command of English, the only common language for all. But the accepted idea was not to separate members of the same national group, and thus to accelerate their acclimatization with the new atmosphere and better organize their free time (weekends and afternoons) activities.

The Observation Period

The participants arrived in Beer Sheva in groups of three or four when the project included only 1 month of observation, and then in pairs in the second part of the project, when the participants were offered a longer period of observation, thus giving each visiting physician a chance to become more familiar with one of the specialty fields: critical care, obstetrical anesthesia, cardiothoracic anesthesia, pain management, etc.

Each participant was integrated in the daily activity of the Division of Anesthesiology at SMC. It started with participation in the 7:00 a.m. meeting, which included the previous night's report, a quick glance into the morning schedule, and a 10-min presentation by one of the residents. A simultaneous translation from Hebrew to English through headphones was provided by one of the staff.

Then members of the group were assigned to the activities of the morning, either in the OR non-OR areas such as the pain clinic, pre-anesthesia assessment clinic, or ICU. They also took part in the consultations on the floor and in any teaching activity involving the anesthesiology residents. When possible, the foreign physicians were given a chance to take part in educational events outside Beer Sheva, such as a national convention or a refresher course in anesthesiology and related domains. Special attention was given to those areas that interested the foreign physicians. Their interest varied from One year to another and from one group to another. The main explanation for varying interest in new knowledge was that gradually, the average Eastern Europe anesthesiologist became accustomed to new achievements in the profession. Hospitals in various countries of the eastern part of the continent started purchasing modern equipment and drugs, and a process of reorganization of the daily activity was evident in many medical centers. Additionally, a new system of continuous education was gradually implemented in many Eastern countries, with the aim of offering young physicians a chance to improve theoretical knowledge and apply it to the daily work.

Table 26.2 shows the gradual changes in the list of some topics of interest among the participants in the project. It reflects the progress made by the profession in various participating countries during the first decade of the free market system and liberation from the communist system limits. The table reveals some interesting points.

Table 26.2 Topics of special interest to the WFSA–Beer Sheva project participants in different years of its existence

Year	Topic
1992	• Oximetry • Capnography • Caudal anesthesia for children
1994	• Neurostimulator • Pulmonary artery catheter • Invasive blood pressure monitoring
1997	• Pencil-point needles for spinal anesthesia • Isoflurane replacing halothane for inhalation anesthesia
2000	• Intracranial pressure monitoring • Postoperative pain relief in children • Hemofiltration in ICU • Pre-anesthesia outpatient clinic
2001	• Fiber-optic tracheal intubation • Pediatric critical care • Organization of a recovery (PACU) room
2002	• Laryngeal mask • Combined spinal-epidural anesthesia • Continuous spinal anesthesia • Percutaneous tracheostomy • Organization of an acute pain service

At no stage of the project did the average participant feel a need for clinical theoretical presentations. The access to electronic information became progressively easier in every country involved in the program and the young specialist was able to improve his/her theoretical knowledge base by a simple process of self-learning.

The specific interest started with items belonging to compulsory monitoring in the OR, a demand difficult to achieve in the absence of the necessary equipment. Once the visiting specialist became accustomed to this basic equipment in his/her own hospital, the general interest switched to more complicated practical items, most of them originating from the personal subspecialty interest. Also some of the foreign specialists had the opportunity to visit and work in other developed medical centers (abroad and even in their own countries and cities). There they encountered modern equipment and all necessary drugs for modern anesthesia. They also were offered the opportunity to participate in international scientific conventions and contact colleagues from more developed countries. Once back home, they could implement some of the things seen and learned.

Table 26.3 Countries and number of participants in the WFSA–Beer Sheva project during 1992–2005

Year/country	1992	1993	1994	1995	1996	1997	1998	1999	2000	2001	2002	2003	2004	2005	*Total*
Romania	2	4	4	4	4	4	2	2						1	27
Moldova						4	4	4	4	4	4	4	4	4	36
Slovakia									4	4	2	2	2	2	16
Bulgaria						4	4	4	3	3	4	4	4	4	34
Slovenia							2	4	2	3					11
Serbia														4	4
Macedonia											2		8		10
Hungary						4	2				3				9
Belarus											1				1
Total	2	4	4	4	4	16	14	14	13	14	16	10	18	15	148

This rather new reality created the basis for changing the direction of the educational process. We felt the obligation to search for other ideas that could better serve the purpose of closing the gap between the two parts of the old continent (vide infra).

During 1992–2005, 148 foreign specialists in anesthesia, from nine countries, all younger than 40 years old, took part in the WFSA–Beer Sheva project, spending between 1 and 6 months, at SMC (Table 26.3). Most of them were allowed only to observe, but those who spent longer time in the hospital got the opportunity to directly participate in the daily activity in the OR and outside it, under continuous supervision. Thus they got more exposure than an average specialist in anesthesia is able to offer his/her patients. The observer was not involved in patient care; he/she just observed the treatment offered to the patient. But when the guest spent at least 6 months at SMC (very few cases), an educational license was issued by the Israeli Ministry of Health, thus the foreign physician was allowed to take part in patient care under direct and permanent supervision of an Israeli physician.

Did this first project significantly contribute to the process of closing the gap between the two parts of Europe? The answer is unclear. The project created a practical base for a young specialist to become familiar with modern equipment and an approach to the specific needs of the surgical patient. Some ethical aspects of our clinical activities and judgment contributed to a better understanding of the limits of healthcare and the rights of the patient.

Once back home, participants transmitted to colleagues concepts learned at SMC and also tried to change practice at home This permanent desire for progress was amplified by a continuous process of improving the Eastern European conditions for work, better equipment, better drugs, availability of disposable items, as well as a much easier approach to information.

On the other hand, a close observation of this improvement process uncovered some of the still existing flaws of the system in the participants' countries. These flaws are partially explained by the reminiscence of old regime obstacles and limits. The residency track was supposed to keep pace with the continuous changes in daily activity in and out of the OR, but in some countries this process was significantly delayed. Parts of the organization of an anesthesia department were still neglected, such as the pre-anesthesia outpatient clinics, acute pain service, or recovery rooms. Finally, the paucity of resources did not allow the involvement of the project "graduates" into clinical and basic sciences research.

Overall, the feedback obtained both at the end of each observation period and during various occasions visiting the involved countries proved, that the WFSA–Beer Sheva project was worthwhile. The demonstrated personal development of the participants and the improvement of care in their home countries were definitely positive and justified the financial cost covered by the world organization.

The project did not include a follow-up system to determine what happened to individual anesthesiologists, but we do know that upon their return home some became directors of anesthesia departments, chiefs of professional units, and organizers of congresses and conventions. We also know that some 20–25 % of them found their way to Western Europe and are currently employed in foreign departments.

The WFSA–Beer Sheva project moved in 2005 to the Wolfson Medical Center in Holon, Israel under the leadership of Prof. Tiberiu Ezri for 7 more years. Up to 2012 it included 23 young anesthesiologists from eastern European countries, such as: Slovakia, Romania, Moldova, Bulgaria, Serbia, the Czech Republic, and Uzbekistan. At the initiative of WFSA, 14 specialists from Africa also joined the project.

The Wolfson leg of the project offered participants a 6-month period of training within the framework of the department of anesthesia. Each participant could select one of the following fields of interest: critical care, pediatric anesthesia, obstetrical anesthesia, and cardiac anesthesia. Foreign physicians were permitted "hands-on" experience by obtaining a temporary educational license from the Israel Ministry of Health and were involved in clinical practice on daily basis, under the close supervision of an Israeli specialist. A small stipend was offered by WFSA and lodging was provided by the host hospital.

A New Direction in the Process of Closing the Gap Between East and West

The WFSA–Israel project was an important step in trying to close the gap between the two sides of Europe. But at the same time, we became aware of two important facts that demanded a change in planning for further projects.

The first was the new reality in the vast majority of the former communist countries. Gradually medicine in general and anesthesiology in particular was changing its characteristics and incorporating some of the features of modern, Western medicine. A new generation of specialists assumed the destinies of the specialty and had already been exposed to new trends in organization of healthcare. They had implemented the principles of patient safety in their places of work. The new generation of anesthesiologists possessed the necessary skills and knowledge to provide a good level of anesthesia practice in the OR and also outside it. But the new atmosphere and enthusiasm that invigorated Eastern Europe anesthesiology lacked one item; educational skills. Internet and easy approaches to electronic information could not offer the young physician the necessary knowledge in experience regarding training in the domain of teaching.

Permanent contact with our profession all over Eastern Europe very clearly showed that one of the weak points of educating the new generation of specialists was the use of old methods to teach new things. Once the need for basic equipment and drugs had been, at least partially, solved and access to up-to-date information ceased to be a problem, we felt that we had to take care of the system of teaching.

During our frequent visits to those countries in the first years of the new millennium, we found that the *teaching system and methods* had been less influenced by the permanent contact with the other part of the continent. A simple example would help demonstrate this statement. How does one teach a clinical item such as acute pulmonary edema? Many years ago teachers would have approached such a subject by defining the disease and its etiology, explaining the pathophysiology, presenting the symptoms, and finally bringing to the attention of the student/resident the methods of prevention and treatment. But today attitudes have changed. In order to facilitate understanding the clinical framework of such an acute situation, we created a clinical scenario, in which a patient arrives to an emergency room with symptoms of dyspnea and cyanosis, and with cardiac pathology in the past, after—let's say—a copious meal that included a too salted main course. The student is asked to discuss the data, inquiring about the clinical examination results, proposing a differential diagnosis, asking for adjuvant tests, such as an X-ray and arterial blood gases, and then gradually reaches the correct diagnosis. From that moment the path to treatment and prognosis becomes an easy one.

In many university centers this kind of teaching was absent, and the so-called "problem-based learning" (PBL) unheard of or not used as a teaching tool. The explanation is simple. The introduction of PBL in undergraduate and postgraduate medical courses necessitates special training of teachers and monitoring of their performance [4]. It demands good teachers, which cannot be obtained by a process of "spontaneous generation," but rather by creating groups of new teachers, who have been taught how to teach and how to use the proper means of teaching for facilitating an easier understanding of the lesson. Creating a good and successful teacher is not a simple task. In some countries, simulation teaching has been successfully used but the expense involved remains prohibitive for many areas.

Azer [5] compiled a list of 12 qualities of a good teacher, among them: commitment to work, an ability to interact and communicate respect, capacity to encourage clinical thinking, a proper teaching environment, interest in teamwork, as well as readiness to accept feedback and criticism. Some recent studies showed the qualities that a clinical teacher should achieve in order to create a proper framework for training other clinicians. Masunaga and Hitchcock [6] studied 205 residents and 148 faculty in family medicine who completed the Clinical Teaching Perception Inventory (CTPI) online between April 2001 and July 2008. The participants ranked 28 single-word descriptors that characterized clinical teachers along a 7-point-scale ranging from "least like my ideal teacher" to "most like my ideal teacher." Their results revealed that both residents and faculty indicated that the ideal clinical teachers should be stimulating, encouraging, competent, and communicative, and should not be conventional, cautious, or controlling. Molodysky [7] emphasized that without specific training in educational methods, clinical teachers may be less efficient and effective in their teaching activity.

The general understanding today is that we are not born teachers, as we are not born car drivers. In spite of the fact that physicians teach all their life, they may not know how to teach. The art of training is to be taught and learned like any other skill.

Of course, young physicians still learn how to teach from other people's experience.

"Reciprocal learning", means that each physician is influenced by his/her colleagues' experiences [1]. But this kind of learning proved to be a slow one. The implicit danger is that the older teacher could be stuck with old methods and would consider the task of teaching a secondary aim of his/her daily work. Thus the idea of learning from another's teaching colleague experience could lead to an undesired effect, that of "teaching without a real teacher"!

Teaching the Teacher

These thoughts created a new project, a European institution (*The International School for Instructors in Anesthesiology—ISIA*) with the aim of preparing, in a limited number of countries outside of Israel, a group of instructors who would be exposed to the modern methods of teaching theoretical and practical subjects, as well as the main aspects of organizing our profession. We considered the idea of preparing experts in clinical teaching a very important task of anesthesiology in the new millennium.

Clinical teaching is important because it improves clinical abilities for effective thinking near the patient's bed. It creates a tradition of bedside and formal transmission of clinical information and expertise. By improving the quality of clinical teaching we expected an improvement in the teaching system in those countries that had been selected to participate in the project.

The project was presented to the Committee of Education of WFSA in 2004, on the occasion of the 13th World Congress held in Paris. The Committee discussed the various aspects of the proposal, decided to sponsor this new European project, and advised the inclusion of a third facet. Besides the PBL items and organizational aspects of the profession, committee members added the basic knowledge of using modern teaching tools. A faculty was appointed and included physicians dedicated to teaching as well as a specialist in the art of teaching, possessing comprehensive experience in teaching education techniques for physicians.

The main aim of the established curriculum was to teach new methods of lecturing on clinical subjects, based on descriptions of real cases, including evidenced base data and basic sciences knowledge. Then the curriculum was enriched by adding a long series of subjects related to educational skills and anesthesia organizational items. The idea of including organizational items derived from an additional scope of the school. The faculty considered the course a good opportunity to prepare students to become leaders of the specialty in their respective countries. Due to their young age, we considered the participants fit candidates to obtain, in the near future, leading positions in their own departments, hospitals, and national societies, as well as in the professional international institutions.

The proposed schedule included 3 weeks for each course, separated by a period of 6 months. The time lapse was due to recognition of the difficulty for a young visiting physician to abandon his/her daily duties and family for a period longer than 1 week. At the same time, we offered the student the opportunity to start and use, even before graduating, the knowledge and skills learned at ISIA's first classes in their own departments, as practical drills. In this way the student could assess the progress attained and become aware of topics that needed more serious effort and attention in the future classes.

Once again we approached the national societies of anesthesiologists in Eastern countries, asking for candidates to take part in the first planned course. We recommended the following criteria for selecting participants to the ISIA course:

- A very good command of English
- Readiness to participate in all three classes
- Commitment to take the task of organizing local similar courses.

This last demand needs further explanation. WFSA and ISIA faculty have opined that we had to avoid the creation of an elite group of young alumni, who would be able use the knowledge and experience accumulated during the classes solely for their own purpose.

The project was supposed to continue after the students graduated. Each national group had to assume the responsibility of organizing similar courses in their own countries, under the auspices of each national society, thus creating the so-called snowball effect, hoping that they would be able to teach other people, also young specialists and residents in the last part of their training, the art of teaching.

The Schedule and Content

Each of the 3 weeks included:

- Five full days
- 10 h per day
- Lectures and presentations by the faculty
- Workshops
- Rehearsals of presentations by students
- Teaching in small groups
- Short presentations by the students (in the last 2 weeks of the course)

As explained above, each of the classes dealt with items belonging to the three components of the program: clinical scenarios and cases, educational skills and methods, and theoretical presentations of organizational aspects of the anesthesiology.

Table 26.4 presents a variety of *clinical topics* that were discussed during the three classes using the PBL format. They covered almost all the domains of activity of the profession and for each item at least one case was prepared and discussed with the students. Discussions followed the presentation of each case and students were encouraged to review the literature and find solutions for managing the case, taking into consideration the availability of equipment, drugs, and organization facilities (recovery rooms, intensive care units, CT scans, etc.).

The second group of items in the curriculum comprised *teaching tools*. It included:

- Plan and develop a curriculum
- Plan a lecture or a course
- How to use the Internet
- How to write multiple choice questions
- Ways to improve power point slide quality
- Use of simulators for teaching purposes
- How to organize interactive sessions

The techniques of dealing with the audience were also included. The student learned how to check the lecture hall before any presentation, to ensure audibility and slide visibility. The

Table 26.4 Examples of clinical cases presented and discussed

1st course	2nd course	3rd course
1. Preop assessment and preparation	1. Pediatric and neonatal anesthesia	1. Management of crisis in anesthesia
2. Critical care	2. Obstetrical anesthesia and analgesia	2. Chronic pain
3. Regional anesthesia	3. Cardiac anesthesia	3. Management of difficult airways
4. Acute pain	4. Neuroanesthesia	4. Outpatient anesthesia
5. Anesthesia for trauma	5. Anesthesia for the elderly	5. Immediate postoperative care

importance of proper body position and language during lecture was emphasized by presenting examples of good and bad habits. The faculty worked hard to enable students to understand the elements of teaching and to improve further practice. Later on, during the last class, students prepared short presentations; each mini-lecture was discussed and critique for improvement was offered, by both the faculty staff and the other Students. Finally, a series of state-of-the-art formal lectures about *organization* of the profession occupied an important place in the students' schedule. Examples of subjects included in this category include:

- Organization of a department of anesthesia
- How to equip an operating room with restricted budget
- Planning a residency track in anesthesiology
- Critical care units and high-dependency units, how do they work together?
- Clinical research—rules and pitfalls
- Sterility in the Operating Room and prevention of ICU cross-infection
- Informed consent for anesthesia
- Introducing new methods into routine practice
- Organization of a pain clinic

The faculty was aware of the wide differences between countries regarding the organization of the profession. Thus discussions and comments of each subject were assigned a special place and time. Students learned how some problems were solved in other countries or departments. The organizational sessions created a framework for exchange of opinions and experience and offered students a different perspective about the situation of anesthesiology in different parts of the continent.

The students received "homework" tasks for each period between classes. They were asked to complete questionnaires regarding their didactic activity "at home" and to emphasize the difficulties still encountered during teaching, as a self-evaluation and reflection report.

Completion of the Course

Three full courses were organized between 2007 and 2012; each included 3 weeks of study. The first took place in Bratislava and Belgrade, the second in Predeal, Romania, and the third on the island of Crete. The last two courses were equally sponsored by WFSA and the European Society of Anesthesiologists (ESA). A fourth course (under a new name of "Teaching the Teacher"—TtT) started in October 2013, in the framework of the ESA Autumn Meeting in Timisoara, Romania.

In order to obtain the final certification the student was expected to fulfill the following criteria:

- Attend all three classes
- Participate fully in all large and small group tasks and presentations using English
- Between courses 1–2 and 2–3 they should:
  - Teach in different styles and on different occasions
  - Produces a self-evaluation and reflection report
- Assignment between the first two classes: reflect on and evaluate a teaching session—planning, content, methods, and delivery
- During the last class:
  - deliver a 30-min case presentation lead a discussion
  - Demonstrate competence in delivering the lecture
  - Proper use of power-point presentation technique
  - Presents three multiple-choice questions related to a case presentation

Sixty specialists in anesthesiology from 16 countries (Table 26.5) graduated the first three courses of ISIA. In addition to the Eastern Europe countries, Greece, Turkey, and Malta, three countries not belonging to the former communist bloc decided to take part in the ISIA project. The acceptance of participants from additional countries was based on the fact that the need for a "Teaching the Teacher" project was global and not specifically restricted to the communist part of Europe. During the three classes of the ISIA third course (2011–2012) we did not feel a significant difference between the background and behavior of the students coming from either part of the continent. All participants shared the same kind of deficiencies in "know-how" in the domain of modern teaching.

Table 26.5 Countries and number of ISIA graduates during the first three courses (2006/2007, 2009/2010, and 2011/2012)

Country	Number of graduates
Bulgaria	4
Croatia	3
Georgia	3
Greece	5
Hungary	4
Latvia	4
Lithuania	4
Macedonia	4
Malta	2
Moldova	4
Poland	4
Romania	4
Serbia	4
Slovakia	3
Slovenia	4
Turkey	4
Total	60

The Feedback

During 2011 and 2013 questionnaires were sent to all 60 ISIA graduates, with the aim of obtaining precise data about the impact that the school had on the development of its participants. Fifty graduates filled out the questionnaire (83 % responders).

Three categories of questions were included in the feedback form and they referred to:

1. Pre-ISIA teaching activities of each participant
2. ISIA impact on their teaching abilities
3. Incidental benefits of the ISIA teachings

Tables 26.6, 26.7, and 26.8 present the results of the feedback. Most of the ISIA alumni did not have any previous training in the art of teaching and thus they lacked confidence in communicating with the audience before taking part in the ISIA first classes. Two-thirds of the responders had never used a modern system of presenting or discussing a case before being exposed to ISIA principles.

Table 26.6 Patterns of pre-ISIA teaching activities—50 responders

Topic	Item	Number of responders	Percentage (%)
A. Source of teaching abilities	1. Specific lectures or lessons	6	12
	2. Other people's experience	34	68
	3. Specific books	6	12
	4. No previous instructions or frontal teaching	17	34
B. Feelings during teaching	1. Fear	25	50
	2. Lack of confidence	30	60
	3. Lack of communication with the audience	35	70
	4. No difficulty at all	6	12
C. Type of presentation	1. "Classical" definition, etiology, etc.	30	60
	2. Use of a case as a starting point	9	18
	3. Special slides for interacting with audience	1	2
	4. Special slides for conclusions	19	38

Table 26.7 The feedback on ISIA alumni teaching abilities after graduating the school, in comparison to the pre-ISIA period—50 responders

Topic	Item	Number reporting better results
A. Presentation details	1. Content	50
	2. Quality of slides	50
	3. Ability to involve audience	50
	4. Personal appearance	48
B. Feelings during presentations	1. Much better personal feeling	49
	2. Possessing greater ability to teach	47
	3. Greater self-confidence as a teacher	47

Table 26.8 Answers to the question: How did the ISIA course change your personal attitude towards the organizational aspects of the profession?—50 responders

Before ISIA course		After ISIA course	
Always interested	25	1. No change	4
Not so interested	17	2. Became alert on this topic	19
Not at all interested	8	3. Significant impact on daily activity	27
		4. Trying to change things in:	
		• Own department	27
		• Own hospital	20
		• Own country	15

Graduating ISIA changed their teaching ability: the graduates stated that they improved the content of their presentations, the quality of slides, the ability to involve the audience in the discussions, and their own personal appearance in front of an audience. They felt better when they taught, were more confident, and related better to the audience during presentations. Most of them became more involved in teaching in their own place of work. Actually, in total, graduates almost doubled their teaching activities after the ISIA course.

Many became involved in a process of changing the organizational aspects of the profession at different levels: anesthesia departments in hospitals as well as at local and national levels. Some have been elected as officers of their own national societies of anesthesiology and other professional organizations, such as WFSA and ESA.

The Post-ISIA National Courses

One of the main objectives of the ISIA courses was to create a number of gifted teachers who, in turn, would organize similar courses in their own countries. The ISIA faculty did not possess the necessary tools for a precise follow up in this direction, but periodic news from different countries reported a long series of courses organized by ISIA alumni. Some of them took responsibility to prepare courses in the framework of the national congresses. Other courses combined topics, in which professional subjects and educational skills have been included in the program. A rough estimation of this post-ISIA activity brings the number of local anesthesiologists (residents in the last year of their training and young specialists) to almost 200.

Conclusions

The two projects presented, the WFSA–Beer Sheva/Israel project and the International School for Instructors in Anesthesiology (ISIA) could be considered unique in the field of medicine, not only in Europe but also all over the world [8]. Both projects involved a large number of trainees.

Whether these projects significantly contributed to closing the professional gap in anesthesiology between the two geographical parts of Europe is unclear for several reasons.

First, the dramatic changes in the political climate in Europe after the fall of the Iron Curtain created a continuous process of clinical training for many Eastern Europe anesthesiologists who have been kept, for decades, away from the progress made in other parts of the continent. This new permanent communication contributed tremendously to the unification of the healthcare systems, utilization of up-to-date equipment and drugs, as well as the use of the same ethical principles that had been implemented in Western Europe in previous decades.

Another difficulty in assessing the real impact for Eastern Europe is that not all the former communist countries have been involved in these educational projects. Progress, if any, produced by the above projects, could not affect all Eastern Europe. None-the-less some conclusions can be drawn from the data. Without any doubt, the WFSA–Beer Sheva project facilitated a first contact with modern anesthesiology and its tremendous progress in the second part of the twentieth century to almost 150 anesthesiologists. The participants could experience how a busy anesthesia department performs, not only in the OR but also in all the other domains of the specialty: critical care, obstetrical analgesia, pain management, sedation, etc.

For most of the participants to the WFSA–Beer Sheva project the time spent at Soroka Medical Center represented a good opportunity once back home, to implement changes in their own departments and hospitals. Things seen for the first time represented a proper start for further activities with the aim of reducing the gap between their own places of work and the typical modern department.

The ISIA idea was born out of the new reality of Eastern Europe. The average anesthesiologist there no longer needed a simple glance at what is done in a modern, well-equipped anesthesia department. Many Eastern Europe anesthesiologists easily reached the western side of the continent where they could use all the opportunities to enrich their knowledge and professional skills. ISIA was supposed to create, in each of the involved countries, a cadre of dedicated and skilled teachers, who learned how to teach and use the new training techniques in their own milieu. In almost all the countries that sent participants to the ISIA courses, the anesthesia national societies offered the ISIA alumni the necessary framework for organizing local courses, in which the new trainees were exposed to those methods taught during the three classes of each ISIA course and thus they, by themselves, could use those experiences in their own further teaching activities. The ISIA graduates are recognized as skillful teachers in their own departments and countries. Some of them were invited to teach in other countries as well as other medical specialties. As recommended by WFSA [9], a group of six alumni of the ISIA 1 and 2 courses alumni [9], from Serbia and Greece, became members of the ISIA 3 course (2011–2012) faculty and they substantially contributed to the teaching program during the three classes.

The optimistic conclusions of this report cannot hide the fact that there is, still, a long way to the final aim of unifying the level of the profession of anesthesiology in Europe. The gap still exists, although it is smaller and progressively less significant.

The brain drain process continues, with many Eastern Europe anesthesiologists looking for positions in the western part of the continent. This reality is a clear proof that we are not witnessing, yet, the complete disappearance of the differences between the two parts of the old continent. Progress is to be made in Eastern Europe in many directions, among them organization of anesthesia departments and creation of solid research centers. But without any doubt the WFSA–Beer Sheva and ISIA projects opened the way towards the unification of anesthesia practice in Europe.

Acknowledgments The author would like to express his gratitude to all those who contributed to the success of both projects: Prof. Mitsugu Fujimori (Japan), Dr. Haydn Perndt (Australia), Dr. Angela Enright (Canada), Dr. Jannicke Mellin-Olsen (Norway), Prof. Paolo Pelosi (Italy), Prof. Eberhard Kochs (Germany), and all the anesthesia national societies' officers who assisted and encouraged the initiative.

References

1. Gurman G, Bar-Lavie Y. The education and teaching anesthesiology in Israel. Tel Aviv: Breirot; 1992. p. 56.
2. Gullo A, Ruprecht J, editors. World Federation of Societies of Anesthesiologists—50 years. New York, NY: Springer; 2004a. p. 171.
3. Kane J. PBS Newshow. October 22, 2012.
4. Barrows HS. Problem-based learning in medicine and beyond. A brief overview. In: Wilkerson L, Gijselaers WH, editors. Bringing problem-based learning to higher education: theory and practice, number 68. San Francisco: Jossey-Bass; 1996.
5. Azer SA. The qualities of a good teacher: how can be they acquired and sustained? J R Soc Med. 2005; 98:67–9.

6. Masunga H, Hitchcock MA. Residents' and Faculty's beliefs about the ideal clinical teacher. Fam Med. 2010;42:116–20.
7. Molodysky E. Clinical teacher training. Maximising the 'ad hoc' teaching encounter. Aust Fam Physician. 2007;36:1044–6.
8. Galeotti G. An Argentinian perspective of the ISIA course. ESA Newsletter. 2013;54:27.
9. Gullo A, Ruprecht J, editors. World Federation of Societies of Anesthesiologists—50 years. New York, NY: Springer; 2004b. p. 201–3.

The Role of the Visiting Anesthesiologist in In-Country Education

27

Julia L. Weinkauf, Marcel E. Durieux, and Lena E. Dohlman

Introduction

Malawi, 2013: This country of 46,000 square miles has about 25 district hospitals and several larger central referral centers (Fig. 27.1), which serve a population of approximately 15 million. There are no local anesthesiologists or nurse anesthetists. All anesthesia care is provided by about 100 clinical officers who are mid-level providers with about 4 years of formal training (in general medical care). A fledgling residency program is run by expatriates. It combines training at a central hospital—where residents are mostly supervised by clinical officers—with a year of experience in South Africa. The program is about to graduate its first anesthesiologist in 2014. Volunteers from Health Volunteers Overseas assist sporadically with training of clinical officers.

Pennsylvania, 2013: This state of 46,000 square miles has more than 250 hospitals, serving a population of about 15 million. There are 1,900 anesthesiologists and 3,600 nurse anesthetists. There are eight accredited residency programs that graduate more than 50 residents per year.

Malawi has approximately one tenth of the number of hospitals, and approximately 1/50th of the number of anesthesia providers as does a US state of similar size and population. In addition, Malawian anesthesia clinical officers train for fewer years and with less clinical apprenticeship than anesthesiologists or nurse anesthetists in high income countries (HICs). The training of Malawian anesthesia clinical officers and residents is largely self-directed and infrequently supervised. Although mid-level providers often have a wealth of clinical experience and are technically skilled, their limited training in physiology, pharmacology, and the principles behind anesthesia practice place severe constraints on their capabilities, and this likely contributes to the high perioperative mortality—approaching 5 % in low- and middle-income countries (LMIC).

With the hospitals overloaded, the providers overworked, those few who are involved in teaching have most of their time taken up by administrative and clinical issues. Compare the Malawian residency program, which has two physicians and no administrative support, to a US residency program with hundreds of clinical faculty and dozens of support staff. As a result, even if qualified students, adequate facilities and appropriate materials are present, training still may not occur simply because there are no teachers available.

In addition, this vicious circle is a critical factor holding back the development of many specialties, including anesthesiology, in many countries. The USA has about 25 physicians per 10,000 population; Malawi, Rwanda, and Tanzania, and about 20 or so other nations make do with less than 1 per 10,000 [1]. The countries with this excessively low ratio are largely in sub-

J.L. Weinkauf, M.D. • M.E. Durieux, M.D., Ph.D. (✉)
Department of Anesthesiology, University of Virginia, Charlottesville, VA, USA
e-mail: durieux@virginia.edu

L.E. Dohlman, M.D., M.P.H.
Department of Anesthesia, Critical Care, and Pain Management, CHA/MGH, Boston, MA, USA

R. Roth et al. (eds.), *The Role of Anesthesiology in Global Health: A Comprehensive Guide*,
DOI 10.1007/978-3-319-09423-6_27, © Springer International Publishing Switzerland 2015

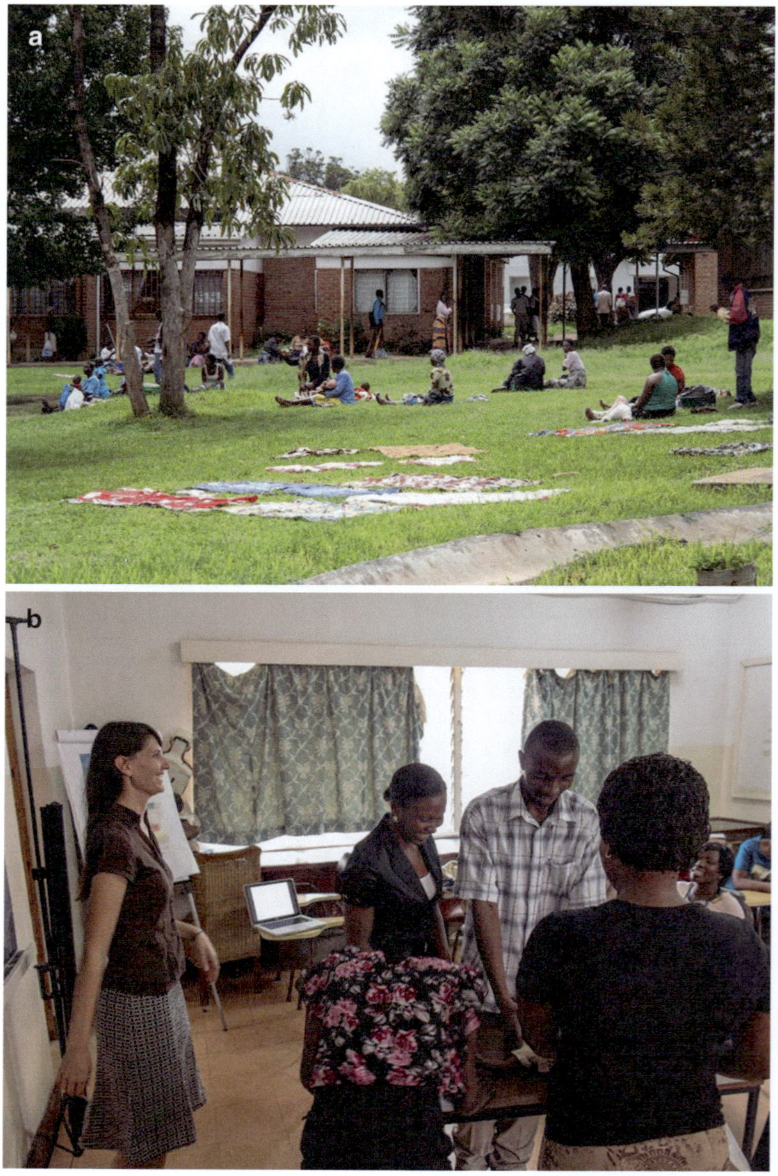

Fig. 27.1 Queen Elizabeth Hospital. (**a**) Queen Elizabeth Hospital in Blantyre, Malawi, is the largest referral hospital in the country, with about 1,000 beds. (**b**) Teaching anesthesia clinical officers in training in pediatric advanced life support at Queen Elizabeth Hospital. Photographs M.E. Durieux

Saharan Africa (Fig. 27.2). In such countries, a critical mass of teachers will have to be established before the cycle can be broken, and this can be done only with outside teaching support. This disparity, the resulting impact on the health of the population, and the clear need for educators demonstrate why anesthesiologists from HICs should become engaged in teaching in LMIC.

In this chapter we provide practical information for anesthesia providers who want to play a role in improving anesthesia education opportunities by volunteering their time to teach overseas. First, we discuss some important practical considerations for volunteers considering teaching work beginning with the difference between service and education focused work and continuing with some considerations for pre-trip planning. This section expands on some material published recently [2]. The subsequent sections focus on pre-departure preparation and practicalities of in-country teaching.

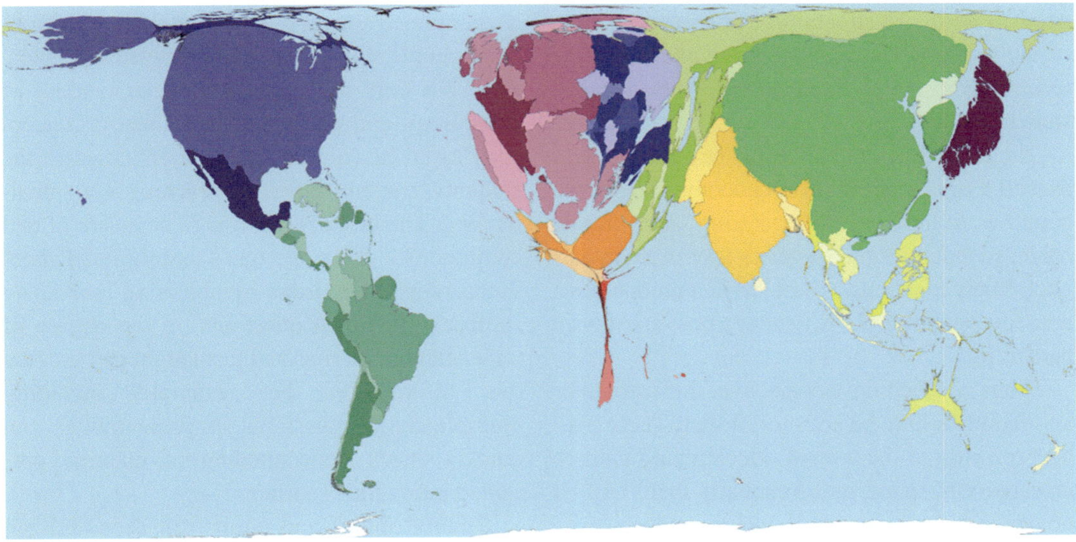

Fig. 27.2 Physicians working around the world. Territory size shows the proportion of all physicians that work in that territory. In 2004 there were 7.7 million physicians working around the world. If physicians were distributed according to population, there would be 12.4 physicians to every 10,000 people. The most concentrated 50 % of physicians live in territories with less than a fifth of the world population. The worst off fifth are served by only 2 % of the world's physicians. Note the disproportionately low number of physicians in Africa (*red*). © Copyright Sasi Group (University of Sheffield) and Mark Newman (University of Michigan). Reproduced under Creative Commons license

A Comparison of the Teaching and Service Volunteer Experience

The primary goal of service-based global health work is to provide medical or surgical care to the local population, while the goal of education-based global health work is to build capacity and train a workforce. When a volunteer commits to service or education, these goals will impact not only the enjoyment of the experience, but the outcome of the work. There are many models of providing service and education, or a mix of the two, but here they are contrasted in their most basic forms.

Facilities, Equipment, and Techniques

Service work focuses on treating the maximum number of patients in the limited available time. For this reason, practitioners will often bring their own equipment and drugs, so as not to be dependent on the local supply. In teaching settings, the trainees will need to be trained on their own equipment with drugs that will be available after the teachers leave. Hence, the visitors will have to make themselves familiar with anesthetic drugs, equipment, and techniques that they may not be used to, or, in fact, may never have seen or heard of before (Fig. 27.3). The volunteer may

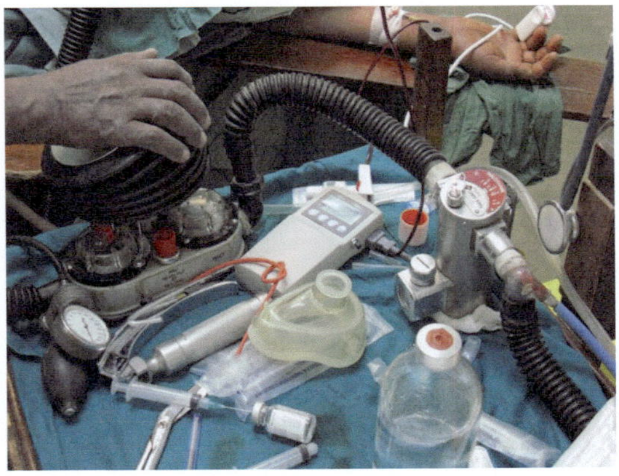

Fig. 27.3 Unfamiliar anesthesia equipment. Material in use at Haydom Lutheran Hospital in Haydom, Tanzania, a large district hospital covering an extensive capture area. An Oxford miniature draw-over vaporizer is used to deliver halothane; Oxford Inflating Bellows are used to ventilate the patient. The pulse oximeter was brought by one of the authors (MED), who was teaching anesthesia medical officers in the hospital. Photograph M.E. Durieux

need to dedicate substantial preparation prior to the teaching trip to familiarize and train her- or himself in the methods and tools used by the students.

The practice setting is likely to be quite different as well. For example, it is not uncommon in some countries to have several operating tables in one room, so that multiple surgeries take place in parallel. Many locations will not have a preoperative area for evaluating the patient or a post-anesthesia care unit.

From a teaching perspective, infrastructure and facilities may be scant or absent. There may be very little in the way of educational facilities or classroom space, and frequently there will be no defined curriculum from which to work.

Workload

The pace of work can be quite different between service and education trips. Again, during service missions, the team attempts to maximize the number of cases done, and that means starting early and often working in the operating room until late at night. Usually, little else is done during the trip. During education work, the volunteer has to adapt to local customary start and end times, which are generally quite different from those in academic medical centers. Even though the hours are different, volunteer educators will work hard. The nonclinical time at the beginning and end of the day is packed with lecture preparation, test writing and grading, and meeting with students. In addition, it is not uncommon to become involved—whether planned or unplanned—in other educational activities such as medical school curriculum development, outside lectures, or teaching for practitioners outside the specialty.

Cultural Considerations

Language barriers can be a major problem during both service and teaching work. For teaching, a good understanding of the level of education of the trainees, and of their background knowledge and clinical experience is required. This information can be difficult to obtain, and at times the teacher may not have worked previously with trainees with this mix of knowledge. For example, as mentioned above, it is not uncommon to work with people who have quite extensive clinical skill, but only a rudimentary understanding of physiology and pharmacology. Even a concept such as "tidal volume" may be unknown to the students, making effective teaching very challenging. The best approach is to be aware of and continuously challenge one's assumptions about the learners' knowledge by obtaining immediate feedback. Frequent questions on the degree of understanding of material just taught can provide this information. For example, including multiple-choice questions in presentations can quickly check understanding of material presented a few slides earlier.

Cultural mores and norms run deep and can challenge and surprise even the most effective teacher. An educator needs to be mentally prepared to find one morning that all of the students are absent because someone's distant relative has died and they all needed to be at the funeral as a sign of respect. A visiting teacher needs to be ready for unexpected pushback during a discussion of ventricular fibrillation, because the students know from experience that none of those patients survive in their hospital, so it is not worth instituting treatment. While it is helpful to prepare by reading on the culture and religion of the area where the teaching will be done, the reality is that the visiting educator will be confronted with unexpected responses and behaviors. The ability to adapt and improvise is an important trait for both the service-based volunteer and teacher; however, a longer duration of a teaching trip means there will be more surprises.

Program Duration

Short- versus long-term involvement will be discussed in more detail later in this chapter, but in the context of a comparison between service and education, it is important to realize that education work will require more time in-country than does a service mission. Unless one commits to a long-term in-country stay, this means that the individual educator will only see a small slice of the whole job. After a service mission of 2 weeks, the volunteer anesthesiologist knows exactly how many patients were operated on and helped; after 2 weeks educating local anesthesia providers, progress may not be quite so visible, and it is easy to become discouraged about long-term prospects. The volunteer can mitigate the natural tendency to become discouraged by understanding the totality of the group's mission, being mentally prepared not to see immediate results, and maintaining contact with people who have previously worked on the same project. On the other hand, educational work often affords practitioners more opportunity and more time for close personal contact and for developing friendships with the local teams, which can be professionally and personally satisfying. Also, educational activities come with the realization that one is adding to capacity, and not in any way taking away from or displacing local professionals.

Program Planning

It is unfortunately only too easy to come into a developing country with the best of intentions yet unprepared to really effectively help with an educational program. For each program, some important considerations need to be addressed. Below we discuss how to define the organizational structure, tailor the message and methods to the intended audience, incorporate technology, and be sensitive to the history of medical education in the country. Incorporating this level of understanding into teaching activities will increase the probability of implementing a successful medical education program.

Program Organization

In-country education programs that are driven by the local clinicians and administration—who are the only people who really understand the local needs and limitations—are more likely to accomplish their goals. Not even the most intense and frequent "scouting trips" and "evaluation visits" can match local knowledge. A formal needs assessment is important and very useful for planning the program, but it cannot replace direct input from local people. Local practitioners are also the people who know if other outside groups are involved in local teaching and can keep well-intentioned organizations with similar goals from duplicating each other's work. In-depth interaction with the local stakeholders will assure that the program is unified and comprehensive, that separate efforts directed at a residency or mid-level training program are aligned, and that all visiting faculty teach according to a defined curriculum. Ideally the local faculty members are in charge of the entire process.

The Audience

Practically, the level of instruction will differ between programs for residents and those geared for anesthesia technicians. Philosophically, many anesthesia educators in HICs feel that anesthesiologists should focus on training more physician providers. Whether efforts and resources should be spent on developing nascent residency programs or whether those efforts are better expended towards improving technician training is a heavily debated question. Physician anesthesiologist and anesthesia technician programs are sometimes at odds within the host country, and the visiting educator may need to negotiate these politics [3]. Because in over half the countries in the world technicians or nurses with an average of 1–2 years of training provide most of the anesthesia care, it is in the best interest of the local patients that technicians are optimally trained, and participation in their training is valuable [4, 5]. At the same time, the goal of having at least one anesthesiologist available in each hospital is an important one—physician anesthesiologists can advance anesthesia care with respect to other medical and surgical services, they can provide subspecialty services, and they can supervise and support technicians and mid-level practitioners. Ideally for the health of the population in LMICs, residencies will be started, and residents and technician education will have to take place simultaneously [6].

Distance Learning

Internet facilities in most parts of the world are by now capable of video uplinks of very acceptable quality, and tele-education can be immensely valuable in many ways. As one important example,

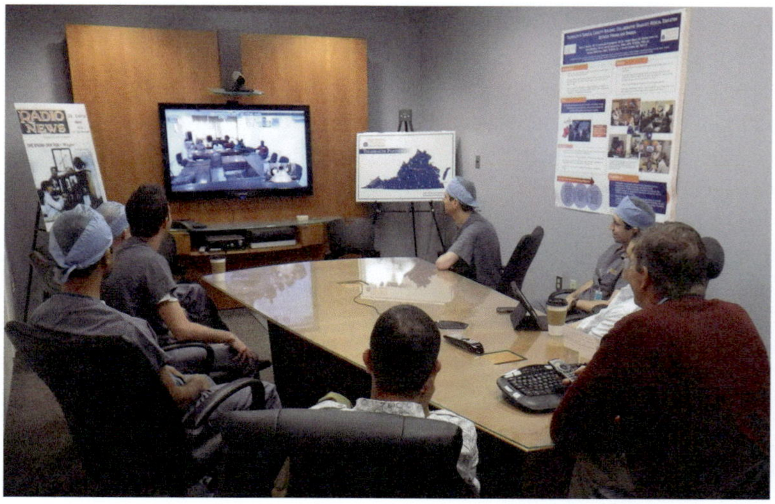

Fig. 27.4 Distance learning. A case teleconference in progress between the anesthesiology departments of the University of Virginia and the University of Rwanda. Photograph C. Lewis, with permission

it allows a variety of specialists, not all of whom would be able or willing to travel to another country, to take part in educational activities. In addition, it allows residents or other learners to see behavior modeled by their counterparts in HIC. Case teleconferences can be an excellent learning tool for residents in LMICs and remote areas of HICs; for example, the University of Virginia runs a monthly case conference with the anesthesiology residency in Rwanda (see Fig. 27.4), and these are being evaluated positively [3]. Although operating room and bedside teaching are an essential part of medical training that cannot be replaced by distance learning, teaching be enhanced through the use of technology for case-based learning or simulation. A program such as the case conferences mentioned above can maximize educational value and minimize cost for training programs in LMICs.

Beyond the Curriculum

When physician educators arrive to teach the curriculum and implement an educational program, they become ambassadors from their home country. What this means is that they are unavoidably a model for many of the trainees, and this may be one of the more important aspects of in-country teaching. A visiting physician educator walks a fine line between capacity building and recruiting anesthesia providers away from the home country.

Many developing countries suffer greatly from "brain drain": For a variety of reasons, local physicians trained, at great difficulty and cost, are at high risk of leaving the country and finding more comfortable and lucrative employment elsewhere [7–10]. To prevent this, it is important that foreign teachers do more than train in technical and cognitive aspects. Working and teaching in the local setting can be a truly interesting job and this needs to be conveyed to the trainees. They also need to be made to feel part of the modern anesthesia world. In some ways, when one talks about techniques, drugs and approaches used in the western world, trainees in LMIC get a glimpse into their future. Our goal as anesthesia educators is for them to be part of that future—in their own country.

Before You Go: Finding a Program and Preparing for Your Experience

Somewhere in sub-Saharan Africa: A woman of 48 years needs surgery for a uterine fibroma. Her husband is a surgeon and she told him she does not want general anesthesia. The husband recommends a surgeon colleague who works in a private hospital famous for its regional anesthesia. In this hospital the surgeon is also the doctor who gives anesthesia. The husband plans to assist his friend in operating on his wife. What happens?

The day of the operation, the surgeon places the single shot epidural anesthesia. Both surgeons prepare themselves for the operation and an assistant trained by the surgeon is charged with taking the blood pressure, and monitoring pulse and oximetry parameters. Before the incision, the husband remarks that his wife is yawning. His friend tells him that she probably wants to sleep and asks his assistant to give 100 mg of propofol intravenously to help her sleep. The propofol is given and the operation begins. After a few minutes, the husband, not hearing his wife, tries to talk to her. She doesn't answer. When the assistant attempts to measure the blood pressure, it is not recordable: the woman is in cardiac arrest. An anesthetist from another hospital is called to come and resuscitate. He arrives 30 min later, but by that time the patient is dead. On site there was equipment to ventilate but the laryngoscope didn't work because of battery failure.

Although the details change, stories of avoidable anesthetic deaths such as the one above are shockingly common in many parts of the world. The high perioperative morbidity and mortality in many LMICs has a number of causes, but a lack of well-trained anesthesia providers is certainly an important one [6, 11]. As we have discussed, an increasing number of anesthesiologists and anesthesia trainees from high-income countries are eager to travel overseas and help. Several practical pre-trip steps can be taken before an educational visit overseas to make it a more productive, rewarding, and safe experience for the visitor, the host, and most importantly for the patients. The following section will review the most critical steps in preparing for an educational trip.

Program or Project Selection

An important first step in contributing to in-country anesthesia training is to search for a reputable aid organization or program that is a good fit with the physician's skills, interests and values. An established program has the advantages of having performed a needs assessment and having worked out relationships between key players at the overseas site. It is important that a visiting anesthesiologist not be a burden to already overworked health care providers by making demands on their time for assistance with orientation, housing and transportation needs. A good organization can help guide the educator with planning, communication, and setting reasonable expectations in order to increase the likelihood of a useful and productive trip.

If the anesthesiologist is not already aware of an educationally oriented organization, how does he/she find one? Fortunately in the past 5–10 years there has been a strong focus on workforce development and education in anesthesia and other specialties by academic institutions, the World Health Organization (WHO), and the US Government [12]. Good places to start looking are within the home institution, on websites such as the American College of Surgeons Operation Giving Back (OGB) [13], the American Society of Anesthesiologists (ASA) Global Humanitarian Outreach (GHO) [14], and subspecialty websites such as the Society for Pediatric Anesthesia [15] and the Society for Education in Anesthesia [16]. Networking with health care workers interested in global health at the home institution and at meetings can also be helpful. Other educationally oriented anesthesia organizations that are useful are the World Federation of Societies of Anaesthesiologists (WSFA) [17], Health Volunteers Overseas (HVO) [18], and Kybele [19], which are all represented in this text. An opportunity for longer involvement in teaching is the newly launched Rwanda Human Resources for Health Program [20].

Many residents are interested in global health and can contribute as well as benefit from an international teaching rotation. Residents can play a special role as peer mentors to local students who may relate better and be more comfortable asking questions of a fellow adult learner. Residents are often technically savvy and innovative which can help to bring new and exciting teaching techniques to a developing country. For example, one SEA HVO traveling fellow taught residents in Peru how to film procedures at their hospital using a cell phone and some inexpensive attachments. These filmed procedures could then be used to teach new residents how the procedure is performed at their hospital. Also, residents may at times be a better source of practical clinical information and clinical "pearls" than the academic faculty.

Some anesthesia residency programs have standing overseas teaching rotations. Residents in these programs are well advised to let their program director know early in their residency if they are interested in global health. Residents who do not find an opportunity within their own institution can apply to receive a month's scholarship with the SEA HVO Traveling Fellowship. Applications can be found on the HVO or SEA websites on December 1st each year for the following academic year. Residents should be aware that traveling with an organization outside their own program may be considered an "out of program rotation" by the country's accreditation body. For example, according to the American Board of Anesthesiology (ABA), international rotations have special requirements including (1) the rotation must occur during the first 9 months of the fourth postgraduate year of anesthesia training and (2) a letter requesting ABA approval must be obtained prior to departure for the rotation. Details on requirements for residents teaching abroad can be found on the SEA website [16].

Next, the anesthesiologist should evaluate his or her skills, values, interests, and needs and decide how these attributes best match with a program. To maximize the chances of a successful visit for the educator and the host, this issue should be addressed when choosing a program—not when in-country. A potential volunteer should take into consideration the following:

- How much time are you willing and able to spend overseas?
- Do you have special health needs or concerns that will limit where you can visit and for what amount of time?
- Do you plan to bring family members with you and will it be safe for them? What will your spouse or partner do while you are working?
- Do you prefer to train anesthesia providers in basic anesthesia techniques or to educate anesthesiologists with more sophisticated concepts? Some sites are more suitable for one or the other.
- Is the anesthesiologist comfortable teaching in a hospital with equipment, drugs and patient conditions that he/she has only read about and is he/she willing to learn from the hosts as well as to teach?
- Would you be willing to work in a country with political, social, or religious values which you don't share? Would it be difficult to resist judging or criticizing their ways? If so, it may be best to choose another program or site.

Anesthesiologists with a flexible, patient, and nonjudgmental approach and an enthusiasm for learning as well as teaching should do well when some effort has gone into finding the most appropriate program and site.

Personal Health and Safety

The health and safety of medical professionals is too often neglected in the enthusiasm for going overseas [21]. Illnesses and injuries—often avoidable—can be a disaster for the educator but can also be a burden for the host. It is a good idea to visit a travel clinic several months before leaving the country to get advice about vaccinations, malaria prophylaxis and how to handle postexposure HIV prophylaxis. Educators who are participating in hands-on teaching in the OR or ICU should be aware that many of the protective barriers and devices used at home as part of universal precautions are in short supply or not available in many low resource countries. Bringing gloves, masks, eye protection and hats will help the visitor maintain universal precautions and will prevent the hosts institution from being further depleted of supplies.

Preparations should also include reviewing coverage under personal health, disability and workers compensation insurance, asking explicitly whether incidents that occur overseas will be covered. The biggest threat to otherwise healthy educators traveling internationally is road safety. Following the advice of knowledgeable locals on how to deal with in country transportation is strongly recommended. According to the Centers for Disease Control (CDC), "Motor vehicle crashes—not crime or terrorism—are the number 1 killer of healthy US citizens living, working, or traveling in foreign countries." [22] Political instability and crime are also factors to consider when picking a country to visit. Checking with the US State Department and with home organizations regarding recent blockades, demonstrations, and interruptions to travel—while remembering that life in one's home country is not without risk—can inform the decision of whether reported risks are worth taking.

Making Trip Arrangements

Trip plans should start several months ahead of travel with passport and visa arrangements since they can take much longer than one might expect. Communication is encouraged with the country site and, depending on the country and program, can be painfully slow when volunteers from HICs are used to instant text, social media, and e-mail messages. Reasons for delays are understandable given the challenges of overworked administrators, loss of internet connections, or bureaucratic barriers.

Although malpractice for educators visiting a developing country is not yet a big concern, it is a good idea to know if and how one is covered, especially if the plan is to teach through demonstration in the operating rooms or ICU. Increasingly, academic hospital's malpractice insurance will cover physicians doing global health work that is supported by or connected to the hospital.

Travel insurance is highly recommended to protect against the catastrophic costs of having to be flown out of the country should one become seriously ill or injured, and is very reasonably priced for the young and healthy. References to travel insurance companies are best obtained from the home academic center, global health program administrator, or by a simple Internet search. Airplane tickets and housing arrangements should ideally be completed 2 months before departure.

Again, there are usually special considerations for anesthesia residents involved in global health education. More information on this process can also be obtained by members of the Society for Education in Anesthesia (SEA) on their website at www.seahq.net. For US residents, the trip must *finish* prior to the last 3 months of residency if it is an outside rotation. Residents must also have the program director send a written and signed application to the ABA for approval *unless* the overseas program is a standing program run by the affiliated department or hospital. The program director's letter must be sent at least 4 months prior to the rotation and should include the following:

- A description of the proposed rotation and the dates.
- Information about the supervision of the resident, including the position and credentials (CV) of the physician overseeing the resident's training.
- Description of how much time the resident has spent training in and away from facilities affiliated or integrated with his/her parent institution.
- Provide assurance that the resident or fellow will remain enrolled in his/her accredited program while training away from the accredited program.
- Provide assurance that the resident or fellow is in good standing at the time of the request.
- Indicate that the resident's or fellow's accredited program will report the training on the semiannual Record of Training/Clinical Competence Committee report filed for the period involved [23].

Educating the Educator

Once a program and country has been chosen, it is essential to do some background work to help better prepare for the teaching experience. Reading about health and population statistics, workforce and economic conditions and country-specific diseases can all be helpful in forming "the big picture" prior to departure. Much of this information can be found on organization websites at the WHO [24] and the Centers for Disease Control [25].

Buying a general travel book for the country can be a good way to get information about what kind of weather, food, clothing expectations, and other cultural differences will be encountered. Many countries have an English language newspaper which can be scanned online for local news before you go.

It is essential to try to determine the educational needs and wants of the colleagues and students overseas in order to make the most appropriate educational plan. The organization or program should be able to provide a curriculum (if there is one), help obtain trip reports or contact information from previous educators, and put volunteers in contact with the in-country director of training. Exchanging e-mails, communicating by text message, or scheduling Skype conversations or phone calls with local practitioners or administrators will be important for gathering information. It is also frequently possible to obtain permission to contact one of the students directly before arrival. This contact can be immensely helpful for determining the students' educational level, the hospital resources and case mix, and types of local equipment used.

However, no matter how carefully one prepares, there will always be unexpected changes and surprises. A common occurrence is to be asked to lecture on a subject for which no lesson has been prepared. This will be part of the adventure! Bringing ASA Refresher Courses or other reviews on a laptop can be useful in this situation.

Planning Lessons, Structuring Curriculum, and Finding Resources

There is a great need for quality anesthesia education and training in the developing world. The enormity of this need can seem daunting. Even with a curriculum in hand, it can be difficult to know what teaching will be welcome and most helpful. It can be useful to remember that although the circumstances might be different, the role of an educator overseas is basically the same as at the home institution. First and foremost educators are obligated to teach anesthesia providers to give safe anesthesia. Anesthetic deaths in countries lacking adequately trained anesthesia providers are reportedly often the result of preventable airway problems and hypovolemia in young, healthy patients [11]. Focusing on the known sources of mortality in basic anesthetic care can be lifesaving. Common sources of morbidity and mortality easily translated into teachable moments include:

- Airway and ventilation management
- Assessing and maintaining intravascular volume and vascular tone
- Preoperative assessment
- Techniques for monitoring and vigilance
- Recognizing and intervening in the case of a total spinal
- Preventing drug and transfusion errors

Introducing the WHO Surgical Safety Check List is proven to decrease morbidity and mortality [26]. It can be useful to bring handouts on monitoring, fluid management, and management of common intraoperative problems. Bringing expired or open and unused airway equipment to run airway management workshops is usually welcome and inexpensive.

As discussed earlier, physician educators are also responsible for being role models for professional and ethical behavior when abroad or at home. This can sometimes be challenging since the standards of care vary greatly internationally. For example, it is not standard practice in all countries for an anesthesia provider to be in the room at all times during an anesthetic. One explanation for this is that there are often more surgeons and surgical procedures than anesthesia providers and the anesthesia provider is forced to cover more than one room at a time. There is no easy solution to such an ethical dilemma, but how it will be handled should be considered before departure.

Anesthesia educators also promote lifetime continuing education for local anesthesia providers. By preparing refresher courses, skills workshops, case-based workshops, and simulation-type courses to bring overseas, the volunteer can reinforce basic safety techniques as well as introduce new techniques to local providers. Teaching how to use ultrasound in ICU diagnosis and regional anesthesia is an example that has been quickly accepted in academic centers overseas (Fig. 27.5). Since recruiting and retaining trained staff is a serious problem in many LMICs it is important to do what can be done to add to a stimulating career and to prevent anesthesiologists from feeling isolated and stagnant [27]. Supporting in-country training programs leading to specialty qualification in fields like anesthesia has been shown to help retain physicians [28]. Teaching current methods (as long as they can be done safely and sustainably) can contribute to a more satisfying and interesting work for the in-country anesthesiologist.

Another role educators take on at home and abroad is to encourage self-education by providing

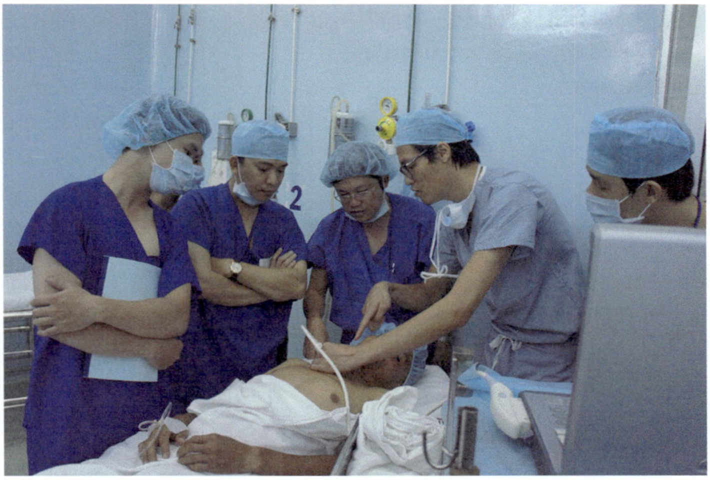

Fig. 27.5 Teaching regional anesthesia. Daniel Vo, a Society for Education in Anesthesia/Health Volunteers Overseas Traveling Fellow in 2011, teaches ultrasound regional anesthesia techniques in the Hospital for Traumatology and Orthopedics in HCMC, Vietnam

references to books, journals, and Internet sites. The internet is increasingly accessible in developing countries and it is recommended to bring a list of favorite anesthesia education internet web sites to share with overseas students. A good example is the free anesthesia education site Open Anesthesia, which is associated with the International Anesthesia Research Society [29]. Open access journal articles and other educational materials that can be put in pdf format and downloaded on students' laptops or the department computers are also often welcome.

First Do No Harm

The role of the physician educator overseas must also include a self-reflection on the actual benefits of his or her teaching as well as possible unintentional harm. Physicians who volunteer to teach in developing countries often comment when they return that they feel they learned more than they taught. This may be particularly true of lessons learned about health care rationing and making do with less. Other lessons are more emotionally challenging. Seeing a baby with correctable congenital deformities die for lack of equipment or a young mother with injuries left to die because it would be "too expensive" to operate can be traumatic for the physician who trained in a high-resource setting. Sometimes the opposite occurs and the visiting anesthesiologist is asked "as an expert from overseas" to participate in cases she or he deems futile. Finding a mentor to contact at home or locally to talk over these ethical dilemmas when they occur can be helpful (see also the section on "On Location: Tips for Teachers, Personal Impact, and Ethical Dilemmas" below).

Many of us who have spent time teaching in developing countries have made our share of cultural missteps over the years. Some lessons learned include the following:

- Avoid comments that may be construed as a criticism of the country, politics, religion, or health care.
- Dress and act with respect for the local norms.
- Listen to the learners as to what they want to be taught. Neither underestimate nor overestimate what local providers know. Some of them struggle with basic concepts but many of us have met some truly brilliant, educated and vastly experienced anesthesiologists who have taught us much more than we taught them.
- Adjust teaching to stay within the usual local working hours. Students may have other jobs or responsibilities they have to attend to.
- Be flexible and accommodating as much as possible.
- Learning the names of the colleagues is very important.
- Be patient—change is slow.

When traveling overseas, an educator becomes a role model and diplomat of the profession, his or her home institution, and native country. The physician educator also becomes a student of another culture and health care system and a new friend to many wonderful and interesting people.

On Location: Tips for Teachers, Personal Impact, and Ethical Dilemmas

You are a visiting teacher doing clinical and classroom teaching in a low-resource setting for the past 6 weeks. You have just finished overseeing a case in the operating theatre with a local resident. Upon arrival to the recovery area, you find a group of local nurses and doctors performing advanced cardiac life support (ACLS) on a patient in cardiac arrest.

You ask about the patient and are told that it is a 20-year-old healthy woman with post-partum hemorrhage who just had a Bakri balloon placed while she is in the recovery room. The bleeding has improved, but she had a pulseless electrical activity arrest just as the procedure was finished, around 5 min ago, and is now in asystole. There is a bag of whole blood running freely into a 16 gauge IV in her antecubital fossa.

You notice that the staff performing chest compressions are not following American Heart Association ACLS guidelines. The compressions are being performed at a rate of around 200 per minute for short bursts of 10–15 s, at which point the compressor looks at the monitor to check the rhythm.

Should you step in and perform the chest compressions yourself? Should you try to instruct the nurse on how to improve the compressions now? Should you say something to the senior physician present? Should you wait until later, after the resuscitation either succeeds or fails? What would be the most effective way to change local practice? What are the ethical implications of not stepping in and thus increasing the potential for a bad outcome for this patient?

Different Situations, Different Opportunities: Short- Versus Long-Term Involvement, Teaching for Your Strengths, and Maintaining Continuity

Short- Versus Long-Term Involvement

Much of the overseas global health work in anesthesiology is done as short-term surgical service trips, or "missions," which can be service-oriented or educational, as mentioned above. Another approach is longer term involvement, including frequent visits to the same location or a long-term placement.

The three elements of education are: knowledge, skills, and behavioral (also known as nontechnical skills in medical education) [30]. Behavioral or nontechnical skills include less concrete but crucial elements of being a good physician, such as communication, knowledge-acquisition skills, and professionalism. Short-term work by its nature is more conducive to the first two elements of training. Knowledge and skills are things that can be taught effectively by practitioners in formats such as lectures, case discussions, and other classroom activities, as well as at the bedside. Expanding classroom activities into simulations and workshops can provide an especially stimulating environment that may result in more retention and absorption (Fig. 27.6).

Anesthesia providers in resource-poor settings are in need of behavioral and non-technical skills just as much as they are in need of knowledge- or even skill-based competencies. This is due to several factors: easier access to knowledge-based learning materials, human resources needs that lead to a lack of mentorship and senior guidance, as well as the fact that developing country training programs often emphasize knowledge-based elements far more than technical or especially nontechnical skills. Doing long-term work (>3 months), or returning to the same site, allows far more opportunity to develop these nontechnical skills among local students. Indeed, repeat volunteers have reported a sense that their regular presence resulted in a greater impact over time [31]. Although there is no clear evidence that any type of outreach is superior to another, there are definite roles for both short- and long-term involvement in the educational process.

Maximizing Education Opportunities

With short-term educational work, it is desirable to have an ongoing organized teaching program that is fulfilled by the short-term visiting teachers. Local audiences often graciously submit to teaching of topics that have been presented to them not so long ago. This type of repetition wastes local practitioners' valuable educational time. Typically clinical care is on hold or at least modified when the staff is attending an educational conference, as there simply are no other

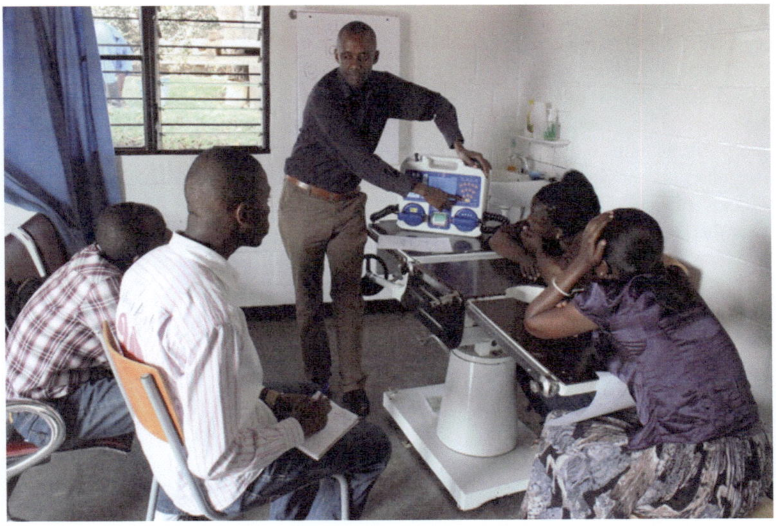

Fig. 27.6 Simulation session. Expanding classroom activities into simulations and workshops can provide an especially stimulating environment that may result in more retention and absorption. Local faculty can learn to teach through these methods at the same time. Rwandan anesthesiologist Kiviri Willy teaching local operating room staff ACLS and defibrillator use. Centre Hospitalier Universitaire de Kigali, Rwanda

practitioners to take over the duties. Thus, having a plan for short-term educators assures that patient care does not suffer for minimal benefit.

It is important to be sensitive to the knowledge base of the local practitioners. Resources for acquiring knowledge are often accessible in the form of online sources and materials that foreigners have left behind or donated. The easy access to knowledge-based learning materials means they may know *more* than many US trainees. Implementing that knowledge into practice is limited more by lack of resources and behavioral techniques than by lack of knowledge base or learning materials per se.

With this is mind, though they may not have the materials or equipment necessary to implement advanced therapies, it may be inappropriate to "dumb down" your teaching presuming that students have a limited knowledge base. By erring on the side of teaching to the highest level of evidence possible within the resources that they have available—appropriate to the audience's level of training, of course—one can then modify or simplify material only if necessary. Appropriately challenging conferences are the ones that have the most impact on a local audience. In general, educators should tailor lectures and programs to the same level as they would at their home institution, but in a resource-appropriate way. A talk intended for a 1st-year anesthesia resident in a developing country should be similar to a CA-1 anesthesia talk in the USA; a presentation for faculty in a developing country should be similar to a presentation for faculty in the USA, if their resources permit. One may want to include a bit less information than normally included to allow time to speak more slowly or with translation to an audience listening to a presentation when English is their second, third or fourth language.

Consideration should be given to passing along a particular skill, rather than general knowledge. For example, if one is an ultrasonographer or an ACLS instructor, perhaps workshops can be arranged to take advantage of that expertise (Fig. 27.7). Other possibilities for specific skill transfer could include difficult airway techniques, flexible bronchoscopy, regional anesthesia techniques, and many more.

Translating Respect into Effect

Physician educators must earn local practitioners' respect—it is not conferred automatically. Many visiting teachers are perplexed or even incensed when the local workers do not quickly believe what they say, listen to them, and start practicing in that way. Realizing that the local practitioners are professionals and colleagues who have not had access to as many opportunities and resources will increase the volunteer's chance

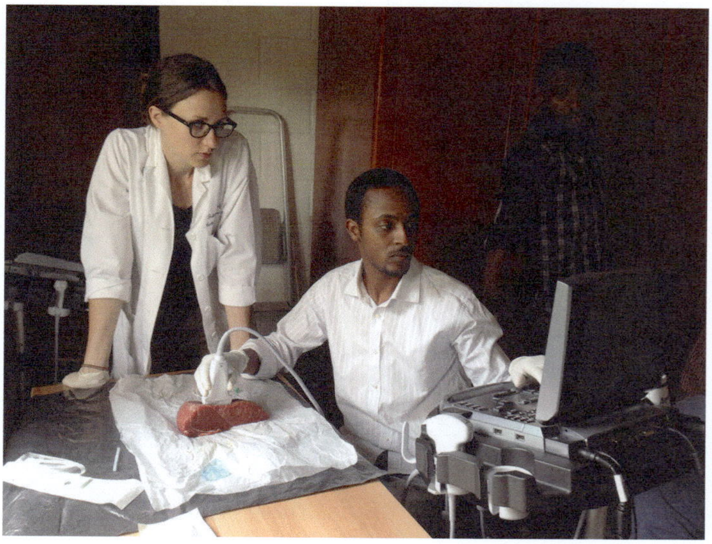

Fig. 27.7 Ultrasound training. Training in particular skills may be at least as useful as transmitting general information; use of ultrasound for diagnosis and nerve blockade is a good example. Julia Weinkauf teaching ultrasound technique to residents Gaston Nyirigira and Benjamin Semakuba, Centre Hospitalier Universitaire de Kigali, Rwanda. Photograph by Denise M. Chan, M.D.

of leaving something real behind. Impact is greater if the teacher is respected, and respect is earned over time. Local practitioners have developed their practice and gained local success for a reason. Expect buy-in to take at minimum weeks or months.

One simple but frequently neglected way to earn respect and attention is to spend time learning peoples' names. One of the biggest barriers to having an impact is earning trust. Learning a person's name has tremendous power in establishing rapport. Physician educators should devote time to learning people's names upon arrival, just as time has been devoted to preparing teaching materials. Many of us have experienced (or have been) a foreigner exasperated by a local practitioner's unwillingness to act quickly or listen to concerns or mobilize something for a sick patient. When then asked who it was they were working with, it turns out the foreigner didn't know the person's name, or sometimes not even what role or service they were with. It then becomes clear why that person would not act on the suggestion of a stranger.

Great teachers often get students to talk more than they talk. In observing visiting educators, one notes a strong tendency to move quickly to announcing the answer to a clinical question, especially when struggling with communication and language barriers. In addition, local practitioners are often so used to visiting educators feeding them information and resources, that they are sometimes comfortable with this one-way flow of information. This approach goes nowhere. Not only does the specific knowledge not transfer well via unidirectional flow, but the educator misses an opportunity to develop communication and approaches to processing materials. Didactic sessions are generally only effective for knowledge acquisition, whereas exchanges between practitioners provide these opportunities to develop non-technical skills. When working with a local colleague, one should initiate a discussion about what they would do or what their practice is. In a discussion between two colleagues, the learner is far more likely to feel empowered to think critically about a situation, ask questions, and integrate new concepts. Using the following question as a test to ask whether one is feeding students or supporting and nurturing them: "Am I doing most of the talking?"

As a foreign worker, going around the local system to improve immediate patient care is tempting. An example of this includes calling other foreigners directly for consults or expedited services. Using influence and connections in this way can make the local health care system worse since there is less drive for improvement if it is possible to detour around dysfunction when desired. Challenging oneself to stay within the system—even though it is slower and frustrating is preferable- and the experience will be richer as a result. If there is initiative for change among local co-workers and time to support the project, a visiting educator can help formulate a system improvement plan.

Projects: From Idea to Continuity

There are endless programmatic and systems-based projects one can consider in a long-term assignment or with repeat visits. Some of these could include:

- Starting a morning case conference or a grand rounds series or journal club series
- Starting a scheduling system for the OR
- Starting an morbidity and mortality conference
- Implementing a preoperative or postoperative evaluation system
- Implementing an anesthesia preparedness checklist
- In the ICU, standardizing rounding, consults, and presentations
- Writing locally appropriate educational guides for anesthesia subspecialties
- Implementing a quality improvement program
- Initiating monitoring or pain control protocols in the PACU
- Organizing an emergency airway box
- Organizing an emergency cart

Waiting at least a month before suggesting or starting working on any of these projects, and talking with the locals about previous attempts is desirable. Chances are that these ideas may have been suggested or tried before. In general, one certainly wants local faculty approval and sincere involvement before embarking on these endeavors. The rule of thumb is: they must want it *at least as much* as the educator does, or it will not be used and will not last.

Finally, consideration should be made as to whether just being a "worker bee" continuing to teach how to work within the system that is in place, might be better for building capacity in the long-run. The pressure to "make a difference" as an educator is enormous, but simple quality teaching and human resource capacity building, role modeling, and setting standards can truly make a difference, especially in the realm of behavioral and nontechnical skills. Not everyone needs to start a project. Many of these will end up forgotten on a shelf anyway. The local practitioners are always the best ones to start and implement projects, whenever possible. Support them. Local oversight is, in reality, the only way to ensure continuity after visiting educators leave.

Personal, Career, and Ethical Issues

Personal and Career Impact

The personal motivations for doing educational work overseas are often similar to the motivations for doing service work. These motivations range from the altruistic desire to "make a difference" and recognition of a global community, to the more selfish ones such as the desire to connect to a social network, and honing of personal skills and knowledge [32]. Volunteers doing educational or development work often stress their desire to leave a more lasting contribution than direct care of a small number of patients, though there is no clear evidence that one form of volunteerism makes more of an impact than another.

Upon return to their home country, most volunteer educators feel that they had a positive experience, including finding it personally rewarding and feeling that they contributed positively to the local conditions. They also report an improvement of their own skills and knowledge [31]. Some reasons for dissatisfaction include a lack of clarity or doubt about the utility of the volunteer's role, a perception that the local health care workers are not motivated themselves for improved conditions, and frustration with lack of resources. First-time volunteers often expect a fast-paced, intense, and tiring experience, and are surprised when they find that keeping business hours is the norm of the local staff. This is an example of the difference between educational work and service work that can contribute to dissatisfaction if not anticipated.

Teaching in a foreign environment provides unique challenges that can improve teaching skills in a way not possible in a home environment. The visiting teacher is obliged to be more sensitive to the reception of the material by local staff, constantly adjusting communication methods, speed of material delivery, as well as the material itself.

Volunteers also report an increased appreciation not only for the resources available in their home country, but the public health infrastructure and hospital safety systems that have been designed to enable practitioners in developed countries to deliver (and patients to obtain) safer, more effective, and efficient care. Visitors in long-term placements who work on implementing systems and public health improvements gain greater insight into the challenges of building such systems from scratch and of the massive benefits they can have when successful. The paperwork we groan over at home can suddenly seem not so onerous when confronted with an environment in which those processes, and their protective benefits are totally absent.

Overseas involvement can also have an impact on a volunteer's professional career. The recent surge in global health interest has led to increased involvement by departments and demand by residents and medical students to have such experiences integrated into their training [12]. This creates demand for faculty with global health experience and connections and the need for departmental support—both financial and in terms of non-clinical time—for volunteers.

Ethical Issues

The visiting teacher will inevitably encounter ethical dilemmas ranging from minor curiosities to situations that concern patients' well-being. Volunteers need to be prepared to navigate difficult unexpected situations.

One easily identifiable ethical dilemma occurs when a visitor perceives delivery of poor care by locals, but is not directly involved, and is tempted to intervene in the moment. When conflicts arise, we think it is preferable to err on the side of allowing the local health workers to direct things, rather than interject our position. A discussion or educational intervention can then be considered after the fact, consistent with one's role as teacher rather than service provider. This arguably will result in increased buy-in from the locals, more so than stepping in the moment, which can quickly create resentment. This is especially true for relatively minor, non-life-threatening questions (such as the best way to close an incision), but can be the best practice for serious situations as well. There is no quicker way to lose the respect and attention of local workers than to disrespect and criticize their practice in the moment without grace and humility.

This position must lead to an acknowledgement that, for the visiting teacher, the patient in front of us may not be our first priority. We are often forced to choose between providing the best care and providing the best educational experience for the teaching audience. The visitor must decide for himself how much he can accept in the way of slow or substandard care, in the hopes of a lasting improvement of local practice.

Another ethical dilemma that presents itself to the visiting teacher is the redirection of the local staff's efforts from their patients to us, the foreigners. Foreign visitors require a lot of attention. Educators of course believe that it is an investment to leave behind a greater benefit, but they should be mindful of minimizing the distraction. Consider carefully what information and attention is actually needed to do the work effectively. Does one really need to visit the laboratory or the blood bank or the pharmacy? Imagine how many times the locals have answered the same questions to people who will not benefit them or their systems or their patients. Imagine how many times they have told foreigners where the restrooms are. Disruption of the local schedule is unnecessary unless a benefit can be foreseen.

Another ethical concern when doing humanitarian work is the fostering of "learned helplessness." Broadly, this refers to the concern that if the needs of a community or organization are supplied by outside sources, there will be no internal impetus for change. This concept has been written about extensively around the topic of foreign aid in general, but can apply in a more microcosmic way to work as foreign teachers as well. If the educator's presence consistently supplies the educational needs of a department, or even the specific answers to clinical questions in the moment, the local practitioners may not have the incentive to teach, develop their teaching skills, or even answer their own clinical questions.

At an extreme, it can create incentive to neglect what would otherwise be their sole responsibility, which is a natural response to being overburdened when someone else will handle matters. There is no clear way to navigate this ethical quandary, but most visitors and programs strive to include the local workers as much as possible, and supplement and support rather than replace their efforts.

One final ethical dilemma is the potential for systems or organizational projects implemented by a visitor to falter after that visitor leaves the country. There are infinite numbers of projects pushed forward hard by visiting educators and physicians that quickly died from lack of local support and resources when the foreigner left. This not only wastes time, but is harmful in that it dilutes local enthusiasm for change. For example, if an Operating Room scheduling system is attempted by many different players, locals will be less and less likely to support the next effort at initiating a system, and subsequent attempts are that much more likely to fail. Failed attempts at projects are inevitable, but we should do our best to achieve local buy-in and support, and initiate things in a carefully organized way in order to minimize these problems.

Conclusion

In-country teaching of anesthesiology is an immensely challenging, long-term job. It can be highly rewarding, but also frustrating. A thorough understanding of what one is getting into, and meticulous preparation on a personal and professional level will help avoid some of the frustrations.

For our specialty all over the world to have the position that it enjoys in western countries, eventually, the same high standards of anesthesia care should apply everywhere. As anesthesiologists we are members of a worldwide community of physicians that should support one another. We should do what is best for patients on a global scale and support well-designed overseas teaching efforts. Without help, it will remain impossible for the few, overworked anesthesiologists in low- and middle-income countries to train enough residents, create the critical mass, and break the vicious cycle of insufficient personnel that prevents each patient from having access to an anesthesiologist when needed.

References

1. http://www.who.int/gho/health_workforce/physicians_density/en/.
2. Durieux ME. But what if there are no teachers …? Anesthesiology. 2014;120:15–7.
3. Zimmerman M, Lee M, Retnaraj S. Non-doctor anaesthesia in Nepal: developing an essential cadre. Trop Doct. 2008;38(3):148–50. PubMed PMID: 18628537.
4. McAuliffe MS, Henry B. Nurse anesthesia practice and research—a worldwide need. CRNA. 2000; 11(3):89–98. PubMed PMID: 11865942.
5. Rosseel P, Trelles M, Guilavogui S, Ford N, Chu K. Ten years of experience training non-physician anesthesia providers in Haiti. World J Surg. 2010;34(3):453–8. PubMed PMID: 19655194.
6. Cherian M, Choo S, Wilson I, Noel L, Sheikh M, Dayrit M, et al. Building and retaining the neglected anaesthesia health workforce: is it crucial for health systems strengthening through primary health care? Bull World Health Organ. 2010;88(8):637–9. PubMed PMID: 20680130, Pubmed Central PMCID: 2908973.
7. Opoku ST, Apenteng BA. Career satisfaction and burnout among Ghanaian physicians. Int Health. 2014;6(1):54–61. PubMed PMID: 24473596.
8. Okeke EN. Brain drain: do economic conditions "push" doctors out of developing countries? Soc Sci Med. 2013;98:169–78. PubMed PMID: 24331896.
9. Brassington I. What's wrong with the brain drain (?). Dev World Bioeth. 2012;12(3):113–20. PubMed PMID: 21790962.
10. Aluttis C, Bishaw T, Frank MW. The workforce for health in a globalized context—global shortages and international migration. Glob Health Action. 2014;7:23611. PubMed PMID: 24560265, Pubmed Central PMCID: 3926986.
11. Enright A. Review article: safety aspects of anesthesia in under-resourced locations. Can J Anaesth. 2013; 60(2):152–8.
12. Dohlman LE. Anesthesia education across borders. Curr Opin Anaesthesiol. 2013;26(6):732–6. PubMed PMID: 24113269.
13. American College of Surgeons. Operation giving back. Resources for the surgical team. http://www.operationgivingback.facs.org. Accessed 12 Mar 2014.
14. American Society of Anesthesiologists. Global humanitarian outreach. https://www.asahq.org. Accessed 10 Mar 2014.
15. Society for Pediatric Anesthesia. Volunteer medical services abroad. http://www.pedsanesthesia.org. Accessed 10 Mar 2014.

16. Society for Education in Anesthesia Global Outreach Committee. http://seahq.net. Accessed 12 Mar 2014.
17. Lo B, Honemann W, Durieux ME. Preemptive analgesia: ketamine and magnesiums reduce postoperative morphine requirements after abdominal hysterectomy. Anesth Analg. 1998;89:A1163.
18. De Oliveira Jr GS, Agarwal D, Benzon HT. Perioperative single dose ketorolac to prevent postoperative pain: a meta-analysis of randomized trials. Anesth Analg. 2012;114(2):424–33.
19. Zeng J, Thomson LM, Aicher SA, Terman GW. Primary afferent NMDA receptors increase dorsal horn excitation and mediate opiate tolerance in neonatal rats. J Neurosci. 2006;26(46):12033–42. PubMed PMID: 17108177.
20. Ling GS, Paul D, Simantov R, Pasternak GW. Differential development of acute tolerance to analgesia, respiratory depression, gastrointestinal transit and hormone release in a morphine infusion model. Life Sci. 1989;45(18):1627–36. PubMed PMID: 2555641.
21. Panosian C. Courting danger while doing good—protecting global health workers from harm. N Engl J Med. 2010;363(26):2484–5. PubMed PMID: 21175310.
22. CDC health information for international travel, travelers' health, injuries and safety. wwwnc.cdc.gov. Accessed 9 May 2014.
23. American Board of Anesthesia (ABA). Training away from the accredited program checklist. www.theba.org. Accessed 9 May 2014.
24. WHO. Global health workforce statistics. http://who.int/hrh/statistics/hwfstats/en/index.html. Accessed 1 Mar 2014.
25. Center for Disease Control. http://www.cdc.gov/. 12 Mar 2014.
26. Walker IA, Newton M, Bosenberg AT. Improving surgical safety globally: pulse oximetry and the WHO guidelines for safe surgery. Paediatr Anaesth. 2011;21(7):825–8. PubMed PMID: 21208335.
27. Mullan F, Frehywot S, Omaswa F, Buch E, Chen C, Greysen SR, et al. Medical schools in sub-Saharan Africa. Lancet. 2011;377(9771):1113–21. PubMed PMID: 21074256.
28. Lavy C, Sauven K, Mkandawire N, Charian M, Gosselin R, Ndihokubwayo JB, et al. State of surgery in tropical Africa: a review. World J Surg. 2011;35(2):262–71. PubMed PMID: 21153818.
29. Open anesthesia. http://www.openanesthesia.org/. Accessed 22 Mar 2014.
30. Larsson J, Holmstrom I. Understanding anesthesia training and trainees. Curr Opin Anaesthesiol. 2012;25(6):681–5. PubMed PMID: 23026803.
31. Pieczynski LM, Laudanski K, Speck RM, McCunn M. Analysis of field reports from anaesthesia volunteers in low- to middle-income countries. Med Educ. 2013;47(10):1029–36. PubMed PMID: 24016173.
32. Philpott J. Training for a global state of mind. Virtual Mentor. 2010;12(3):231–6. PubMed PMID: 23140874.

Letters from Around the World 28

Ram Roth

Introduction

As Paul Pomerantz, the CEO of the American Society of Anesthesiologists, noted in his report in the June 2014 issue of the Newsletter of the ASA, Marshall McLuhan, the Canadian philosopher of communication, described earth as a "global village" over 50 years ago. McLuhan also predicted the World Wide Web some 30 years before it came into reality. Since then as technology has increased and heightened our awareness of the advantages and plights of other countries, it seems almost as though the world has shrunk. We are moving in the direction of a universal model of team-based care that may not be realized by identical means throughout all nations but quality, ethical standards, and availability of basic resources are the goals. A growing number of volunteers in anesthesiology, from medical students to qualified professionals, are seeking ways in which these ideal models can be met. As the concept of the Perioperative Surgical Home (PSH) grows, with the emphasis on team-based care, anesthesiologists are well positioned as leaders of that team. Thus it is hardly surprising that anesthesiologists at every level of training are anxious to be at the forefront of these exciting ventures where they not only provide care but also learn valuable lessons.

But it is not always smooth sailing! Shortly after we embarked on this book project, we began to hear many stories from physicians returning from missions as well as from anesthesiologists in visited countries. Some spoke of accomplishments and successes while others described pitfalls and how they might be avoided. We felt it important that their voices also be heard. Thus the following vignettes, or letters, voice some of the lessons they have learned.

R. Roth, M.D. (✉)
Icahn School of Medicine at Mount Sinai,
New York, NY, USA
e-mail: ram.roth@mountsinai.org

R. Roth et al. (eds.), *The Role of Anesthesiology in Global Health: A Comprehensive Guide*,
DOI 10.1007/978-3-319-09423-6_28, © Springer International Publishing Switzerland 2015

Letter 1: New York to a Mission

Ram Roth

It is Monday morning, warm even at this early hour. By midday it will be a scorcher. I hope the air conditioner in the OR is working, but you never know. I was given a brief description of this OR by a colleague who had worked there; "they have everything you need… you will be fine." The space is cramped with lots of equipment, some of it older than I am. I look for the capnograph on the monitor and realize it appears to be missing one. The anesthesia machine is a Drager Narkomed®; there is a circuit, a bag, and an isoflurane vaporizer but no ventilator. It is like a dinosaur but without a heart. I rifle through the drawers of the cart and scavenge a few items so I can set up for a case. A woman I have never seen before hands me a liter of normal saline and asks if there is anything else I will need, "and the first patient is waiting to see you," she says. Who among us has not experienced the stress and excitement of working in a new environment?

The OR described above is a back room of a fancy Park Avenue plastic surgery office in Manhattan. The sentiment described above is only a fraction of the intensity of emotions experienced when one is on a mission in a foreign setting. As anesthesiologists we endeavor to control our environment and maintain homeostasis in our patient. Yet by definition, we face the unknown every day.

When I recruit and prepare anesthesia attendings and residents for international missions, I encounter the same cycle of emotions and anxiety. The most honest advice I can offer to new volunteers is this: "No matter how well you prepare for this mission, you will be surprised and challenged in ways you cannot imagine. No matter how hard you feel you have worked on any given day, you will work harder while on a mission… and you will love every minute."

R. Roth
Icahn School of Medicine at Mount Sinai,
New York, NY, USA

But back to the mission: You arrive to your destination and explore your new work environment. The immediate task is to prepare the available tools and equipment for any eventuality that may present itself. In both examples of new environments, the ORs on Park Avenue and in the lower and middle income countries (LMIC), the anesthesiologist feels isolated. Alone he/she has to set up for a safe and successful anesthetic with the resources at hand. In a sense, all small surgical groups travelling abroad undergo a learning process, improving efficiency with the acquisition of experience.

While leading the anesthesia team during a university medical school surgical trip organized by second and fourth year medical students, I was required to assign each of the three available operating rooms to our anesthesiologists. Each room had its advantages and disadvantages. One was small and cramped, without windows for the scavenging tube. Another was large and spacious but had three individual monitors for electrocardiography, pulse oximetry, and blood pressure. In an effort to be fair, we planned to rotate anesthesiologists through the rooms. Toward the end of the week, we realized that fairness was not as important as "owning the room." Each rotation meant that the anesthesiologist had to ascertain the nuances of a new space. On subsequent missions to the same location we planned for each anesthesiologist to stay in his/her own room for the duration of the trip. Once the room was set up with equipment as desired, anesthesiologists were able to stock the drawers and shelves, as they preferred, creating a familiar work environment.

We decided that on each surgical trip we would create a guide or "playbook" in order to record vital practical information about the experience. It included lists of equipment and drugs carried from the USA, identifying surplus and what was lacking. It contained information about personnel at the site, contact information, and assistance provided. We described rooms, equipment and workflow, so that good processes could be repeated and others improved. This guide provided a vertical transition of information from year to year. Each group learned from the experience of their predecessors.

An early group realized that local staff members, after having worked with our team for a few days, brought in patients who were friends or relatives for procedures. They were not screened on our first day and we did not recognize them. We were told that we *had* screened them and must have lost the records. It was a compliment to our work that the staff was bringing us patients, but suddenly accommodating an additional patient was disruptive to our workflow and planning. The next year our team secured an ID band on each patient assigned to have surgery as the final step in the screening process. Patients were told not to remove the wristband until after they were discharged from our care.

Another group complained that in order to contact our team on the wards, they had to ask the head nurse in the OR suite to notify the ward nurse who may or may not have time to find someone. On subsequent trips we brought walkie-talkie sets which improved our communication efficiency.

Our approach to surgical trips was developing and maturing over time, but the evolution was slow. It would take a year to implement a new idea and see the result. Our "playbook" information was 11 months old. Even if were returning to the same site, many changes may have occurred. Changes such as new building, a new OR, recently donated equipment from another group or a construction project which might disrupt our power supply could occur during our absence. Communication with our hosts by phone or email was poor. At best we managed to set a date of arrival, but not much information was shared about the changing conditions.

We knew that other groups visited the same site throughout the year. There was a schedule on the wall of the OR office. We recognized some names of organizations listed. Had there been a forum to share information about a particular location among the volunteer caregivers, our information could be "horizontal." We could potentially learn from others who used the facility and provided care the week before our arrival. We could be updated with the latest information. If they wrote a "playbook" of their mission and shared it, we could be much more effective. We could implement strategies they had contemplated and report back to them and the group following us for the benefit of all.

To date, there exists no such forum. Journal articles appear with increasing frequency. Greater organization of effort and research of surgical missions is becoming a focus of many medical institutions [1]. Guidelines for success have been proposed [2]. Global health institutes are popping up and are endeavoring to standardize the approach to travel medicine or "medical tourism."

References

1. Fisher QA, Fisher G. The case for collaboration among humanitarian surgical programs in low resource countries. Anesth Analg. 2014;118(2):448–53. PMID: 24445642.
2. Grimes CE, Maraka J, Kingsnorth AN, Darko R, Samkange CA, Lane RH. Guidelines for surgeons on establishing projects in low-income countries. World J Surg. 2013;37(6):1203–7. PMID: 23474858.

Letter 2: Challenges in Delivering Care to a Pediatric Patient with a Difficult Airway in a Resource-Poor Setting

Grace Hsu

Located in the horn of Africa, Ethiopia is home to 92 million people. It is one of the world's poorest countries, with a per capita GDP of $410. The Black Lion hospital in the capital, Addis Ababa, is one of Ethiopia's major referral hospitals. Of the 1,421 physicians in the country, 106 are surgeons and 14 are anesthesiologists [1]. Nurse anesthetists administer anesthesia for the rest of the country. Access to surgical care is poor—thus limiting most surgery to emergent or late presentations.

It was my third day in Ethiopia. I was at the Black Lion Hospital in Addis Ababa to teach students in the Master's of Science in Nurse Anesthesia program. I arrived at the hospital and crowded around the operating schedule board at 7:00 am with a large group of other hospital staff to see the assignments for the day. I was to cover two rooms, a pediatric and a urology room. The first pediatric case was removal of a cervical lymphangioma in a 7-month-old boy.

With one of the students I went to the preoperative holding area to see the pediatric patient. A very large mass distorted the boy's right jaw, face, and neck. His face, lips, and neck were swollen to a point beyond recognition. The parents gave us the history: The baby was born with a right neck mass but was otherwise healthy. At around 2 months of age, the mass began increasing in size. By 5 months, he had extreme difficulty eating and was failing to thrive. He drooled constantly, and was unable to swallow saliva effectively. One week prior, he came to the hospital for the first time in his life, with pneumonia. He was in respiratory distress and required oxygen 2 l/min to maintain adequate saturation. The pediatric surgeon recommended surgery immediately as development of complete airway obstruction was imminent.

On exam, the infant was thin and listless. The mass and swelling had stented his mouth open to its maximum, but with little patent area in his oropharynx. He was tachypneic and had decreased breath sounds in the right upper lung fields. A CT scan film indicated that the mass compressed his upper trachea and appeared to extend beyond the thoracic inlet and into the anterior mediastinum. Portions of his right lung were whited-out from pneumonia.

I expressed concern about a difficult airway to the pediatric surgeon, given the severe degree of swelling. We expected difficulty ventilating, especially with positive pressure, given the small opening in the oropharynx and the potential for the mass encroaching into the anterior mediastinum. Even if we were successful in passing an endotracheal tube through the patient's vocal cords, we might not be able to pass beyond the tracheal narrowing. The surgeon felt she would not be able to provide an emergency surgical airway, given the neck distortion and high likelihood of numerous collateral vessels in the region. The only airway adjuncts in the hospital were supraglottic airways, an adult-sized gum elastic bougie and an adult bronchoscope.

I asked a Norwegian anesthesiologist who was there teaching residents for 6 weeks, and another recent graduate of the Ethiopian residency program at the Black Lion Hospital to be present for induction. I outlined a plan for a group of students: start with an inhalation induction to preserve spontaneous ventilation and allow the anesthesia student two attempts to secure the airway. If she was unsuccessful, an anesthesiologist would then take over. Our only size-appropriate airway adjunct was a supraglottic airway. We planned to use a small 3.0 cm cuffed endotracheal tube in anticipation of tracheal narrowing.

Induction and intubation proved difficult. The nurse anesthesia student induced anesthesia with halothane via mask. With loss of muscle tone in the oropharynx, the patient began to obstruct and oxygen saturation dropped rapidly.

G. Hsu
Department of Anesthesiology and Critical Care Medicine, The Children's Hospital of Philadelphia, Philadelphia, PA, USA

Despite earlier discussion of the plan, under stress, the student began to apply positive pressure. Although ventilation was not adequate, it was sufficient to keep the patient unconscious with inhalational anesthesia but also weak enough to obstruct. The nurse (anesthesia student) attempted to intubate the patient twice—but was unable to see the larynx. Next, the Ethiopian anesthesiologist attempted direct laryngoscopy. With a shoulder roll and laryngeal pressure, she obtained a grade III view and placed a 3.0 endotracheal tube successfully through the narrowed portion of the trachea. Although there was no air leak around the deflated cuff, we decided to continue the case with this tube. We gave a single dose of dexamethasone to minimize swelling (Figs. 28.1 and 28.2).

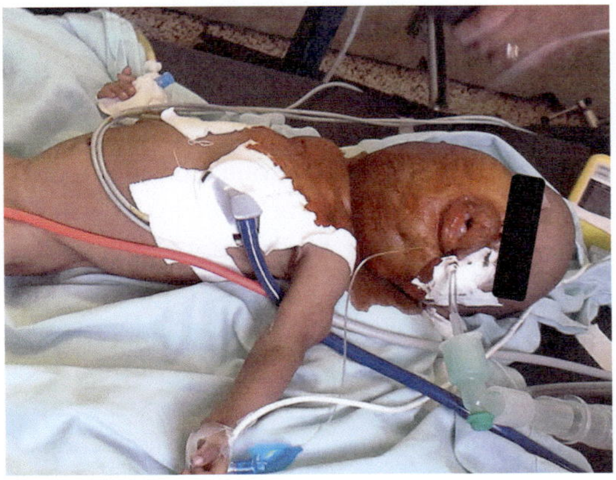

Fig. 28.1 The cervical lymphangioma made both mask ventilation and laryngoscopy difficult in a setting with limited airway adjuncts (supine view)

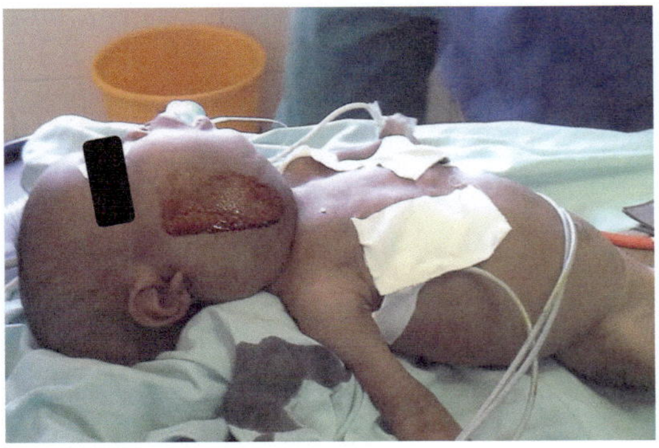

Fig. 28.2 Lymphangioma lateral view

The surgical portion of the case went smoothly, other than significant blood loss from the venous collaterals draining the head and neck. A full blood volume was replaced. While considering postoperative care, I learned that the hospital did not have a pediatric-sized ventilator. The 6-bed intensive care unit had two adult ventilators that would likely cause volutrauma if used for a child. Limited medical and nursing staff overnight meant that no one would be available to manually support the baby's ventilation. Thus, the patient would need to breathe spontaneously through the small endotracheal tube without any support until extubated. I again enlisted the help of the Norwegian and Ethiopian anesthesiologists. The Ethiopian anesthesiologist explained that it was extremely rare for a pediatric patient to be intubated and ventilated in the hospital. We also discussed the possibility that the patient would weaken throughout the night, breathing through a long, narrow tube. Acute airway obstruction the night after surgery was also a significant risk [2]. We decided to extubate the child—again, preparing for a difficult reintubation. The 30 min that followed proved that the patient could not tolerate extubation—the swelling from surgical manipulation was too great. The patient did not appear to have recurrent laryngeal nerve deficits as he was phonating; however, he quickly obstructed. We reintubated him—again, a difficult task.

Transfer to the intensive care unit itself was a feat. There were no fully functioning bag-valve masks with tubing to attach to an oxygen source. We improvised with intravenous fluid tubing to connect the bag-valve mask to an oxygen tank. After traveling 20 ft down the hallway in a metal crib with a large oxygen tank lying at the foot, one wheel of the crib broke off and nearly caused the crib and patient to topple. The elevator ride from the fourth floor operating rooms to the sixth floor intensive care unit was also precarious. (The rubber mat on the floor of the elevator car was ineffectively covering a hole one-foot in diameter).

The baby did well and was extubated by the ICU team on post-op day 1 and discharged home on post-op day 6.

The key learning points of this case were the following:

- The history and physical exam are key for the anesthesiologist in formulating a plan and in determining the most likely things that will harm a patient perioperatively. In this case the three major considerations were a difficult airway, intraoperative hemorrhage and postoperative ventilation.
- In resource-poor settings, where airway adjuncts are extremely limited, human resources may be just as important in a difficult situation. In this circumstance, the only airway adjunct appropriate for this 7 kg patient was a supraglottic mask airway. It is important to involve other airway experts and team members in the case early and discuss a plan.
- Especially when there are language and cultural barriers, it is important to have a clear plan that all team members understand. In this case, it would have been prudent to not attempt mask ventilation after obstruction during induction. One should allow the patient to emerge from general anesthesia.
- Given that this patient required this surgery for survival, there seemed to be little choice in performing the operation. Some might argue that such high-risk cases should not be undertaken because a bad outcome may jeopardize future missions. However, this decision falls more to the surgeon than to the anesthetic team. Consideration of postoperative resources and availability of adequate support is crucial to the decision.

References

1. Chao TE, Burdic M, Ganjawalla K, Derbew M, Keshian C, Meara J, McQueen K. Survey of surgery and anesthesia infrastructure in ethiopia. World J Surg. 2012;36:2545–53.
2. Ameh EA, Nmadu PT. Cervical cystic hygroma: pre-, intra-, and post-operative morbidity and mortality in Zaria, Nigeria. Pediatr Surg Int. 2001;17:342–3.

Letter 3: Great Planning: But Not Everything Works

Ram Roth

For many years, anesthesiologists have embarked with surgical teams from Mount Sinai Medical Center in New York on short-term missions to underserved countries. Not only have we been able to help hundreds of people in these countries but we have also garnered considerable satisfaction and experience for ourselves. The stories of successful missions abound. On one recent mission, however, the outcome did not go according to plan and the results were disastrous.

Background

Perioperative care for patients at a mission site is in many ways similar to that provided in the USA with some adjustments or local availability of resources. A preoperative evaluation of all potential patients allows the surgical team to be able to prioritize candidates for surgery. Local physicians make the initial evaluation and selection. The teams of surgeons and anesthesiologists then have the opportunity to evaluate the need for surgery, cardiac risk indices, comorbidities, medications, and airway management considerations.

Standard preoperative evaluation is based on the guidelines of the mission site, the external organization involved, and/or hospital of mission origin. The mission site we visited had more stringent rules than apply at our institution in New York regarding preoperative evaluation, and requires cardiac clearance on all patients over the age of 40. This is possibly due to a shorter life expectancy and generally less prophylactic care received

R. Roth
Department of Anesthesiology,
Icahn School of Medicine at Mount Sinai,
New York, NY, USA

by potential surgical candidates. Alternatively, it may be included to ensure that all visiting surgical groups are satisfied with their screening process. Patients are usually "cleared for surgery" by local cardiologists before they come to the center. All patients are admitted the night before surgery in order to minimize transportation problems and ensure preoperative fasting. Anesthesia screening also includes assessment of the availability of appropriate support following surgery and determination that the patient will recover within the time frame of the mission with sufficient support mechanisms in place.

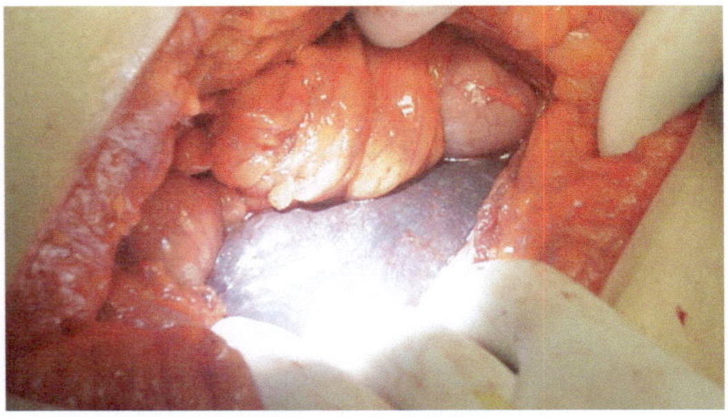

Fig. 28.3 Congested liver

Case

A 60-year-old woman presented with a longstanding history of severe gastroesophageal reflux disease and upper abdominal pain. An open cholecystectomy was scheduled after the finding of multiple gallstones. She had a history of diabetes and hypertension. She repeatedly denied any cardiac symptoms, despite questioning by several health care workers at different levels. Medication included metformin, propranolol, enalapril, and glyburide, all of which she took regularly. She reported that her diabetes was well controlled. She had undergone two cesarean sections in the distant past under spinal anesthesia. She did not smoke or drink. There was no history of allergies.

On physical examination she was found to weigh 100 kg with a height of 161 cm (BMI 39). While not taking her medication her blood pressure was 144/91 and heart rate 78 and regular. No murmurs were identified and her lungs were clear to auscultation. A cardiologist had seen her in the recent past and she reported that all was well. The plan was to schedule her operation later in the week.

On the penultimate surgical day of our mission, 3 days before our departure, the patient was transported to the operating room at 16:40 after having fasted for 23 h. Standard monitors were applied and an intravenous infusion started. Induction and intubation proceeded uneventfully. Medications included fentanyl 100 ugm, propofol 200 mg, morphine 8 mg, rocuronium 20 mg. Anesthesia was maintained with sevoflurane in oxygen. Vital signs remained stable for about 30 min into the operation (BP 110/70, heart rate 80). Thereafter, oxygen saturation fell to the 80 s and the blood pressure was unobtainable. Phenylephrine, epinephrine and atropine were administered. As the surgeon exposed the gallbladder, he noted that the liver appeared congested (Fig. 28.3). After 10 min the vital signs stabilized. Ventilation continued with oxygen 100 % while the gallbladder was exposed and resected. Subsequently, blood pressure was unobtainable and she was resuscitated with crystalloid and vasoactive agents. The pulse returned and the surgery proceeded with only 5 min remaining in the case. The patient continued to require repeated boluses of phenylephrine and vasopressin for episodes of hypotension. Attempts to gain additional intravenous access were not successful. She was given a total of 1 liter of crystalloid and was breathing spontaneously via the endotracheal tube as the bandages were applied. However, she remained unstable; blood pressure continued to decrease despite vasopressor therapy and additional crystalloid via a groin central line. Pulseless electrical activity developed and full ACLS protocol was instituted in the cramped operating room. She regained her pulse on several occasions but the rhythm could not be sustained. After more than 1 h of cardio pulmonary resuscitation she was pronounced dead.

Discussion

An event such as this is devastating, not just to the family but also to the entire team of health care providers, both visitors and local. We held debriefing sessions with the local doctors that night and with the operating room staff the next day.

After returning to our guesthouse, the entire mission team participated in an emotional debriefing. Members of the team described how the experience affected them. Medical students and attendings openly cried, the former for having experienced their first death in the operating room and the latter for having experienced one so unexpected.

The next day was originally planned to be the last day of surgery. The team felt that doing the few small cases scheduled would be inappropriate and those cases were cancelled to be performed on a subsequent mission. We began the day with a debriefing for the nursing and operating room staff. Educationally, they were most curious about our teamwork during cardiopulmonary resuscitation. They had never seen a "code" except on TV shows. We explained how we all undergo ACLS training and practice responding and appreciated that this was an area of focus for future missions. This certainly left us with the idea that our next mission would include an program on cardiopulmonary resuscitation for the staff.

We also explained that in our practice we investigate every detail of any death or major complication. We arranged for a full review of all past records and spoke with the family. Some relevant pages from her prior cardiac studies had been removed and were determined to be "lost." Eventually, the local director of anesthesiology learned that the patient had been diagnosed with severe heart disease, which had been revealed to previous visiting teams and to local surgeons. Surgery had been ruled out in the past. Since her colic symptoms were intensifying, she determined, in consultation with her family, not to admit to any heart problems to our team. She was rehearsed in screening questions and her previous answers that would not allow her surgery to proceed.

We were anxious to determine the pathology and suggested an autopsy in the public city hospital. The family refused for religious reasons. The hospital administrator then beneficently made arrangements to cover funeral expenses. Even though we could not determine the cause of this tragic outcome we worked to obtain all additional information. The remainder of the day was spent in obtaining as much information as we could and taking care of the patients in the ward and bonding with our friends and colleagues in the hospital.

Upon returning to our institution, we conducted a formal mortality review chaired by the Dean of Global Health. All members of the mission team were interviewed and the patient's records as well as perioperative surgical and anesthetic charts were reviewed. We reexamined our protocols and concluded that little could be done to uncover information that was deliberately withheld. Students and residents were given another opportunity to discuss the emotional impact of the tragic event. A review panel added a cardiac risk assessment and a mini-stress test to the preoperative evaluations for all missions. The Global Health office reviewed the institute's malpractice coverage to ensure that missions were protected for claims brought at home and in countries we visit.

Our next mission to the site is anticipated and we were assured that we would be welcomed to continue our work there.

Conclusion

Despite the best intentions and due to circumstances beyond our control, poor outcomes may still occur. That is the nature of medicine and surgery in the developing world. Cooperation with the host countries should be in place for success. There must exist some degree of trust in the local physicians and belief that patients will give accurate information, as most do. Patients must be evaluated carefully by skilled clinician and rejected if necessary when their physical findings or history is not compatible with obvious objective clues (e.g., morbid obesity). An understanding of attitudes and what may be considered reasonable and acceptable behavior in other countries is very hard for many, especially young health care workers from our modern institutions. Counselling should be made available to the team, recognizing the tragedy of the case at several levels and also acknowledging that global surgical missions are a beneficial endeavor.

Letter 4: Life-Saving "The Magic" Wire

Miodrag Milenovic

Difficult airway workshops are often highly attended and the most popular events at international congresses and regional meetings. Serbian anesthesiologists, just like others, are very keen to attend them and later on their return home to give a "hard time" to the hospital management asking them to buy all those hi-tech, often very expensive devices for difficult airway management. Should devices be obtained, not all of us are practiced to use them, because there is no official obligation to do so and it is time consuming.

There are a number of clinical situations when the anesthesiologist and intensivist cannot completely visualize entrance into the trachea. Very often this was the moment when we realized that not so many of us are skillful enough to properly use the bronchoscope or other techniques available to us.

One of the international scholars and an AAF alumnus returned from the Postgraduate Assembly in New York with a few pieces of long gum elastic bougies, or Eschmann Stylets. These are tracheal tube introducers, a flexible device that is 60 cm (24 in.) in length, and 15 French (5 mm diameter) with a small "hockey-stick" angle at the far end. It can be a useful adjunct for the persistent epiglottis-only-view situations. Although this product has been on the market for almost 30 years now, probably because of the small population in Serbia and the low cost, we have not been offered it by medical industry representatives in our country. It was not on the market in the region.

From that time 10 years ago, when the department was given several pieces, as a gift from the colleague who came back from abroad, long gum elastic bougies have became the necessary equipment for difficult airway management and for re-intubation of an already difficult intubated patient. My colleages (anesthesiologists and nurses) call it "the blue wire" or even "the magic stick," because it has saved a number of lives over the last decade, especially before we became more efficient in bronchoscope use.

A case in point: A 66-year-old man had been hiding out in a tree for several hours, hoping to shoot a deer. He had drunk some beer and, feeling rather feverish, had ingested some cold remedy. He was soon fast asleep and fell to the ground, dislocating his neck at C7. In the hospital he was initially stabilized in a collar but over the next 24 h, his sensory level rose to C5. The decision was made to take him to the operating room for surgical stabilization. He had no history of prior surgery. A plan was made to perform rapid sequence induction as he had not eaten in 30 h with in-line stabilization. Immediately after induction, large amounts of fluid and undigested food were regurgitated. The larynx could not be visualized. Finally, with fiber-optic scope, the airway was secured. Surgery proceeded without incident. He appeared to be awakening, and was trying to remove the endotracheal tube. We placed a bougie through the tube prior to extubation. Some 4 h later, he experienced some respiratory distress and we were able to quickly secure the airway this time over the bougie. He was successfully extubated 30 h later.

Being a part of the moderately developed medical system but still less affluent world, there is no doubt that our hospitals need to renew medical equipment, but the professionals need to be more realistic, pragmatic, and skilful to be able to deal with difficulties, not relying only on the latest generation of hi-tech devices, because we may need some time to achieve much.

From the moment we become aware of such simple but excellent adjuncts as gum elastic bougies, it is part of our official demands and we still do not have suppliers of such simple and cheap airway adjuncts. It is still not on the market. So, a number of such easy-to-carry, inexpensive, and simple-to-use adjuncts should be necessary as disposable equipment for all outreach medical missions, because small things like gum elastic bougies can change anybody's life.

M. Milenovic
Department of Anesthesiology and Intensive Care Medicine, Clinical Center of Serbia, Belgrade, Serbia

Letter 5: Transfusion Conundrum

Erin Gertz

It was the third day of a 5-day short-term surgical trip in the Dominican Republic (D.R.). The final procedure, a vaginal prolapse repair under epidural anesthesia, was uncomplicated and had just finished (Fig. 28.4). Although, a middle-income country, the medical infrastructure in the D.R. is limited and the local community was extremely grateful for our surgical mission work.

As the patient was transferred into the recovery room, the PACU nurse was standing beside another patient taking a manual pulse. That patient, a 45-year-old woman with uterovaginal prolapse and no other significant medical history, had undergone an uncomplicated vaginal hysterectomy under general anesthesia. The estimated blood loss (EBL) was 300 ml and she was given 2.5 l of crystalloid during the case. The nurse was concerned and asked the anesthesia team to evaluate the patient (Fig. 28.5). The blood pressure was 92/50, pulse 114, and O_2 saturation 99 % on room air and the patient was complaining of nausea. She did not look toxic, but was pale and occasionally retched into a small basin. A review of the chart showed the patient had obtained preoperative testing and her hematocrit 2 days ago was 38 %. After discussing the case, the anesthesia team suspected hypovolemia and vasodilation. Most patients come to surgery quite dehydrated and this patient had also just received a small dose of fentanyl for pain. Therefore a bolus of crystalloid 500 ml was ordered and vital signs were checked every 10 min. The in-country liaison was asked to obtain a complete blood count (CBC). Since there was no laboratory at this facility, the liaison explained that to obtain a "stat" CBC, the nearest private lab would send a tech who would draw blood, return to the lab, run the test and call back with the results. The process would take over an hour.

Thirty minutes later, the patient's blood pressure was 82/47 and pulse was 125 bpm despite the fluid bolus. She continued to complain of nausea

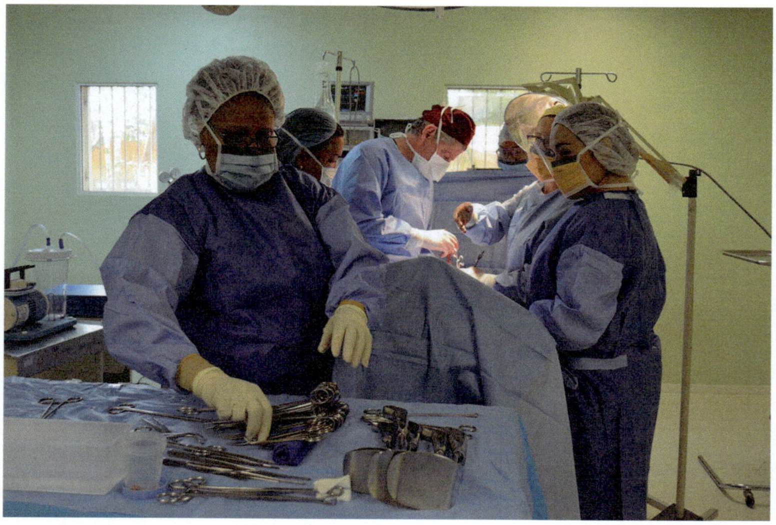

Fig. 28.4 Our operating room in the Dominican Republic

E. Gertz
Global Women's Health Division, Department of Obstetrics, Gynecology and Reproductive Sciences, Icahn School of Medicine at Mount Sinai, New York, NY, USA

and now had increasing abdominal pain and drowsiness. The surgeons were alerted and on examination found abdominal distention, tenderness to palpation, rebound and guarding. There was no vaginal bleeding. The team decided to return to the OR for an exploratory laparotomy for suspected intra-abdominal bleeding. The patient's trachea was reintubated and upon opening the abdomen, approximately 800 ml of blood clot was evacuated. A small bleeding vessel was found and ligated. Total estimated blood loss from both procedures was 2 l. The in-country liaison was asked to order blood for transfusion and to coordinate possible transfer to a hospital with an ICU facility. He said delivery of blood should take no more than one half hour. There was no reliable national ambulance service for a transfer, so a private company would have to be hired to transport the patient to the local hospital. The team discussed who should accompany the patient. An anesthesiologist and one of the surgeons were chosen. A curious medical student on our team asked what the ICU is like in the hospital that would accept the transfer and who exactly would take over the patient's care. No one was able to answer these questions. The team discussed whether transfer would actually be in the patient's best interest. The lab technician then arrived to draw the CBC. Three hours had passed since the blood test was ordered.

Intravenous hydration was continued and the patient's vital signs stabilized. Though she remained obtunded and tachycardic, she was extubated without difficulty. The reason for her altered mental status remained unclear. After waiting for almost 2 h, the team realized that both the arrival of blood and the transfer to another hospital might not happen (Fig. 28.6). One of our surgeons, known to be blood type O negative, offered to donate blood. After a discussion about the consent signed prior to the surgery – we decided that the patient had understood the consent well-enough regarding a transfusion, the team decided to proceed (Fig. 28.7).

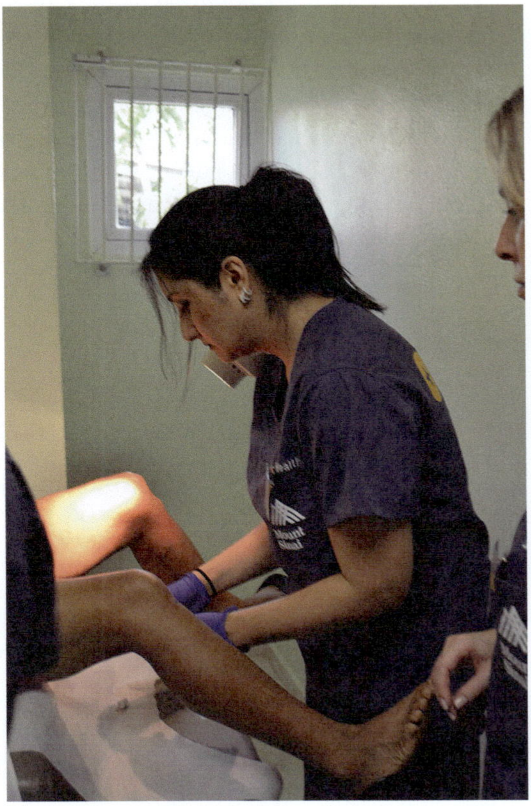

Fig. 28.5 Examination of the patient

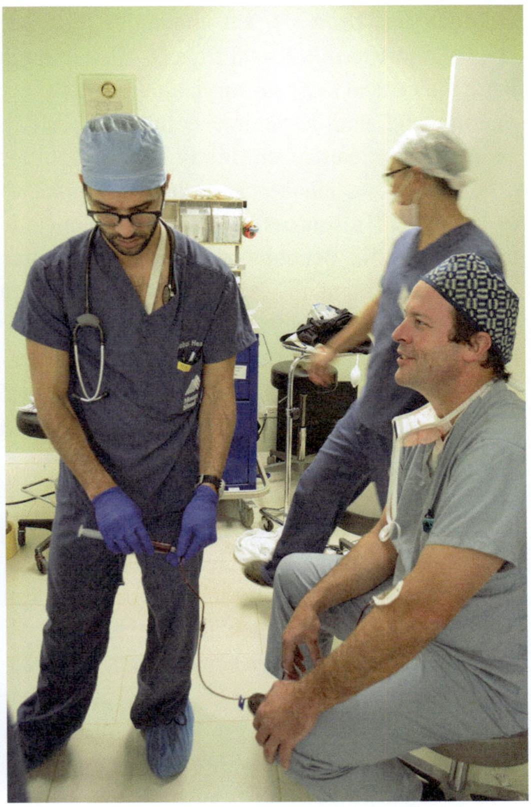

Fig. 28.6 The surgeon is donating his own blood

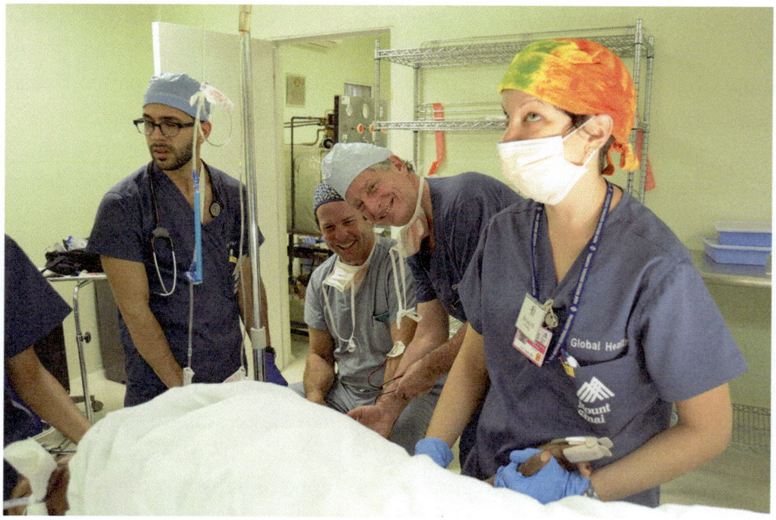

Fig. 28.7 Blood being transfused in the patient

Discussion

This case highlights a number of important issues to consider.

Much has been written about the pros and cons of short-term surgical trips [1–3]. Although there is a critical need for surgical/anesthesia care in low- and middle-income countries (LMIC), short trips by teams from high-income countries may not be sustainable and can undermine or overtax local resources. Capacity building and transfer of skills depends on cultural or resource appropriateness of the procedures, buy-in from local practitioners and availability of resources. Postoperative care, follow-up, and management of delayed complications depend on the length of the trip, the relationship with local partners and availability of both human and material resources. However, besides the obvious benefits for individual patients, short-term trips can fill specific gaps in care while LMICs build surgical infrastructure.

Practitioners struggle for true informed consent with every procedure. When traveling abroad, cultural differences, language barriers, lack of education, and limited biomedical health literacy further complicate this issue [4]. Prior to the procedure, this patient had been consented to both the surgery to be performed and all other necessary procedures, including blood transfusion. However, the team had to consider whether this included or implied consent for direct transfusion from a member of the team, without testing for infectious disease and without cross matching.

Patient outcomes are improved through effective teamwork of the entire operating room staff. Incorporating local liaisons in the team can be challenging due to cultural and language differences. Collaborative decision making between anesthesiologists, surgeons, nursing, and the local partners led to a creative solution and fortunately a good patient outcome.

References

1. Farmer PE, Kim JY. Surgery and global health: a view from beyond the OR. World J Surg. 2008;32:533–6. doi: 10.1007/s00268-008-9525-9. PMID: 18311574.
2. Wright IG, Walker IA, Yacoub MH (2007) Specialist surgery in the developing world: luxury or necessity? Anaesthesia. 62(Suppl 1):84–9.
3. Shrime MG, Sleemi A, Ravilla TD. Charitable platforms in global surgery: a systematic review of their effectiveness, cost-effectiveness, sustainability, and role training. World J Surg. 2014. [Epub ahead of print] PubMed. PMID: 24682278.
4. Krogstad DJ, Diop S, Diallo A, Mzayek F, Keating J, Koita OA, Touré YT. Informed consent in international research: the rationale for different approaches. Am J Trop Med Hyg. 2010;83(4):743–7. doi: 10.4269/ajtmh.2010.10-0014. PubMed PMID: 20889858; PubMed Central PMCID: PMC2946735.

Letter 6: Notes so as Not to Make the Same Mistake Twice

Clifford Gevirtz

Case 1: A 15-year-old Vietnamese male with a cleft lip presented for repair under general anesthesia. The anesthesia equipment consisted of an older anesthesia machine with Russian writing and a copper kettle, a portable monitor with EKG, pulse oximeter and noninvasive automatic blood pressure. There was no oxygen analyzer in the circuit. There was no capnometry or agent analyzer available. A twitch monitor was also utilized. The oxygen source was an H-cylinder with a two-stage pressure reducing valve in place. The labeling on the tank and valves was in Russian. The needle indicated approximately 70 kPa pressure. The anesthetic plan was induction with thiopentone, use succinylcholine for paralysis and then place a RAE endotracheal tube. A Mapleson D circuit was to be utilized with a table mounted Halothane vaporizer that had been brought in from the United States. An American anesthesiologist was paired with a local "senior," who had checked the anesthesia machine that morning.

After induction with thiopentone, a mask was placed on the patient to prove the ability to ventilate and the flush lever was turned to fill the bag on the circuit. However, no oxygen flowed to the circuit. The backup Oxygen tank on the machine was then turned on, but the needle dropped to zero within 20 s. Mouth-to-mouth ventilation was then performed as there was no Ambu bag present. After five breaths, the patient was intubated and mouth to tube ventilation continued until another tank was brought into the room. Anesthesia was maintained with thiopentone until the new H cylinder arrived. The case proceeded uneventfully thereafter.

C. Gevirtz
LSU Health Sciences Center, New Orleans, LA, USA

Lessons learned:

1. When using anesthesia equipment where the labelling is in another language, try out the machine with a backup in place along with another experienced anesthesia provider. The reducing valves may not function or be inaccurate. Here some oil was apparently applied and the needle was stuck on 70 kPa. Apparently, it had been functioning this way for a considerable length of time with the need for a sudden change out not unusual event.
2. Clarify the training level of the person you are working with; a senior medical student is not a senior anesthesia resident. The hosts had given me a "senior" to work with; I didn't realize that he was a senior medical student.
3. Mouth-to-mouth respiration would not be acceptable practice today but at the time it seemed the only way to support the patient, clear mouth shields are now available which provide a safer alternative, mouth to mask could also be utilized. Once intubated mouth to endotracheal tube could be utilized in an emergency.
4. Awakening the patient could also have been considered, if no further tanks were available.

Case 2: In this particular institution, there were two OR tables per room with a small moveable screen between the tables. The plan was for one surgeon to start a case with two anesthesia providers present and after the case was stable, a second case would be started on the other side of the screen. This had the advantage of there being two surgeons and two anesthesiologists within shouting distance should any complication arise.

During a cleft palate repair, a surgeon had gastrointestinal distress and had to leave the OR. This resulted in two patients being asleep at the same time. A senior surgeon took over after completing one case and then finished the other. The rest of schedule in that room was performed alternating between tables.

Lessons learned:

1. One physician in the group should be designated as the team physician for the entire group. Complete medical histories of all team members should be available and reviewed by

the team physician before embarking. When someone takes ill, that person needs to be relieved without delay. Heroics such as trying to operate or perform anesthesia while ill can cause serious harm both to patients as well as to the physician.

2. When traveling into malaria infested areas, it is important to ascertain which species is most prevalent and which antimalarial is most effective. Yellow fever, hepatitis A and B, tetanus, diphtheria, and pertussis vaccines should also be considered before joining a mission (note it may a week before sufficient levels of antibodies are produced). A complete physical exam by the participant's primary care physician at home should also be considered prior to volunteering for a mission, to evaluate suitability for working in the lesser developed country (LCD) environment. Team members with serious preexisting conditions such as coronary artery disease should seriously reconsider their participation. In general, if a physician would be graded an ASA 3 then it is probably not a wise idea to embark on a mission. In the one team member death I observed (an obese woman (approximate BMI 40) with hypertension and prediabetes), the issue in retrospect was whether she should have been allowed to come on a mission in the first place.

A separate supply of medications should be held in reserve to treat medical emergencies amongst the team members. Backup supplies including a wide range of antidiarrheals, antibiotics, and non-narcotic analgesics are suggested. Emergency IV fluids, angiocaths should be reserved and then can be left behind when leaving the country.

Case 3: Bleeding diathesis: A 3-year-old 11 kg child underwent a cleft palate repair with mobilization of two flaps. Both during the procedure and in the post-operative period diffuse oozing was noted with significantly more blood loss than expected even with infiltration with epinephrine containing local anesthetic. The patient had an initial hematocrit of 32 %. A spun hematocrit in the recovery room was 23 %. The patient was markedly tachycardic with a narrowing pulse pressure. Additional intravenous access was obtained, crystalloids and a single unit of albumin was administered (only one 200 cc vial was available) and a Foley catheter was placed. There was no blood bank in the facility. The patient was brought back to the OR for re-exploration but there continued to be diffuse bleeding. Another spun hematocrit was performed and it was 15 %. A direct father to child whole blood transfusion was started after performing a field compatibility test. However, the oozing continued and the child arrested approximately 12 h after the end of surgery.

Lessons learned:

1. In this case, the parents were grateful for the efforts of the team. However, that may not always be the case. It is important to clarify what happens if there is a serious complication or a death. In some countries, e.g., in the People's Republic of China, medical malpractice claims are treated more like a labor union dispute than as a tort claim. In other countries, e.g., Libya, health care personnel can be arrested if there are complications. Registering with your embassy to make sure they are aware of your location is very helpful in case of altercations with local authorities.

Bring tubing along with stop cocks and large syringes to perform a person to person transfusion.

The etiology of this bleeding diathesis was never fully explained. There was no family history or history of easy bruising in the child. The surgical field was reviewed by three separate surgeons on the mission and no surgical source was detected.

Case 4: During induction of a cleft lip, there was a power failure with total loss of light; there were no emergency backup lights as one would find in the USA. Using a flashlight and the surgeons head-light the induction was completed. The hosts assured us that power would be back on within 20 min, which it was. The case proceeded safely and uneventfully thereafter.

Lesson learned:

Always have a backup laryngoscope with a working bulb as well as flashlight. An iPhone with a flashlight application can also be very helpful.

The electricity supply is unreliable in many LDC countries and backup plans should be in place. In many LDCs there are windows directly into the OR which may prevent total darkness, but the natural light provided may be insufficient to continue with the planned surgery.

Make sure that all the team members know where the backup flashlights are stored.

Case 5: During a cleft palate and mandibular advancement case, the surgeon kept turning the patient's head from side to side rather abruptly. This child had a nasal intubation and the airway resistance decreased abruptly as did the breath sounds. There was no capnograph on this case. The patient was spontaneously breathing but they were shallow breaths. The surgeon was informed that the patient appeared to be extubated but the surgeon said he only needed a few more minutes to finish the case and the oxygen saturation was holding at 95 %. A rather heated discussion ensued and while I turned up the oxygen flow, my local assistant kept turning it back down. The case was finished within 8 min.

The mouth was suctioned and the patient awakened without serious sequelae.

Lessons learned:
Clear communication amongst the team is essential. The surgeon who was from the local community did not understand what I meant by extubation and thought I was just asking him to hurry up. Similarly, my local assistant thought I was wasting oxygen as the oxygen saturation was stable. When working with a mostly local team, it is important to have an interpreter present at all times (Figs. 28.8 and 28.9).

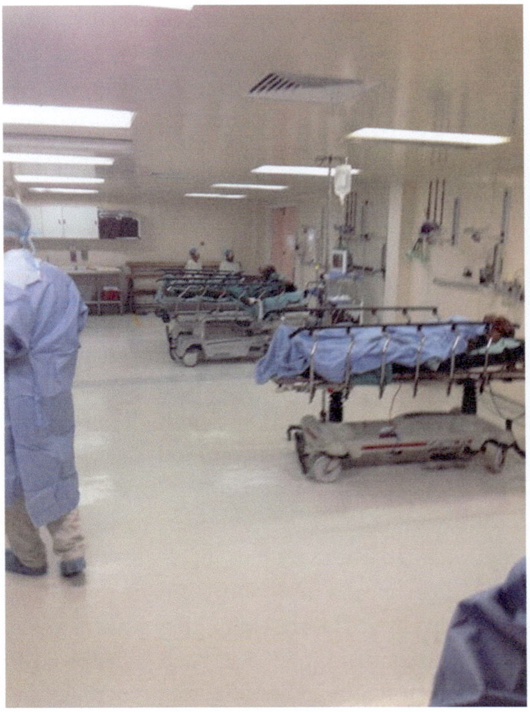

Fig. 28.8 Holding area in Guyana, note 1980s equipment with few monitors

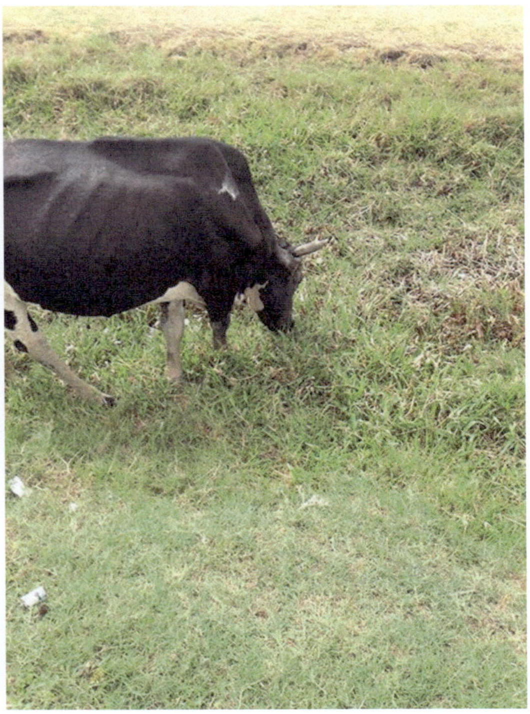

Fig. 28.9 A local source of milk for morning coffee

Letter 7: The Leonardo Martinez Valenzuela Hospital and the Medical Brigades

Maria Portillo

The Leonardo Martinez Valenzuela Hospital (San Pedro Sula) is one of the busiest hospitals in Honduras and has also important social projects. The institution hosts national and international medical brigades (missions) year-round that help decrease the surgical waiting list at the rest of the hospitals in the western part of the country.

The hospital has a maternity ward equipped with three operating rooms and a separate general surgery building equipped with four operating rooms. Basic monitoring, such as ECG, O_2 Sat, and NIBP, is available in all of the operation rooms. Arterial blood pressure monitoring and capnography are available in only one of the operating rooms. The staff, consisting of 6 anesthesia technicians and 3 anesthesiologists, perform on average 15 orthopedic, general surgery, and gynecologic cases a day. In the maternity ward some 10–15 obstetrical surgeries are done daily. This high workload, combined with a relative lack of resources, while still maintaining high standards of care, greatly increases the difficulties of the anesthesiologist's job.

Every year we welcome approximately 6 visiting brigades that perform up to 50 surgical cases a day. They are divided into ear nose and throat, gynecology (GYN), general surgery and podiatry. The advantage of these brigades is that we learn the techniques that are employed in hospitals around the world, not only from the surgical but also from the anesthetic point of view. Implementing new techniques helps us better manage postoperative pain and reduce hospital stay while improving hospital through put. The medical personal involved in these brigades is devoted to teaching new surgical techniques and appropriate drug use to the local medical personal.

But there are few disadvantages we must acknowledge. The foremost is the difficulties in communication, given that not all the people involved speak English and Spanish. This deficiency sometimes leads to delays in the cases or miscommunication, and requires that additional personal become involved in the brigades to help with communication. Ideally, local medical students would help with translation, since they are familiar with the medical terminology but this is not always possible.

Although the help provided by these medical brigades is invaluable, there have been complications, possibly due to the lack of time and/or resources. These complications include: wound dehiscence, bleeding, and infection. Sometimes these problems have required additional surgical interventions performed overnight when the brigade's personnel are no longer available.

For example an interesting case occurred during one of the GYN brigades. The patient was a 46-year female with a history of hypertension and uterine myoma, but with no other significant or medical history. On physical exam she was in good general appearance; vital signs were within normal limits: blood pressure (BP) 140/80, heart rate (HR) 72 bpm; height 5′2″, and weight 230 lb. Routine lab work was within normal limits. The patient underwent total abdominal hysterectomy under spinal anesthesia, with an estimated blood loss of 600 cc. Both the intra and immediate postoperative period were uneventful, and the patient received non steroidal analgesics and morphine for pain control.

Twenty-four hours into the postoperative period, after the patient has been transferred to the surgical floor and upon initiating ambulation, she immediately complained of difficulty breathing, diaphoresis and pallor. She became uncon-

M. Portillo
Hospital Leonardo Martinez Valenzuela, San Pedro Sula, Honduras

scious. The medical team on call immediately administered additional oxygen. Vital signs were: BP 100/70, HR 140 bpm, and O_2 Sat 85 %. At this point perioral cyanosis was also observed. Due to the acute deterioration a decision was made to intubate the patient. Immediately after intubation there was no detectable pulse and cardio pulmonary resuscitation (CPR) was initiated and maintained for an hour, unfortunately without success. Although the patient had received two subcutaneous doses of low molecular weight heparin, the probable cause of this unfortunate outcome was pulmonary embolism.

Despite receiving available thromboembolic prophylaxis, the patient likely developed a thrombus and subsequently a pulmonary embolism due to other associated risks factor, such as obesity. Our practice was to wrap the lower extremities with ace bandages perioperatively.

As a consequence of this case, there was a revision in the surgical prophylaxis protocols and use of donated sequential compression devices (SCD) was initiated with subsequent medical brigades. The implementation of perioperative thromboembolic prophylaxis based on low molecular weight subcutaneous heparin and SCDs has helped significantly decrease the incidence of this serious complication.

This was admittedly a rare but devastating complication, highlighted because it followed surgery performed during a brigade when the surgical team had left. Had more education regarding perioperative thromboembolic prevention and SCDs been available, it might have been avoided. But we have learned from the event and been able to identify techniques that we need to prevent pulmonary embolism occurring postoperatively especially in obese patients presenting for gynecologic surgery.

Letter 8: From Medical Student to Resident: A Student Perspective on International Health Care Delivery

Kate Liberman

A doctor's first foray into international medicine is frequently as a young medical student. Filled with hope and excitement at their initial interview, some premedical students inquire about an institution's international hospital interactions. Once accepted to medical school, students are willing to apply for medical missions by completing arduous applications. They then painstakingly fundraise, devise curricula, and spend extra hours after medical school classes preparing. They sacrifice vacation for a week or two of rigorous medical and surgical experience without reimbursement. What motivates someone to give up their time and put forth tremendous energy for this type of philanthropy?

Students may be driven by the desire to see another system of healthcare, appreciate cultural differences in the approach to health, make an impact where resources are scarce, research a special interest for a master's degree, learn a language, or perhaps travel. Everyone has different reasons. Data from the Accreditation Council for Graduate Medical Education (ACGME) shows a steady increase in interest in global health among medical students in the USA over the last three decades. It is likely that today's doctors who had international experiences as students continue to

K. Liberman
Department Anesthesiology, Perioperative and Pain Medicine, Brigham and Women's Hospital, Boston, MA, USA

seek them out in their career. Given the trending popularity among students and physicians, it is crucial to discuss the implications of early global health exposure on medical careers.

My experiences providing medical care and anesthesiology abroad as a student and then as a resident have been formative in shaping my career path. Nelson Mandela said that "a good head and good heart are always a formidable combination. But when you add to that a literate tongue or pen, then you have something very special." In this vein, I share my personal perspective that will hopefully provide others—who are in medical school or post-graduate training—insight into the lessons learned and the motivation found through delivering patient care in an international setting.

As a medical student at Mount Sinai School of Medicine in New York City, I traveled to San Pedro Sula, Honduras, for two medical outreach missions. The first was a 1-week trip during winter vacation. It was 2007, my first year of medical school. The administration in the global health department designed a program for ten interested students to learn about primary care in a developing country. In small teams, our group worked with the Ministry of Health's national vaccination campaign and volunteered in a public hospital's emergency department.

My most formative experience in Honduras that first year started on one already-hot morning in a grassy parking lot. I squeezed into the back of a cream-colored station wagon with four Honduran nurses. One of them strapped speakers to the roof of the car to announce our arrival in the rural neighborhood. We slowly rambled along on a road that led into the mountains. On my lap, I held a Styrofoam box filled with dry ice and vaccines. We drove with these vaccines an hour on unpaved, and sometimes muddy, roads to a group of residences constructed of little more than sheets and sticks. I ducked under low-hanging electrical wires and avoided open fire pits in order to stop at every home to collect yellow vaccine cards. After checking the name and birthday on the cards, I administered the appropriate intramuscular injections and oral vaccines.

At one home, a mother came to the entryway with her two sons. As they approached us, it was clear that one child had yellow sclera and a large belly. She beckoned me and a nurse through her home and out behind the house, where she pointed out his pale stool in a small dirt ditch. Her son had hepatitis. He had stayed home from school for weeks, and she was fretful about his well-being, nutrition, and future. That day, we took him to the nearest hospital for blood tests and treatment. As I vaccinated his brother against hepatitis A and B, the power of preventive medicine struck me. For the first time, I was able to make a real impact, helping these children and their parents to avoid disease.

This positive experience prompted me to look for more international opportunities. I returned to Honduras 3 years later on a surgical mission with Medical Students Making Impacts (MSMI) supervised and mentored by anesthesiologists. By this point in my career, I had matched for a residency in anesthesiology. As a future resident, I was curious about the role of surgical subspecialties in the developing world. I read papers written by Paul Farmer, and I studied the World Health Organization's (WHO) and World Federation of Societies of Anesthesiologists' (WFSA) websites. I began to understand that anesthesiologists are underrepresented in medicine worldwide. Many countries lack organized training and application of evidence-based practice. I embarked on this surgical mission hoping that soon I could fulfill a need by working in a medically-underserved and resource-poor country.

I took a leadership role preparing for the surgical trip. My classmates and I convened in a large storage closet and planned for the number of surgical supplies and amount of medication we would need. We wrote fundraising letters to companies asking directly for supplies or requesting funding to buy them ourselves. At the same time, I created a curriculum that included a journal club, simulation, workshops, lectures and travel planning (Fig. 28.10). After weeks of preparation, we were excited to finally be able to deliver medical care—preoperative assessments, deliv-

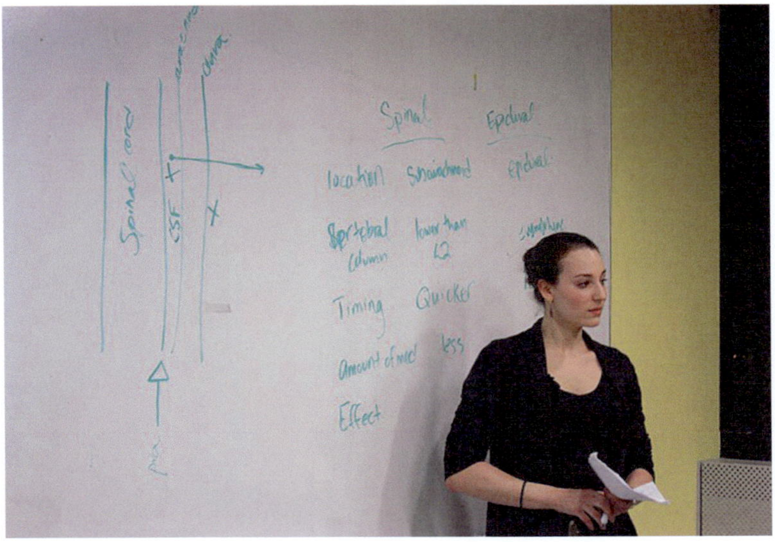

Fig. 28.10 Teaching pre-trip curriculum

ery of anesthesia, pain management and perioperative medicine. Despite this intense preparation, my experiences on this trip made me realize how much more I needed to grow. The basics of medicine are not enough.

The first patient interaction I had on this second trip to Honduras was with broken Spanish. After taking beginner language classes as an extracurricular activity and completing two discs of computer language lessons my vocabulary and syntax left much to be desired. A translator was assigned to provide me with assistance. I practiced some sentences with the interpreter. I was trying to understand and master words, and I wanted the independence to speak on my own. I meant to tell a patient that "I was going to put bandages on her legs to reduce her swelling." However, I accidentally substituted a vulgarity for the Spanish word "vendaje," meaning "bandage." The patient was offended, the translator was amused, and I was oblivious—I did not realize what I had said until later.

Understanding the importance of clear communication with my patients prompted me next to sign up for a Spanish immersion program, during which I lived with a family in Costa Rica and focused on language study. Now proficient in medical Spanish, I fully appreciate the importance of understanding a medical history and expressing nuances of medical care in the patients' native language. One of the most crucial jobs of a physician is to communicate. Without a fluid understanding, it is difficult to be a excellent doctor.

Another interaction that expanded my understanding of international medicine took place in the recovery unit. I was visiting a middle-aged patient who had undergone a total abdominal hysterectomy (Fig. 28.11). After an uncomplicated surgery, she was recovering well. Her parents and children surrounded the bed, encouraging her to drink water and take her pain medication. After asking the usual questions, I was shocked to see a plastic pathology bag with her uterus on the bedside table. Her son stepped forward and questioned if the organ needed to be taken for a biopsy. When I told him it did not, he explained that he intended to plant it in their yard underneath a new tree. He explained that the organ had been his "home" for 9 months, and he wanted to honor it and his mother by merging it with a new living organism. This situation was entirely new to me and significantly different from patient encounters in the United

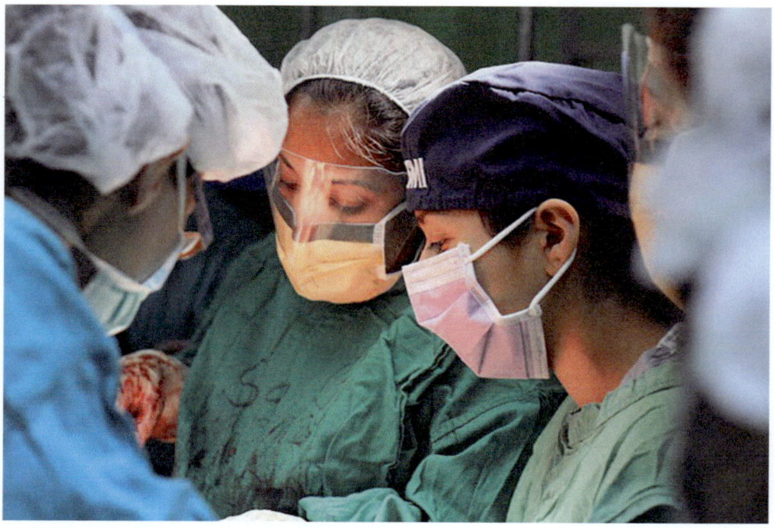

Fig. 28.11 Total abdominal hysterectomy

States. It gave me insight to the barriers of medical care in the Honduran system. The onus and cost of having a pathologist examine surgical tissue fell on the patient. There was no internal hospital system to have pathologic study of the tissue. I considered how most patients in North America do not know what happens to their specimens after being surgically removed. I was also unaccustomed to patients wanting to interact with their surgically-removed parts. Most importantly, I was moved by the tender gesture of gratitude from the son to his mother. While it was culturally different from the social practices that I knew, it showed a love and honor of family. That was a feeling I understood from my own family. Since this experience, I have tried to reflect on how the perception of different behaviors can actually point towards cultural commonalities.

A factor in creating my rank list for residency match was the ability to participate in international medicine. I selected to do my preliminary year of training in internal medicine at the Lahey Clinic Medical Center in Burlington, MA. This program allowed me to travel to Cochabamba, Bolivia with Project Pacer International, a Boston-based, nonprofit organization that provides modern cardiac therapy to indigent patients. As a senior resident in anesthesiology at Brigham and Women's Hospital in Boston, MA, I will be traveling to Kigali, Rwanda, to teach anesthesiology.

In 2012, The Project Pacer International group arrived at a tertiary care center, Viedma Hospital, with 60 pacemakers that were donated by large corporations. There were hundreds of people waiting patiently in a line that snaked through the main lobby and extended through the cafeteria and into the courtyard. Many were dressed in traditional garb with brimmed hats, full skirts, and thick dark braids and had deep wrinkles that attested to years of manual labor under the sun. Patients had come from distant areas in the country, some traveled for multiple days to be seen by our team.

Due to the prevalence of Chagas disease, many patients were in complete heart block. Because of frequently untreated strep pharyngitis, patients also presented with rheumatic heart disease. The most common complaint was shortness of breath and low exercise intolerance that prevented patients from working on farms for family income. I saw patients in a small, hot exam room that had a ceiling fan circling below the room light. It cast a strobe effect over every patient as I scrutinized the history, physical exams, EKG, and echocardiogram (ECHO) to determine if they would benefit from a pacemaker insertion or a valvuloplasty.

One patient was escorted into the exam room by the chairman of the cardiology department. She had no chart, but the physician explained that she was in her first trimester of pregnancy and having respiratory difficulty. She had a severely stenotic mitral valve and as her blood volume continued to increase with her gestational age, she was likely to experience worsening pulmonary edema unless she had a valvuloplasty. During the procedure, we covered her gravid uterus with a lead shield fashioned from multiple thyroid shields such that it would not obscure her groin, the entry point for the cardiologists' wires and dilators. This enabled the team to maintain a sterile field and simultaneously protect the fetus. The team successfully carried out a venous transseptal approach to the valve with minimal radiation to the lower abdomen. The adaptability of the cardiologists, protecting the baby from radiation in a less than ideal situation with few resources, piqued my interest. They were able to repurpose technology in the operating room to achieve excellent patient care. Since then, I have developed an interest in looking at the use of common OR equipment in unique ways to arrive at inexpensive, practical and highly effective solutions to deliver care. Ingenuity in the operating room has become one of my research interests.

My experiences in providing international healthcare have helped me grow as a doctor and a person. I have learned the power of applying simple medical knowledge, the need for effective communication in a foreign language, the role of cultural sensitivity and the necessity of ingenuity when resources are scarce and the stakes are high. I have cared for a diversity of patients, and they have trusted me to treat them and their families. I have—in small and large ways—made people's lives better. It is with humility that I realize how privileged we are to have the resources available to us in the developed world. I am confident that I will travel abroad again, and I encourage other students and doctors to also explore these opportunities.

Letter 9: Burnout of Anesthesiologists in a War-Torn Environment

Miodrag Milenovic

Growing interest of the scientific community over the past decade in burnout syndrome identified problems of emotional exhaustion, depersonalization, and lack of personal fulfillment for anesthesiologists. The syndrome is the result of hard work, mental and physical exhaustion, stress, chronic unresolved interpersonal relations among other factors [1].

Anesthesiologists perform highly responsible and stressful jobs, with patients whose treatment, recovery, or a better quality of life depends in large measure on their work and decisions. Several studies have shown that anesthesiology is one of the most stressful specialties in medicine and as such, anesthesiologists may be at higher risk of Burnout Syndrome [2]. Burned-out anesthesiologists may have a higher rate of job turnover, marriage issues, drug and alcohol abuse, caffeine and nicotine addiction, suicidal ideas, and shorter life expectancy [3].

Some studies suggest that chairpersons of anesthesiology in the USA are prone to Burnout Syndrome because of the very stressful and responsible job [4]. Preliminary and unpublished research results from Serbia shows exactly the opposite, which is strongly related to personal accomplishment and the financial situation of the heads of anesthesiology departments.

Although several former Eastern and South European nations made great efforts train sufficient numbers of anesthesiologists and to improve the working environment, long period of political instability, military conflicts, and economic crisis would seem to work against these goals. Moreover, lack of control, unfairness, community breakdown, value conflict, and insufficient personal incomes in the Ex-Yugoslavia countries probably exert a cumulative effect on the health of anesthesiologists. Also, opening of the

M. Milenovic
Department of Anesthesiology and Intensive Care Medicine, Clinical Center of Serbia, Belgrade, Serbia

European borders and professional migration caused local manpower shortages in anesthesia [5].

We conducted a study to determine the impact of many of these factors on anesthesiologists in Serbia. Voluntary and anonymous questionnaires were completed and a cross-sectional study was conducted, with a legally acquired battery of instruments that included the Maslach Burnout Inventory—Human Services Survey (MBI-HSS). The research population was Belgrade anesthesiologists (272), employed in tertiary level public hospitals, and who constituted almost 50 % of the members of the Serbian Association of Anesthesiologists and Intensivists (SAAI).

According to preliminary results, the percentage of high and moderate levels of burnout among staff anesthesiologists is disturbingly high: emotional exhaustion up to 80 % (high level 52.7 % and moderate level 26.8 %); feeling of lack of personal accomplishment up to 70 % (low level 42.4 % and moderate level 28.8 %); and depersonalization in 12 %. Nearly 40 % admitted that at some stage they are cynical, without empathy and not interested in patient outcome.

Departments and societies with a high percentage of burnout may become resigned, stagnant, and visionless. Patients are in danger of receiving poor quality and life-threatening care. It is very important for anesthesiologists and health care authorities in less affluent environments to understand the concept of burnout and to be aware of its signs and symptoms. Recognition of the problem, strategies to cope, and suggestions for improvements should be developed.

References

1. Maslach C, Leiter MP. Early predictors of job burnout and engagement. J Appl Psychol. 2008;93(3):498–512.
2. Rama-Maceiras P, Parente S, Kranke P. Job satisfaction, stress and burnout in anaesthesia: relevant topics for anaesthesiologists and healthcare managers? Eur J Anaesthesiol. 2012;29(7):311–9.
3. Lindfors PM, Meretoja OA, Luukkonen RA, Elovainio MJ, Leino TJ. Attitudes to job turnover among Finnish anaesthetists. Occup Med (Lond). 2009;59(2):126–9.
4. De Oliveira GS Jr, Ahmad S, Stock MC, Harter RL, Almeida MD, Fitzgerald PC et al. High incidence of burnout in academic chairpersons of anesthesiology: should we be taking better care of our leaders? Anesthesiology. 2011;114(1):181–93.
5. Statistical Office of the Republic of Serbia (2012). Statistical yearbook of Serbia, 2012. Belgrade, Serbia.

Letter 10: A Reverse Mission: Education, Observation, and Opportunity

Elizabeth Frost

During the World Congress in The Hague in 1992 and at European meetings 2 years prior, Dr. Alex Gotta and I remarked on the style of teaching and presentations; mainly that group sessions such as problem-based learning were not offered. We were attending the conventions as representatives of the New York State Society of Anesthesiologists (NYSSA) to introduce the Postgraduate Assembly, our annual meeting in New York, and encourage attendance. It became clear that while we might have a lot to offer, many young anesthesiologists would not have the resources to participate. So the idea of an International Scholars program was generated. Unclear as to what financial resources we might have but confident we would have at least seed money from the NYSSA, we devised a program that would invite young anesthesiologists, offering registration, hotel accommodation in New York for the duration of the meeting along with some travel expenses. Our plan was to expose these physicians to what we were doing in the USA and allow them to realize what they could reasonably incorporate into their programs at home.

In 1993, we entertained nine scholars mainly from Eastern Europe (Hungary, Lithuania, the Czech Republic, Poland, Ukraine, and one from Brazil). The following year, we had almost twice as many applicants. We formed a committee to attempt to identify those who would most gain from the program.

The program has evolved over the past 21 years. In that time we have hosted 319 anesthesiologists from 58 countries for the 6-day program (Table 28.1). Funding depended at first on private donations and contributions from the NYSSA, none of which were tax deductible. In 2010, we

E. Frost
Department of Anesthesiology, Icahn School of Medicine at Mount Sinai, New York, NY, USA

Table 28.1 International scholars: history (1993–2014)

Country	Year attended
Argentina (3)	2001–2008
Armenia (1)	2004
Austria (2)	2000–2006
Bangladesh (1)	2013
Bhutan (3)	2004–2009
Brazil (4)	1993–2009
Bulgaria (2)	1995–2005
Chile (3)	1995–2000
China (1)	2002
Colombia (3)	1998
Croatia (12)	1999–2013
Cuba (7)	1997–2008
Czech Republic (18)	1993–2013
Egypt (1)	2011
Estonia (1)	2011
Finland (1)	2004
France (1)	2005
Germany (1)	2011
Greece (2)	2009–2011
Honduras (2)	2011–2012
Hungary (15)	1993–2009
India (8)	1995–2013
Israel (3)	2001–2013
Italy (5)	2000–2005
Jamaica (1)	2011
Kazakhstan (2)	1993–2007
Kyrghyz Republic (1)	1993
Latvia (1)	2000
Lebanon (9)	1997–2004
Liberia (1)	2009
Lithuania (5)	1993–2002
Mexico (4)	2007–2013
Mongolia (2)	2008
Nepal (23)	2001–2013
Netherlands (2)	2013
Nicaragua (1)	2013
Nigeria (1)	2013
Peru (14)	2005–2013
Poland (11)	1993–2013
Romania (25)	1994–2009
Russia (2)	1994–2003
Serbia/Montenegro (17)	2004–2013
Slovak Republic (13)	2005–2013
Slovakia (25)	1994/2012
Slovenia (9)	1998–2013
South Africa (1)	2004
Spain (6)	1999–2013
Syria (1)	2001
Tanzania (1)	1997
Tenerife (1)	2013
Thailand (26)	1998–2013
Turkey (2)	2012–2013
Ukraine (4)	1993–2005
United Kingdom (1)	2011
Uruguay (1)	2012
Vietnam (3)	2005–2008
West Africa (1)	2009
Yugoslavia (4)	1994–2002
Since program inception (1993)	
Total number of scholars	*319*
Total number of countries	*58*

Intl. scholars history as of 1/2014

successfully petitioned the Government for tax exempt (501c3) status as the Anesthesia Foundation of New York. The foundation awards scholarships and grants to enhance the training and education of the most enthusiastic, dedicated, and committed anesthesiologists working in the developing world.

The program has also grown in its educational offerings. Whenever possible, scholars are offered the opportunity to participate in mini-workshops, workshops and problem based learning discussions. They are encouraged to participate, gratis, in pharmaceutically sponsored symposia in the vicinity of the meeting. In addition, the NYSSA and its officers organize a welcome reception on the first day to introduce the scholars to each other and to learn about the organization of the NYSSA. Attendees discuss what they hope to gain from their involvement and express their individual interests. At a final breakfast on the last day, an informal discussion reviews how well we fulfilled the expressed aspirations. This event is often spectacular in that many pharmaceutical companies donate large quantities of equipment (mostly airway devices) and publishers gift dozens of textbooks. A visit to a local medical center is also arranged for those who are interested.

The NYSSA has essentially two arms; an academic aspect and a political function. The annual meeting of the House of Delegates of the Society is held during this week and the scholars are welcomed. The president and officers of the American Society of Anesthesiologists attend these sessions giving the scholars the opportunity to hear about anesthesiology on a national level in the USA.

Not infrequently, the home University or Department will help to defray some travel costs if the anesthesiologist presents a poster of his/her work. Not only do we encourage such participation, but special consideration is given to including these exhibits. These participants are usually required to give a formal presentation on their return to their own departments.

The selection process occurs several months in advance to allow for acquisition of appropriate documents. Scholars are recommended by senior anesthesiologists in the United States or overseas or by previous participants. They receive different financial awards, determined by their application, ranging from free registration to shared hotel accommodation and some meals, workshop, and mini-workshop attendance, all of which are reimbursed after arrival. Reimbursement for airfare is usually not possible although individual members of the NYSSA and the sponsors often provide airport transportation costs and offer other features such as walking tours or introduction to cultural events in New York City. The program is used as an award at the European Anesthesia Meeting. While almost all anesthesiologist who are selected attend the meeting, there still remain problems of war, lack of finances, inability to get time away, and visa restrictions, all of which can arise at the last moment and restrict travel.

Measurable advances have occurred in the several countries involved including introduction of examinations and standardization, improved monitoring, expansion, and in some instances, introduction of obstetrical anesthetic services, and organization of residency training programs, using especially, problem-based learning discussions. Participants have gone on to become program directors, organizers of local assemblies and leaders at national meetings.

Typical of many of the comments we have received from the scholars are the following:

> It was a great experience for me …. I attended for the first time such a big anaesthesiology meeting… I made comparison how Slovenian anaesthesiologists and anaesthesiologists from all over the world approach problems and solve them. Of great importance for me was attending the workshop for difficult airway management and practicing with all devices available.

> I deeply appreciate the possibility to see how anesthesia is being performed overseas, and the chance to compare my experiences in the Czech Republic with those of other International Scholars. All lectures have brought me valuable knowledge. Not all things were new to me but it is important to know someone is doing same or similar way. I will use my newly gained knowledge in both my medical and teaching practice.

> I return to my country full of great knowledge. Anesthesiologists of Central American countries really need this kind of support. I give three books in the service of anesthesia. A dream come true.

> This was a unique opportunity to bring something back home to Spain. I found that mini-meetings (PBLD's) were far beyond more interesting than any other formula. We could interact directly with experts in the topic and get to know different points of view from other anaesthesiologists, all over the world… we can all benefit of sharing experiences and knowledge.

> It was a great opportunity to follow new approaches and share experiences with my colleagues from other countries. And I believe we will keep in touch with my new friends and continue to share our knowledge and experiences in our practice in Turkey.

> Attending PGA in NYC as International Scholar from the Netherlands provided me with the opportunity to meet other anesthesiologists from around the world. I hope you can maintain this Program for many years to come!

> I learned a great deal and it was really valuable for my everyday anesthesiology practice and my research in Romania. I am doing my best to apply knowledge particularly from acute pain management, obstetric anesthesia and intensive care.

> Immediately after coming back to my hospital in Croatia we did changes in our local difficult airway protocol and included two new pieces of equipment that I acquired from PGA meeting industry fair. I have established several contacts with colleagues from abroad and hope that will

> result in stronger cooperation (scientific work with publishing and professional visits). The meeting enhanced my professional knowledge and skills from which my department is already having benefits.

> It has been one of the best experiences ever for my life. ...learned a lot. ....open a new era for me... I will disseminate my experiences to our post-graduate Anaesthesiology students in Bangladesh.

> The day after I returned to Thailand I was on call. A large man required emergency surgery. The airway was difficult. I had been given a big LMA at the PGA and I was able to save his life. We did not have one at my hospital.

While the majority of attendees availed themselves of the many educational opportunities, one might imagine that some might be distracted by the activities of New York City during the December holiday season. Ahead of participation in the Assembly, scholars are advised that failure to attend the sessions might result in adverse reports back to their departmental chairs and might negatively impact future selection of their colleagues. Thus, absence is uncommon.

Benefits have accrued not only to the international scholars but also to members of the NYSSA and to the society itself. The program has afforded us tremendous admiration and given us much publicity overseas as well as cementing lasting relationships. Participants write warmly of their experiences and of what they have learned and many lasting friendships have been formed. The thorough and careful evaluations which they send to us both at the conclusion of the meeting and some weeks and months later not only help with planning of future postgraduate assemblies but are also included in the documentation necessary for formal accreditation for continuing medical education.

The International Scholars program has been a worthwhile endeavor and one that we hope will continue for many years.

The Future of Anesthesiology and Global Health in a Connected World

29

Carrie L.H. Atcheson

Mobile communications offer major opportunities to advance human and economic development – from providing basic access to health information to making cash payments, spurring job creation, and stimulating citizen involvement in democratic process.

Rachel Kyte, World Bank Vice President for Sustainable Development.

Definitions

App Shorthand for "application." An application is software that is used for business, lifestyle, or entertainment. The word application can refer to almost any software created for a task from the Flash media player to a functional Excel spreadsheet to games like Angry Birds, but it specifically excludes a device's operating system [1].

eHealth Health care information systems that maintain and transmit information specifically online. These systems include epidemiological tracking databases, medical guidelines, patient information websites, online communities, and health care administration mechanisms.

Massive Online Open Course (MOOC) An instructional curriculum offered online, free of charge, with open enrollment. A MOOC syllabus may utilize audio, video, gaming, readings, problem sets, tests, and individual or group projects to teach content and may offer evaluation or a certificate of participation for adequate work. The largest providers are Coursera and edX (free) and Udacity (paid).

mHealth The use of mobile device applications and or basic mobile device technology to improve health care access, quality, information systems, or behavioral norms. The term also applies to the private, nongovernmental organization (NGO), and government projects that utilize them.

Phishing scam The perpetrator creates an open public network in a location where victims would expect to find one (coffee shop, public square, building lobby), and when victims connect their personal devices to this network, the perpetrator can access personal information (passwords, credit card information) with the intention of committing fraud.

Platform The built environment within which a software application runs. This may involve a particular piece of hardware (in the case of an app, a particular brand of smartphone), the operating system that governs the function of the hardware and software (e.g., iOS, Android OS, Windows, or Google), a web-based environment (e.g., the functional course webpages at edX.org or the online pharmaceutical library of Lexicomp Online), or the look, feel, and function of a mobile app.

419 Scam Named after a section of the Nigerian penal code (section 419) and also known as the "Nigerian Letter" scam, the victim receives an email or letter requesting an advance payment for the purpose of taxes, fees, bribes, etc. to assist a Nigerian Government official in laundering large sums of money in exchange for a promised large percentage of the money laundered. The pleas are often very detailed and factual, with authentic-looking fraudulent documents

C.L.H. Atcheson, M.D., M.P.H. (✉)
Oregon Anesthesiology Group, Department of Anesthesiology, Adventist Medical Center, Portland, OR, USA
e-mail: unchamby@gmail.com

R. Roth et al. (eds.), *The Role of Anesthesiology in Global Health: A Comprehensive Guide*, DOI 10.1007/978-3-319-09423-6_29, © Springer International Publishing Switzerland 2015

included to enhance authenticity [2]. This scam has been running successfully through the postal service, then over the internet since the 1980s, and it is estimated that $5 billion has been extracted from victims internationally.

Smartphone A handheld mobile device that possesses the capabilities for mobile phone calls, SMS messaging, as well as Internet access over a Global System for Mobiles (GSM) or Code Division Multiple Access (CDMA) network.

SMS Short message service (SMS) provides transmission of a 160-character text message from one mobile phone to another or from a mobile phone into a web-based database.

Introduction

We live in a world where more people have access to a cell phone than to clean water and sanitation services [3]. By 2013, mobile telecommunication penetration was 96 % worldwide (see Fig. 29.1)—with 89 % of households in the developing world having access to mobile communication (see Fig. 29.2) [4]. The mobile telecommunications industry doubles its bandwidth every year and a half and is quickly expanding into rural areas. Most people in the world have access to mobile technology, and more impor-

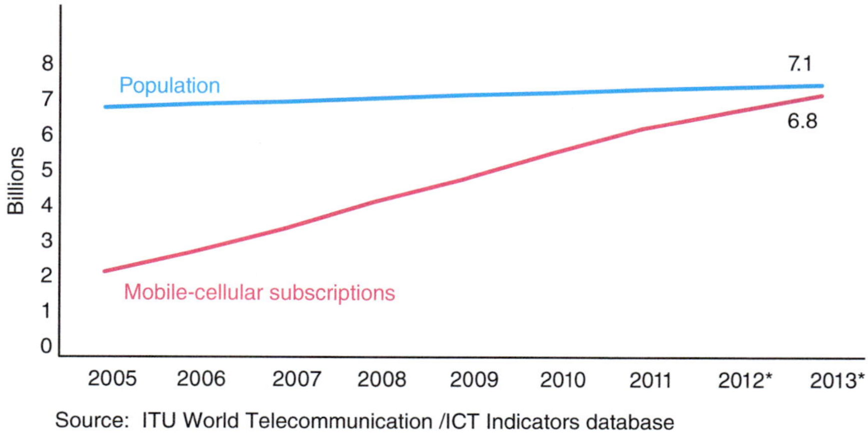

Fig. 29.1 Worldwide mobile cellular subscriptions relative to population. Worldwide, the number of mobile cellular subscriptions approaches the population, demonstrating the increasingly universal access to cellular technology. *Source*: International Telecommunications Union (Branch of United Nations)

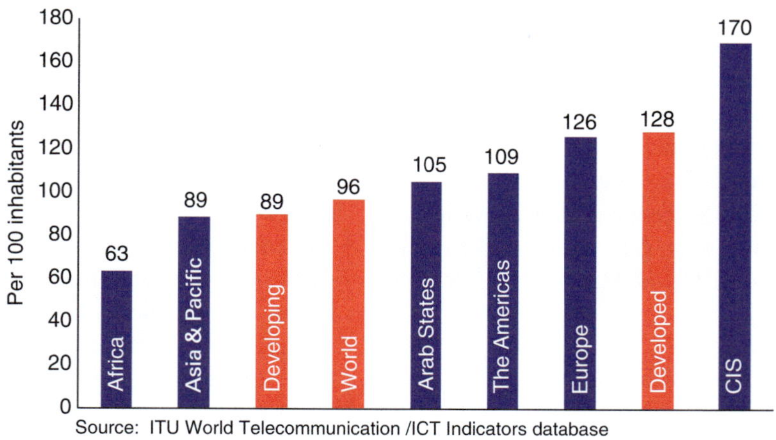

Fig. 29.2 Mobile subscriptions per 100 inhabitants by region. In some countries, it is common for people to hold more than one cellular subscription (e.g. one for personal use and one for business use), while in other countries, families, or communities may share a subscription or a device. *Note*: Commonwealth of Independent States (CIS). *Source*: International Telecommunications Union (Branch of United Nations)

tantly, people stay within a several foot proximity to their mobile devices 83 % of their lives [5].

Because of the accessibility of mobile technology, industries such as banking that provide exclusively mobile services are growing exponentially in the lowest income countries. In 2013, 52 % of mobile money accounts were located in sub-Saharan Africa, and there were nine countries in sub-Saharan Africa where citizens held more mobile money accounts than bank accounts [6]. This technology can and is being applied in the health care industry in the form of mHealth initiatives. Mobile devices can be used to monitor heart rate and oxygen saturation, and inroads are being made in other diagnostic and imaging modalities. Indeed the use of mHealth tools is one area where the gap between high income countries (HICs) and low and middle income countries (LMICs) is narrow—the World Health Organization (WHO) noted in 2011 that 77 % of LMICs and 87 % of HICs had implemented mHealth initiatives [3]. According to Google Trends, interest in mHealth is increasing and is highest outside of high income countries (See Figs. 29.3 and 29.4) [7]. The first section in the chapter explores the application of mHealth to surgical quality and perioperative medicine.

Personal computing and internet access lag behind access to mobile technology—especially in low- and middle-income countries (LMICs). For example only 7 % of households in Sub-Saharan Africa have internet access allowing 16 % of the population to be online [4]. The biggest barrier to expanding internet access in LMICs is cost; internet access costs 31 % of the gross national income per capita (GNI p.c.) in LMICs versus 1.7 % of GNI p.c. in high income countries [4].

However, because of Facebook, Google, and other internet giants, "poorer countries in Asia, Africa, and Latin America represent the biggest opportunity to reach new customers" [8]. The industry is poised to change. With its $19 billion purchase of WhatsApp, a platform that uses the internet to send information via smartphones, and their participation in the Internet.org initiative, Facebook made an investment in expanding Internet access in LMICs via smartphones in 2013 [9]. As Internet costs continue to decrease and mobile Internet access continues to increase, Internet educational platforms such as Massive Open Online Courses (MOOC) and real-time data-gathering become more accessible. The second section in this chapter addresses the global health applications of Internet-based learning and public health surveillance.

Finally, the flipside of transparency and access is lack of privacy. In the last section the emerging issues of digital professionalism and privacy in a global health context are explored.

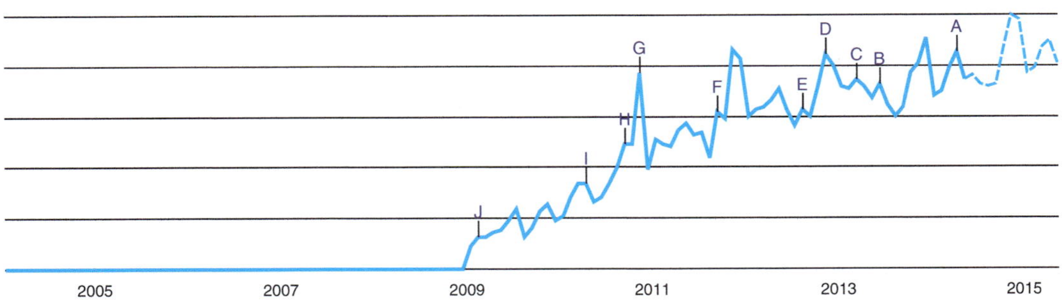

Fig. 29.3 Google Trends Search Index shows interest in mHealth is growing. The Google Trends search index shows the relative number of searches for a given term relative to the maximum number of searches for that term. For example, if the term "health" was searched 10,000 times in 2010 that would correspond to a search index of 100. It demonstrates growing or waning international interest in a given topic. For the term "mHealth" interest spiked after 2009 and has been growing steadily. Trend prediction for the year 2015 is included

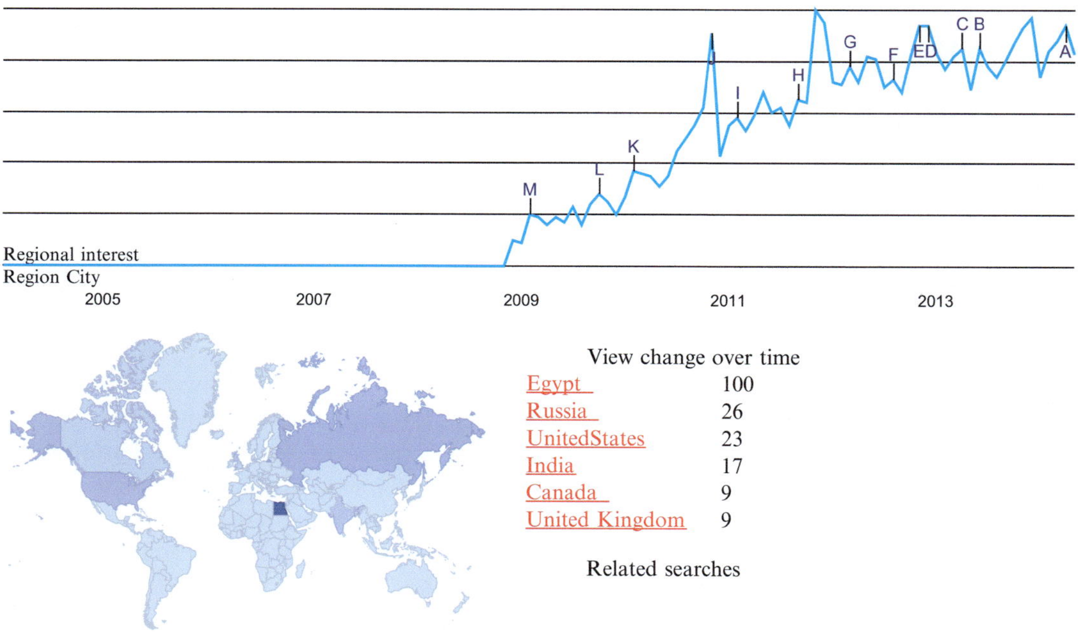

Fig. 29.4 Google Trends Search Index of mHealth by country. The Google Trends Search Index by country shows the relative number of searches for the term mHealth worldwide. The country with the most searches is indexed as 100

mHealth: What Is It, and How Does It Apply to Surgical Care in Global Health?

The mHealth Landscape

Mobile communication-based health care applications, programs and technologies are collectively known as mHealth. According to the World Bank, mHealth applications run on any mobile device from a cellphone to a smartphone to a tablet and fulfill one or more of the following health care functions:

- Improving management and decision making by health care professionals.
- Real-time and location-based data gathering.
- Provision of health care to remote and difficult-to-serve locations.
- Fostering learning and knowledge exchange among health professionals.
- Promoting public health.
- Improving accountability.
- Improving patient health self-management [3].

mHealth programs can take a variety of forms—from SMS messaging feeding real-time data into a national database in India to mobile applications helping patients count calories in the US or keep track of drug therapies in Haiti to reminders for appointments at a hospital in Kenya [3, 10, 11]. As described in Fig. 29.5, a variety of stakeholders contribute to the development and implementation of mHealth initiatives. Often mHealth initiatives are joint public and private ventures [3, 10, 12, 13].

The majority of mHealth programs initiated thus far focus on communicable diseases, health care systems, and behavioral health. Of the projects registered with the mHealth Institute at Johns Hopkins University, only 7 of the 118 address surgical diseases and none specifically address perioperative medicine (see Table 29.1) [14]. A similar pattern holds true for the 2014 mHealth Summit, a joint industry-government conference hosted by the Health Information and Management Systems Society (HIMSS) in conjunction with the National Institutes of Health (NIH). Panels will separately address the role of mHealth in programs and policy in

Table 29.1 mHealth projects registered at Johns Hopkins University Global mHealth Initiative, grouped by area

Content area	Number of projects
Systems, education, and behavior	50
Communicable diseases	43
Noncommunicable diseases	18
Surgical diseases	7

Based on a count taken from the projects registered with the Johns Hopkins University Global mHealth Initiative (JHU GmI), mHealth applications designed to address surgical diseases are underrepresented relative to the global burden of surgical disease. From www.jhugmi.org accessed April 13, 2014.

domestic hospital medicine and initiatives for different populations in global health, but no sessions specifically address surgical diseases in global health [15]. Thus far surgical care and perioperative medicine have been in the periphery of the larger mHealth conversation with projects such as:

- RapidSMS helps local officials in remote areas who have low technical literacy monitor UNICEF supply chains through SMS messaging. In the transition from paper-based data collection to SMS-based data collection, the data quality improved—discrepancies decreased from 14.2 to 2.8 % [3].
- The medAfrica app created by a Kenyan company Shimba Technologies, Ltd. aims to "increase access to health related content and services to save lives and build healthy populations with the aim of reaching every household in Africa." Through this app, patients with surgical diseases can find location-based screening or consultation services with one of Kenya's 7,000 doctors [16].
- Anyone in the world can have a dermatology consultation within 24 h through the iDoc24 iOS, Android, or web platform. The user takes a picture of his/her skin issue, uploads the picture, describes associated symptoms, pays the $39.00 USD fee, and receives a response from a remotely located dermatologist within 24 h [17]. Though this fee is out of the reach of most citizens of LMICs, given that 90 % of patients with HIV will have skin manifestations, climate change will make skin cancer more prevalent, and that most of the lowest income countries have few if any dermatologists, iDoc24 offers an interesting model for increasing access [18].

These projects just scratch the surface of what is possible in surgical care and perioperative medicine through mHealth. Using eHealth and mHealth technology, local and visiting surgeons and anesthesiologists in low-resource settings can enhance education and support for health care providers, strengthen infrastructure and data management systems, and offer actual health care services such as pre-procedure evaluation and postoperative follow-up. In the next two sections we address some of the mHealth technologies available for anesthetic care in a low resource setting and offer examples of possible applications.

SMS Messaging in mHealth: Low Tech, Cheap, and Versatile

Every cellular device manufactured for use over current commercial networks has the ability to use the Send Message Service (SMS) to send or receive a 160-character text message. SMS messages can also be sent or received by a computer. It is a push technology, which means that SMS messages are received by the user's device without any action from the user [10]. Though SMS messaging was designed for person-to-person communication, it can also be used by outside entities to connect with customers or, in the case of health care, patients. Because SMS messages can be sent to and processed by a computer with larger data management capabilities, SMS messages can be easily turned into data for logging behaviors, physiologic data, or operations information.

SMS messaging has been used by mHealth programs and applications for sending appointment reminders and personalized health tips or education materials, documenting supply chains, and, in its most advanced form, goal tracking [10]. Goal tracking incorporates both the data gathering function, wherein a patient sends an SMS message noting behavior, symptoms, or physiologic parameters to a computer application which processes this information in the context of the patient's health goals, and sends an SMS

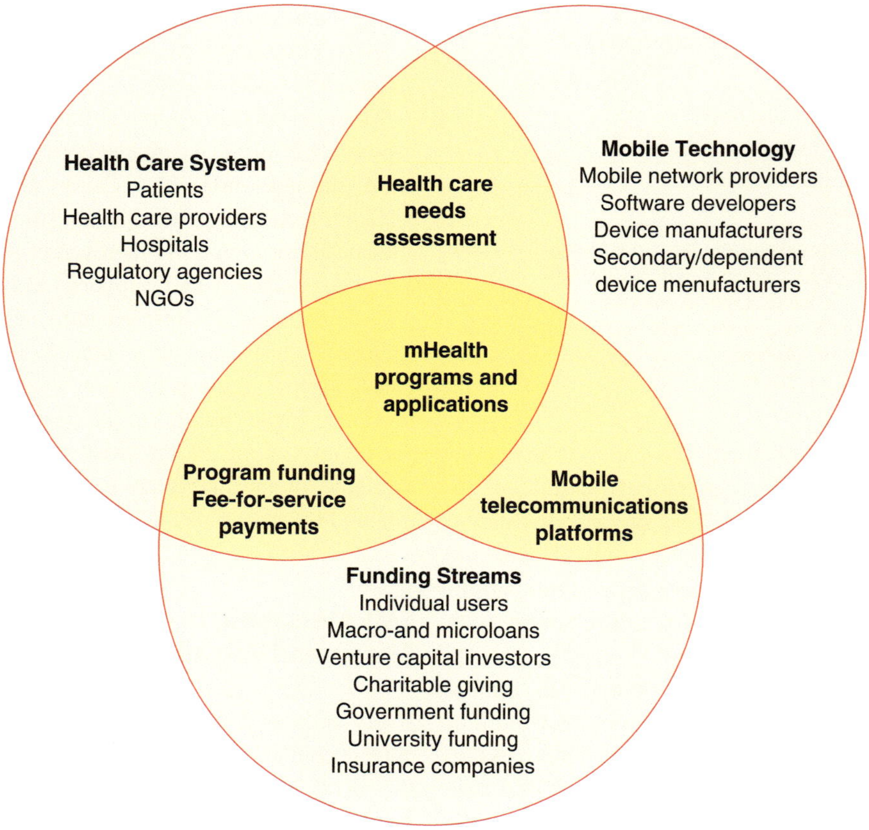

Fig. 29.5 The mHealth landscape [3, 11, 12]. mHealth applications and programs depend equally on the needs of stakeholders in the health care system, the interests of those controlling funding streams, and the developers of the mobile technology that supports the applications. *Sources*: References [3, 10, 11]

message advancing or affirming these goals. SMS message goal tracking has been applied in the context of smoking cessation [19], but because smartphone technology lends itself well to goal tracking, SMS-based mHealth initiatives in perioperative medicine are not found in the literature. Several mHealth programs for goal tracking and medication compliance in solid organ transplant patients or free-flap patients in the U.S. have been designed for use with smartphones [20]. But, in areas like sub-Saharan Africa where SMS messaging is a high penetrance technology and smartphones are a low penetrance technology, these types of initiatives could be undertaken with SMS. For patients, an SMS message goal tracking application might be useful in encouraging rehabilitation exercises for orthopedic surgery patients in areas where outpatient physical therapy is not available or feasible. For providers, studies in Kenya and Uganda have shown improvement in health care workers' compliance with medical guidelines after use of SMS-based mHealth applications [21], and this could be used to encourage compliance with evidence based guidelines for perioperative care.

Physiologic Monitoring and Diagnostics via Smartphone

In the 2009 blockbuster movie Star Trek, which takes place in the twenty-third century AD, the starship's flight doctor points a device that looks remarkably similar to a handheld retail store barcode scanner at a crew member's forehead to accurately measure several physiologic variables and diagnose an infectious disease within seconds. In real life, mobile mHealth diagnostics moves closer to science fiction every day. Currently smartphone and Bluetooth compatible pulse oximeters, heart rate monitors, spirometers and ultrasound machines are on the market. Some of the devices currently available, their compatibility, and current uses are detailed below.

There are several smartphone compatible pulse oximeters on the market. Masimo released the iSpO2™ device and companion app for iPhone in late 2013 and expanded to the Android platform in 2014. iSpO2™ is a dual wave pulse oximeter, and the app provides the pulse rate as well as a perfusion index and can trend, store, and transmit 12 h of data. It weighs under a pound and currently retails on Amazon.com for $149–139 USD. There are several personal-use grade pulse oximeters available such as the iChoice™ from ChoiceMed (compatible with iOS, retails for $69 USD) and the iOximeter™ from SafeHeart (compatible with iOS and Android platforms, retails for $69 USD).

Recognizing the potential global health benefits of smartphone compatible pulse oximeters, the Government of Canada partnered with Canadian angel investor and entrepreneur Irfhan Rajani to expand the development and manufacture of the smartphone-, tablet-, and computer-compatible Kenek O2™ (its prototype was the Phone Oximeter™) from LionsGate Technologies for use in global health settings. The Kenek O2 pulse oximeter, like the iSpO2™ has been validated across a range of peripheral blood oxygen saturation values versus traditional stand-alone oximeters [22]. LionsGate Technologies has developed a full line of mobile device compatible monitors (see Fig. 29.6) including blood pressure cuff, heart rate, and temperature probe, each of which are designed for a global health setting [23]. Such large scale investment in smartphone compatible monitors coupled with the upcoming production of cheaper smart phones aimed at LMIC markets by the Mozilla Foundation could translate to increased availability of standard anesthesia monitors in global health settings [9]. The combined cost of the Mozilla smartphone and the LionsGate Technologies Kenek O2™ would be $65 USD, which is 1/100th of the cost of a stand-alone portable pulse oximeter.

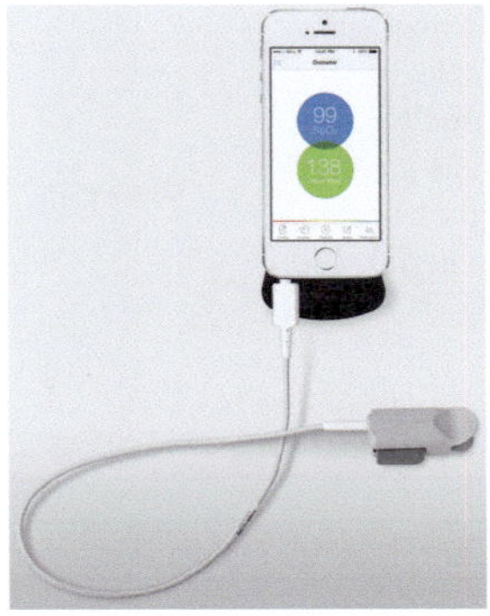

Fig. 29.6 The Phone Oximeter™ was designed by Lionsgate Technologies and is being developed for global health uses through a $2 million USD grant from the Government of Canada and a private investor. *Source*: Lionsgate Technologies

Other devices with potential applications for anesthesiology providers in global health settings that are currently on the market include:

- The MobiUS™ SP1 smartphone compatible ultrasound by MobiSante was approved for patient use by the U.S. Food and Drug Administration (FDA) in 2012. The MobiUS™ probe runs off of the auxillary port of a specialized smart phone (they come as a package) and can store and transmit the 8 MB ultrasound images over a WiFi connection [24]. While the device portability will appeal to anesthesiologists looking to offer regional anesthetics or invasive vascular access in remote settings, the price point is less appealing at $7500 USD.
- SpiroSmart is a smartphone application that uses a specialized microphone attached to a smartphone to measure the forced expiratory volume in 1 s (FEV_1), forced vital capacity (FVC), and peak expiratory flow (PEF) with 5.1 % mean error as compared to traditional spirometry [25]. Developed by researchers at the University of Washington, the cost is less than $100 USD compared to the cheapest traditional portable spirometry apparatus at $1,000 USD or stand-alone module at $5,000 USD.
- Researchers at the Henry Samueli School of Engineering and Applied Science at the University of California in Los Angeles

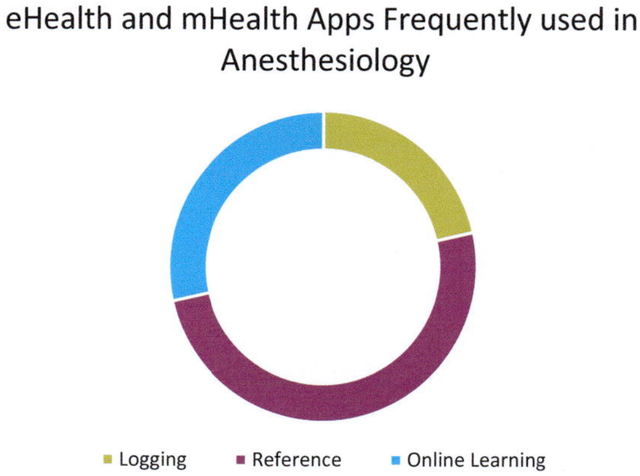

Fig. 29.7 The majority of eHealth and mHealth applications used by anesthesiologists are used for logging, quick access to reference material, and online learning

(UCLA) have developed a smartphone-based wide-field microscope and flow cytometer [26], which could help improve access to pathology services in the diagnosis of surgical diseases and could have implications for cheap end-tidal gas sampling.

eHealth and mHealth for Anesthesiology Education and Data Management

We [Coursera] have close to 2 million students world-wide right now. A third of them are in the United States, and two-thirds are outside, including many in developing countries where this is really the only access to education that they are ever likely to have. Daphne Koller, Co-founder of Coursera and Professor of Computer Science at Stanford University, in testimony before The President's Council of Advisors on Science and Technology (PCAST).

mHealth refers to health care efforts utilizing mobile technology and eHealth refers to health care activities utilizing the Internet. Because eHealth applications may be accessed via personal computer or mobile devices and because smartphones are gaining functionality and personal computers are shrinking in size, the boundary between these fields is ever-changing. In the following section emerging platforms and technologies for education and data management in global health, fields that both find a natural home on mobile and web-based platforms are discussed.

Apps and MOOCs: The New Teachers Are Online

Many educators debate whether the "age of the sage" is over—in other words, they are wondering how our relationship to personal mobile devices, the ease of audio and video processing and distribution, and more open access to teachers and learning institutions on the internet are going to affect the logistics and economics of education [27]. In anesthesia education, online and mobile learning tools have increased access to up-to-date information for students and life-long-learners as well. Reference and resource applications dominate the anesthesia education eHealth and mHealth niche (see Fig. 29.4) [28, 29]. A list of commonly used anesthesiology reference and teaching applications is provided in Table 29.2—these might be useful to local providers and trainees at global health sites. Another useful resource to assure colleagues in LMICs have access to is OpenAnesthesia, an iPhone, iPad, and web-based application for residency and continuing education that was released in 2013 by the International Anesthesia Research Society (IARS) and is accessible from most countries in the world.

Each of these eHealth and mHealth applications is small in scale, complements traditional lecture-based education, and does not amount to a revolution, however, the nature of higher education may have changed forever with the widespread adoption of the Massive Open Online Course (MOOC). The principles of open access and remotely connected educational

Table 29.2 mHealth and eHealth applications most frequently used in anesthesiology

Functionality	Logging	Reference	Teaching and learning
Applications	iGas Log	Epocrates	OpenAnesthesia
	GoogleForms	Oxford Handbook of Anesthesia	ECG Guide
	ACGME Caselog	Paeds ED	SonoAccess by SonoSite
		MedCalc	NYSORA
		Johns Hopkins ABX	
		Stoelting's Anesthesia of Coexisting Diseases	
		Anesthesia Drug Handbook	

Note: Table 29.2 These currently available eHealth and mHealth applications have use in anesthesiology education for logging, reference, and teaching. Current as of May 2014, the market is constantly expanding and this list is constantly growing.

communities did not begin in 2011 when the first Stanford University MOOC achieved enrollment of over 100,000 students—these principles have been in use in traditional education for a century. From radio broadcasts of lectures during the early twentieth century to sites such as Blackboard that have allowed "executive" degree programs to rely exclusively on online interaction, teachers have always used the newest available technology to reach learners outside of the university environs [27]. However the viral spread of open-access online education and the organizations and companies that are streamlining the use of online platforms to provide students with the ability to interact, access, and create photo, audio, and video and rapidly give and receive feedback have forever changed the way future generations will learn. And—because the learning takes place, not in Cambridge, Massachusetts, or Cambridge, England in series between 200 paying students and one tenured professor but online between one user, one computer, and one instructor in parallel with possibly hundreds of thousands of other student, device, and instructor couplings and is (for now) free—the majority of the world has access to this new learning model.

Though MOOCs have yet to be actively applied in medical education, the model certainly has application. The Robert Wood Johnson Foundation, Stanford University, and Khan Academy began a multimillion dollar effort to build the structure that massive online medical education will eventually take. Throughout 2014, faculty at the medical schools at Stanford University, Duke University, University of Washington, University of California at San Francisco, and University of Michigan are working to create a map of critical medical knowledge that will guide the construction of Khan Academy content, content that will surely be used all over the world [30]. MOOCs, by their nature, apply the educational techniques that the authors of Chap. 24 of this text advocate as most effective for anesthesia education in global health: real-time feedback, scalability of learning groups, and continuous improvement of content [31].

Big Data in Low-Resource Settings: Innovations in Compatibility and Quality

In the short term, eHealth and mHealth applications offer opportunities for improved efficiency, improved quality of outcomes data, and reduction in time spent or staff required for health care programs. These process measures can be used as markers to evaluate efficacy of eHealth and mHealth programs [11]. Highlighted earlier in the chapter was RapidSMS, a UNICEF program that teaches local people to use SMS messaging to monitor UNICEF supply chains. This program shows that a simple mHealth program can improve the quality of data collected and reduce the number of person-hours required for that administrative function [3]. The same high quality of data is generated by RapidSMS-CMC, an application that populates a maternal health and morbidity dataset in Liberia directly from text messages sent by local midwives [21]. There are limitations and biases to data gathered in real-time by mHealth applications that must be explored going forward; however, the benefits of this technology are substantial. Low literacy levels are not a limitation to the use of mHealth technology for data gathering [11, 18]. Gathering data by mobile device is efficient [3]. One study showed a 93 % reduction in time required to process public health data gathered by an mHealth application, as compared to the standard paper and pencil methods [32].

In the long term, eHealth and mHealth applications will be used to increase portability of medical information across state, national, and language barriers. A joint effort between Zhejiang University in China, Kyoto University, and Miyazaki University, Project Dolphin created a medical markup language (MML) specifically for medical records, which translates into the receiver's language [33]. There are currently one million participants in the BlueButton® project, which allows home access to electronic medical records for patients at the United States Department of Veterans Affairs, which is 40 times the number of participants they had expected [34]. The ID Ecosystem Steering Group (IDESG) is looking for ways to validate cyber-identity to make all of these transfers of health care data secure [35].

Transparency, Privacy, Physician Professionalism, and Patient Autonomy in the Digital Age

Unlike previous advances in communication, such as the telephone and email, the inherent openness of social media and self-publication, combined with improved online searching capabilities, can complicate the separation of professional and private digital personae. [36].
Arash Mostaghimi, MD, MPA and Bradley H. Crotty, MD, MPH

Nowhere is this statement more true than when a physician is engaging in a short term surgical trip, a medical mission, or a career in global health. The physician's motivations are part professional and part personal, so his or her publication or sharing of those experiences will, by their nature, fall into both the personal and professional spheres. mHealth and eHealth platforms present a special challenge to patient privacy and autonomy because digital interactions occur via a personal mobile device, where (rightly or not) people are used to sharing personal data without thinking about privacy. And finally, there are a great many government, private for-profit, and private not-for-profit stakeholders interested in the huge amount of personal health data becoming available through mobile and internet sources. Physicians and patient advocates are the gatherers of personal information, so by default, it often ends up in their hands for safekeeping. Assuredly, the patients and the communities that physicians serve do not have the resources, literally the big computers, needed to make sense of and profit by their own data. The question then becomes the following: How do physicians handle their own and their patients' information responsibly? In this section, these issues of digital professionalism and big data and health information privacy in a global health context are briefly reviewed.

Digital Professionalism in Global Health

Through social media one can hear voices and perspectives not previously accessible, and activity on social media platforms translates into actions and events. Researchers at the University of Washington confirmed that *Twitter*, blog posts, and Facebook® group activity shaped political debates, foreshadowed political events on the ground, and spread revolutionary ideas across international borders during the 2011 wave of protests for democracy across the Arab world known as the Arab Spring [37]. Social media helps nonprofit organizations and universities—like those organizing short term surgical trips—recruit and maintain a network of supporters [38,

39]. However, every new technology comes with new responsibilities, or, as noted philosopher and author of *The Original Accident* and *The Information Bomb* Paul Virilio put it: "inventing the ship amounts to inventing the shipwreck, when you invent the plane you also invent the plane crash; and when you invent electricity, you invent electrocution…Every technology carries its own negativity, which is invented at the same time as technological progress" [40].

The widespread use of social and digital media by usually well-intentioned people has wrought many digital shipwrecks. A recent report from the United States Institute of Peace implicates Western reporters' and policymakers' use of English language blogs and *Twitter* feeds in the spread of misinformation during the Civil War in Syria [41]. Courtesy of mainstream media coverage, most people in the medical community are familiar with the fate of doctors and nurses who commit gross breaches of professional conduct via using social media or mobile technology. Even though she used no identifying information, an online community of expectant mothers requested the firing of Dr. Amy Dunbar after the OB-Gyn resident posted on Facebook® about her frustrations with a patient's chronic lateness to prenatal appointments [42]. Mayo Clinic Chief Resident Dr. Adam Dubowick was fired after he took a photo of a humorous tattoo on a patient's penis while the patient was anesthetized during gallbladder surgery [43]. Dr. Patrick Yang placed stickers on the face of a colleague and took a photo as a practical joke while the colleague was under anesthesia for a minor surgical procedure at the hospital where they both worked. The victim of the practical joke did not see the humor and brought suit against the hospital and Dr. Yang [44].

Various institutions have implemented digital privacy or social media policies, but these infractions have occurred at institutions with and without such policies. Commonly, a digital and social media privacy policy includes stipulations on timing (can it be used during the work day), location (can it be used on hospital computers), content (distinguishing personal from official communication), affiliation (can the practitioner attach the hospital's name or their work email address to their account). The extreme bad digital behavior reported on the nightly news may or may not be mitigated by digital privacy policies just as not all criminals feel morally bound by laws. In health care, digital and social media policies are designed to help well-intentioned practitioners maintain the professionalism online that they display in face-to-face interactions. Indeed the Massachusetts General Hospital social media guidelines reminds employees and faculty: "when using social media, be aware that existing hospital policies apply" [45].

As discussed in Chap. 24 of this text, global health practitioners carry with them a standard of professional conduct and ethics even though there is often not an entity providing a high degree of professional oversight. For universities, nonprofit organizations, and hospitals conducting medical missions, implementing a social and digital media policy can help remind well-intentioned physicians, nurses, and volunteers that ultimately every on- and off-line action taken while on location will be judged as a professional action.

Health Care Data Privacy in an International Setting

Practitioners on short-term surgical trips and medical missions handle issues of privacy differently than they would in their home country. We take pictures with patients and coworkers in medical settings. Medical records are kept in a cardboard box, backpack, or personal laptop. We leave messages with family members, text from our personal cell phones, and show up at patients' homes. And we often make assumptions that all of these things are acceptable to our patients and the governments of the countries we are visiting. Some of these actions are necessitated by the logistics of providing medical care outside of a hospital setting—it would be entirely impractical to carry a locked file cabinet for medical records to a rural community. The urgency of information and action—e.g., the need to reschedule a surgery before the team leaves or to convey serious abnormal test results requiring a follow up plan—sometimes requires the involvement of the patient's family and community members. And there is no hospital risk management hotline or ethics committee to call upon for guidance.

So how do practitioners stay on the right side of protecting patient privacy? The practitioner should begin by assuming that patients in a global health setting, regardless of custom, culture or other experts' assurances or previous experiences have the same desire for privacy as patients at home. It is, in medicine, best practice to adhere to the highest level of evidence available, and nascent data suggests that people everywhere have the same concerns for internet privacy and that people from LMICs live in the same confusing climate of digital privacy as people in HICs.

One study of populations in Taiwan, Hong Kong, and the USA showed that culture was not associated with differences in desire for privacy safeguards of personal information in different internet settings (social media, banking, etc.) [46]. Indeed patients from LMICs may have a heightened desire for Internet privacy out of necessity—even though only 2 % of the world's Internet traffic comes from sub-Saharan Africa, this region accounts for 10 % of the world's cybercrime (e.g., phishing scams and 419 scams) [47]. Recognizing this growing threat, the South African Government enacted the Protection of Personal Information Act of 2013 (PoPI), which requires consent for digital processing of personal information, puts limits on direct marketing via phone, fax, or SMS message, and requires industry oversight of customer privacy [48]. With actions like the PoPI Act, the governments of LMICs may protect citizens' personal information from corporations, but, like the US National Security Administration, they may also be using questionable tactics vis a vis citizen's online personal information in matters of national security. When Facebook® released the list of governments that had inquired about activity on citizens' accounts, the governments of Botswana, South African, and Egypt had all made requests, and Google's 2013 Transparency Report noted "a worrying upward trend" in government requests for user information and removal of political content globally, with a markedly high number of requests from the governments of Russia and Turkey [47, 49].

The answer then is to apply the spirit of usual professional standards of patient privacy while in a novel setting—be it in a different culture or an online community—and to safeguard the control over data obtained from patients [50]. If access to a locked file cabinet is not an option, records should be kept in a locked backpack or on a password protected memory key. When working with industry or local government partners, enquiry should be made about data privacy policies and how information gathered as a result of the practitioner's efforts is to be used. Sensitivity is essential when contacting patients via a third party. Such attitudes must extend also to community health workers dealing with personal health information. Finally, as one classic ethical postulate goes: give it the "gut test." If posting photos of patients on a university or nonprofit website feels uncomfortable it should not be done. Research shows that people do the right thing more often when they use their "gut feeling" rather than deliberate decision making [51].

Indeed, Büschel et al. note that there is a "privacy paradox," a discrepancy between "individual's motivation for the consented processing of personal data and their fears about unknown disclosure, transferal and sharing of personal data via information and communication technologies" [50]. So though consent for use of photographs or personal information may be obtained during a service trip, patients almost certainly still have unvoiced concerns about use of their image and personal information. As demonstrated in this section, research and international law on digital privacy is in its earliest stages of development, and there is very little concrete guidance for a practitioner in many situations, so the best policy is to have the same safeguards one would in one's home country and home institution. And, for now, the best guide may be the gut, the practitioner's internal moral compass.

References

1. The Computer Language Company Inc. PC magazine encyclopedia. www.pcmag.com/encyclopedia. Accessed 18 Apr 2014.
2. Federal Bureau of Investigation and U.S. Department of Justice. Common fraud schemes. 2014. http://www.fbi.gov/scams-safety/fraud/fraud#419. Accessed 28 Apr 2014.
3. Federici N, Hulin C, Yamamichi M. Information and communications for development in 2012: maximizing mobile. Washington, DC: World Bank; 2012. p. 45–59.
4. Telecommunications and development sector. ICT facts and figures. Geneva, Switzerland. 2013:1–8. www.itu.int/en/ITU-D/Statistics/Pages/facts/default.aspx.
5. Patel S, Keintz J, Hayes G, Bhat S, Abowd G. Farther than you may think: an empirical investigation of the proximity of users to their mobile phones. In: Dourish P, Friday A, editors. UbiComp 2006: ubiquitous computing. Berlin: Springer; 2006. p. 123–40.
6. Penicaud C, Katakam A. State of the industry: mobile financial services for the unbanked. London; 2013:727–9. doi:10.1016/j.jacr.2013.05.035.
7. Google trends – Web search interest: mHealth – 2004 to present. http://www.google.com/trends/explore#q=mhealth. Accessed 12 May 2014.
8. Scott M. Zuckerberg says WhatsApp deal was a bargain. The New York Times. 24 Feb 2014.
9. Ngo N. 4 Takeaways for developing countries from mobile world congress 2014. TechChange. 2014. www.techchange.org/2014/03/04/-4takeaways-for-developing-countries-from-mobile-world-congress-2014/. Accessed 15 Mar 2014.
10. Klasnja P, Pratt W. Healthcare in the pocket: mapping the space of mobile-phone health interventions. J Biomed Inform. 2012;45(1):184–98. doi:10.1016/j.jbi.2011.08.017.
11. Leon N, Schneider H, Daviaud E. Applying a framework for assessing the health system challenges to scaling up mHealth in South Africa. BMC Med Inform Decis Mak. 2012;12:123. doi:10.1186/1472-6947-12-123.
12. Qiang C, Yamamichi M, Hausman V, Miller R. Mobile applications for the health sector. Washington, DC: World Bank; 2012.
13. Rosendale D, Cassells SW, Goldman JM, et al. Road map for mHealth innovation road map for mHealth innovation. San Antonio, TX; 2014:1–3.
14. Johns Hopkins University. Global mHealth initiative. www.jhumhealth.org. Accessed 28 Mar 2014.
15. HMISS Media. 2014 mHealth Summit. www.mhealthsummit.org. Accessed 28 Mar 2014.
16. medAfrica. medAfrica demo. 2012. www.medafrica.org. Accessed 10 Apr 2014.
17. iDoc24 AB. iDoc 24 | Skin advice on any device. 2014. www.idoc24.com. Accessed 7 Apr 2014.
18. McCoy K. The importance of dermatology in global health. Burlington, MA; 2011:1–3.
19. Haug S, Meyer C, Schorr G, Bauer S, John U. Continuous individual support of smoking cessation using text meassaging: a pilot experimental study. Nicotine Tob Res. 2009;11(8):915–23.
20. McGillicuddy JW, Weiland AK, Frenzel RM, et al. Patient attitudes toward mobile phone-based health monitoring: questionnaire study among kidney transplant recipients. J Med Internet Res. 2013;15(1):e6. doi:10.2196/jmir.2284.
21. Aranda-jan CB, Mohutsiwa-dibe N, Loukanova S. Systematic review on what works, what does not work and why of implementation of mobile health (mHealth) projects in Africa. BMC Public Health. 2014;14(1):1–15. doi:10.1186/1471-2458-14-188.
22. Petersen C, Chen T, Ansermino JM, Durmont GA. Design and evaluation of a low-cost smartphone pulse oximeter. Sensors. 2013;13(12):16882–93.
23. LionsGate Technologies Inc. Mobile vital signs monitoring: everyone everywhere. Vancouver, BC.
24. Mobisante. The MobiUS SP1 system. 2014. www.mobisante.com/products/product-overview/. Accessed 1 May 2014.
25. Cohn G, Gupta S, Lee T, et al. SpiroSmart: using a microphone to measure lung function on mobile phone. Proceedings Ubicomp 2012. 2012.
26. Zhu H, Ozcan A. Wide-field flourescent microscopy and flourescent imaging flow cytometry on a cellphone. J Vis Expr 2013;74. www.jove.com.
27. President's Council of Advisors on Science and Technology. Letter to the President of the United States. Washington, DC; 2013:1–9.
28. Ruskin KJ. Mobile technologies for teaching and learning. Int Anesthesiol Clin. 2010;48(3):53–60.
29. Dasari K, White S, Pateman J. Survey of iPhone usage among anesthetists in England. Anaesthesia. 2011;66: 630–1. doi:10.1111/j. 1365-2044.2011.06735.x.
30. Painter M. TED 2014: grandmother avatar with TB Beckons medical education her way. 2014. www.thehealthcareblog.com/blog/2014/03/21/ted2014-grandmother-avatar-with-tb-beckons-medical-education-her-way/. Accessed 10 Apr 2014.
31. President's Council of Advisors on Science and Technology. Harnessing technology for higher education. 2014. www.whitehouse.gov/share/technology-for-higher-ed. Accessed 13 Apr 2014.
32. Yu P, de Courten M, Pan E, Galea G, Pryor J. The development and evaluation of a PDA-based method for public health surveillance. Int J Med Inform. 2009;78(8):523–42. http://www.ncbi.nlm.nih.gov/pubmed/19369114.
33. Js L, Ts Z, Chu J, Araki K, Yoshihara H. Design and development of an international clinical data exchange system: the international layer function of the Dolphin Project. PubMed commons. J Am Med Inform Assoc. 2014;18(5):683–9. doi:10.1136/amiajnl-2011-000111.
34. The United States Department of Health and Human Services. The BlueButton connector. http://www.healthit.gov/bluebutton. Accessed 30 Apr 2014.

35. Gropper A. IDESG is a glimpse of our digital future. The Health Care Blog. 2014. http://thehealthcareblog.com/blog/2014/01/26/idesg-is-a-glimpse-of-our-digital-future/#more-69251. Accessed 23 Mar 2014.
36. Mostaghimi A, Crotty BH. Ideas and opinions professionalism in the digital age. Ann Intern Med. 2014; 154(8):560–3.
37. Howard P, Duffy A, Freelon D, Hussain M, Mari W, Maziad M. Opening closed regimes: What was the role of social media during the Arab Spring? Seattle, WA; 2011:1–30
38. Convivio. Going social: tappling into social media for nonprofit success. Austin, TX: Convivio; 2010. p. 1–37.
39. Barnes NG, Lescault AM. College presidents out-blog and out-Tweet Corporate CEOs as higer education delves deeper into social media to recruit students. Dartmouth, MA. 2013. www.umass.edu/cmr/social-media/collegepresidentsaboutblog/.
40. Virilio P. Politics of the very worst. New York, NY: Semiotext(e); 1999.
41. Lynch M, Freelon D, Aday S. Blogs and bullets III: Syria's socially mediated civil war. Washington, DC; 2014:1–38.
42. Browning W. OB-GYN's Facebook Rant leads to calls for her firing. Yahoo! News. www.news.yahoo.com/ob-gyn-facebook-rant-leads-calls-her-firing-193400733.html. Published 5 Feb 2013.
43. Turley J. Mayo doctor fired for photographing patient's penis during surgery. http://jonathanturley.org/2007/12/22/mayo-doctor-fired-for-photographing-patients-penis-during-surgery/. Accessed 15 Apr 2014.
44. Knowles D. Woman sues hospital after anesthesiologist puts stickers on her face and nurse takes pictures during surgery. The New York Daily News. www.nydailynews.com/news/national/anesthesiologist-put-stickers-patient-face-surgery-article-1.1447041#ixzz2zZRkoXua. Published 5 Sept 2013.
45. Massachusetts General Hospital. Guidelines for Massachusetts General Hospital employees and faculty who use social media. 2014. www.massgeneral.org/notices/socialmediapolicay_employees.aspx.
46. Yao M, Liang T-H. Understanding privacy concerns: a cross cultural perspective. Proceedings of the International Communication Association. 2014.
47. Maboja W. Blurring lines of security and surveillance. CNBC Africa. http://www.cnbcafrica.com/insights/special-reports/world-economic-forum/the-blurring-lines-of-security-and-surveillance/. Published 3 Feb 2014.
48. Minister of Justice and Constitutional Development. Protection of personal information act. South Africa: Government Gazette; 2009:1–52. http://www.justice.gov.za/legislation/bills/B9-2009_ProtectionofPersonalInformation.pdf.
49. Google. Transparency report: government removal requests continue to rise. Google off blog. 2013. http://googleblog.blogspot.com/2013/12/transparency-report-government-removal.html. Accessed 2 May 2014.
50. Büschel I, Mehdi R, Cammilleri A, Marzouki Y, Elger B. Protecting human health and security in digital Europe: how to deal with the "privacy paradox"? Sci Eng Ethics. 2014. doi:10.1007/s11948-013-9511-y.
51. Zhong C-B. The ethical dangers of deliberate decision making. Adm Sci Q. 2011;56:1–25.

Appendix

Contact Information for Medical Groups Providing Services in LDCs

Please note: This listing of some groups providing care in LDCs does not imply endorsement or concurrence by the editors with the organization's policies and procedures. It is incomplete and is provided for information only.

Medical Missions.org
www.medicalmissions.org
2655 Northwinds Pkwy
Alpharetta, GA 30009, USA
Contact Phone: 866-204-3200
(This website acts as a clearinghouse for organizations looking for medical volunteers for overseas missions.)

Medicin sans Frontier/Doctors without Borders
www.doctorswithoutborders.org
333 7th Avenue, New York, NY 10001–5004
212-679-6800

Orbis International Headquarters
520 8th Avenue, 11th Floor
New York, NY 10018
USA
Tel: 1-800-ORBIS-US (1-800-672-4787)
www.Orbis.org

Operation Smile
www.operationsmile.org
3641 Faculty Boulevard
Virginia Beach, VA 23453, USA
1-888-OPSMILE (888-677-6453)

ReSurge International
www.resurge.org
145 N. Wolfe Road
Sunnyvale, CA 94086
408-737-8743
Fax: 408-737-8000
info@resurge.org

Project HOPE
www.projecthope.org
255 Carter Hall Lane
PO Box 250
Millwood, VA 22646
E-mail: HOPE@projecthope.org

Medical Mission International, Inc.
500 Old Country Road, Suite 304
Garden City, NY 11530
T: (516) 741–3434, (516) 874–4346 • F: (516) 741-3436
info@medicalmissioninternational.org

International Medical Relief
1151 Eagle Drive Suite 457
Loveland, CO. 80537
Phone: (970) 635-0110
Fax: (970) 635-0440
contact@imrus.org

R. Roth et al. (eds.), *The Role of Anesthesiology in Global Health: A Comprehensive Guide*,
DOI 10.1007/978-3-319-09423-6, © Springer International Publishing Switzerland 2015

International Healthcare Volunteers
ihcvinfo@gmail.com
P.O. Box 8231, Trenton, New Jersey 08650
Phone: 609-259-8807
Fax: 609-259-6108

Refuge International
P.O. Box 3586
Longview, TX 75606–3586
Tel 903-234-8660 | Fax 903-234-8664

Samaritan's Purse
P.O. Box 3000
Boone, NC 28607
Phone (828) 262-1980
Fax (828) 266–1056
www.medicalstudentmissions.org

International surgical mission support
225 Windmill Lane Southampton, Suite 1, NY 11968 | Phone: +1 (631) 287–6202
www.Ismission.org

Surgical Volunteers International
65712 E. Mesa Ridge Ct,
Tucson, Az 85739
Phone: +1 832-434-1593
Fax: +1 832-415-2814
E-mail: tflood1431@gmail.com
www.internationalmedicalrelief.org

Mercy ships
www.mercyships.org
P.O. Box 2020
Lindale, TX 75771
903.939.7000
1.800.772.SHIP (7447)

World Surgical Foundation
P.O. Box 1006
Camp Hill, PA 17001-1006
Tel: 717-232-1404
E-mail: info@worldsurgicalfoundation.org

Index

R. Roth et al. (eds.), *The Role of Anesthesiology in Global Health: A Comprehensive Guide*,
DOI 10.1007/978-3-319-09423-6, © Springer International Publishing Switzerland 2015

MIX
Papier aus verantwortungsvollen Quellen
Paper from responsible sources
FSC® C105338

If you have any concerns about our products,
you can contact us on
ProductSafety@springernature.com

In case Publisher is established outside the EU,
the EU authorized representative is:
Springer Nature Customer Service Center GmbH
Europaplatz 3, 69115 Heidelberg, Germany

Printed by Libri Plureos GmbH
in Hamburg, Germany